Child and Adolescent Psychiatry

Savita Malhotra · Paramala Santosh
Editors

Child and Adolescent Psychiatry

Asian Perspectives

Springer

Editors
Savita Malhotra
Post Graduate Institute of Medical Education and Research (PGIMER)
Chandigarh
India

Paramala Santosh
Centre for Interventional Paediatric Psychopharmacology and Rare Diseases (CIPPRD)
National and Specialist Child and Adolescent Mental Health Services, Michael Rutter Centre
Maudsley Hospital
London
UK

and

Department of Child and Adolescent Psychiatry
Institute of Psychiatry, Psychology and Neuroscience (IoPPN), King's College London
London
UK

ISBN 978-81-322-3617-7 ISBN 978-81-322-3619-1 (eBook)
DOI 10.1007/978-81-322-3619-1

Library of Congress Control Number: 2016950746

Printed on acid-free paper

This Springer imprint is published by Springer Nature
The registered company is Springer (India) Pvt. Ltd.
The registered company address is: 7th Floor, Vijaya Building, 17 Barakhamba Road, New Delhi 110 001, India

Foreword

"Perspective," from the Latin *perspicere*, or "to see through," is a particular attitude toward or way of regarding something, in the present instance, child and adolescent psychiatry in Asia. In essence, this "perspective" offers a point of view or frame of reference for this rapidly emerging scientific and clinical discipline in the most populated region of our globe. While Asia has an extraordinary intellectual and cultural history, the study of child development and developmental psychopathology has been relatively neglected until recently and it remains a relatively new and, as Malhotra and her colleagues demonstrate, an eagerly nourished element of medical practice in this rapidly growing and changing region.

Before proceeding further, one must take note that "perspective" has an alternative meaning that may be even more important to this volume of work. "Perspective" also means the art of using a two-dimensional medium or surface to present objects that that appear to be three-dimensional and have height, width, depth, and position in relation to each other when viewed from a particular point. Perspective was a hard earned skill for human beings. Despite the human urge to draw spanning a period 20,000 years or more (see the caves at Lascaux), it was not until about 500 years ago, in the fifteenth century, that our forbearers mastered the ability to truly represent objects in perspective; and, it took many more years of work to refine this ability and then transfer it to books, movie theaters, television and, now, the internet. This serves to point out that true perspective is hard earned and requires considerable craftsmanship. Furthermore, to provide the full dimensionality of perspective takes the hearts and minds of many distinguished individuals who are willing and able to put themselves and their own work to the test of careful scrutiny, as was done at the conference preceding this volume as well as in the preparation of this book. Indeed, this volume ably presents the multidimensionality of child and adolescent psychiatry, and hence its richness, on a flat page (or computer screen) but with a depth, height, and breadth that offers an impressive vision of the field. With this "perspective" the authors allow us to peer through the complexities of childhood and human development to understand its variation and perturbations we now know as developmental psychopathology.

When I first saw the title of this work, I was struck by the concept of "Asian perspectives." Indeed, I initially found the idea disquieting. How can there possibly be an "Asian perspective" on anything? After all, Asia may be the most incredibly diverse and disparate region of our world. By some estimates it includes about one-third of the Earth's land surface and two-third of the world's population in more than 50 countries. It is the birthplace of the world's major religions and the home to innumerable languages, as well as social and cultural traditions. Even without the hand of a skilled artist, Asia is surely multidimensional and cannot be fully captured without a richly developed capacity for perspective. And, that is what we see in this interesting volume.

So, what do we learn about the "Asian perspective?" First of all, we learn that to provide such a perspective it takes the efforts, minds, and hearts of many distinguished individuals because there are so many topics to address. Second, Malhotra and her colleagues teach us that while there are many unique elements to the "Asian perspective," at its very heart, children, adolescents, and their families share a great deal with their brothers and sisters around the world proving that we are all more alike than different. But, "more alike" does not mean the same. The authors help us understand these similarities and differences.

While there are many examples of the unique elements of the Asian perspective, several are quite striking. Certainly, the challenges of applying diagnostic systems that were developed in the West is but one of them. It is striking how culture changes perspectives on developmental psychopathology. This struggle is clear in many forms but not clearer than ADHD that Sood et al. (Chap. 3) so nicely illustrate. Another culturally sensitive perspective is provided in Benegal and Jayarajan's "reframing" of addiction (Chap. 6). And, while the description and treatment options for psychopathology are challenges, the lack of resources in this vast region is brought clearly into focus by Konar and Balachander's discussion of psychopharmacology (Chap. 17) and Kapur's effort to identify "low cost solutions for learning disabilities" (Chap. 22). In these chapters, we can all learn how to do much more for children in need with much less. This is impressive, especially for those of us in relatively resource-rich nations.

Equally striking in this volume is the authors' willingness to address environmental factors that cross cultures and continents. Hong's chapter on the impact of rapid sociocultural change on child-rearing (Chap. 8) is a cogent reminder to all of us on how the pressures of globalization and the "cyber" era (also covered by Boon and Fung in Chap. 10) are creating an enormous impact on how parents and children are managing in an increasingly complex world. We are also reminded that economic disparity may have the greatest impact on our youth with a very poignant description in Banaag's chapter (Chap. 9) on "street children."

So, with so many points of view, do we have a clear "Asian perspective" on child and adolescent psychiatry? The answer is a resounding, "Yes!" From Asia, we have much to learn from our incredibly determined and thoughtful colleagues about how to understand the challenges facing children and families in a very rapidly changing world. We can also admire the courage and commitment of our colleagues in Asia who are creatively providing care to as many youth as possible with limited resources. The challenges are great but so are the opportunities.

But, perhaps, what we have learned most from the "Asian perspective" is that the Earth is a very small planet and that while we must recognize our diversity and differences, we have so much more in common and so many lessons to learn. In children and families, we can find both need and hope. In diversity, we can find strength. In the face of adversity, we can find creativity and courage. And, in Asia, we find wonderful colleagues who are very much a part of the worldwide community of professionals, who are determined to understand, prevent, and treat child and adolescent psychiatric disorders wherever and whenever we find them. This is a good perspective for all.

Prof. Bennett L. Leventhal, MD
Child and Adolescent Psychiatry
The University of California
San Francisco, USA

Preface

Child and Adolescent Psychiatry: Asian Perspectives is a compilation of resources in child mental health from a perspective applicable to Asia. There are differences in many areas of child and adolescent mental health such as child-rearing practices, societal acceptance of psychopathology, resilience, availability of newer treatments, and professionals between Asia and the West. Fundamentally, most of the knowledge guiding the theory and practice of child psychiatry in the world has been derived from studies done in Europe and America. In this context, we attempted to gather available information from within Asia that could provide a strong evidence base to inform professionals in the field during the 7th Asian Society for Child and Adolescent Psychiatry and Allied Professions (ASCAPAP) Congress held in New Delhi, India in September 2013. Leading experts in child and adolescent psychiatry from Asia and other parts of the world discussed their research and provided valuable insights into various issues of contemporary importance in child mental health and psychiatry. We decided to capture this information in its updated form for purposes of this book.

The majority of neurodevelopmental disorders persists along the entire lifespan of the individual and can have a deleterious impact on the quality of life of the individual and their families. To manage this in part, where there are limited resources, treatment strategies ought to involve comprehensive and multidisciplinary approaches. In recent years, there has gradually been some pertinent literature emanating from Asia. There are, however, at present no major child psychiatry books from this region.

There is a pressing need to make available resources that are credible in order to provide perspectives for professionals to interpret and adapt knowledge that will benefit their patients in routine clinical practice. We hope that this volume will allow readers to take a more considered approach when treating and managing children with mental health problems in Asia. To a certain extent, extrapolating principles and guidelines from developed countries is useful; however, information regarding prevailing child psychiatry theories and practices, and their applicability across populations, taking into account the local sociocultural context, need to be contextually examined and evaluated.

This volume focuses on several child psychiatry disorders and mental health issues from an Asian perspective, as applicable. The contributors are leading authorities from Asia and other parts of the world in their respective fields.

The book has 26 chapters divided into 7 parts. Part I deals with some of the major psychiatric disorders seen in children and adolescents, including pediatric bipolar disorders (Chap. 1), dissociative disorders (Chap. 2), attention deficit hyperactivity disorder (Chap. 3), affective disorders, highlighting current status and controversies (Chap. 4) and suicide (Chap. 5). Part II deals with substance abuse disorders (Chap. 6) and tobacco use amongst children and adolescents (Chap. 7), and focuses on the impact that these substances might have on the developing brain. Part III focuses on the role of environment and cultural issues in shaping the growing brain and emerging personality of children. The chapter on parenting and child-rearing practices in the globalizing world (Chap. 8) highlights contemporary issues in parenting and consequences for child development. There is also a chapter on resilience among street children (Chap. 9). Cyberage and child mental health is also discussed (Chap. 10) as is child sexual abuse (Chap. 11). The chapter on parental loss (Chap. 12) provides a psychoanalytic view of long-term consequences of early childhood parental loss. Early diagnosis and intervention is dealt with in Part IV, focusing on early diagnosis and intervention, underscoring the importance of infancy and early childhood in recognizing and treating psychopathology (Chap. 13). Chapters on temperament (Chap. 14) and childhood antecedents of personality disorders (Chap. 15) provide insights into developmental trajectories leading on to the evolution of personality and adaptation patterns through childhood experiences. Part V includes pharmacological and biological treatments in children. The chapters in this part deal with the paradigm shift in child psychopharmacology (Chap. 16) and from a low resource country perspective (Chap. 17). It also includes a lucid discussion and review of psychopharmacology of neurodevelopmental disorders in children (Chap. 18); which provide valuable insights into web-based health monitoring and wearable sensor technology for managing neuropsychiatric symptoms in rare diseases. The last chapter in this part (Chap. 19) discusses electroconvulsive therapy for severe mental disorders in children and adolescents. Part VI on non-pharmacological interventions includes chapters on play therapy (Chap. 20), psychosocial interventions in poor scholastic performance (Chap. 21), and low cost solutions in learning disabilities (Chap. 22). The last part, Part VII, refers to services and policy for children and focuses on the progress and promise of mental health policy (Chap. 23) and describes an innovative model of telepsychiatry service developed in India for treating children and adolescents, using nonspecialists, in remote areas (Chap. 24). Following on from this, mental health gaps between needs and resources in Asia are discussed (Chap. 25) and finally, teaching of child psychiatry from a transcultural perspective is discussed (Chap. 26).

We hope that mental health professionals, students and researchers in Asia and other parts of the world with sizeable Asian communities will find this book to be a useful addition to the literature. Students of child psychiatry and psychology will also benefit from exploring the chapters in an analytical and an adaptive manner in particular sociocultural issues that are relevant to child mental health. We would be happy if this volume serves this purpose.

Chandigarh, India Savita Malhotra
London, UK Paramala Santosh

Acknowledgements

We are grateful to all the contributors for their faith and trust in us. We are indebted to Dr. Jatinder Singh, a senior researcher at the Centre for Interventional Paediatric Psychopharmacology and Rare Diseases (CIPPRD) at the National and Specialist Child and Adolescent Mental Health Services, Michael Rutter Centre, Maudsley Hospital, London, UK, and the Institute of Psychiatry, Psychology and Neuroscience (IoPPN) at King's College London, UK, whose critical review of chapters for important intellectual oversight and content is much appreciated. We also thank Dr. Soumya Jhanda, a DM student in Child and Adolescent Psychiatry at the Postgraduate Institute of Medical Education and Research, Chandigarh. We would like to offer our deep appreciation and thanks to these colleagues who assisted in compilation, correspondence, and editorial work. Their selfless and painstaking contribution is gratefully acknowledged.

We also thank Ms. Shinjini Chatterjee and her team in Springer for bearing with us while we prepared the chapters. Thanks are due to Springer for accepting the proposal and agreeing to publish the book.

Contents

Editors and Contributors

About the Editors

Savita Malhotra MD, Ph.D., FAMS, is Professor of Psychiatry, Dean and Head, Department of Psychiatry, Drug Deaddiction and Treatment Center, and Child and Adolescent Psychiatry at the Postgraduate Institute of Medical Education and Research (PGIMER), Chandigarh, India. She has over four decades of experience in psychiatry and child psychiatry in India. She has made pioneering contributions to the development and establishment of services and the academic discipline of child psychiatry in India through teaching, research, and advocacy. She is a recognized leader and resource person in mental health and child mental health in India and the world. Her areas of expertise include temperament of children, epidemiology of child psychiatric disorders, childhood disintegrative disorders, and telepsychiatry. She is a recipient of many academic awards and recognitions at the national and international levels. Dr. Malhotra has published over 250 research papers and book chapters, and eight books. She is a Life Fellow of the Indian Psychiatric Society, Indian Association for Social Psychiatry, and Indian Association for Child and Adolescent Mental Health. She is a Life President Indian Association for Child and Adolescent Mental Health, and Past President of Indian Association for Social Psychiatry. She is also the immediate Past President of the Asian Society for Child and Adolescent Psychiatry and Allied Professions, and Board Member of the Child Psychiatry Section of the World Psychiatric Association.

Paramala Santosh MBBS, Dip NB (Psych), MD, Ph.D., FRCPsych, is a Consultant Child and Adolescent Psychiatrist who has dually trained in psychiatry from India and the UK. He has developed and heads the Centre for Interventional Paediatric Psychopharmacology and Rare Diseases (CIPPRD) at Maudsley Hospital, London, UK and is a Honorary Reader at the Institute of Psychiatry, Psychology and Neurosciences (IoPPN), King's College London, UK. He also runs a clinic at Tadworth Children's Trust, England, for Pediatric Neurorehabilitation, and is recognized as an international expert on developmental psychopharmacology, neuropsychiatry, attention deficit and hyperactivity disorder (ADHD), autism spectrum disorders (ASD), intellectual disability, pediatric neurodegeneration, suicidality, and digital health technology. He has conducted research into the overlap of ASD, ADHD, and bipolar disorder; psychopharmacology and rare diseases in the context of Rett syndrome, mucopolysaccharidoses, septo-optic dysplasia, and other rare diseases. He is also recognized as an expert in the field of assessment and management of complex treatment-resistant co-occurring disorders. He has been involved in developing eHealth platforms such as the HealthTracker™ and has demonstrated the use of wearable sensor technology in routine clinical care. He is a principal investigator in multiple ongoing multinational and national research projects funded by the European Union, and the National Institute of Health Research, UK. He is a regular internationally invited speaker and has over 100 research publications.

Contributors

Dr. Salman Akhtar, MD, is Professor of Psychiatry at Jefferson Medical College, and Training and Supervising Analyst at the Psychoanalytic Center of Philadelphia. He has served on the Editorial Boards of the *International Journal of Psychoanalysis, Journal of the American Psychoanalytic Association,* and *Psychoanalytic Quarterly*. His 77 books include 17 solo-authored, the most prominent of these are: *Immigration and Identity* (1999), *Comprehensive Dictionary of Psychoanalysis* (2009) and *Psychoanalytic Listening* (2013). He also has 52 edited books in psychiatry and psychoanalysis to his credit. He has received numerous awards, the most recent being the prestigious Sigourney Award (2012) for outstanding contributions to psychoanalysis. He has also published eight volumes of poetry and is Scholar-in-Residence at the Inter-Act Theatre Company in Philadelphia.

Dr. Alan Apter is Professor of Psychiatry at the Sackler School of Medicine at the University of Tel Aviv. He graduated from the University of Witwatersrand Medical School in Johannesburg and did his child psychiatry fellowship at Children's Hospital in Washington DC. He also was a Belfer scholar in Biological Psychiatry at the Albert Einstein College of Medicine in New York. In 2016 he received the Distinguished Research Award from the American Foundation for Suicide Prevention.

Dr. Srinivas Balachander did his MD in Psychiatry from the Postgraduate Institute of Medical Education and Research (PGIMER), Chandigarh and is currently working as a Senior Resident in the Department of Psychiatry, National Institute of Mental Health and Neuro Sciences (NIMHANS), Bengaluru.

Dr. Cornelio G. Banaag, Jr. MD, is Professor Emeritus, University of the Philippines College of Medicine; President, Philippine Mental Health Association. He was responsible for setting up training programs in child and adolescent psychiatry in the Philippines and currently directs the three existing child and adolescent psychiatry training programs in Manila.

Dr. Aniruddha Basu, MD, PDF, (Addiction Medicine) is a DM student in Addiction Psychiatry at Postgraduate Institute of Medical Education and Research in Chandigarh India. His main area of interest is addiction psychiatry. He had been associated with the tobacco cessation services of National Drug Dependence and Treatment Centre (NDDTC) at AIIMS, New Delhi and NIMHANS, Bangalore.

Dr. Myron Belfer is Professor of Psychiatry Harvard Medical School and Senior Associate in Psychiatry, Boston Children's Hospital. He was Senior Advisor for Child and Adolescent Mental Health at the World Health Organization in Geneva from 2000 to 2005. He was president of the International Association for Child and Adolescent Psychiatry.

Dr. Vivek Benegal is Professor of Psychiatry at the Centre for Addiction Medicine, Department of Psychiatry, NIMHANS. His research interests include vulnerability to substance use and externalizing disorders, the epidemiology of substance use in India, and interventions for substance use disorders.

Dr. Astrid Berg is a Psychiatrist, Child and Adolescent Psychiatrist as well as a Psychoanalyst. She is an Emerita Professor at the University of Cape Town and A/Professor Extraordinary at the University of Stellenbosch. She consults to and teaches at the Parent–Infant Mental Health Services and Child Psychiatry Divisions at both Universities.

Dr. Yuval Bloch is the head of the Child and Adolescent Outpatient Clinic in "Shalvata" Mental Health Center in Israel. He is a senior lecturer in Sackler's School of Medicine, Tel Aviv University. His research on ECT in treating adolescents contributes to the field and received competitive academic grants (NARSAD).

Dr. Jillian Sok Teng Boon is a Senior Educational Psychologist in the Neuro-Behavioral Clinic (ADHD Services), under the Department of Child and Adolescent Psychiatry, Singapore. Jillian's research interest and publications are mostly in improving psychological treatment through the use of technology and gamification as a population-based approach.

Dr. David C. Call, MD, is a Child and Adolescent Psychiatrist in the Department of Psychiatry and Behavioral Sciences at Children's National Medical Center in Washington D.C. and is an Instructor of Pediatrics at the George Washington University School of Medicine & Health Sciences.

Dr. Rakesh Kumar Chadda is Professor of Psychiatry at the All India Institute of Medical Sciences, New Delhi. He is a Fellow of the Royal College of Psychiatrists of the UK and the National Academy of Medical Sciences (India) and Distinguished International Fellow of the American Psychiatric Association. He has about 200 publications to his credit including four books.

Dr. Subho Chakrabarti is currently professor at the Department of Psychiatry, PGIMER, Chandigarh. He is a Member of the National Academy of Medical Sciences (India) and a Fellow of the Royal College of Psychiatrists (UK). He has over 250 publications spanning adult psychiatry, mood disorders, family caregiving, liaison psychiatry, ECT, and telepsychiatry.

Dr. Prabhat Kumar Chand, MD, DNB, MNAMS, his main area of interest is intervention, outcome and training in the area of addiction and mental health. He has been part of the Tobacco Cessation Centre (TCC) NIMHANS, a resource center for South India. With the NIMHANS team, he has developed a weekly virtual, i.e., synchronous (LIVE) and asynchronous (e-learning module), training platform to mentor and handhold the health professionals in providing the best practice care in their own community on tobacco cessation and various other addictive disorders.

Dr. Lisa M. Cullins, MD, is the Training Director for the Child and Adolescent Psychiatry Fellowship Program and the Director of Outpatient Psychiatry at Children's National Medical Center. Dr. Cullins is an Assistant Professor of Psychiatry, Behavioral Sciences and Pediatrics at George Washington University School of Medicine in Washington, DC.

Dr. Daniel Shuen Sheng Fung is the Chairman Medical Board of Singapore's Institute of Mental Health. He is an Adjunct Associate Professor at the Yong Loo Lin Medical School, Duke-NUS Medical School, National University of Singapore and Lee Kong Chian School of Medicine, Nanyang Technological University.

Dr. Neera Ghaziuddin, MD, MRCPsych, (UK) is an Associate Professor of Psychiatry at the University of Michigan, Ann Arbor. She is the Director of the Treatment Resistant Disorders clinic. Her publications include the AACAP Practice Parameters for the use of ECT in minors and a book, *Use of Electroconvulsive Therapy in Children and Adolescents* (OUP).

Dr. Yari Gvion, Ph.D., is a supervising clinical psychologist who has worked for many years in a psychiatric hospital with adolescents and in private clinic. She is a staff member at Bar-ILan University and Tel Aviv—Yafo College. Her main fields of research include risk factors for suicide attempts, severity of suicide attempts, and self-destruction in adolescent psychiatric patients.

Dr. Gordon Harper was trained in Pediatrics, Psychiatry, and Child Psychiatry in Boston; he teaches at Harvard Medical School. He has served as Director of Inpatient Psychiatry at Boston Children's and as Medical Director of Child/Adolescent Services for Massachusetts' Department of Mental Health. He writes about treatment planning and mental health policy.

Dr. Kang-E. Michael Hong is Professor Emeritus, College of Medicine Division of Child Psychiatry, Seoul National University Bundang Hospital, South Korea Founding President of Korean Academy of Child and Adolescent Psychiatry, Past President of the Asian Society of Child and Adolescent Psychiatry and Allied Professions, and Past Vice President of International Association of Child and Adolescent Psychiatry and Allied Professions.

Dr. Rajeev Jairam is the Clinical Director ICAMHS and Senior Lecturer (conjoint) UNSW and UWS, ICAMHS, Mental Health, SWSLHD, Campbelltown Hospital, Therry Road, Campbelltown, Australia. Pediatric Bipolar Affective Disorder has been his major area of interest with numerous national and international publications.

Dr. Deepak Jayarajan is an Assistant Professor in the Department of Psychiatry, NIMHANS. He works in the Psychiatric Rehabilitation Services unit, and his research interests include substance use disorders, adolescent mental health, comorbidities and rehabilitation in chronic mental illnesses.

Dr. Soumya Jhanda is MD in Psychiatry and a student of DM in Child and Adolescent psychiatry at the Post Graduate Institute of Medical Education and Research at Chandigarh India.

Dr. Paramjit T. Joshi, MD, is the Distinguished Endowed Professor and Chair of Psychiatry at the Children's National Medical, Washington DC and Immediate Past President of AACAP. She completed her training in adult and child psychiatry at Johns Hopkins. Her areas of interest are depression, bipolar disorder, global mental health and childhood trauma.

Dr. Kandasamy Preeti is Assistant Professor of the Department of Psychiatry, JIPMER, Puducherry, India. Anxiety Disorder and Autism Spectrum Disorder have been her major areas of interest.

Prof. Dr. Malavika Kapur is a Visiting Professor at the National Institute of Advanced Studies, Bangalore. She has 13 books to her credit that deal with her work in the clinic and the community especially in schools. She is a Fellow of several professional associations in India and abroad. She has been a consultant for national and international organizations such as NCERT, ICSSR, UGC and the WHO. She has explored child care in the Indian indigenous health systems, namely Ayurveda, Unani, Siddha, and the Tibetan medicine from a developmental perspective.

Dr. Palvi Kaukonnen is a Child Psychiatrist, Consulting Officer at the Department for Social and Health Services, Ministry of Social Affairs and Health, Finland and Chief Medical Officer, Department of Child Psychiatry, Tampere University Hospital, Tampere, Finland. Executive Director of the World Association for Infant Mental Health (WAIMH).

Dr. Miri Keren, MD, is a Child and Adolescent Psychiatrist, Director of Infant Mental Head Unit, Geha Mental Health Center, Head of Infant Psychiatry Course and Faculty Member at Tel Aviv University Sackler Medical School, and Past WAIMH President.

Dr. Devashish Konar is a General Psychiatrist with special interest in Child Mental Health, Director and Consultant Psychiatrist of Mental Health Care Centre, Burdwan and Kolkata, Visiting consultant to Woodlands Multispecialty Hospital, Kolkata and Bellevue Clinic, Kolkata. Currently, he is also Chairman, Specialty Section, Child and Adolescent Psychiatry, Indian Psychiatry Society, India.

Dr. Saurabh Kumar is working as a senior resident in the Department of Psychiatry and National Drug Dependence and Treatment Center at the All India Institute of Medical Sciences (AIIMS). He graduated from Maulana Azad Medical College, New Delhi and completed his postgraduation in Psychiatry from AIIMS, New Delhi.

Dr. Pratima Murthy, MD, DPM, FRCP (Glasg), is at the Centre for Addiction Medicine, NIMHANS, Bangalore. She has developed training manuals on cessation for health professionals for the WHO SEARO, pioneered setting up of tobacco cessation services in India; been involved in framing national guidelines for cessation and in developing content for mobile tobacco cessation in India.

Dr. Jared Ng completed his medical and psychiatric training in Singapore, and is the consultant-in-charge of the child and adolescent inpatient services at the Institute of Mental Health, Singapore. He obtained his Masters of Public Health from Harvard University and also completed his international observership at Boston Children's Hospital.

Dr. Anula Nikapota, FRCPsych (UK) has a wide experience teaching, training, and working clinically in South East Asia particularly Sri Lanka, and the UK. Special interests include service planning, cross cultural issues, postgraduate training and development of teaching material.

Dr. Susanta Padhy is Associate Professor in Child and Adolescent Psychiatry in the Department of Psychiatry at PGIMER, Chandigarh, India. Has experience of more than 13 years in Psychiatry, has 51 international and national publications, has been awarded ICMR international fellowship for young biomedical scientists for the year 2015–2016.

Dr. Bichitra Nanda Patra is Assistant Professor of Psychiatry at the All India Institute of Medical Sciences, New Delhi. He has about 20 research publications to his credit. He has been a recipient of Bhagwat award (as a coauthor) of the Indian Psychiatric Society and Dr. B.B. Sethi award of the Indian Association for Social Psychiatry.

Dr. Peter Parry trained in child and adolescent psychiatry in Adelaide, South Australia. He has worked in child and adolescent mental health services in South Australia, Wales (UK), and Queensland, Australia. He is medical director of mental health services at the Queensland Children's Hospital, Brisbane. He is affiliated with University of Queensland and Flinders University.

Dr. Sathya Prakash is currently working as a senior resident at the Department of Psychiatry at All India Institute of Medical Sciences, New Delhi. He has a keen interest in various aspects of Psychiatry including clinical, teaching, and research. He has authored many papers in peer reviewed scientific journals.

Dr. Rachel Z. Ritvo, MD, is an Assistant Clinical Professor of Psychiatry and Behavioral Sciences, George Washington University School of Medicine and Health Sciences, Washington, D.C., USA. She teaches psychodynamic psychotherapy and play technique in the child and adolescent psychiatry training program at Children's National Medical Center and is on the faculty of the Baltimore Washington Center for Psychoanalysis.

Dr. Shekhar Seshadri is Professor and Head, Department of Child and Adolescent Psychiatry, National Institute of Mental Health and Neuro Sciences (NIMHANS),

Bangalore. Besides core child and adolescent mental health including developmental disabilities, he is actively involved with areas of gender, trauma, and children in difficult circumstances, juvenile justice, Pal methodologies, community/school mental health and qualitative research.

Dr. Ruchita Shah is Assistant Professor of Psychiatry at the Post Graduate Institute of Medical Education and Research, Chandigarh, India. She is working in the area of CAMH in capacities of a clinician, an academic (DM resource faculty) and a researcher. She has published 33 research papers and authored four book chapters. She has received a medal for her postgraduate academic performance and three national awards for research.

Dr. Pratap Sharan is a professor at the All India Institute of Medical Sciences. He is a Member of the WHO International Advisory Group for the Revision of ICD-10 Mental and Behavioural Disorders. His main areas of interest are public mental health, cultural issues in psychiatry, personality disorders, and classification of mental disorders.

Dr. Aakanksha Singh is MD in Psychiatry and a student of DM in Child and Adolescent Psychiatry at the Post Graduate Institute of Medical Education and Research at Chandigarh, India.

Dr. Jatinder Singh, MSc, Ph.D., is a Senior Researcher in the Centre for Interventional Paediatric Psychopharmacology and Rare Diseases (CIPPRD) at the Maudsley Hospital, London, UK and the Institute of Psychiatry, Psychology and Neurosciences (IoPPN), King's College London, UK. Dr. Singh's research interests include different aspects of child and adolescent neuropsychiatry and rare neurodevelopmental disorders.

Dr. Aradhana Bela Sood, MD, MSHA, FAACAP, is Professor of Psychiatry and Pediatrics, and Senior Professor of Child Mental Health Policy at Virginia Treatment Center for Children, Virginia Commonwealth University, Richmond, VA.

Dr. Ashvin R. Sood is a fourth-year medical student at Virginia Commonwealth University in Richmond, VA. Ashvin is planning to practice in the field of psychiatry. Ashvin helps lead both the student psychiatric society at VCU as well as serves as a volunteer counselor for bereavement amongst children and adolescents.

Dr. Shoba Srinath is Senior Professor of Department of Child and Adolescent Psychiatry, NIMHANS, Bangalore, India with more than three decades of academic and clinical experience. Autism Spectrum Disorder and Pediatric Bipolar Affective Disorder have been her major areas of interest with numerous national and international publications.

Dr. Kai von Klitzing, MD, is Professor of Child and Adolescent Psychiatry, University of Leipzig, Germany, psychoanalyst for adults, adolescents, and children, Editor of the German language journal *KINDERANALYSE* (Child Analysis), Associate Editor of the *Infant Mental Health Journal*, and President of the World Association for Infant Mental Health. His scientific interests are: Developmental psychopathology, early triadic relationships (mother–father–infant), children's narratives, psychotherapy (individual and family), childhood maltreatment and neurobiology. He has several books on attachment disorder, children of immigrant families, and child psychotherapy.

List of Figures

List of Tables

Part I
Current Understanding of Psychiatric Disorders

Chapter 1
Pediatric Bipolar Disorders: Current Understanding and Management

Lisa M. Cullins, David C. Call and Paramjit T. Joshi

Abstract There is no question that when a youngster develops bipolar disorder, it can severely affect the normal development and psychosocial functioning of the child or adolescent and significantly increase the risk for suicide, substance abuse, academic, social and legal problems. Despite the diagnostic criteria being so well delineated, there has been much debate and interest in how bipolar disorder presents in pediatric populations, how professionals assess and diagnosis bipolar disorder in children and adolescents, and how this impacts treatment. This chapter will aim to not only discuss the epidemiology, risk and genetic factors, assessment and treatment of bipolar disorder in children and adolescents but also highlight recent trends, advancements, and research to better understand pediatric bipolar disorder.

Keywords Bipolar disorder · Mania · Children · Risk factors · Assessment · Treatment

L.M. Cullins · D.C. Call · P.T. Joshi (✉)
Department of Psychiatry and Behavioral Sciences,
Children's National Medical Center, George Washington
University School of Medicine, Washington, DC, USA
e-mail: PJOSHI@childrensnational.org

L.M. Cullins
e-mail: lcullins@cnmc.org

D.C. Call
e-mail: dcall@childrensnational.org

L.M. Cullins · D.C. Call · P.T. Joshi
Immediate Past President (AACAP), American Academy
of Child and Adolescent Psychiatry, Washington, USA

S. Malhotra and P. Santosh (eds.), *Child and Adolescent Psychiatry*,
DOI 10.1007/978-81-322-3619-1_1

1.1 Case Example

Billy is a 15-year-old adopted male with a history of attention deficit hyperactivity disorder and learning disorder who presents with a decline in functioning in school setting. Billy has always been a good-natured, well-mannered young teenager who was kind and thoughtful. Billy struggled with his social interactions and appeared to be slightly more immature than his same age peers. When Billy entered high school, although he was ready for this new educational milestone he struggled from the start in his large high school setting. Billy's mood appeared depressed and he was withdrawn and isolative at times. With the support of his individualized educational plan (IEP), Billy was able to do the work, but he had significant difficulty with his decision-making strategies and navigating social constructs. Billy began to follow negative behaviors of his peers. The peers with whom he was spending time had conflict with another group at school to the point that they began to be verbally aggressive and even threatened physical harm to Billy and his associates. Thus out of fear, Billy brought a knife to school for protection. A female peer noticed it in his backpack and notified school officials and Billy was subsequently placed in an alternative school setting. After a month of settling into his new school placement, more incidents began to occur. Billy began to leave home for long periods of time. He was supposed to take out the trash but would be gone for 2 h. His mother would drop him off at school but then he would wander off school grounds and be marked absent for the day. Billy even was detained shortly for shoplifting after he was "dared" by his peers to steal some speakers from a store. Other electronics would appear in his possession over time, which he would explain as either someone gave them to him or he bought them off of another person. Billy stated that he was able to purchase these electronics with his own money from the "candy business" he had recently started. Billy denied rapid thoughts, disturbed sleep, and pressured speech but during this time felt that he had unique skateboarding techniques that no one else could do. He also felt that he could teach the lessons in school better than his teachers. He felt a thrill of adrenaline when he was dared to do something and did it even though he knew it was wrong "I felt good. I felt powerful." He also felt that if anyone tried to take his possessions he would fight them and protect himself. As mentioned previously, Billy was adopted but when family history was further explored it was discovered that his biological father with whom he has no contact has a history of bipolar disorder. One night Billy left his home for 24 h. When he finally came back home he was taken to the emergency department for assessment and was subsequently hospitalized. Billy was started on a low dose atypical antipsychotic medication and the hypomanic/manic symptoms began to remit.

1.2 Introduction

There has been much debate and interest on how bipolar disorder presents in pediatric populations, how professionals assess and diagnosis bipolar disorder in children and adolescents, and how this impacts treatment. There is no question that when bipolar disorder strikes, it can severely affect the normal development and psychosocial functioning of the child or adolescent and significantly increase the risk for suicide, substance abuse, academic, social, and legal problems.

The diagnostic criteria for bipolar disorder is quite clear in the Diagnostic Statistical Manual of Mental Disorders—DSM-5 (American Psychiatric Association 2013). The one critical manic episode upon which this diagnosis is paramount requires that there is a distinct period of abnormally and persistently elevated, expansive, or irritable mood lasting at least 1 week (4 days for hypomania) and be present most of the day, nearly every day. It also requires a distinct period of abnormally and persistently increased goal-directed activity or energy, lasting at least 1 week (4 days for hypomania) and be present most of the day, nearly every day. In addition, there must be the presence of at least 3 (4 if the mood is only irritable) symptoms that include grandiosity, decreased need for sleep, pressured speech, racing thoughts, distractibility, psychomotor agitation or increased goal-directed activity, and involvement in high-risk activities (American Psychiatric Association 2013). Despite the diagnostic criteria being well delineated, much interest has gone into how bipolar disorder presents in pediatric populations, as the DSM criteria do not differentiate between how these symptoms might manifest in children compared to adults. This chapter will aim to not only discuss the epidemiology, risk and genetic factors, assessment and treatment of bipolar disorder in children and adolescents but also highlight recent trends, advancements, and research to better understand pediatric bipolar disorder.

1.3 Epidemiology

Multiple prevalence studies have been done to try to examine rates of bipolar disorder in pediatric populations, although most of the literature examines adolescent populations and not pre-pubertal children. The prevalence of pediatric bipolar disorder is approximately 1.8 % (Van Meter et al. 2011). This finding is further supported by the fact that approximately 60 % of adults with bipolar disorder had the onset of their symptoms prior to age 20 (Birmaher 2013). Prevalence rates can be as high as 5–6 % in subsyndromal pediatric bipolar disorder. Subsyndromal bipolar disorder is characterized by a distinct period of abnormal or persistently elevated, expansive, or irritable mood plus one or more symptoms of mania; but not meeting full criteria for bipolar disorder (Lewinsohn et al. 2000). Interestingly, being categorized as having subsyndromal bipolar disorder in adolescence was more greatly associated with developing a major depressive episode in young adulthood compared to meeting criteria for bipolar disorder in young adulthood. Further, having diagnoses of bipolar disorder or subsyndromal bipolar disorder was associated with greater psychosocial impairment, poorer global functioning, and being more likely to utilize mental health care as adults. *Billy appears to fall into either one of these diagnostic categories.*

Recent studies in the United States show a trend of increasing rates of diagnosis of bipolar disorder in pediatric populations. One study showed that in outpatient office-based settings, the number of youth with a diagnosis of bipolar disorder increased 40-fold during these time periods (1994–1995 and 2002–2003 survey data), while only increasing twofold in the adult populations (Moreno et al. 2007).

To further the importance of recognizing that individuals with bipolar disorder may start to have onset of symptoms in childhood, another study looked at adults with a diagnosis of bipolar disorder and used self reports to group them into three categories: those with the symptom onset in childhood (<13 years of age), adolescent onset(13–18 years), and adult onset. Individuals that had child onset bipolar disorder were more likely to have experienced more prolonged manic episodes, non-remitting courses (<2 months without symptoms) and greater risk of having diagnosis of antisocial personality disorder in adulthood. Childhood and adolescent onset type also had higher prevalence of substance use disorders (Goldstein and Levitt 2006).

1.4 Risk Factors

Research has looked into what factors may predispose children to develop bipolar disorder in their lifetime. The best established early marker of bipolar disorder risk remains family history. This factor has ben widely accepted in clinical practice, despite the fact that the majority of the high-risk offspring of individuals with mood disorders do not develop bipolar disorder in particular. However, a large proportion of offspring develop other mental disorders (Paaren et al. 2014). A meta-analysis of offspring studies where at least one parent has a diagnosis of bipolar disorder showed that 52 % of their offspring had a mental disorder in childhood compared to 29 % of offspring of parents with no mental disorder diagnosis. Those offsprings of a parent with bipolar disorder were four times more likely to develop a mood disorder, including bipolar disorder (DelBello and Geller 2001). A more recent longitudinal study that looked at 129 offspring (aged 16–26-years old) that had at least one parent with a diagnosis of bipolar disorder over a 5 year period found that there was an increase in diagnosis of bipolar disorder in the offspring from 3 to 10 % over the 5 year period. Prevalence rates of any psychiatric disorder increased from 44 to 59 %, showing that a positive family history of bipolar disorder is a risk factor for developing bipolar disorder and should be taken into consideration in evaluations of children (Hillegers et al. 2005). Another study that examined potential biological risk factors for development of pediatric bipolar disorder found rates of positive family history of a bipolar disorder diagnosis in first-degree relatives to be significantly higher in children diagnosed with bipolar I disorder. It also found there to be a positive association with the presence and number of perinatal risk factors, such as in utero medication exposure prescribed for medical reasons, illegal drug use during pregnancy or birth complications, and children diagnosed with bipolar disorder; suggesting family history and perinatal risk factors as potential risk factors for bipolar disorder in children (Pavuluri et al. 2006).

From the case example, there could much debate on whether Billy's clinical presentation was classic bipolar disorder or a subsyndromal type. The most compelling element that favors a bipolar process is Billy's first-degree family history of bipolar disorder.

Family studies show potential genetic and environmental links to the development of pediatric bipolar disorder. Strober et al. showed increased rates of bipolar disorder and major depressive disorder in first-degree relatives of bipolar disorder patients. Interestingly, they found an even higher prevalence of bipolar disorder in first-degree relatives of pediatric bipolar disorder patients, compared to adult onset cases (29.4 % vs. 7.4 %) (Strober et al. 1988). Another study showed that relatives of bipolar disorder patients that had onset before the age of 21 years of age were twice as likely to have bipolar disorder than those patients with onset after the age of 21 (Neuman et al. 1997). Twin studies to better understand the genetic heritability of bipolar disorder has primarily been on adult onset cases, but one study looked at pediatric twins using data from the Child Behavior Checklist (CBCL) and identifying cases with potential bipolar disorder through a profile of elevated scores on attention problems, aggressive behavior, and anxious/depressed subscales. This study showed there was a shared genetic and environmental component in the children that met the profile through the CBCL suggestive of pediatric bipolar disorder, but was limited in that the children were not interviewed and assessed to meet DSM criteria for bipolar disorder (Hudziak et al. 2005).

Premorbid psychiatric problems are common in pediatric bipolar disorder. Numerous studies have demonstrated high rates of developing mania in children and adolescents who are experiencing difficulties with disruptive behavior disorders, irritability, depressive, and anxiety symptoms. Approximately 20 % of children and adolescents with major depression go on to experience manic episodes in adulthood. Factors that predict the eventual development of mania in depressed children and adolescents include: (1) a depressive episode characterized by rapid onset, psychomotor retardation, and psychotic features; (2) a family history of affective disorders, particularly bipolar disorder; and (3) a history of mania or hypomania after treatment with antidepressants (McClellan et al. 2007).

Genetic studies have been an area of interest in better understanding the etiology and potential risk for development of bipolar disorder and a number of potential genes that are implicated in bipolar disorder include COMT (catechol-O-methyltransferase), MAO (monoamine oxidase), the dopamine transporter, and BDNF (brain-derived neurotrophic factor) (Althoff et al. 2005). Genetic studies looking at juvenile bipolar cases have been more limited, but include one small study that showed a polymorphism in the BDNF gene, suggesting that there could be a shared gene in both pediatric and adult onset bipolar disorder cases (Geller et al. 2004).

There is a growing consensus that bipolar disorder can be a progressive disease process in children and adolescents. Neuroscience findings thus far underscore the importance of tracking the progression of the underlying processes from early manifestations of the disease onward. This step is considered necessary to clarify neurophysiology prior to the confounding effects of medication exposure and illness course. Several thought provoking hypotheses have been suggested such as: increase cortical volume might represent failed pruning and white matter abnormalities may exist prior to the illness onset. These alterations in neurodevelopment may lead to affective dysregulation and eventual onset of the first manic episode (Fristad and Algorta 2013).

1.5 Diagnostic Challenges

Early studies suggested that children with bipolar disorder tend to have presentations that have a mood disturbance characterized by irritability, rather than euphoria; and have a course that is more chronic as opposed to episodic (Wozniak et al. 1995). There has been debate about the presentation of chronic irritability and if this is a true presentation of bipolar disorder in youth versus being a separate diagnostic category altogether, or a presentation of an alternative diagnosis characterized by the non-specific symptom of irritability. This led to the idea of identifying different phenotypes of mania in children for research purposes, which included a narrow phenotype that fits the criteria and definition of discrete hypomanic or manic episodes for the duration of 7 days or more (or 4 days for hypomania); intermediate phenotypes consisting either of the episodes with hallmark symptoms of mania, but lacking the duration criteria or episodes meeting the duration criteria but not meeting enough of the hallmark or "cardinal" symptoms of bipolar disorder; and a broad phenotype consisting of a more chronic course of irritability and hyperarousal that does not meet the discrete episodic nature of the narrow phenotype. Because of the uncertainty at the time of whether the broad phenotype is truly a presentation of bipolar disorder, it was termed 'severe mood dysregulation' (SMD) (Leibenluft et al. 2003). Further studies, regarding SMD suggested higher prevalence rates compared to bipolar disorder (3.3 % in a sample of 9–19-year old), and also suggested an association between meeting criteria for SMD in childhood and being diagnosed with a depressive disorder when followed prospectively. Surprisingly, the study did not show an association with meeting criteria for bipolar disorder in the future (Brotman et al. 2006). Other studies include a longitudinal community-based study that examined 776 youth at three different time points (mean ages 13.8–22.1-years old) and found that *chronic* irritability at the first time point was associated with meeting criteria for ADHD at the second time point and major depressive disorder at the third time point. In contrast, having *episodic* irritability at the first time point was associated with simple phobias and mania at the second time point. The study also showed that the type of irritability (chronic versus episodic) was likely to be stable when following it through the longitudinal course (Leibenluft et al. 2006). Yet another longitudinal study looked at children who met criteria for SMD followed them over a 2-year period to determine if there was an increased risk of developing the more classic hypomanic or manic presentations of bipolar disorder when compared to children meeting criteria for bipolar disorder. The study found that only 1 out of 84 subjects identified at the start of the study with SMD went on to develop a hypomanic or manic episode during the follow up period, contrasted with a more than 50 times greater probability of developing a hypomanic or manic episode in those children that met criteria for bipolar disorder at the start of the study (Stringaris et al. 2010).

Given that much of the evidence have shown that children presenting with the more chronically irritable phenotype seem to follow a different course than children with the more narrow, classic phenotype of bipolar disorder; a new diagnostic category was created and included in the DSM-5: disruptive mood dysregulation disorder (DMDD), to capture this phenotypic presentation. This was listed under the depressive disorder category and not the bipolar disorder section in the DSM-5. Criteria for DMDD include severe recurrent temper outbursts that are out of proportion to the situation, occurring three or more times/week and our inconsistent with the child's developmental level; presence of a persistently irritable or angry mood for most of the day nearly every day, presence for greater than 12 months without a 3 month period of absence of the above symptoms, and presence of the above symptoms in 2 out of 3 settings with the level of impairment being severe in at least one setting and at least mild-moderate in the other setting. The diagnosis should not be made for the first time before 6 years of age or after 18 years of age, and the onset be before 10 years of age. The child should not have had a distinct period of more than 1 day where the full criteria (besides duration) of hypomania or mania have been met, the behaviors do not occur exclusively in the context of a major depressive episode and are not better explained by an alternative mental disorder, or are attributable to effects of a substance or a medical condition. Given these recent changes in the diagnostic classifications, clinicians should be attentive in interviewing patient to get a good history of the time course of irritability in addition to the standard symptoms of mania. In addition, clinicians should be attentive to the overlap of some of the DMDD symptoms with ODD, but differentiating the two by the severity of the impairment, presence of severe, frequent outbursts, and presence of persistent mood disturbance in between outbursts. If the child meets both criteria for DMDD and ODD, only the diagnosis of DMDD is given (American Psychiatric Association 2013).

Another significant change in the DSM-5 criteria from DSM-IV for bipolar disorders, was that the "A" criterion now requires the combination of both the period of change in mood (euphoric, expansive, or irritable) and a change of increased goal-directed activity or energy; as opposed to these being two independent criterion. In applying the DSM-5 criterions to children and adolescents, a number of challenges arise: the symptom of irritable mood is commonly found in many other psychiatric disorders that affect children; including anxiety disorders, major depressive disorder, ADHD, developmental disorders, ODD, and PTSD. In particular, a number of symptoms such as increased rate of speech, distractibility, and increased energy can be seen in ADHD as well as bipolar disorder. A comparison study between children with ADHD versus bipolar disorder, showed that rates of irritability, hyperactivity, distractibility, and accelerated speech were similar between groups making their use for differentiating the groups challenging. Symptoms that were shown to be more specific for mania were elated mood, grandiosity, racing thoughts, hypersexuality, and decreased need for sleep that do not overlap with ADHD (Geller et al. 2002). This has led some to believe that elated mood and grandiosity should be considered "cardinal" symptoms of mania, as they appear to be more specific to bipolar disorder.

In terms of common symptoms of mania (not to be confused with the "cardinal" symptoms), (Kowatch et al. 2005) completed a meta-analysis of the phenomenology of bipolar disorder to determine what symptoms were most commonly found in children with bipolar disorder. The most common symptoms were increased energy (89 %), distractibility (84 %), pressured speech (82 %), irritability (81 %), and grandiosity (78 %). Interestingly, hypersexuality, which is one of the more specific symptoms for pediatric bipolar disorder was found to be the least commonly found symptoms (38 %) and psychosis, which does not always accompany manic episodes was found to occur at a rate of 42 % (Kowatch et al. 2005). Care must also be taken to differentiate what types of behaviors in children are developmentally appropriate versus a symptom of mania. Examples include differentiating the elation a child may feel at a party or holiday event versus elation without any clear reason to be; or the roles children may take in imaginative play such as pretending to be a superhero versus behaving in this way outside of the context of play (Geller et al. 2002). Further detailed histories must be taken to help differentiate other potential causes for what is seen as irritability, such as a major depressive episode; or what is perceived to be racing thoughts, which may actually be a manifestation of frequent ruminations and worries—as seen in a patient with an anxiety disorder.

In Billy's clinical presentation the main diagnostic challenge is discerning which part of his clinical presentation is secondary to normal adolescence in which Billy is attempting to develop his sense of self and self-identity and be autonomous and independent with his new found freedom and expansion of social network in his school setting versus understanding these events and his decision-making strategies as secondary to a disease process and representing a stark change from his baseline level of functioning. Given the persistence of the symptoms, impairment of functioning in both the home and school setting and the stark change from being a more isolative withdrawn youth to one who is thrilled by a dare, it appears that Billy's symptomatology is more accurately understood as part of an underlying mood disorder such as bipolar disorder or DMDD.

1.6 Assessment

In order to make the diagnosis of bipolar disorder, a comprehensive diagnostic assessment must be completed. This includes a parent–child interview, child interview, and interviewing the parents alone. The illness represents a marked departure from baseline functioning and it should be reflected in the level of impairment in different realms of the child's life. Normal social/emotional development, contextual framework (i.e., family, peers, school and other psychosocial factors), and cultural implications are extremely important to integrate as symptomatology is being assessed and understood in children and adolescents. The pattern of illness, duration of symptoms, and association with psychomotor, sleep and cognitive changes are important diagnostic clues given that manic like symptoms of irritability and emotional reactivity for instance may be found in a variety of childhood disorders (McClellan et al. 2007). Collateral information should be obtained from schools, primary care physician, etc. Structured diagnostic interviews and questionnaires are available that may be helpful for diagnosing bipolar disorder in children and adolescents such as the KSADS and the WASH-U-KSADS. The Young Mania Rating Scale is commonly used to assess the severity of manic symptoms and assess treatment response. However, the YMRS is not a diagnostic instrument. To date there are no biological tests such as imaging or genetic studies that are helpful in making the diagnosis of bipolar disorder in children and adolescents (McClellan et al. 2007). The clinical interview is the gold standard and the child usually needs to be seen over a period of time as symptoms often fluctuate and are episodic.

Billy's clinical presentation unfolded over the course of the school year in a fluctuating episodic nature. The integration of collateral information from parent and school and monitoring the symptom emergence over a period of time aided in understanding the disease process and accurate diagnosis.

1.7 Course of Illness

The clinical course of bipolar disorder in a child or adolescent diagnosed with this disorder can often times be an undulating and tumultuous one. Most studies have shown that at least 70–100 % of children and adolescents will recover (i.e., no significant symptoms within 2 months). However, of those who recover, up to 80 % will experience one or more recurrences in a period of 2–5 years (Birmaher et al. 2009). It has been found that these youth may suffer multiple hospitalizations, psychosis, suicide attempts and completion, substance abuse, unemployment, legal problems, and poor academic, and psychosocial functioning, which have a negative impact of multiple realms in the global level of functioning and interpersonal relationships (Martin and Volkmar 2007). In fact, the World Health Organization (WHO) reported that bipolar disorder is the fourth leading cause of disability among adolescents globally (Birmaher 2013).

The course of the illness is characterized with multiple fluctuations between syndromal and subsyndromal symptoms. Recent studies have shown that approximately 60 % of youth experience both syndromal and subsyndromal symptoms including both depressive and mixed states, which seems to be much more common in children and adolescents than adults (Martin and Volkmar 2007). Studies have shown that youth with bipolar disorder spent approximately 20 % of their follow up treatment course with full syndromal symptoms, 40 % of the time with subsyndromal symptoms and 40 % of the time euthymic (Birmaher 2013). The fluctuations in symptomatology are often rapid which contribute to the difficulty in diagnosing bipolar disorder in children.

The literature has demonstrated that early age of onset, long duration of illness, low socioeconomic status (SES), mixed or rapid cycling episodes, psychosis, subsyndromal symptoms, comorbid disorders, exposure to negative life events, and family psychopathology are associated with worse outcome (Birmaher et al. 2009; Martin and Volkmar 2007).

Furthermore, youth with subsyndromal mania (BP-NOS), especially those with a family history of bipolar disorder, are at risk to convert to BP-1 or 2 with rates of conversion of 45 %. And youth with BP-NOS have been shown to have just as much psychosocial impairment and risk for suicidality and substance abuse as the children with full syndromal bipolar type 1 (Birmaher et al. 2014).

1.8 Treatment

Treatment can usually be divided into phases: acute, continuation, and maintenance. A comprehensive treatment plan that is culturally sensitive, combining both medications and psychotherapeutic modalities should be considered to address both the frank symptoms and the psychosocial sequelae in children and adolescents with bipolar disorder. The goal of this comprehensive treatment plan is to improve symptoms, provide education about the illness, and promote treatment compliance in order to prevent relapse, reduce long-term morbidity, and promote normal growth and development (McClellan et al. 2007).

Psychoeducation and supportive therapy are essential during all of the phases of treatment. Given the significant psychosocial impairment and poor long-term prognosis associated with pediatric bipolar disorder, psychosocial intervention is imperative for a multimodal treatment approach (Weinstein et al. 2013). The unique symptoms of bipolar disorder in children and adolescents are associated with significant psychosocial impairment in several domains across development. Academically, youth with bipolar disorder demonstrate neurocognitive deficits and academic underperformance as well as disruptive school behaviors. Social functioning is influenced by limited peer networks, peer victimization, and poor social skills. Further, families of bipolar youth experience frequent sibling and parental conflict, lower levels of warmth, family adaptability and cohesion, and chronic stress in the context of family life. Children and adolescents with bipolar disorder also struggle internally with low self-esteem, hopelessness, and maladaptive coping skills (Weinstein et al. 2013).

Over recent years, there has been burgeoning research on evidence-based psychosocial interventions for pediatric bipolar disorder. Based on the literature, family psychoeducation plus skill building has the most empirical support and are considered first-line psychosocial interventions for pediatric bipolar disorder. These treatment modalities include multi-family psychoeducational psychotherapy (MF-PEP) and family-focused treatment for adolescents with bipolar disorder (FFT-A and FFT) (Fristad and MacPherson 2014). MF-PEP is a manualized intervention for children with depressive and bipolar spectrum disorders and their parents that combine psychoeducation with family therapy and cognitive behavioral therapy techniques. FFT-A consists of psychoeducation, communication enhancement training, and problem-solving skills training with adolescents, parents, and siblings. Child- and family-focused CBT as well as dialectical behavioral therapy with both a psychoeducation and skills building component have also demonstrated promising results, but more randomized controlled trials are needed. Interpersonal and social rhythm therapy that primarily targets medication compliance, interpersonal stress, and circadian rhythm dysregulation demonstrated preliminary positive findings in the current literature (Fristad and MacPherson 2014). It is important to note the similarities in all of the therapeutic approaches. The common active ingredients that should be included in the treatment of pediatric bipolar disorder should include: family involvement, psychoeducation about etiology, symptoms, course, medications, risk and protective factors, and effective treatment of bipolar disorders; skill building (especially communication, problem solving, CBT, and emotion regulation skills); and relapse prevention (Fristad and MacPherson 2014). Theses studies have also shown that clinicians should focus on improving parents' knowledge of mood disorders and beliefs about treatment, and equipping them with skills to be effective advocates and coordinators of services for their child. Lastly, youth who are the most impaired, or come from negative familial environments, will benefit the most from implementation of family psychoeducation plus skill building interventions (Fristad and MacPherson 2014).

Pharmacotherapy primarily targets symptom improvement but often does not address the associated social, academic, and family difficulties that compromise quality of life and long-term outcomes. Thus, adjunctive psychosocial treatment has been indicated as a critical component of optimally effective treatment for pediatric bipolar disorder (Weinstein et al. 2013).

In the acute phase of treatment, stabilization of symptoms is the goal. Until recently, for mania or mixed states monotherapy with either a mood stabilizer such as lithium, valproate, or carbamazepine or an atypical antipsychotic was first-line treatment. Over the past few years, pharmacologic trials have increased rapidly and have led to updated treatment algorithms, placing atypical antipsychotics ahead of mood stabilizers as a first-line treatment choice (Fristad and Algorta 2013). Although atypical antipsychotics as a group are more effective in reducing manic symptoms, they are fraught with more metabolic side effects

(Peruzzolo et al. 2013). Atypical antipsychotics have been shown to have a more rapid response and highly effective in reducing manic symptoms (Geller et al. 2012). If monotherapy fails and/or there is a partial response then the combination of two mood stabilizers or a mood stabilizer and an atypical antipsychotic must be considered. For children and adolescents who has mania with psychosis an atypical antipsychotic is considered first-line treatment. In bipolar youth with depression, mood stabilizers including lamotrigine and lithium in particular or atypical antipsychotics are still first-line treatment. However, often times, there is a partial response and the addition of an antidepressant such as a selective serotonin reuptake inhibitor or bupropion is needed. For youth with bipolar disorder in particular, cognitive behavioral therapy, interpersonal therapy, and dialectical behavioral therapy have been shown to be helpful in addition to psychoeducation and supportive therapy.

At times, adjunctive medications are needed to target severe agitation, insomnia, or aggression. In those circumstances, benzodiazepines such as lorazepam or clonazepam have been efficacious. In cases of severe illness, which has been treatment refractory, ECT in adolescents can be considered (Martin and Volkmar 2007). Once acute symptoms have been stabilized, the continuation and maintenance treatment phase goal is to prevent new mood episodes. Relapse can be as high as 92 % in children and adolescents who stop taking their medications. Thus, most youth require at minimum monotherapy for maintenance treatment (Martin and Volkmar 2007).

In regards to the case example, *Billy responded very well to monotherapy with an atypical antipsychotic and has been maintained on the same dose without any further mood episodes.*

It is clear that pharmacotherapy can be quite effective. Thus, choosing the right medication is very important. The most influential factors are efficacy, the long-term side effect profile and practicality. Lithium has been shown to be quite an effective medication for youth with bipolar disorder in both manic/mixed states and depressive states. However, from a practical point of view, given that lithium levels will need to be drawn on a regular basis, consideration must be given for the patient if he/she can sustain recurrent blood draws. In regards to atypical antipsychotics, the metabolic side effects are the most problematic and must be taken into account in the decision-making process. If the patient is already overweight and/or prediabetic these factors become even more important when contemplating treatment with these medications.

With comorbid illnesses, it is very important to treat both the bipolar disorder and the comorbid disorders; because if left untreated (i.e., ADHD), it will worsen the prognosis of bipolar disorder. It is recommended that the treatment for bipolar disorder be optimized first and then subsequently address the comorbid symptoms. Since there is overlap in the symptoms of bipolar disorder and ADHD such as impulsivity and short attention span—often when the underlying bipolar disorder is successfully treated—the patient may no longer have the symptoms of ADHD suggesting that ADHD was not a comorbid condition in that case.

1.9 Future Directions

Given the growing consensus that bipolar disorder is a progressive disease, obtaining real-time psychologic and self-report measures is extremely helpful to both understand the disease process but also to ascertain efficacious real-time coaching or other interventions in order to provide highly personalized and timely interventions to children and adolescents with bipolar disorder (Fristad and Algorta 2013). Technology can pave the way for this and children and adolescents have already demonstrated in the burgeoning telepsychiatry literature that they actually like using technology in the scope of treatment. Utilizing novel technological devices such as smartphones or higher definition, more sophisticated devices for daily monitoring of mood changes could permit identification of individual disease patterns, which could possibly provide new avenues to early detection of full episodes, as well as guide treatment adjustments. These technological advances have the potential to lead to the development of precise prognostic models and personalized, timely treatment, which may ultimately include the prevention of suicide and long-term disability. These new treatment strategies also have the potential to reach populations with poor access to services and reduce costs associated with the provision of care. Treatment might include modules on: compliance to pharmacological and psychosocial treatment modalities; sustaining a regular sleep pattern; identifying mood features; developing cognitive restructuring strategies; enhancing relaxation techniques; and could include real-time personalized feedback. It may also be possible via technology to improve communication strategies with family members and other supports in a child's life (Fristad and Algorta 2013). This type of work has already been implemented with adults, and by initial accounts appear to be quite promising in youth. There has been only one feasibility study to date in pediatric samples (Fristad and Algorta 2013).

As research has examined the benefits of both pharmacological and psychosocial interventions in pediatric bipolar disorder, the importance of nutrition in the treatment of bipolar disorder in youth has recently been empirically investigated. Recent studies have examined the role of Vitamin D and mood impairment suggesting that Vitamin D deficiency may be associated with severity of mood symptoms and psychosis. Studies have also looked at the role of omega-3 fatty acids in mood stabilization (Fristad and Algorta 2013).

Further more, machine-learning approach has been utilized in emerging research to help diagnose children and adolescents with bipolar disorder. Several studies have used pattern recognition and neuroimaging to decode present and future symptom severity in behaviorally and emotionally dysregulated youth (Mwangi et al. 2014; Mourão-Miranda et al. 2016).

Lastly, although the emergence and efficacy of evidence-based psychosocial treatment interventions have been promising more work needs to be done in the development of treatment and psychosocial approaches to be utilized in the school setting and also for dually diagnosed children and adolescents with drug and alcohol use/abuse (Fristad and Algorta 2013).

1.10 Case Outcome

Although Billy had a fluctuating episodic course, it was eventually discerned that had bipolar disorder and was promptly started on a low dose atypical antipsychotic medicine. Billy responded well to the medication and his hypomania/manic symptoms dissipated. However, Billy continued to struggle with his decision-making strategies and navigating social constructs. With ongoing individual therapy and family therapy over time, Billy has demonstrated improvement in these areas as well and has made it through his sophomore year in high school without incident.

1.11 Conclusion

Bipolar disorder can be a devastating illness, which is associated with significant morbidity and sadly at times mortality due to suicide. However, it is a treatable illness and if a child or adolescent is provided the appropriate and timely pharmacotherapy and psychotherapeutic interventions symptoms can be alleviated and the patients stabilized so they can do well and enjoy a healthy emotional life. Bipolar disorder in children and adolescents provides an added level of complexity diagnostically due to a number of factors: the rapid fluctuation in mood symptoms, developmental issues that impact the clinical picture, the difficulties that youth have in articulating how they feel and the high rates of comorbid disorders. Recent research has emerged that has shed light on symptom presentation and treatment efficacy in children and adolescents with bipolar disorder. But there remains much more to learn about risk/genetic factors and a better understanding of the biological underpinnings, cognitive development and changes in the brain. Further, we do not currently fully appreciate all of the long-term effects and efficacy of the treatment modalities and their long-term impact. Several studies are underway examining the role of social/environmental factors such as: parental lifetime and current psychopathology, level of psychological support, and exposure to negative life events (abuse, poor school or neighborhoods, and ongoing family conflict). Without question, combination treatment that includes pharmacotherapy, family involvement, psychoeducation about etiology, symptoms, course, medications, risk and protective factors, skill building (especially communication, problem solving, CBT, sleep hygiene, emotion regulation skills), and relapse prevention can reduce symptoms and improve overall level of functioning. However, much more needs to be learned to improve treatment response and ultimately prevent and/or cure bipolar disorder in children and adolescents.

References

Althoff, R. R., Faraone, S. V., Rettewe, D. C., Morley, C. P., & Hudziake, J. J. (2005). Family, twin, adoption, and molecular genetic studies of juvenile bipolar disorder. *Bipolar Disorders, 7*(6), 598–609.

American Psychiatric Association. (2013). *Diagnostic and statistical manual of mental disorders* (5th ed.). Arlington, VA: American Psychiatric Publishing.

Birmaher, B. (2013). Bipolar disorder in children and adolescents. *Child and Adolescent Mental Health, 18*(3), 140–148.

Birmaher, B., Axelson, D., Goldstein, B., Strober, M., Gill, M., & Hunt, J. (2009). Four year longitudinal course of children and adolescents with bipolar spectrum disorder. *American Journal of Psychiatry, 166*(7), 795–804.

Birmaher, B., Gill, M. K., Axelson, D. A., Goldstein, B. I., Goldstein, T. R., Yu, H., et al. (2014). Longitudinal trajectories and associate baseline predictors in youths with bipolar spectrum disorders. *American Journal of Psychiatry, 171*(9), 990–999.

Brotman, M. A., Schmajuk, M., Rich, B. A., Dickstein, D. P., Guyer, A. E., Costello, E. J., et al. (2006). Prevalence, clinical correlates, and longitudinal course of severe mood dysregulation in children. *Biological Psychiatry, 60*(9), 991–997.

DelBello, M. P., & Geller, B. (2001). Review of studies of child and adolescent offspring of bipolar parents. *Bipolar Disorders, 3*(6), 325–334.

Fristad, M., & Algorta, G. (2013). Future directions for research on youth with bipolar spectrum disorders. *Journal of Clinical Child and Adolescent Psychology, 42*(5), 734–747.

Fristad, M., & MacPherson, H. (2014). Evidence-based psychosocial treatments for child and adolescent bipolar spectrum disorders. *Journal of Clinical Child and Adolescent Psychology, 43*(3), 339–355.

Geller, B., Badner, J. A., Tillman, R., Christian, S. L., Bolhofner, K., & Cook, E. H., Jr. (2004). Linkage disequilibrium of the brain derived neurotrophic factor Val66Met polymorphism in children with a prepubertal and early adolescent bipolar disorder phenotype. *American Journal of Psychiatry, 161*(9), 1698–1700.

Geller, B., Luby, J. L., Joshi, P., Wagner, K. D., Emslie, G., Walkup, J. T., et al. (2012). A randomized controlled trial of risperidone, lithium or divalproex sodium for initial treatment of bipolar 1 disorder, manic or mixed phase, in children and adolescents. *Archives of General Psychiatry, 69*(5), 515–528. doi:10.1001/archgenpsychiatry.2011.1508

Geller, B., Zimerman, B., Williams, M., DelBello, M. P., Bolhofner, K., Craney, J. L., et al. (2002a). DSM-IV mania symptoms in a prepubertal and early adolescent bipolar disorder phenotype compared to attention-deficit hyperactive and normal controls. *Journal of Child and Adolescent Psychopharmacology, 12*(1), 11–25.

Geller, B., Zimerman, B., Williams, M., DelBello, M. P., Frazier, J., & Beringer, L. (2002b). Phenomenology of prepubertal and early adolescent bipolar disorder: Examples of elated mood, grandiose behaviors, decreased need for sleep, racing thoughts and hypersexuality. *Journal of Child and Adolescent Psychopharmacology, 12*(1), 3–9.

Goldstein, B. I., & Levitt, A. J. (2006). Further evidence for a developmental subtype of bipolar disorder defined by age at onset: Results from the national epidemiologic survey on alcohol and related conditions. *American Journal of Psychiatry, 163*(9), 1633–1636.

Hillegers, M. H., Reichart, C. G., Wals, M., Verhulst, F. C., Ormel, J., & Nolen, W. A. (2005). Five-year prospective outcome of psychopathology in the adolescent offspring of bipolar parents. *Bipolar Disorders, 7*(4), 344–350.

Hudziak, J. J., Althoff, R. R., Derks, E. M., Faraone, S. V., & Boomsma, D. I. (2005). Prevalence and genetic architecture of child behavior checklist-juvenile bipolar disorder. *Biological Psychiatry, 58*(7), 562–568.

Kowatch, R. A., Youngstrom, E. A., Danielyan, A., & Findling, R. L. (2005). Review and meta-analysis of the phenomenology and clinical characteristics of mania in children and adolescents. *Bipolar Disorders, 7*(6), 483–496.

Leibenluft, E., Charney, D. S., Towbin, K. E., Bhangoo, R. K., & Pine, D. S. (2003). Defining clinical phenotypes of juvenile mania. *American Journal of Psychiatry, 160*(3), 430–437.

Leibenluft, E., Cohen, P., Gorrindo, T., Brook, J. S., & Pine, D. S. (2006). Chronic versus episodic irritability in youth: A community-based, longitudinal study of clinical and diagnostic associations. *Journal of Child and Adolescent Psychopharmacology, 16*(4), 456–466.

Lewinsohn, P., Klein, D., & Seeley, J. (2000). Bipolar disorder during adolescence and young adulthood in a community sample. *Bipolar Disorders, 2*(3Pt2), 281–293.

Martin, A, Volkmar, F. (2007). *Lewis' child and adolescent psychiatry. A comprehensive textbook* (4th ed.). USA: Lippincott Williams & Wilkins.

McClellan, J., Kowatch, R., & Findling, R. (2007). Practice parameter for the assessment and treatment of children and adolescents with bipolar disorder. *Journal of the American Academy of Child and Adolescent Psychiatry, 46*, 1.

Moreno, C., Laje, G., Blanco, C., Jiang, H., Schmidt, A. B., & Olfson, M. (2007). National trends in the outpatient diagnosis and treatment of bipolar disorder in youth. *Archives of General Psychiatry, 64*(9), 1032–1039.

Mourão-Miranda, J., Oliveira, L., Ladouceur, C. D., Marquand, A., Brammer, M., Birmaher, B., et al. (2016). Pattern recognition and functional neuroimaging help to discriminate healthy adolescents at risk for mood disorders from low risk adolescents. *Journal of Affective Disorders, 192*(1), 219–225.

Mwangi, B., Spiker, D., Zunta-Soares, G. B., & Soares, J. C. (2014). Prediction of pediatric bipolar disorder using neuroanatomical signatures of the amygdala. *Bipolar Disorders, 16*(7), 713–721.

Neuman, R. J., Geller, B., Rice, J. P., & Todd, R. D. (1997). Increased prevalence and earlier onset of mood disorders among relatives of prepubertal versus adult probands. *Journal of the American Academy of Child and Adolescent Psychiatry, 36*(4), 466–473.

Paaren, A., Bohman, H., von Knorring, L., & Olsson, G. (2014). Early risk factors for adult bipolar disorder in adolescents with mood disorders: A 15 year follow up of a community sample. *BMC Psychiatry, 14*, 3638.

Pavuluri, M. N., Henry, D. B., Nadimpalli, S. S., O'Connor, M. M., & Sweeney, J. A. (2006). Biological risk factors in pediatric bipolar disorder. *Biological Psychiatry, 60*(9), 936–941.

Peruzzolo, T., Tramontina, S., Rohde, L., & Zeni, C. (2013). Pharmacotherapy of bipolar disorder in children and adolescents: An update. *Revista Brasileira de Psiquiatria, 35*(4), 393–405.

Stringaris, A., Baroni, A., Haimm, C., Brotman, M., Lowe, C. H., Myers, F., et al. (2010). Pediatric bipolar disorder versus severe mood dysregulation: Risk for manic episodes on follow-up. *Journal of the American Academy of Child and Adolescent Psychiatry, 49*(4), 397–405.

Strober, M., Morrell, W., Burroughs, J., Lampert, C., Danforth, H., & Freeman, R. (1988). A family study of bipolar I disorder in adolescence. Early onset of symptoms linked to increased familial loading and lithium resistance. *Journal of Affective Disorders, 15*(3), 255–268.

Van Meter, A. R., Moreira, A. L. R., & Youngstrom, E. A. (2011). Metaanalysis of epidemiologic studies of pediatric bipolar disorder. *Journal of Clinical Psychiatry, 72*(9), 1250–1256.

Weinstein, S., West, A., & Pavuluri, M. (2013). Psychosocial intervention for pediatric bipolar disorder (PBD): Current and future directions. *Expert Review of Neurotherapeutics, 13*(7), 843–850.

Wozniak, J., Biederman, J., Kiely, K., Ablon, J. S., Faraone, S. V., Mundy, E., et al. (1995). Mania-like symptoms suggestive of childhood-onset bipolar disorder in clinically referred children. *Journal of the American Academy of Child and Adolescent Psychiatry, 34*(7), 867–876.

Chapter 2
Dissociative Disorder in Children and Adolescents

Susanta Padhy, Soumya Jhanda and Savita Malhotra

Abstract Conceptually, the term dissociation means alteration of subjective experiences in perceptual, affective, memory, and identity functions in response to stress. The presentations of dissociative disorders may include distorted sensory perceptions, altered time perception, amnesia, conversion symptoms, derealization, depersonalization, fugue states, and multiple personality disorder, in isolation or in combination. Dissociation has also shown to serve major defensive roles; has psychoanalytic and neurobiological underpinnings. It has been shown that dissociation has a developmental basis beginning right from infancy (as seen in relation to attachment theory). Until recently there has been little research in this area. In this chapter we shall focus on how the concept of dissociation has evolved, addressing the defensive functions of dissociation, neurobiological characteristics particularly the developmental basis of dissociation.

Keywords Dissociative Disorder · Defense mechanisms · Neurobiology · Development · Attachment Disorders

S. Padhy (✉) · S. Jhanda · S. Malhotra
Department of Psychiatry, Post Graduate Institute of Medical Education and Research, Chandigarh 160012, India
e-mail: susanta.pgi30@yahoo.in

S. Jhanda
e-mail: soumyajhanda86@gmail.com

S. Malhotra
e-mail: savita.pgi@gmail.com

S. Malhotra and P. Santosh (eds.), *Child and Adolescent Psychiatry*,
DOI 10.1007/978-81-322-3619-1_2

Abbreviations

DID	Dissociative Identity Disorder
MPD	Multiple Personality Disorder
ICD	The International Classification of Diseases
DSM	Diagnostic and Statistical Manual of Mental Disorders
MRI	Magnetic Resonance Imaging
FDG-PET	Fluorodeoxyglucose-Positron Emission Tomography
PTSD	Posttraumatic Stress Disorder

2.1 Introduction

In a normal child, the consciousness, memory, identity, emotion, perception, body representation, motor control and behavior are integrately organized; there is a considerable degree of conscious control over the memories and sensations that can be selected for immediate attention and the movements to be carried out. However, in a child with dissociative disorders is a partial or complete loss of integration between memories of the past, awareness of identity, immediate sensations, and control of bodily movements; and ability to exercise a conscious and selective control is impaired, to a degree that can vary from day-to-day or even hour-to-hour (ICD 10). When memories are poorly integrated, the resulting disorder is dissociative amnesia; fragmentation of identity results in dissociative identity disorder; disordered perception yields depersonalization/derealization disorder.

Dissociative disorders represent more disturbances in the organization or structure of mental contents than a disturbance in the contents themselves. Memories in dissociative amnesia are not so much distorted as they are segregated from one another; the aspects of the self that are fragmented in Dissociative Identity Disorder (DID) are two-dimensional aspects of an overall personality structure. The problem is the failure of integration of information, rather than the contents of the fragments. Hence, all types of dissociative disorders have in common a lack of immediate access to the personality structure or mental content in one form or another. As neuropsychiatric disorders, they have much to teach us about the way humans adapt to traumatic stress and about information processing in the brain. In this chapter we will discuss how dissociation has evolved as a concept to serve certain functions, with associated neurobiological underpinnings and developmental dimensions.

2.2 The Evolution of a Diagnosis

The dissociative disorders were classified as Psychoneurotic Disorders in DSM-I, which described that anxiety either "directly felt and expressed or unconsciously and automatically controlled by various defense mechanisms". This was, to a large extent, influenced by the psychoanalytic theory.

DSM-II (1968) classified these disorders as Hysterical Neurosis, with two subtypes, i.e., conversion type and dissociative type. In conversion type, the special senses were described to get affected, causing symptoms such as blindness, deafness, anaesthesia, paraesthesia, ataxia, and dyskinesias. In the dissociative subtype, alteration was described to occur in patient's state of consciousness or in his identity, to produce symptoms such as amnesia, somnambulism, fugue, and multiple personality.

DSM-III (1980) and its revision DSM-III-R (1987) included it under the diagnostic categories of psychogenic amnesia, psychogenic fugue, multiple personality disorder (MPD), depersonalization disorder, and atypical dissociative disorder. DSM-III-R stated that the essential feature of the dissociative disorders was "a disturbance in the normally integrative functions of identity, memory, or consciousness." in the absence of brain insult, injury, or disease.

DSM-IV (1994) and DSM IV-TR (2000) included under the dissociative disorders: the categories of dissociative amnesia, dissociative fugue, dissociative identity disorder, depersonalization disorder, and dissociative disorder NOS. Cases resembling DID, but without amnesia, was moved to the new category of "Dissociative Disorder Not Otherwise Specified" (DDNOS).

Major changes in dissociative disorders from DSM IV-TR to DSM-5 include the following: (1) derealization has been included in the name and symptom structure of what previously was called depersonalization disorder and is now called depersonalization/derealization disorder, (2) dissociative fugue is now a specifier of dissociative amnesia rather than a separate diagnosis, and (3) the criteria for dissociative identity disorder have been changed to indicate that symptoms of disruption of identity may be reported, as well as, observed, and those gaps in the recall of events may occur for everyday and not just traumatic events. Also, experiences of pathological possession in some cultures are included in the description of identity disruption.

2.3 Dimensions of Dissociation

Dissociation is a complex process composed of a number of related domains. In addition to the disruptions of memory and identity that are a core feature of dissociative disorders, dissociation involves experiences of intense absorption (Bernstein and Putnam 1986). Measures of absorption such as the Tellegen Absorption Scale (Tellegen and Atkinson 1974) correlate significantly with measures of hypnotizability and with measures of pathological dissociation (Nash et al. 1993).

Dissociation is often discussed from another perspective, that of entry into a specific state of consciousness, the dissociative state. The concept of dissociative state of consciousness was present in the earliest writings of hypnosis and dissociative disorders. Dissociative states were a core feature of Janet's thinking about dissociative disorders and continue to be routinely invoked in discussions of hypnosis and the dissociative disorders today (Putnam 1991). From this perspective, an individual experiencing dissociation enters into a unique state of consciousness—the dissociative state that has certain specific features—(a) isolation of memory and affect from normal states of consciousness (b) disturbance in sense of identity or sense of self (c) intense absorption of focused concentration and in the case of hypnotic state and increased suggestibility.

Dissociation is thus conceptualized as a specific state of consciousness with certain properties that individuals enter into with different frequencies and/or for different lengths of time, thereby creating a continuum distribution of the degree of dissociation (Saxe et al. 1993). Those individuals who enter into a dissociative state more often and/or for longer periods, experience significantly more dissociative phenomena. An individuals' dissociativity can be defined as a function of the frequency and duration with which the individual spontaneously enters into a dissociative state of consciousness in naturally occurring situations (Putnam 1991).

2.3.1 The Defensive Mechanisms of Dissociation

Dissociation is widely regarded as a defensive operation invoked by individuals caught in situations they wish to escape or avoid. From Janet (1920) onward, it has been recognized that dissociation serves to defend an individual against unacceptable psychological or physical experiences. Ludwig (1983) proposed a set of adaptive and defensive functions performed by dissociation including automatization of certain behaviors, efficiency, and economy of effort, escape from the constraints of reality and isolation of catastrophic experiences and cathartic discharge of feelings. Additional defensive operations such as analgesia and detachment from the self have been identified by others (Putnam 1991).

These aforementioned defense functions can be broadly classified into four defensive operations: (a) automatization, (b) compartmentalization, (c) alteration of identity, (d) protection from unbearable pain. These dissociative subprocesses work independently and in combination to produce the psychological and clinical phenomena identified as dissociative behavior. It should be kept in mind that dissociation is commonly present in a variety of minor forms in everyday life and it is in many respects a last effort psychological defense response.

2.3.1.1 Automatization

Many of the examples of "everyday" normal dissociative behaviors involve automatization of complex actions such as driving a car in high-speed traffic. Automatization involves a redirection of conscious awareness away from an activity. Usually attention is withdrawn from a repetitive or procedural activity that can be done by rote. Conscious awareness is frequently redirected from external activities to internal preoccupations. The ability to divide attention, particularly in situations where the individual is facing a boring but potentially demanding task, increases the ability to accomplish necessary mental chores such as planning and problem solving.

Automatization may occur in varying degrees, with a dynamic waxing and waning of conscious awareness of the activity depending on changing circumstances. Automatized activities may range from complex tasks like driving an automobile to minor mental overflow activities like doodling while talking on the telephone. Return of conscious awareness to the automatized task may be rapid and abrupt.

2.3.1.2 Compartmentalization

A second, critical component of defensive dissociation is compartmentalization, the partitioning off of areas of conscious experiences from each other. Defensively, compartmentalization permits the isolation of catastrophic experiences. Overwhelming perceptions, sensations, affects and ideation can be walled off from everyday waking consciousness, allowing the individual to function in other areas of life. The dissociation of traumatic experiences from normal consciousness, however, impedes their psychological resolution so that walled-off trauma remains "raw" and psychologically fresh despite the passage of time. Dissociated traumatic material often seems to have a life of its own, periodically intruding into awareness through dreams and nightmares, flashbacks, intrusive images, affects, and memories. The induction of altered states of consciousness by alcohol, drugs, hypnosis, or other procedures frequently increases the leakage of dissociated material into conscious awareness (Ludwig 1983). In addition to sequestering traumatic material, compartmentalization can act to preserve sensitive psychological functions and capacities by rigidly isolating them from disruptive and intrusive material.

2.3.1.3 Alterations and Estrangements of Self

Dissociative defensive alterations of identity take a variety of forms. In psychogenic amnesia, the individual may "forget" who and what he is in a global and selective way as necessary to protect himself from the effects of a traumatic event. While in a psychogenic fugue, an individual may elaborate another identity, remaining largely amnesic for his original identity and its problems. In multiple personality disorder, the individual switches among a series of alter identities that personify specific functions, capacities or experiences. In depersonalization, the individual experiences a loss of or a distortion in his or her sense of reality of self, often accompanied by feelings of detachment and "numbness".

Profound alterations of identity in concert with compartmentalization, can effectively, if only transiently, isolate catastrophic psychological experiences. The withdrawal of investment in self that accompanies traumatically induced depersonalization acts to protect the individual from the loss or annihilation of self in the face of death.

The alter personalities of MPD represent complex disturbances of identity and self that contain conflicts, preserve functions, and express forbidden impulses. The partial or complete obliteration of identity in psychogenic amnesia often serves to "stop time" until the individual can safely process the overwhelming event. Dissociative alterations in self and identity transform the denial process from "its not happening" to "its not happening to me".

2.3.1.4 Protection from Unbearable Pain

Most of the defensive operations of dissociation act to spare the individual from overwhelming psychological and physical pain. Analgesia or even complete anaesthesia for pain is commonly reported during traumatically induced dissociative reactions. Protection from physical pain, together with depersonalization of self, permits some individuals to endure horrible experiences such as rape or torture in a detached manner (Nash et al. 1993).

2.3.2 Neurobiology of Dissociation

2.3.2.1 Neurobiology of Amnesia

Less is known about the neurobiology of amnestic states, as these are often difficult to capture as they are occurring, and their dissociative nature may not be firmly established before they resolve. Nonetheless, fMRI has been used to study laboratory paradigms of memory suppression or repression using nonpsychiatric participants instructed to either think or not think of the second member of a pair of words previously seen (Shmuelof and Zohary 2005). Subsequent cued recall of suppressed words was inferior to recall of baseline words. This suppression response perhaps involved the circuits involving prefrontal cortex, paralimbic, subcortical, and parietal integration areas accompanied by bilateral reduced activation of hippocampal areas (Milner 1959; Shmuelof and Zohary 2005). However, Hippocampal activation patterns differed between individuals with ordinary forgetting versus suppression-induced forgetting. Moreover, there is suggestion of involvement of dorsolateral prefrontal cortex, hippocampus, anterior cingulate cortex, medial temporal lobe, dorsal pre-motor cortex, presupplementary motor area, and intraparietal areas which might support a neurobiological model for memory control in response to trauma, and the duration of amnesia.

There are very few neurobiological studies of individuals with dissociative amnesia. In a paper in which glucose-PET data from 14 patients with dissociative amnesia and severe episodic-autobiographical memory deficits were analyzed in combination, it was found that again the right temporo-frontal region was hypometabolic in a significant number of patients, with a significant reduction in the right infero-lateral prefrontal cortex (Brand et al. 2009). This finding has possible therapeutic implications. It suggests that if the brain regions of the right temporo-frontal cortex, which are interconnected by the uncinate fascicle, were brought to normal metabolic activity via environmental manipulations, the patients' ability to recollect personal events from the past might be reinstated. A kind of confirmation and extension of these results came in same year from the work of Tramoni et al. (2009), who in a patient with dissociative ("functional") amnesia performed magnetization transfer ratio measurement and MR spectroscopic imaging—methods sensitive to microstructural and metabolic brain changes. They found evidence of significant metabolic changes and subtle structural alterations of the white matter in the right prefrontal region. A recent review of these studies (Staniloiu et al. 2012) suggested that disruptions or functional disconnections between major neural networks might be etiological in dissociative amnesia syndromes.

2.3.2.2 Neurobiology of Depersonalization

Depersonalization disorder involves a dissociation of perceptions (feeling detached from own body or mental activity, like in a dreaming state or like an outside observer), in the absence of significant impairment of reality testing. It is characterized by an alteration of the subjective experience of self.

While several imaging studies of depersonalization focused on targeting the neural correlates of depersonalization as a symptom of other disorder (Lanius et al. 2005) or a symptom that was induced via various environmental manipulations (Stone et al. 2006; Blanke and Metzinger 2009) only a few studies looked at the neural correlates of depersonalization disorders. Simeon et al. (2000) investigated 8 subjects with depersonalization disorder and 24 healthy matched controls with both structural (MRI) and functional imaging (FDG-PET). During the PET scanning the subjects were given a variant of California Verbal Learning Test modified for use in imaging study. The depersonalization disorder group showed significantly lower metabolic rates in areas belonging to the right superior temporal gyrus and middle temporal gyrus. In addition, they showed higher metabolic rates in parietal lobe in comparison to normal probands. In occipital lobes, left Brodmann area 19 was significantly more active in the depersonalization group. The authors concluded that depersonalization disorder is associated with functional abnormalities in sensory cortex (visual, auditory and somatosensory) as well as areas that are important for body schema (such as parietal cortex).

2.3.2.3 Imaging the Symptom of Dissociation

Various dissociative symptoms can accompany a number of psychiatric diagnostic entities (other than dissociative or conversion disorders) and have been targeted by several functional imaging studies (Kraus et al. 2009; Ludascher et al. 2010). For example dissociative amnesia can occur as a symptom in certain anxiety disorders, such as acute stress disorder and posttraumatic stress disorder (PTSD) or in the DSM-5 described somatization disorder or in borderline personality disorder (Horowitz 1979; Zanarini et al. 2008). PTSD conditions which are accompanied by "positive" dissociative symptoms such as flashbacks and intrusions seem to engage different neural networks than PTSD conditions that are accompanied by "negative" dissociative symptoms such as amnesia (Oakley 1999). Lanius (2005) found that in general a network of prefronto-temporoparietal are as was engaged in all patients, but that the group with "positive" symptoms had compared to normal subjects—in addition a greater covariation with the right insula and right visual association cortex (compared to the reference in the left ventrolateral thalamus). Between the two groups, that with "negative" symptoms of dissociation showed—compared to the "positive" (flashbacks) group—a more significant covariation in the left inferior frontal gyrus, while vice versa the "positive" symptoms group had more significant covariations with posterior cingulate/precuneus regions, the right middle temporal and the left inferior frontal gyri. In a recent review arguments were made for a mechanism of under modulation of emotion via failure of prefrontal inhibition of limbic regions (such as amygdala) underlying the reexperiencing/hyperarousal PTSD subtype and one of over modulation of the emotional limbic reactions in the ("negative") dissociative PTSD subtype (Lanius et al. 2010).

2.4 The Developmental Basis of Dissociative Disorders

2.4.1 Normative Dissociation in Children

Very little is known about the developmental basis of dissociation and the dissociative disorders. Potentially relevant domains of knowledge include (a) research on the developmental basis of hypnotizability (b) studies of behavioral states in infants (c) the array of diverse theoretical perspectives and empirical data on the nature and development of imagination and fantasy in children (d) research on attachment and attunement, particularly as it relates to dissociative behavior between the mother and child and, (e) studies of the development and integration of self.

Most authorities believe that children are normatively more dissociative than adults (Kluft and Loewenstein 2007; Putnam 1991). This is based more on clinical experience than on empirical data (Deka et al. 2007). Experimental knowledge about one form of normal dissociation comes from the studies of hypnotizability, a modern correlate of clinical dissociation in adults and only a presumed correlate of clinical dissociation in children. A second and source of data comes from research with the Child Dissociative Checklist (Putnam et al. 1993). In sum, these data lend support to the clinical conceptualization that children are more dissociative than adults. They also indicate that dissociative capacity declines over the course of childhood and adolescence. Beyond these general impressions, however, virtually nothing is known for certain about the developmental trajectory of normative dissociation.

Data on hypnotizability in children show a curvilinear relationship with age, initially rising to a peak at about 9–10 years of age and then declining during adolescence (Putnam 1991). Cross-sectional studies of adults reveal that hypnotizability continues to decline over the life cycle, though the slope becomes more gradual by the third decade (Jans et al. 2008).

2.4.2 Imagination and Fantasy

One of the most important areas in the development of dissociative disorders comes through the study of imagination and fantasy. Much has been learned about the range and course of imagination and fantasy capacities over development. Role playing, fantasy, and other aspects of make-believe have received periodic attention by developmental psychologists (Bretherton 1989). These activities have been studied primarily in play or storytelling contexts with samples of normal children, typically preschoolers. Investigation of pretend play reveals a great deal of complexity and richness in young children. Of particular relevance to the dissociative disorders is the identity shifts that children manifest during pretend play. In addition to being "actors" in their make-believe play, children are also "playwrights" and "stage directors". Children switch back and forth among these roles so seamlessly and it is only rarely that they become confused about which role they or their partner are in at a given moment. A better understanding of role playing and role exchanging capacities in normal and traumatized children may shed light on dissociative disturbances in the modulation of identity transformation.

A second area of developmental research has focused on the ability of children to distinguish between reality and fantasy. With age, children develop an increasing ability to distinguish between these domains. Even three year olds can reliably differentiate between real and mental representations of same objects (Harris 1991). It has been postulated that children develop the concept of a boundary between fantasy and reality realms that becomes more sophisticated with time. Children appear to have more difficulty making this differentiation in the area of fantasies about monsters, ghosts, and other scary beings. The studies of children's wary reactions to a box that contain an imagined monster which convincingly demonstrates that even six-year olds can become frightened by their own fantasy creation.

An extention of Harris (1991) hypothesis is that perhaps monsters, ghosts, and scary creatures represent a special class of mental objects that differ from mental representations of common physical objects (cup, toothbrushes, etc.) used in other studies of reality testing. It may be imagined that "living" entities, be they good or evil, are more real for children (and adults) than are imagined physical objects.

A third related area of research concerns the nature of imaginary companionship. Most developmental studies use definition of an imaginary companion as "an invisible character, named and referred to in conversation with other persons or played with directly for a period of time, having an air of reality for the child but no apparent objective basis". Imaginary companionship is relatively common normative phenomena, beginning about the age of four. Parents are often unaware of the existence of number of imaginary companions their child have. A variety of purposes have been proposed for imaginary companions. Psychoanalytic writings concentrate on association with stress, loneliness, or discharge of forbidden impulses, the developmental literature emphasizes on socialization. Firstborn and only children are more likely to have imaginary companions, and children with imaginary companions are more adept at talking and interacting with adults and score higher on measures of socialization (Manosevitz 1973).

Imaginary companionship has been identified as a possible developmental substrate for the creation of alter personalities in MPD patients (Hilgard 1977; Lynn 1988). Many adult MPD patients report that their alter personalities first existed as externalized imaginary companions created for companionship during times of loneliness or physical confinement. Congruent with adult reports, the alter personality in children with MPD are sometimes externalized by the children as vivid imaginary companionship rather than internalized alter personalities (Putnam 1991). Clinical evidence suggests that these externalized alter personalities are later internalized around puberty.

The developmental literature views imagination and fantasy capacities as normative and more likely to be associated with socialization and creativity, whereas, the psychoanalytic literature regards these processes as serving defensive purposes. Among the defensive functions ascribed to fantasy are escape, wish fulfillment, restitution of self-esteem and revenge. It seems reasonable that if adults retreat into imaginary worlds during times of isolation and maltreatment, that traumatized children, with their developmentally heightened imaginary capacities, must also make use of this escape route (Feinstein 2011).

One branch of research on hypnosis has concentrated on the identification and study of "fantasy-prone individuals". Fantasy prone individuals denote a group of persons who "live much of their time in a world of their own making- a world of imagery, imagination and fantasy". It is estimated that about 4 % of the population are fantasy prone. These individuals tend to hallucinate vividly, experience fantasy as reality, and to have difficulty in differentiating fantasy events from real experiences. Fantasy prone individuals report a variety of identity alteration processes including, believing that they become someone else while in fantasy and having out of body experiences. Fantasy prone individuals are also highly hypnotizable. Of particular interest is the observation that fantasy prone individuals generally share a childhood background of abuse, neglect, and hardship (James 1984; Lynn 1988). In addition to being highly hypnotizable, fantasy prone individuals are also highly dissociative.

In summary, several lines of evidence connect dissociation with imagination and fantasy capacities.

2.4.3 Dissociation and Attachment Theory

The concept of attachment has proven to be a powerful construct driving much research in the field of developmental psychology and developmental psychopathology. The impact of maltreatment on attachment behavior in children has been investigated. Histories of insecure attachment are significantly related to self-destructive behaviors in adults abused or neglected as children (Van der Kolk 1991). High levels of dissociation were predictive of self-mutilation and suicide attempts in the above study sample. Significant levels of dissociation, on the part of the child and/or caretakers, are likely to influence the display of attachment behaviors in certain contexts and to influence the quality of attachment relationship.

Although no formal studies of attachment behavior exist for dissociative patients, clinicians have invoked attachment theory in explanations of MPD. Barach (1991) equates the detachment phase of separation response described by Bowlby with dissociation in that the abandoned child is sequestering information and behavior related to attachment stimuli. It has been viewed the detachment response as a "deactivation of the attachment behavioral system that excluded from awareness signals, arising from both inside and outside the person, that would activate their attachment behavior and that would enable them both to love and to experience being loved". The dissociative memory disturbances could serve as a mechanism for screening out attachment cues or for decoupling attachment behavior from attachment stimuli. Clinically, detachment from self and surroundings, usually manifest in depersonalization and derealization, a common feature of dissociative disorder and evoked by overwhelming trauma.

At present, the strongest line of evidence supporting the argument that MPD involves significant disturbances in attachment comes from interpretations of the typical transferential responses of MPD patients in psychotherapy. Early in treatment, MPD patients characteristically "test" their therapists with frequent emergencies, demands for extra sessions and requests for special treatment. At the same time they usually make threats and attempts to leave treatment citing the therapist's failure to meet their needs as justification. Barach (1991) interprets these behaviors as evidence for the activation/deactivation of attachment behaviors. One of the core principles of treatment for MPD is that the therapist provides a constancy of demeanor and behavior in counterresponse to the perturbations in the therapeutic relationship resulting from alters personalities' differential transference responses (Lyons-Ruth et al. 2006).

One potential area of investigation is the effects of dissociation on the integration of the internal representational models that are postulated to underlie the meaning and organization of attachment responses. A pathologically dissociating child could be expected to have several different working models of an attachment relationship with his/her abuser—each associated with a specific set of dissociatively compartmentalized memories. The dissociative barriers would act to impede the integration of different attachment representations. Consequently, the child would show very different attachment behaviors depending on which set of memories and representational model is currently being activated (Spitzer et al. 2006).

In MPD, clinicians often find within the same individual alter personalities that hate the abusing parent, alter personalities that idealize the same parent, and alter personalities that disclaim any relationship, positive or negative, with the parent. The ability of abused children to maintain strong attachments to their abusers may reflect some form of dissociation of their internal representational models.

2.5 Conclusions

After reading the chapter it is evident dissociative disorders constitute a complex manifestation of mental processes of which emotional trauma seems to play a primary role. They have been understood both in terms of psychoanalytic principles and have also been shown to have neurobiological underpinnings. The set of adaptive and defensive functions performed by dissociation include automatization of certain behaviors, efficiency and economy of effort, escape from the constraints of reality and isolation of catastrophic experiences, and cathartic discharge of feelings. It has shown to be related to attachment theory, and has a strong developmental basis in children. Hence, to be able to understand the phenomena, one has to evaluate in detail the history since early childhood and environmental modulators; and the significant interaction between them.

References

American Psychiatric Association. (1952). *Diagnostic and statistical manual of mental disorders* (1st ed.). Washington, DC: APA.

American Psychiatric Association. (1968). *Diagnostic and statistical manual of mental disorders* (2nd ed.). Washington, DC: APA.

American Psychiatric Association. (1980). *Diagnostic and statistical manual of mental disorders* (3rd ed.). Washington, DC: APA.

American Psychiatric Association. (1987). *Diagnostic and statistical manual of mental disorders* (3 Revised ed.). Washington, DC: APA.

American Psychiatric Association. (1994). *Diagnostic and statistical manual of mental disorders* (4th ed.). Washington, DC: APA.

American Psychiatric Association. (2000). *Diagnostic and statistical manual of mental disorders* (4 Text Rev ed.). Washington DC: APA.

Barach, P. M. (1991). Multiple Personality Disorder as Attachment Disorder. *Dissociation, 4*, 117–123.

Bernstein, E. M., & Putnam, F. W. (1986). Development, reliability, and validity of a dissociation scale. *The Journal of Nervous and Mental Disease, 174*, 727–735.

Blanke, O., & Metzinger, T. (2009). Full-body illusions and minimal phenomenal selfhood. *Trends in Cognitive Sciences, 13*, 7–13.

Brand, M., Eggers, C., Reinhold, N., Fujiwara, E., Kessler, J., Heiss, W. D., et al. (2009). Functional brain imaging in 14 patients with dissociative amnesia reveals right inferolateral prefrontal hypometabolism. *Psychiatry Research, 30*, 32–39.

Bretherton, I. (1989). Attachment: The parental perspective. *Infant Mental Health Journal, 10*, 203–221.

Cardeña, E. A., & Gleaves, D. H. (2003). Dissociative disorders: Phantoms of the self. In M. Hersen & S. M. Turner (Eds.), *Adult psychopathology and diagnosis* (4th ed., pp. 476–505). Hoboken: Wiley.

Deka, K., Chaudhury, P., & Bora, K. (2007). A study of clinical correlates and socio-demographic profile in conversion disorder. *Indian Journal of Psychiatry, 49*, 205–207.

Feinstein, A. (2011). Conversion disorder: Advances in our understanding. *CMAJ, 183*, 915–920.

Harris, P. (1991). Monsters, ghosts and witches: Testing the limits of the fantasy - reality distinction in young children, *British Journal of Developmental Psychology, 9*,105–123.

Hilgard, E. R. (1977). *Divided consciousness: Multiple controls in human thought and action.* New York: Wiley-Interscience.

Horowitz, M. J. (1976). *Stress response syndromes*. New York: Jason Aronson.

James, W. (1984). William James on exceptional mental states. In E. Taylor (Ed.), *The 1896 Lowell lectures*. Amherst, MA: The University of Massachusetts Press.

Janet, P. (1920). *The major symptoms of hysteria* (p. 332). New York: Macmillan.

Jans, T., Schneck-Seif, S., Weigand, T., Schneider, W., Ellgring, H., Wewetzer, C., et al. (2008). Long-term outcome and prognosis of dissociative disorder with onset in childhood or adolescence. *Child and Adolescent Psychiatry and Mental Health, 2*, 19.

Kluft, R. P., & Loewenstein, R. J. (2007). Dissociative disorders and depersonalization. In G. O. Gabbard (Ed.), *Gabbard's treatment of psychiatric disorders* (4th ed., p. 547). Washington, DC: American Psychiatric Publishing.

Kraus, A., Esposito, F., Seifritz, E., Ruf, M., Valerius, G., Ludaescher, P., et al. (2009). Amygdala deactivation as a neural correlate of pain processing in patients with borderline personality disorder and co-occurrent posttraumatic stress disorder. *Biological Psychiatry, 65*, 819–822.

Lanius, R., Williamson, P. C., Bluhm, R. L., Densmore, M., Boksman, K., & Neufeld, R. W. (2005). Functional connectivity of dissociative responses in posttraumatic stress disorder: A functional magnetic resonance imaging investigation. *Biological Psychiatry, 57*, 873–884.

Lanius, R. A., Vermetten, E., Loewenstein, J., Brand, B., Schmahl, C., Bremner, J. D., et al. (2010). Emotion modulation in PTSD: Clinical and neurobiological evidence for a dissociative subtype. *American Journal of Psychiatry, 167*, 640–647.

Ludascher, P., Valerius, G., Stiglmayr, C., Mauchnik, J., Lanius, R. A., & Bohus, M. (2010). Pain sensitivity and neural processing during dissociative states in patients with borderline personality disorder with and without comorbid posttraumatic stress disorder: A pilot study. *Journal of Psychiatry and Neuroscience, 35*, 177–184.

Ludwig, A. M. (1983). The psychobiological functions of dissociation. *Am J Clin Hypn, 26*, 93–99.

Lyons-Ruth, K., Dutra, L., Schuder, M. R., & Bianchi, I. (2006). From infant attachment disorganization to adult dissociation: Relational adaptations or traumatic experiences? *The Psychiatric Clinics of North America, 29*, 63.

Lynn, S.J. (1988). Fantasy proneness. Hypnosis, developmental antecedents, and psychopathology. *Am Psychol, 43*, 35–44.

Manosevitz (1973). Individual and family correlates of imaginary companions in preschool children. *Developmental Psychology, 8*, 72–79.

Milner, B. (1959). The memory defect in bilateral hippocampal lesions. *Psychiatric Research Reports, 11*, 42–52.

Nash, M. R., Hulsey, T. L., Sexton, M. C., Harralson, T. L., & Lambert, W. (1993). Long-term sequelae of childhood sexual abuse: Perceived family environment, psychopathology, and dissociation. *Journal of Consulting and Clinical Psychology, 1993*(61), 276–283.

Oakley, D. A. (1999). Hypnosis and conversion hysteria: A unifying model. *Cognitive Neuropsychiatry, 4*, 243–265.
Putnam, F. W. (1991). Dissociative disorders in children and adolescents. A developmental perspective. *Psychiatric Clinics of North America, 14*, 519–531.
Putnam, F. W., Helmers, K., & Trickett, P. K. (1993). Development, reliability, and validity of a child dissociation scale. *Child Abuse and Neglect, 17*, 731–741.
Saxe, G. N., van der Kolk, B. A., & Berkowitz, R. (1993). Dissociative disorders in psychiatric patients. *American Journal of Psychiatry, 150*, 1037–1042.
Shmuelof, L., & Zohary, E. (2005). Dissociation between ventral and dorsal fMRI activation during object and action recognition. *Neuron, 47*, 457–470.
Simeon, D., Guralnik, O., Hazlett, E. A., Spiegel-Cohen, J., & Hollander, E. (2000). Feeling unreal: A PET study of depersonalization disorder. *American Journal of Psychiatry, 157*, 1782–1788.
Simeon, D., Knutelska, M., Yehuda, R., Putnam, F., Schmeidler, J., & Smith, L. M. (2007). Hypothalamic-pituitary-adrenal axis function in dissociative disorders, post-traumatic stress disorder, and healthy volunteers. *Biological Psychiatry, 15*, 966–973.
Spitzer, C., Barnow, S., Freyberger, H. J., & Grabe, H. J. (2006). Recent developments in the theory of dissociation. *World Psychiatry, 5*, 82–86.
Staniloiu, A., Vitcu, A., Markowitsch, H. (2012). Neuroimaging and dissociative disorders. In *Advances in brain imaging* (pp. 11–34).
Stone, J., Smyth, R., Carson, A., Warlow, C., & Sharpe, M. (2006). La belle indifférence in conversion symptoms and hysteria: Systematic review. *The British Journal of Psychiatry Journal of Mental Science, 188*, 204–209.
Tellegen, A., & Atkinson, G. (1974). Openness to absorbing and self-altering experiences ("absorption"), a trait related to hypnotic susceptibility. *Journal of Abnormal Psychology, 83*, 268–277.
Terr, L. C. (1991). Childhood traumas: An outline and overivew. *American Journal of Psychiatry, 148*, 10–20.
Tramoni, E., Aubert-Khalfa, S., Guye, M., Ranjeva, J. P., Felician, O., & Ceccaldi, M. (2009). Hypo-retrieval and hyper-suppression mechanisms in functional amnesia. *Neuropsychologia, 47*, 611–624.
Van der Kolk, B. (1991). Hypnotizability and dissociation. *Am J Psychiatry, 148*, 1105–1106.
World Health Organization. (1993). The ICD-10 classification of mental and behavioural disorders: Diagnostic criteria for research.
Zanarini, M. C., Frankenburg, F. R., Jager-Hyman, S., Reich, D. B., Fitzmaurice, G. (2008). The course of dissociation for patients with borderline personality disorder and axis II comparison subjects: A 10-year follow-up study. *Acta Psychiatrica Scandinavica, 118*, 291–296.

Chapter 3
Attention Deficit Hyperactivity Disorder and DSM 5: What's New?

Aradhana Bela Sood and Ashvin R. Sood

Abstract The diagnostic and statistical manual (DSM) serves as a guide for the clinical practice of psychiatry internationally. The newest version, the DSM 5 was published in 2013. In this version, the diagnostic criteria for attention deficit hyperactivity disorder (ADHD) have undergone significant changes. This chapter focuses on the current criteria for diagnosing attention deficit disorder (ADD) and provides a synopsis of the changes in the criteria set for ADHD/ADD in the DSM 5 in comparison to DSM IV R. This chapter frames the new/revised criteria for ADHD/ADD by comparing them with the DSM IV TR and provides the reader with the theoretical rationale for the changes. The impact that these new criteria may have on the prevalence and incidence rates of ADHD/ADD and the manner in which the diagnosis in adults and children is arrived at are discussed. The role of culture on similarities and differences, and the manner in which these syndromes present in the USA and India are covered. A brief overview of broad assessment techniques and treatment strategies focusing primarily on the child and adolescent population are also discussed. Clinical vignettes are used to illustrate how these changes potentially affect clinical practice.

Keywords Attention deficit disorder and DSM 5 · ADHD and diagnosis in children and adolescents · ADHD and assessment · ADHD and treatment · Culture and ADHD

A.B. Sood (✉)
Child Mental Health Policy, Division of Child and Adolescent Psychiatry, Virginia Commonwealth University, Richmond, VA, USA
e-mail: Bela.sood@vcuhealth.org

A.R. Sood
Virginia Commonwealth University School of Medicine, Richmond, VA, USA
e-mail: Ashvinsood1@gmail.com

S. Malhotra and P. Santosh (eds.), *Child and Adolescent Psychiatry*,
DOI 10.1007/978-81-322-3619-1_3

3.1 Introduction

Attention deficit hyperactivity disorder (ADHD), or attention deficit disorder (ADD), is globally recognized as a disorder with an onset in childhood. Over the years, the nomenclature of this neurobiological disorder has changed and the use of a collapsing or expanding set of criteria has influenced how the diagnosis is made and coded in various versions of the diagnostic and statistical manual (DSM) of psychiatric diagnoses. The DSM taxonomy has been criticized for its categorical and nondimensional approach in describing symptoms that occur in the normal continuum of human behavior. Attention span, impulse control, and varying levels of energy are common variables in human behavior that become difficult to categorically define as normal and abnormal. Yet the DSM remains a major reference for an international nomenclature for psychiatric illness. In mid-2013, the new DSM 5 was published and currently acts as a guide for the clinical practice of psychiatry. The focus of this chapter will be to present the current understanding of ADD and a synopsis of what the changes in the criteria set for ADHD/ADD are in the DSM 5 in comparison to DSM IV R.

This chapter examines the new and revised criteria for ADHD/ADD and provides the reader rationale for the changes in DSM 5 while providing a brief overview of assessment treatment strategies focusing primarily on the child and adolescent population. Clinical vignettes will help illustrate how these changes will influence practice.

Although international studies conducted to look at the incidence of ADHD worldwide show that the prevalence of the disorder is similar across cultures, there may be a difference in the way ADHD/ADD are viewed in the South Asian subcontinent versus Western cultures. This perspective will be explored using a vignette demonstrating how an ADHD/ADD diagnosis and treatment plan differs and is similar in two cultures.

ADHD is a well-established psychiatric disorder beginning in childhood, which persists into adulthood. During the aftermath of World War I and after epidemics of encephalitis, symptoms which would be indistinguishable from ADHD today were described by Kramer and Pollnow (1932) including inattention and hyperactivity in children and adults. Bradley (1937) accidently discovered that Benzedrine, the most potent stimulant available at that time used to treat headaches in neurologically impaired children arising from pneumoencephalographic studies, did little to cure the headaches but significantly reduced motor restlessness such as that described by Kramer and Pollnow (Rafaelovich 2001; Rothenberger and Neumacher 2005). Benzedrine was replaced by methylphenidate as an agent to reduce hyperactivity as early as 1944 (Morton and Stockton 2000; Rothenberger and Neumacher 2005) and remains the mainstay of modern day treatment of ADHD.

This syndrome has been conceptualized in varying ways as evident from its nomenclature over the past century: minimal brain dysfunction, hyperkinetic reaction of childhood, etc. The DSM has been the most influential source for psychiatric classifications internationally and the five preceding versions have been a singular influence on the clinical usage of psychiatric terminology as well as in education and scientific research.

However, there have been many criticisms raised about the prior DSM classifications. There is recognition that human behavior is a complex phenomenon and it can be described better on a dimensional continuum rather than the categorical scale the DSM uses. Most human behavior is determined to be aberrant based on subjective experiences and although extreme behavioral aberrations can be classified as being abnormal, minor variants are subjective and anchored in the concept of social and occupational functionality, which is usually difficult to quantify and is thus open to criticism. In addition, the DSM has worked well for describing behavior but with minimal emphasis on the etiology or the phenomenology of a disorder. Despite these criticisms, it still serves as a common and unifying language to catalogue psychiatric disorders that allow mental health practitioners across the globe to communicate and conduct ongoing clinical research.

The DSM 5 (the new nomenclature abandoned the Roman numerals) published by the American Psychiatric Association (APA) in the summer of 2013 was the first revision since 1994 and was eagerly awaited, as there was general consensus that the DSM IV (IV Revised) had poor validity; was based on clustering of symptoms that clinicians were following inflexibly but often inconsistent with clinical presentations; and had unexplained and excessive comorbidity creating confusion. Overall, there were too many disorders listed with questionable scientific validity (Reigier et al. 1998). This revision was based on the work of a multiyear task force appointed by the APA that worked in the form of study and work groups. They organized their work around diagnostic spectra, lifespan and development of disorders, effect of gender and culture, psychiatric and medical issues, degree of impairment and assessment mechanisms, and also aligned it to the International Classification of Disease-11 (ICD 11) system of medical disorder classification. The work groups took into consideration scientific evidence and attempted to balance it against clinical utility and experience.

Irrespective of agreement or disagreement with the manner in which the changes in the nomenclature have occurred, it is imperative to become familiar with them and how they impact changes in practice. In addition, it would be interesting to examine how these changes affect clinical work in this area globally and how ADD is similar or different in Asian countries versus the United States. Illustrative examples of how the syndrome may differ and be similar in South East Asia versus the western diaspora will be provided as vignettes. Etiology and treatment considerations for ADHD will also be discussed.

3.2 DSM 5 Changes

Metastructure and place in classification:

The DSM 5 metastructure aligned its classification system with the ICD 11 within which the F-0 subsection is the neurodevelopmental disorder category. For the first time, ADHD was shifted from the group of frequently comorbid disorders of conduct, oppositional and disruptive disorders to the neurodevelopmental disorder category. This category includes Intellectual Disability, Autism Spectrum Disorder, Communication Disorder, Developmental Motor Coordination disorder, and Specific Learning Disorder.

Clinical criticism of the DSM IV TR classification of ADHD (Willcutt et al. 2012):

1. Lack of scientific basis for age-at-onset criterion
2. Questionable validity of subtypes
3. Developmental insensitivity of symptoms and thresholds for adults, including inadequate coverage of impulsiveness
4. Presence of autism/pervasive developmental disorder (PDD) as diagnostic exclusion

The following section will elaborate on the fundamental differences introduced into the DSM 5.

1. **Age at onset of criteria for ADHD**

The previous understanding of when and how ADHD presents was strongly focused on childhood. There was the general assumption that if the disorder had not been identified by age 7, later onset of symptoms ought to be explained by other disorders or secondary to psychosocial events that the child may be reacting to. Not too far back, ADHD as a disorder of adulthood was likewise not recognized. However, in the past two decades there is an increasing appreciation for the adult manifestations of the disorder. As part of the diagnosis, the previous age criteria would send clinicians on an appropriate but frustrating mission to establish early onset of the disorder while obtaining data from adults who were clearly impaired but could not recall when they began to show symptoms. Other investigations of subjective recall of when symptoms of ADHD began and a meta-analysis of the literature (Keiling et al. 2010) did not support the 7-year age in criteria B which stipulates that "Some hyperactive-impulsive or inattentive symptoms that caused impairment were present before age 7 years," as having scientific merit. This loosening of the age criteria caused concern that this would increase the prevalence of ADHD incorrectly. However, further analysis of the implication for prevalence rates due to less stringent age criteria indicated that there would be no increase in base rates (Polanczyk et al. 2010). Hence, the new age threshold has been increased to 12 years.

Summary: Age by which a formal diagnosis of the disorder must be made has been raised from 7 to 12.

Below is a vignette of the adult form of ADHD.

Case 1: *JJ is a 27-year-old referred to the University Counseling Center (UCC). He is a fellow in cardiology but is having a tough time completing his work, is often late to rounds and is frustrating his training director who cannot understand why such a bright individual can be so unpredictable in his performance. On interview, the UCC Child and Adolescent Psychiatrist (CAP) decides that he is not depressed, has always done very well academically (as his admission to medical school proved) and ADHD could not possibly be in the differential diagnosis.*

On a further detailed history, his tested IQ is 140 and although constantly "on the move" as a child, he was charming and managed to do well in grade school. In high school he took five Advanced Placement courses and struggled through them but yet made it into a prestigious undergrad college. It was in medical school that he became progressively more erratic in his performance. When focusing on one area he would get behind in others. Finally residency, with its demanding schedule and multitasking, took its toll and he became paralyzed into inaction with poor attention to detail, often late, and missing deadlines. The CAP understood this history as that of a highly compensated individual who had managed his ADHD until now.

Family history was positive for ADHD in paternal uncle.

A trial of stimulant medications produced steady improvement and removal from probation.

2. **Validity of subtypes of ADD in DSM IV**

The DSM II description of ADD separated the classic triad of attention, hyperactivity, and impulsivity, while the DSM III lumped them all together. In the DSM IV and IV-R, ADD was subtyped into either inattentive or hyperactive/impulsive or a combination of the two. In anticipation of the DSM 5, a meta-analysis of 431 studies (Willcut et al. 2012) lead the authors to conclude that the DSM–IV ADHD subtypes provide "a convenient clinical shorthand to describe the functional and behavioral correlates of current levels of inattention and hyperactivity/impulsivity symptoms, but do not identify discrete subgroups with sufficient long-term stability to justify the classification of distinct forms of the disorder." In the face of this study and clinical experience of experts, it did not appear justified that these subtypes became lifetime diagnoses. As a result, the current criterion for subtypes is renamed "specifiers" of current functioning: either the inattentive or hyperactive/impulsive or combined presentation but stipulates that these descriptors merely describe the most current presentation and that this could change with time. In addition, these symptoms are rated as mild, moderate, or severe.

Summary: In DSM 5, there are no more subtypes but specifiers, which are the inattentive, hyperactive/impulsive or combined reflecting current presentation. These specifiers have a potential for change over time. The severity of the specifiers has to be coded as mild, moderate, or severe.

3. **Developmental insensitivity of symptoms and thresholds for adults, including inadequate coverage of impulsiveness, severity thresholds and impairment**

The development of the diagnostic criteria for ADD goes back to the 1950s when this was considered a disorder of children and considered to dissipate by puberty. Hence, examples of what constituted inattention, hyperactivity, or impulsivity were reflective of commonly observed aberrations that were developmentally related to childhood. With the recognition that ADD persists into adulthood, often with disabling symptoms that are distinct to adulthood, there has been a push to include adult examples of inattention, hyperactivity, and impulsivity as well as reduce the threshold of symptoms to meet diagnosis from six to five.

The DSM 5 provides examples of how these symptoms manifest across age ranges, including ways they would appear in older adolescents and adults. Thus, although the symptom list remains the same, the inclusion of developmentally appropriate examples helps guide clinicians evaluating older adolescents and adults (Keiling et al. 2010).

The nine inattentive symptoms are:

- Often fails to give close attention to details or makes careless mistakes in schoolwork, work, or during other activities (e.g., overlooks or misses details, work is inaccurate).
- Often has difficulty sustaining attention in tasks or play activities (e.g., has difficulty remaining focused during lectures, conversations, or lengthy reading).
- Often does not seem to listen when spoken to directly (e.g., mind seems elsewhere, even in the absence of any obvious distraction).
- Often does not follow through on instructions and fails to finish schoolwork, chores, or duties in the work place (e.g., starts tasks but quickly loses focus and is easily sidetracked).
- Often has difficulty organizing tasks and activities (e.g., difficulty managing sequential tasks; difficulty keeping materials and belongings in order; messy, disorganized work; has poor time management; fails to meet deadlines).
- Often avoids or is reluctant to engage in tasks that require sustained mental effort (e.g., schoolwork or homework; for older adolescents and adults: preparing reports, completing forms, reviewing lengthy papers).
- Often loses things necessary for tasks or activities (e.g., school materials, pencils, books, tools, wallets, keys, paperwork, eyeglasses, and mobile telephones).
- Is often easily distracted by extraneous stimuli (e.g., for older adolescents and adults may include unrelated thoughts).
- Is often forgetful in daily activities (e.g., doing chores, running errands; for older adolescents and adults: returning calls, paying bills, keeping appointments).

The nine hyperactive-impulsive symptoms are:

- Often fidgets, taps hands, or squirms in seat.
- Often leaves seat in situations when remaining seated is expected (e.g., leaves his or her place in the classroom, in the office or other workplace, or in other situations that require remaining in place).
- Often runs about or climbs in situations where it is inappropriate (e.g., in adolescents or adults, may be limited to feeling restless).
- Often unable to play or engage in leisure activities quietly.
- Is often "on the go" acting as if "driven by a motor" (e.g., is unable to be or uncomfortable being still for extended time, as in restaurants, meetings; may be experienced by others as being restless or difficult to keep up with).

- Often talks excessively.
- Often blurts out answers before questions have been completed (e.g., completes people's sentences; cannot wait for turn in conversation).
- Often has difficulty waiting turn (e.g., while waiting in line).
- Often interrupts or intrudes on others (e.g., joins into conversations, games, or activities uninvited; may start using other people's things without asking or receiving permission; for adolescents and adults: may intrude into or take over what others are doing).

In addition, the threshold for diagnosis of ADHD has been reduced for individuals 17 or older in recognition of the clinical observation that many of the symptoms decrease with maturity and that a reliable diagnosis can be made by fewer positive symptoms in older individuals. The 6/9 criteria remains for the below 17 year age individuals while it is five or more for 17 and older.

Overall, the explanations for comparable symptoms in adults are a helpful addition to clarify how the criteria are applicable to adults.

The criteria for impairment has been reduced to "…clear evidence that the symptoms *interfere* with, or reduce the quality of, social, academic, or occupational functioning." This reduction in stringency could increase the rates of a diagnosis of ADHD. Decisions regarding functional impairments are often subjective and value judgments that clinicians routinely make that heavily affect the ultimate diagnosis. However, future research data will be the only way to determine if the base rates of the diagnosis increase. These examples underscore the need for multi-informant information and use of rating scales that are normed over large populations such as the ADHD-IV Rating Scale (DuPaul et al. 1998) or the Vanderbilt Rating Scale (Wolraich et al. 2003).

DSM-5 also requires clinicians to specify the severity level of a client's ADHD as Mild, Moderate, or Severe.

Mild is restricted to cases where there are few, if any, symptoms beyond those required to make the diagnosis and no more than minor impairment in functioning.

Moderate is simply defined as symptoms or functional impairment between "mild" and "severe."

Severe is a term reserved for cases with many symptoms in excess of those required for the diagnosis, or several symptoms that are especially severe, or marked.

DSM-IV had a category called ADHD Not Otherwise Specified (NOS) for individuals who displayed prominent symptoms but who did not meet required criteria.

In DSM-5, this has been changed to Other Specified ADHD and Unspecified ADHD. The former is used when full criteria are not met, symptoms that are present create clinically significant distress or impairment in functioning, and the clinician chooses to convey why full criteria are not met, for example "Other specified ADHD with insufficient inattention symptoms."

4. **Presence of autism/PDD as diagnostic exclusion**

As one recalls from the past, the diagnosis of ADHD could not be made with a concurrent diagnosis of autism. The assumption was that hyperactivity was a part of the autism spectrum disorder and did not reflect a separate disorder. The DSM

IV stated, "The symptoms do not occur exclusively during the course of a PDD, schizophrenia, or other psychotic disorder and are not better accounted for by another mental disorder." In DSM 5 this has been changed to "The symptoms do not occur exclusively during the course of schizophrenia or other psychotic disorder and are not better accounted for by another mental disorder."

Overall, this is a positive change to the criteria and appears clinically sound. It acknowledges the clinical approach to treatment of inattention and impulsivity often seen in conjunction with autism and is reflective of the neurodevelopmental pathogenesis of the symptoms. Below is a case vignette demonstrating how these changes may be utilized in clinical practice.

Case 2: AD is a 6-year-old child with a diagnosis of autism since age 2. For the past seven months he has had troubling temper tantrums. The behavior has curtailed the parent's ability to take him to any public place. In the special school he attends, his teachers have noted that he is "busy" and despite their best efforts cannot be redirected. He strikes other children. When more detailed information is obtained about the triggers and antecedents to the behavior, it becomes clear that he does so when he cannot get his way or when he is stopped from engaging in any activity. He is noted to jump from activity to activity and cannot sit still. Overall he is not moody or angry except during these episodic events. If prepared adequately, he handles transitions appropriately. The most likely explanation to these "new tantrums" is emerging impulsivity (and hyperactivity) rather than impairment arising from mood or transition difficulties. When he has the need to do something or acquire something he is not able to curb the impulsive need to fulfill that desire and gets disruptive. Use of redirection and behavioral interventions is partially successful but a trial of a stimulant produced marked compliance and improved adjustment in the classroom. The importance of recognizing the etiology of the "tantrums" has implications for the choice of somatic treatments.

Brief Summary of Etiology:

From the multiple elements that contribute to the etiology of ADHD, it is reasonable to assert that it is a disorder uniquely multifactorial and has its origins in genetics, familial and environmental factors, and (multiple) neurotransmitters. This complexity makes predictions about developmental trajectory and response to treatment complicated at best.

Genetics: Family and twin studies have strongly and consistently supported that ADHD runs in families (Freitag and Retz 2010) Twin studies suggest that ADHD has a high heritability factor and attribute about 80 % of the etiology of ADHD to genetic factors (Larsson et al. 2004). Adoption studies of ADHD also implicate genes in its etiology. In addition, the correlation of DRD4 and DAT transporter genes and ADHD (LaHoste et al. 1996) reinforce the neurobiological foundation of the disorder.

Neurotransmitters

Structural and functional imaging studies consistently implicate catecholamine-rich fronto-subcortical systems in the pathophysiology of ADHD (Volkow et al. 2007). Given the mode of action of stimulants and their effectiveness in the management of ADHD, catecholamine disruption as at least one source of ADHD brain dysfunction (Berridge et al. 2006) is a plausible neurotransmitter-based model to understand ADHD. Although not entirely sufficient, changes in dopaminergic and noradrenergic function appear necessary for the clinical efficacy of pharmacological treatments for ADHD, providing support for the hypothesis that alteration of monoaminergic transmission in critical brain regions may be the basis for therapeutic action in ADHD (Berridge et al. 2006). However, as not all individuals with ADHD respond well to stimulants, there are perhaps additional neurotransmitters implicated in the disorder. A review of 50 studies by Spencer et al. (2014) supports the role of glutamate in ADHD. Increases in Glutaminergic metabolites in the anterior cingulate cortex (ACC), prefrontal cortex and striatum in youth with ADHD, normalize with stimulant treatment. Magnetic resonance spectroscopy (MRS) detects these changes.

Environmental Factors
There are periods in development when the brain is exquisitely sensitive to exposure to noxious stimuli that influences neurogenesis and synaptogenesis and functionality of the central nervous system (Knudsen 2004). Prenatal exposure to nicotine (Gatzke-Kopp and Beauchaine 2007), alcohol (Godel et al. 2000), and psychosocial adversity (Counts et al. 2005) all have the potential to alter neuronal synaptogenesis and neurotransmitter development resulting in a phenotypic presentation that mimics ADHD such as impulsivity, motoric hyperactivity (Godel et al. 2000), disorganization and inattention along with learning disabilities. Hence, environmental factors that have the potential to affect brain architecture and neurotransmitter systems are risk factors for ADHD.

Assessment:
Although ADHD is now officially a neurodevelopmental disorder, the use of neuro-diagnostic tools such as single-proton emission computed tomography scans (SPECT) are not traditionally available in clinical practice (Schneider et al. 2014). The diagnosis of ADD/ADHD is primarily clinical. A comprehensive history should be obtained that elicits and explores symptoms that several individuals in the child's life report (parents, teachers, relatives, peers, neighbors) and the extent to which the symptoms are impairing. In addition, a medical history and work up of medical symptoms if indicated may be necessary, i.e., seizures may mimic inattention/blanking out spells. Rating scales such as the ADHD IV RS or the Vanderbilt (among many others) are effective means of getting standardized information about the child from varying observers but must never be the only data point for making the diagnosis. Psychiatric comorbidity such as a mood disorder and substance abuse in older children should be explored. Continuous performance tests (CPT) should only be used as supplements to the clinical interview and must not replace it. CPT provides the clinician with cross-sectional data but does not provide context for the data, i.e., inattention may be in the clinical range of abnormality but arising from a significant trauma and not ADHD.

A history of academic performance should explore the child's innate capabilities versus what they are achieving currently; is the underperformance shifting from subject to subject (more consistent with ADHD) versus stable underperformance in one or two arenas (consistent with a learning disability). This will assist in making recommendations to further test for learning disability or try classroom behavioral accommodations and somatic therapies.

Clinicians should be aware of variations in parenting style: a permissive parenting style (Piotrowski et al. 2013) may lead to impairment in behaviors. Often why a child misbehaves in the presence of one adult versus another can be mystifying to the clinician; however, a good clinical interview will reveal information about familial culture, power structure and gender roles. As an example, gender typical roles can lead to differences in behavior. Mothers will traditionally report a tougher time setting limits but their communication style (less authoritarian, more explanation-based commands) assists children in learning problem solving and reasoning while fathers may get better compliance by short authoritarian commands that help children attain quicker behavioral control. Culture may play an important part in how discipline is instituted. In the South Asian culture where mental disabilities are relatively more stigmatized than even the west, adjectives used to describe the behavior are: "naughty" or "spoiled" (overindulged) suggesting that these are behaviors and not disorders and may come from deficiencies in parenting, etc. (Hong 2008; Lee 2008; Lee and Neuharth-Pritchett 2008). This view of dysfunction may delay seeking help. Help seeking is more likely to occur when the behavior impedes academic success, which is relatively strongly emphasized in the Asian culture (Singh 2008). Culturally competent care is delivered when there is an understanding and respect for the healthcare practices, values/beliefs, and needs of a community. When we understand the cultural background of a family and are nonjudgmental about the culturally driven attitudes toward help seeking, then there is an improvement in compliance and outcomes (NIH 2014). Temperamental mismatch between a parent and child or a teacher and child may also produce defiant behavior. It must be differentiated from ADHD related disruptive behavior that occurs across situations regularly but in varying intensities (classroom, home, with relatives, neighborhood, with peers). Familial or environmental chaos can also produce ADHD like symptoms. Although time and resource intensive, when replaced with a consistent, predictable, and orderly life style, this will dissipate disorganized behavior unlike true ADHD, which will persist. This differentiation is essential because of the implications for treatment.

It is extremely important to understand the context of the behaviors, i.e., the role of stressors and life events as they may produce phenotypic expressions of distress that mimic ADHD symptoms (Fisher 1998). However, once removed, the symptoms remit. Ruling out metabolic etiologies such as hyperthyroidism, medication-induced hyperactivity, or subclinical seizures should be part of the initial evaluation (Harber 2000). The role of psychological assessments is hampered by the length of time it takes to complete them. In uncomplicated ADD (i.e., without Learning Disabilities, Sensory Integration Disorder, etc.) a thorough clinical interview can yield adequate data to confirm a diagnosis. However, psychological testing can be helpful when used to support educational interventions and shed light on cognitive styles, deficits, and strengths. Rating scales can be helpful to provide quantifiable data on behavior at baseline and throughout the cycle of treatment. As stated earlier, these rating scales should supplement clinical interview data and not the other way round. Unfortunately, this is becoming a disturbing trend in busy clinical practices. A thorough and detailed assessment is a good investment for both the clinician and the patient.

In summary, an assessment should include a clinical interview that includes a history of presenting problems, temporal chronicling of past and current problems, connection or lack thereof to stressors, familial or environmental chaos, temperamental styles, genetic diathesis, parenting styles, academic performance, comorbid psychiatric or medical diagnoses. As much as feasible multi-informant data, particularly from teachers, is recommended. Supplemental data should include rating scales such as the Vanderbilt or ADHD IV RS or the Conner RS, intelligence and achievement testing when indicated, CPT (if available) and follow up on suspected medical conditions.

Treatment

Treatment of ADD/ADHD is often determined by the degree of impairment that the symptoms produce. Parents seek help for children while adults seek treatment themselves.

A holistic treatment approach is the most successful (Damico and Armstrong 1996).

- Based on large multisite studies (MTA), it is clear that medications have a significant and superior impact in comparison to placebo and behavioral interventions on the triad of impulsivity, inattention, and hyperactivity (MTA Cooperative Group 2004).
- Stimulants are the first line treatment of ADHD. The two major stimulant groups are methylphenidate and mixed amphetamine salts, with both immediate and extended release preparations. The goal of therapy is improvement of symptoms with minimal side effects. Narrative feedback from supervising adults should be used to titrate the dose. Side effects such as appetite suppression, irritability or withdrawal, gastritis, and insomnia can be rate limiting in the titration of these medications and lead to the trial of the non-stimulants such as the alpha-2 agonists, atomoxetine, and bupropion. It is common for parents to be concerned that stimulants lead to substance abuse. Stimulants, however, have been shown to reduce the development of drug and alcohol use disorders later in life (Wilens et al. 2002). The most plausible explanation is that stimulants serve to reduce impulsive decision-making and theoretically reduce the possibility of risk taking behaviors such as substance abuse.
- However, medications may not be effective in addressing the social adjustment issues seen in individuals with ADHD. Behavioral interventions such as Behavior Parent Therapy and Social Skills Training improve a child's overall functioning and their ability to form positive relationships and negotiate life situations. Behavioral interventions that involve parents, teachers, and care givers assist in altering the structure of a child's environment, maximizing positive and minimizing negative behaviors (Kaiser et al. 2011).

- Skills training approaches that target deficits in social, life, and other organizational skills involve providing children directly with small group didactics (Pfiffner et al. 2007) and assist them in practicing those at home/school and social situations.
- Bibliotherapy is also useful and gives parents and children the tools to use on their own (Forehand et al. 2010).

Cross-cultural studies in ADHD do indicate that ethnic and cultural factors have an important role in causal model of symptoms (medical versus nonmedical), defining severity of the disorder, family, and societal tolerance toward deviance and disciplinary practices, and definitely in threshold for treatment seeking. Culturally, in South Asia, respect for adults, compliant behavior, submissiveness, and academic success are highly valued. Within the Asian diaspora, the presence of ADHD symptoms can become a major source of discomfort. Although the fallout from the behavioral syndrome is enormous, help seeking behavior may not be swift. Several researchers have examined the differences in these variables by studying ethnic minorities who reside in countries other than where they originated from, such as Asians (e.g., Chinese, Indian Gujaratis) in the US or UK (Soorkia et al. 2011). In a study from Goa, India, cc conducted in-depth interviews with 24 parents recruited from a list of children who had been diagnosed with ADHD at a community-based child development center (CDC). The most frequent reasons for consulting the CDC were *educational difficulties*. Despite having received an ADHD diagnosis and reporting significant adverse impact of the child's behavior, most parents were reluctant to accept the biomedical explanatory model or even consider their child's difficulties as an illness. Instead, parents most commonly attributed *causality to psychological models, learning and memory difficulties*, and to models that emphasized either the volitional or non-volitional nature of the problem, or to attribute blame to self or spouse. Interventions most commonly used were educational and religious; consultation with the CDC was the last resort for many parents.

Malhotra and Shah (Personal Communication, 2015) indicate that children given a diagnosis of ADHD at their clinic in India were commonly referred from school due to scholastic and/or disciplinary problems. Though on detailed history, parents acknowledge that there had been problems related to hyperactivity, inattention, and impulsivity since early childhood, they had no prior knowledge that these problems could be a "psychological illness" or "medical illness" until teachers referred them to a Child Psychiatry Clinic. Also, overall, they would have never considered seeking any kind of help for these problems, considering them as simply problems attributable to lack of motivation of the child, other family members being too liberal or critical, or blaming self or spouse/spouse's family. The other parent generally shares this perception, albeit reversing the blame. Thus, difficulties encountered in school and complaints from teachers are the main motivating factors for bringing a child to medical attention. In many of the joint families (nuclear and extended family living together) to which several of these children belong, grandparents are either too liberal or too critical, with an opposite pattern in the parent (especially the mother who either tries to discipline or protect the child). Mothers in joint households have major family responsibilities toward which they are expected to devote more time than toward their children. Thus, quality of "*grand parenting*" plays a major role in the evolution and attitude toward these symptoms.

The barriers that prevent help seeking behavior within families are related to two enormous burdens that exist worldwide but are particularly exaggerated in developing countries: the first of which is stigma associated with psychiatric diagnoses. Stigma is quite common in western culture. One study noted that college students tended to view individuals who claimed that they received help when suffering from depression as more emotionally unstable than those who were depressed but refused to seek treatment (Ben-porath 2002). Examples of stigmatization in India are also quite evident. Malhotra and Shah (Personal Communication, 2015) indicate that once the diagnosis is communicated to the parents, the reactions are varied. There is usually some relief that it is an illness, or complete dismissal of a medical model (though enmeshed in bio-psycho-social model). Most parents are reluctant to start medications and insist on non-drug measures, unless problems are very severe and disruptive especially at school (impending suspension from school).

The second burden stems from the lack of access to somatic therapies, as there is limited availability of pharmacological agents in developing countries. Only small portions of the mental health physicians reside in areas of where over 90 % of the global population lives and the majority of the 400 million people with a mental health disorder are not being treated (Patel et al. 2006). In recent years, referrals from schools have increased in India (Malhotra and Shah, Personal Communication, 2015), which might be reflective of teachers' increasing sensitivity toward this problem. However, most schools and parents continue to use punitive measures most commonly. Also, most schools do not seem to be equipped with resources to engage such children in more structured environments, though are receptive to professional suggestions.

Medication also has its complications. Specific dose and timing of medication for each child or adult suffering from ADHD must be carefully titrated and monitored until proper dose has been achieved for optimum functioning with minimal side effects (National Resource Center on ADHD 2008). For example, methylphenidate only has a 55 % efficacy when used in low or medium doses (Elia et al. 1991). Additionally, side effects of amphetamines include anorexia, insomnia, irritability, nervousness, and anxiety (Efron et al. 1997), which may lead to noncompliance.

To understand fully the similarities and differences between how ADHD is seen from both an American and Indian psychiatric perspective, we compared the history of present illness from two psychiatrists treating a child with ADHD.

The US Perspective:

John is a 5-year-old Caucasian male who is brought to this evaluation by his parents who have had a third child just recently. John is the middle child.

John did not make it into any of the kindergartens in the private schools in the town and the schools cited immaturity as well as a problem in attention, impulsivity, and inability to deal with prescribed tasks during the screening for kindergarten. Parents are concerned as they have placed several interventions such as occupational therapy and speech therapy, and they have a social coach for him through a private foundation. John has been identified as having problems particularly in the social and emotional arenas as well as motor lags early on in life. He was identified as having these problems through the Early Intervention Services and has received an intervention program through the preschool that he attends. According to parents, he is somewhat delayed in his milestones and he has always been rather distracted. His distractibility as well as impulsive behavior tends to get in the way of his academic achievements and he really has a tough time in-group situations. He does not follow through with instructions in class. Transitions are extremely difficult; 80 % of the time he has difficulty adjusting to the requests which have made by the adults around him. He gets easily frustrated because of that. The other prominent part of his presentation is that if he cannot get his way or feels that he is being pushed in one direction, he will dig his heels in and refuse to respond to the instructions. Examples of these are if he is asked to take a shower or get dressed in the mornings. He will have a major temper tantrum as this would mean that he has to stop whatever he was doing and follow adults' instructions. Often times, he has a hard time handling social situations such as harassing his 6-year-old sister enough to make her cry. Given that she does respond to him negatively, John is somehow satisfied. Furthermore, his parents note that he takes great pleasure in watching his actions produce a reaction in others. Parents sometimes feel that they have to walk on eggshells simply because they do not know if he will emotionally regress. As far as his inattentiveness and distractibility, parents indicate that he follows through with tasks only halfway and will often be found standing with his pants around his ankles when he has been told to get into his pajamas. He genuinely forgets what the instructions were and at other times they feel that he can be just oppositional. On the positive side, he is seen as being a happy extrovert who has zest for life, and he has a lovely demeanor. He also has a good appetite. He sleeps well and is generally described as someone with a happy mood. Often times he tends to wake up early in the morning. They have noted phases of constipation. He has been identified as having a sensory processing problem, the sensory seeking issues have to do with hyperacusis, running into people and clinging to them in a socially inappropriate fashion. He is a tactile child who likes to "horse play" and then does not know how to stop that behavior, ending up in tackling other children leading to social ostracism. Psycho-educational testing shows functioning in the low average range of IQ.

In summary, the problems appear to be present despite the fact that several services through early intervention have been put into place, but he has trouble with distractibility and impulsive behavior. This is functionally impairing his ability to learn and progress Parents are ready to try medications.

3.3 The South Asian/Indian Perspective

An 8-year-old boy Ganesh, from a Hindu joint family of middle socioeconomic background was brought to the clinic as a referral from school. Ganesh's father ran a family business and mother was a homemaker. Ganesh's grandparents and a younger paternal uncle and his family resided in the same household. His mother and his paternal aunt had to take turns in carrying out various household chores (as decided by grandfather). When mother would have to cook the evening dinner for the whole family, she would not find any time to spend with Ganesh. He was the first male child in the family and was pampered by the grandparents.

The school teachers repeatedly complained to the parents during parent–teacher meeting that Ganesh just did not obey them, seemed very disinterested in his studies, would often not complete his work, make careless mistakes ("but of course, at times he does his work alright"), did not sit at one place, was extremely naughty, would keep fiddling with other children's belongings. Ganesh would very often leave the classroom without permission. They advised the parents that a child psychiatrist or a counselor should see him. Parents had earlier received similar complaints from the previous school. At home, Mother faced difficulties in even dressing him, feeding him, making him sit to study. She felt "I'm always running after him. If I don't keep an eye on him for a minute, something would happen…he might fall or break something." She found it more difficult to care for him since the birth of his younger sister (for last 4 years). She would often lose her temper with Ganesh and beat him for which she was severely criticized by her father-in-law. Ganesh's father would return home only at night and would usually ignore the child's behavior, but occasionally suddenly get very angry and beat him. Grandfather maintained that he was a little naughty and parents were overreacting. In fact, when they received complaints from the previous school, he advised them to change the school. Three years have passed since the first complaint from school. This time around, the parents brought the child to us without the knowledge of the grandparents. After detailed history and examination/observation, when the parents were told that Ganesh is most likely suffering from a medical disorder ADHD and that even his apparent disobedience is stemming from that, they were surprised. They immediately requested the doctors to counsel Ganesh "to behave well." When pharmacological options were given, they were extremely reluctant and chose to go ahead with counseling.

By comparing both histories side by side, we see several differences emerge. Initially, it can be noted that both John and Ganesh demonstrate hyperactive and impulsive behavior, which is evident in both their classroom and home environment. However, Ganesh's parents took much longer to seek treatment and once evaluated, emphasized his inability to perform in school (via feedback from his teachers) as a critical flaw. This point was not nearly as emphasized in John's history, which focused more on his social interactions with his peers and family as deficits in his behavior. Access to care is also a major difference seen between both cases. John has had speech therapy, occupational therapy, and social coaching prior to his initial assessment by a psychiatrist. However, both teachers and parents have only counseled Ganesh prior to his assessment. While access to different behavioral counseling techniques may have been available in the area, the parents did not know what therapy was available. Grandparental influence on "normalizing the behavior" is seen not only in South Asian cultures but in the West too but the eastern culture is more permissive in allowing that to be the decision-making voice rather than the parents. This is secondary to the deference given to the "elders" within Southeast Asian cultures (Singh 2008). Hence, conceptualization of dysfunctional behavior, threshold for seeking help, the type of help utilized and the lag time between diagnosis and treatment may be quite different from a cultural standpoint.

An awareness of these differences and similarities across continents is helpful as we embark on the new era of using the revised/new criteria per the DSM-5 to diagnose ADHD. Whether these changes that have placed ADHD as a neurobiological disorder while simultaneously broadening diagnostic criteria will serve the field well will be evident from prospective design studies that determine how well these criteria capture the construct of the disorder, how stable is the diagnosis over time, what predictive validity do these criteria have, and whether they are better able to assist the practitioner in the field. Future studies that provide a head-to-head comparison of psychopathology in countries in the Western and the Eastern hemispheres, i.e., culturally dissimilar but using similar classification systems, would be helpful in order to constantly, consistently, and thoughtfully refine the DSM for the betterment of children and adults who suffer from mental disorders like ADHD.

References

Ben-Porath, D. D. (2002). Stigmatization of individuals who receive psychotherapy: An interaction between help-seeking behavior and the presence of depression. *Journal of Social & Clinical Psychology, 21*(4), 400, 413.

Berridge, C. W., Devilbiss, D. M., Andrzejewski, M. E., Arnsten, A. F., Kelley, A. E., Schmeichel, B., et al. (2006). Methylphenidate preferentially increases catecholamine neurotransmission within the prefrontal cortex at low doses that enhance cognitive function. *Biological Psychiatry, 60*(10), 1111–1120.

Bradley, C. (1937). The behavior of children receiving benzedrine. *American Journal of Psychiatry, 94*, 577–585.

Counts, C. A., Nigg, J. T., Stawicki, J. A., Rappley, M. D., & Von Eye, A. (2005). Family adversity in DSM IV ADHD combined and inattentive subtypes and associated disruptive behavior problems. *Journal of the American Academy of Child and Adolescent Psychiatry, 44*(7), 690–698.

Damico, S. K., & Armstrong, M. B. (1996). Intervention strategies for students with ADHD: Creating a holistic approach. *Seminars in Speech and Language, 17*(1), 21–35.

DuPaul, G. J., Power, T. J., Anastopoulos, A. D., & Reid, R. (1998). *ADHD rating scale-IV: Checklists, norms, and clinical interpretation*. New York, NY: The Guilford Press.

Efron, D., Jarman, F., & Barker, M. (1997). Side effects of methylphenidate and dexamphetamine in children with attention deficit hyperactivity disorder: A double-blind, crossover trial. *Pediatrics, 100*(4), 662–666.

Elia, J., Borcherding, B., Rapoport, J., & Keysor, C. (1991). Methylphenidate and dextroamphetamine treatments of hyperactivity: Are there true nonresponders? *Psychiatry Research, 36*(2), 141–155. doi:10.1016/01651781(91)90126-A

Fisher, B. (1998). *Attention deficit disorder misdiagnosis: Approaching ADD from a brain behavior/neuropsychological perspective for assessment and treatment.* Boca Raton, Louisiana: CRC Press.

Forehand, R. L., Merchant, M. J., Long, N., & Garai, E. (2010). An examination of parenting the strong willed child as bibliotherapy for parents. *Behavior Modification, 34*(1), 57–76.

Freitag, C. M., & Retz, W. (2010). Family and twin studies in attention-deficit hyperactivity disorder. In W. Retz & R. G. Klein (Eds.), *Attention-deficit hyperactivity disorder (ADHD) in Adults. Key issues in mental health* (Vol. 176, pp. 38–57). Basel: Karger.

Gatzke-Kopp, L. M., & Beauchaine, T. P. (2007). Direct and passive prenatal nicotine exposure and the development of externalizing psychopathology. *Child Psychiatry and Human Development, 38*(4), 255–269.

Godel, J.C., Lee, B.E., McCallum, D.E., Lee, S.L., Macneil, C.W., Liddell, G.A., & Shea, D.R. (2000). Exposure to alcohol in utero: Influence on cognitive function and learning in a northern elementary school population. *Paediatric Child Health, 5*(2), 93–100.

Haber, J. S. (2000). *ADHD: The great misdiagnosis*. Dallas, Texas: Taylor Pub. International Classification of Diseases (ICD) Revision. WHO. N.p., n.d. Web. February 01, 2015.

Hong, Y. (2008). Teachers' perceptions of young children with ADHD in Korea. *Early Child Development and Care, 178*(4), 399–414.

Kaiser, N. M., McBurnett, K., & Pfiffner, L. J. (2011). Child ADHD severity and positive and negative parenting as predictors of child social functioning: Evaluation of three theoretical models. *Journal of Attention Disorders, 15*(3), 193–203.

Kieling, C., Kieling, R. R., Rohde, L. A., Frick, P. J., Moffitt, T., Nigg, J. T., et al. (2010). The age at onset of attention deficit hyperactivity disorder. *The American Journal of Psychiatry, 167*(1), 14.

Knudsen, E. (2004). Sensitive periods in the development of the brain and behavior. *Journal of Cognitive Neuroscience, 16*(8), 1412–1425.

Kramer, F., & Pollnow, H. (1932). Über eine hyperkinetische Erkrankung im Kindesalter. Ausder Psychiatrischen und Nerven-Klinik der Charité in Berlin (Direktor: Geh. Med.-Rat Prof. Dr. Bonhoeffer). *Mschr Psychiat Neurol,* 82, 21–40.

LaHoste, G. J., Swanson, J., Wigal, S. B., Glabe, C., Wigal, T., King, N., et al. (1996). Dopamine D4 receptor gene polymorphism is associated with attention deficit hyperactivity disorder. *Molecular Psychiatry, 1*(2), 121, 124.

Larsson, J. O., Larsson, H., & Lichtenstein, P. (2004). Genetic and environmental contributions to stability and change of ADHD symptoms between 8 and 13 years of age: A longitudinal twin study. *Journal of the American Academy of Child and Adolescent Psychiatry, 43*(10), 1267–1275.

Lee, K. (2008). ADHD in American early schooling: From a cultural psychological perspective. *Early Child Development and Care, 178*(4), 415–439.

Lee, K., & Neuharth-Pritchett, S. (2008). Attention deficit/hyperactivity disorder across cultures: Development and disability in contexts. *Early Child Development and Care, 178*(4), 339–346. doi:10.1080/03004430701321501

Malhotra, S., & Shah, R. Personal email Communication, April 29, 2015.

Morton, W. A., & Stockton, G. G. (2000). Methylphenidate abuse and psychiatric side effects. *Primary Care Companion to the Journal of Clinical Psychiatry, 2*(5), 159–164.

MTA Cooperative Group. (2004). National Institute of Mental Health Multimodal Treatment study of ADHD follow-up: Changes in effectiveness and growth after the end of treatment. *Pediatrics, 113*(4), 762–769.

National Institutes of Health (NIH). (2014). Cultural competency. Accessed 25 March 2015. Retrieved from http://www.nih.gov/clear%20communication/cultural%20competency.htm

National Resource Center on ADHD. (2008). Retrieved May 9, 2015, from http://www.help4adhd.org/index.cfm?varLangen

Patel, V., Saraceno, B., & Kleinman, A. (2006). Beyond evidence: The moral case for international mental health. *American Journal of Psychiatry, 163*(8), 1312–1315.

Pfiffner, L. J., Mikami, A. Y., Huang-Pollock, C., Easterlin, B., Zalecki, C., & McBurnett, K. (2007). A randomized, controlled trial of integrated home school behavioral treatment for ADHD, predominantly inattentive type. *Journal of the American Academy of Child & Adolescent Psychiatry, 46*(8), 1041–1050.

Piotrowski, J. T., Lapierre, M. A., & Linebarger, D. L. (2013). Investigating correlates of self-regulation in early childhood with a representative sample of English-speaking American families. *Journal of Child and Family Studies, 22*(3), 423–436.

Polanczyk, G., Caspi, A., Houts, R., Kollins, S. H., Rohde, L. A., & Moffitt, T. E. (2010). Implications of extending the ADHD age-of-onset criterion to age 12: Results from a prospectively studied birth cohort. *Journal of the American Academy of Child and Adolescent Psychiatry, 49*(3), 210–216.

Rafalovich, A. (2001). The conceptual history of attention deficit hyperactivity disorder: Idiocy, imbecility, encephalitis and the child deviant, 1877–1929. *Deviant Behavior, 22*, 93–115.

Regier, D. A., Kaelber, C. T., Rae, D. S., Farmer, M. E., Knauper, B., Kessler, R. C., et al. (1998). Limitations of diagnostic criteria and assessment instruments for mental disorders: Implications for research and policy. *Archives of General Psychiatry, 55*(2), 109–115.

Rothenberger, A., & Neumärker, K. J. (2005). *Wissenschaftsgeschichte der ADHS*. Steinkopff, Darmstadt: Kramer-Pollnow im Spiegel der Zeit.

Schneider, H., Thornton, J. F., Freeman, M. A., McLean, M. K., van Lierop, M. J., & Schneider, J. (2014). Conventional SPECT versus 3D thresholded SPECT imaging in the diagnosis of ADHD: A retrospective study. *The Journal of Neuropsychiatry and Clinical Neurosciences, 26*(4), 335–343.

Singh, I. (2008). ADHD, culture and education. *Early Child Development and Care, 178*(4), 347–361.

Soorkia, R., Rosemary, S., & Swamy, S. (2011). Factors influencing attitudes towards seeking professional psychological help among South Asian students in Britain. *Mental Health, Religion and Culture, 14*, 613–623.

Spencer, A. E., Uchida, M., Kenworthy, T., Keary, C. J., & Biederman, J. (2014). Glutamatergic dysregulation in pediatric psychiatric disorders: A systematic review of the magnetic resonance spectroscopy literature. *The Journal of Clinical Psychiatry, 75*(11), 1226–1241.

Volkow, N. D., Wang, G. J., Newcorn, J., Telang, F., Solanto, M. V., Fowler, J. S., et al. (2007). Depressed dopamine activity in caudate and preliminary evidence of limbic involvement in adults with attention deficit/hyperactivity disorder. *Archives of General Psychiatry, 64*(8), 932–940.

Wilens, T., Faraone, S., Biederman, J., & Gunawardene, S. (2002). Does stimulant therapy of attention deficit/hyperactivity disorder beget later substance abuse? A meta-analytic review of the literature. *Office Journal of the American Academy of Pediatrics, 111*(1), 179–185.

Willcutt, E. G., Nigg, J. T., Pennington, B. F., Solanto, M. V., Rohde, L. A., Tannock, R., et al. (2012). Validity of DSM-IV attention deficit/hyperactivity disorder symptom dimensions and subtypes. *Journal of Abnormal Psychology, 121*(4), 991–1010.

Wolraich, M. L., Lambert, W., Doffing, M. A., Bickman, L., Simmons, T., & Worley, K. (2003). Psychometric properties of the Vanderbilt ADHD diagnostic parent rating scale in a referred population. *Journal of Pediatric Psychology, 28*(8), 559–568.

Chapter 4
Affective Disorders—Current Status and Controversies

Kandasamy Preeti, Rajeev Jairam and Shoba Srinath

Abstract Affective disorders are common during childhood and adolescence and often pose a challenge in clinical settings. The clinical presentation of affective disorders varies with the developmental age of the child and the classical symptoms increase with age and severity. From a developmental perspective, the disruptive mood dysregulation disorder as a new diagnostic category in DSM 5 addresses this concern as well as the unparalleled increase in pediatric bipolar diagnoses. Use of developmentally appropriate assessments has helped address some of the controversies centred around diagnosis of depression in the young. However, there is sparse evidence of effectiveness of pharmacological and psychological means of treatment and controversies continues to exist regarding effective management of affective disorders in children and adolescents in bringing about a more favourable outcome. This chapter focuses on the current status and particularly controversies related to diagnosis of preschool depression, disruptive mood dysregulation disorder, pediatric bipolar and the differences in pattern of comorbidities across western and Indian literature; current insights into the course and outcome of affective disorders and controversies regarding management of affective disorders.

K. Preeti · S. Srinath (✉)
Department of Child and Adolescent Psychiatry, National Institute of Mental Health and Neurosciences, NIMHANS, P. O. Box 2900, Bangalore 560029, Karnataka, India
e-mail: shobasrinath@gmail.com

K. Preeti
e-mail: preetikandasamy@gmail.com

R. Jairam
ICAMHS, Mental Health, SWSLHD
Campbelltown Hospital, Therry Road, Campbelltown, NSW 2560, Australia
e-mail: rajeev.jairam@sswahs.nsw.gov.au

S. Malhotra and P. Santosh (eds.), *Child and Adolescent Psychiatry*,
DOI 10.1007/978-81-322-3619-1_4

Keywords Affective disorders · Depression · Bipolar disorder · Controversies · Children · Adolescents

4.1 Introduction

Affective disorders are a group of disorders with pervasive mood disturbance as the predominant presentation. They are common during childhood and adolescence and the functional consequences of the disorder can interfere with social, emotional and cognitive development. With significant developmental differences in presentation and comorbidities (Demeter et al. 2013; Axelson et al. 2006), controversies centred around diagnosis and pharmacological interventions, affective disorders often pose a challenge in clinical settings.

4.2 Current Status and Controversies in Diagnosis

Clinical presentation of affective disorders varies with the developmental age of the child and classical symptoms increase with age and severity. For example, younger children with depression express more irritability, frustration, temper tantrums and other behaviour problems with poor verbalization of feelings while adolescents present with sleep and appetite disturbances, somatic complaints, social withdrawal, school refusal, suicidal ideation and attempts, with greater impairment in functioning and with fewer melancholic symptoms and delusions (Rao and Chen 2009).

4.2.1 Preschool Depression

Over the past few years, studies have begun to systematically investigate depression among preschool-aged children and have shown that depressive syndrome can present in this population (Stalets and Luby 2006). Although the controversy regarding diagnosis of depression in young children still exists, age-appropriate mental status evaluation and age-adjusted symptom translations can facilitate diagnosis of depression in young children (Luby 2010).

Longitudinal prospective studies examining the trajectories and continuity of preschool depression have found that even after accounting for other risk factors including maternal depression, preschool depression predicted major depressive disorder in later childhood highlighting the importance of early interventions (Luby et al. 2014).

4.2.2 Disruptive Mood Dysregulation Disorder and Related Controversies

Disruptive mood dysregulation disorder (DMDD) was introduced in DSM-5 to describe children with chronic, severe and persistent irritability and frequent episodes of extreme behavioural dyscontrol. The introduction of this concept as a disorder has been controversial with the primary aim being to address the astronomical increase in pediatric bipolar diagnoses over the past two decades. This rise in diagnosis was largely fuelled by researchers considering severe, non-episodic irritability as a characteristic of bipolar disorder in children (American Psychiatric Association 2013; Tourian et al. 2015). Preliminary, largely post hoc, research has so far demonstrated that children with DMDD usually do not go on to have bipolar disorder in adulthood but are more likely to develop depressive or anxiety disorders. Its placement under depressive disorders emphasizes the disorder's mood component and its distinction from bipolar disorder (Roy et al. 2014).

DMDD have symptoms that overlap with many other disorders including Attention deficit hyperactivity disorder (ADHD), anxiety disorder, depressive disorder and bipolar disorder and poses difficulties in diagnosis. In a recent study, the 3-month prevalence of DMDD was found to be 8.2 % among 6-year-old children. DMDD co-occurred with behavioural and emotional disorders in about 60.5 % of children. Some of the predictors of DMDD at age 3 years included ADHD, oppositional defiant disorder (ODD), temperamental factors such as high urgency, negative emotional intensity and lower effortful control, parental lifetime substance use and higher parental hostility. At age of 6 years, there was association with depression and ODD apart from temperamental and parental factors (Dougherty et al. 2014).

While the DSM 5 criteria has addressed the concern for better diagnosis both for clinical and research purposes, management of DMDD is still a concern as there is paucity of literature in terms of interventions. Current treatment plans are often individualized based on the target symptoms. Treatment options include selective norepinephrine reuptake inhibitors, mood stabilizers, psycho-stimulants, antipsychotics and alpha-2 agonists (Tourian et al. 2015).

Notwithstanding the controversies surrounding its validity, the criteria when applied to a cohort of children followed through to adulthood revealed DMDD to be a hetero-typically continuous disorder with poor outcomes and significant psychosocial morbidity in adulthood (Copeland et al. 2014).

4.2.3 Pediatric Bipolar Disorder

More articles have been published on pediatric bipolar disorder than any other topic in child psychiatry over the last 20 years. Major controversies have been regarding its diagnosis, comorbidities and management. Prominent irritability and difficulty in differentiating it from other disorders (which are sometimes comorbid), the high rates of comorbidities, chronicity and rapid cycling makes diagnosing pediatric bipolar in the young challenging. Indian studies on pediatric bipolar have revealed a lesser prevalence of comorbidities with conditions like Attention deficit hyperactivity disorder, conduct disorder and substance abuse (Jairam et al. 2004) as compared to western literature (Yen et al. 2015). Studies have also found that Bipolar II disorder is often misdiagnosed as Major depressive disorder in about 20 % of children (Bhargava Raman et al. 2007).

4.3 Comorbidities

A thorough assessment of comorbid disorders as part of evaluation is essential, as they can influence treatment decisions and also help understand possible long-term course. 40–70 % of children with depressive disorder suffer from another psychiatric disorder and many have two or more comorbid diagnoses (Rao and Chen 2009; Angold et al. 1999; Essau et al. 2008). Common comorbid disorders include Disruptive behaviour disorders 21–83 %, attention deficit hyperactivity Disorder 0–57 %, anxiety disorder in 20–75 %, substance abuse in 20–30 % (Angold et al. 1993, 1999). While western studies shows an increased prevalence of comorbid behavioural disorders, studies from Indian subcontinent shows an increased prevalence of Anxiety disorder—18 % and obsessive compulsive disorder—7 % and lesser comorbidity with disruptive behaviour disorders and attention deficit hyperactivity disorder (Krishnakumar et al. 2006). Conduct symptoms comorbid with depression can sometimes be misdiagnosed as irritable mania in children and treating the depressive illness can reduce conduct symptoms (Srinath et al. 2008).

4.4 Current Status and Controversies in Treatment

4.4.1 Depressive Disorder

Standard treatment guidelines provided by AACAP practice parameter (2007) and NICE Guidelines (2005) recommend that management of a child and adolescent with mild depressive disorder should include psycho-education and supportive therapy for 4–6 weeks. Both child and parents must be taught to develop concept of depression as an illness, identify and label the affect, learn importance of compliance and reduce feelings of stigmatization. Children and adolescents with moderate to severe depression should be provided the cognitive behavioural therapy, interpersonal therapy or short-term family therapy for at least 3 months duration. Antidepressants are indicated to treat those children who do not respond to first line psychotherapeutic interventions or whose level of risk warrants the use of medication; even in these instances, it should be used in combination with psychotherapy.

Studies on psychotherapy for depressed youth have shown modest effect. Duration of therapy did not affect outcome indicating brief interventions may be as efficacious and cost-effective (Weisz et al. 2006).Other forms of therapy that have been reported to be helpful include attachment therapy (Diamond et al. 2002) and contextual emotion-regulation therapy (Kovacs and Lopez-Duran 2012).

Choice of therapeutic modality depends on severity, number of previous episodes, chronicity, subtype, comorbidity, age, contextual issues, previous treatment and response, child's and family's motivation and therapist's orientation and expertise. Choice of treatment may also be dependent on availability of trained professionals and patient and family preference. Children who are actively self harming or suicidal, agitated/psychotic or have low motivation, poor concentration, sleep disturbances or with comorbid developmental disorders may have difficulty in participating in psychotherapy and may need medication in the first instance.

Fluoxetine is approved by US FDA for children 8 years and older and Escitalopram is approved in youth 12 years and older. Fluoxetine is the most studied SSRI and recent reviews indicate that Fluoxetine should be considered as the first line drug treatment for adolescents with Major depressive disorder. In children who cannot tolerate Fluoxetine, Sertraline can be considered.

Treatment of Adolescents with Depression Study (TADS) found that combination of Fluoxetine and CBT was superior to monotherapy at 12 and 36 weeks (March et al. 2007) as shown in Table 4.1.

It also found that suicidal ideation decreased with treatment, but less so with fluoxetine therapy than with combination therapy or CBT. The study concluded that adding CBT to medication would enhance the safety of medication.

Continuation therapy for at least 6–12 months is recommended for all patients. Children and adolescents who have experiences at least two episodes or one severe/chronic episode require maintenance for more than one year. Children and adolescents with double depression may need to continue medication indefinitely. Trial discontinuation when considered should be during a stress free period (AACAP 2007).

Treatment of resistant depression in adolescents (TORDIA) study found that with use of alternate SSRI or combined therapy 38.9 % remission rate was achieved by 24 weeks. Remission was higher (61.6 % vs. 18.3 %) and faster among those who had shown clinical response by week 12. Factors that predicted remission includes lower severity rates of depression, hopelessness, anxiety, suicidal ideation, family conflict and absence of comorbid dysthymia, drug/alcohol use, anxiety and impairment (Emslie et al. 2010).

Table 4.1 Treatment of adolescents with depression study

TADS	Fluoxetine + CBT (%)	Fluoxetine (%)	CBT (%)
12 weeks	73	62	48
36 weeks	86	81	81

Electroconvulsive therapy (ECT) is reserved for children and adolescent with severe, persistent depressive symptoms, disabling or life-threatening symptoms, associated with catatonic symptoms or when there is lack of treatment response (AACAP 2004). Independent evaluation by a psychiatrist who is knowledgeable about ECT is suggested and ECT can be given to children and adolescents only after approval by the Mental Health Review Boards per current recommendations of Mental health care bill, India, 2013 (Narayan and Shekhar 2015). Cognitive assessment and written informed consent should be part of the ECT protocol.

4.4.2 Controversies Regarding Selective Serotonin Reuptake Inhibitor (SSRI) and Suicidality

US FDA in 2004 issued a black box warning to all antidepressant's labelling, that children taking these medications are at increased risk for suicidality. Further review showed suicidal ideation with few attempts and no completed suicide in 4300 subjects. The number needed to harm (NNH) was found to be 125 as compared to the number needed to treat (NNT) 10. The Risk: Benefit has been found to be 1:14.

The possible increase in suicidality could be attributed to roll back phenomenon—decreasing psychomotor retardation, akathisia, induction of anxiety and panic attacks and insomnia, behavioural activation or stage shifts as antidepressants may lead to a switch from depression into mixed states in bipolar depressed patients. However, paradoxical worsening of depression is quite a rare effect.

Evidence that favours administration of SSRI is that SSRIs continue to be the first line pharmacotherapy for depression in children. A declining trend in suicide rates was noted after widespread availability of SSRI and it ended with the decrease in antidepressant prescriptions following official warnings (McCain 2009). Warnings are therefore not meant to decrease the use of SSRIs in children but to emphasis on proper education and regular monitoring.

Clinical recommendations to address safety issues includes (Cheung et al. 2006)

1. Patients and their families need to be fully informed about the risks and benefits.
2. History of suicidal behaviours to be clarified and monitored at all subsequent visits.
3. To start at a low dose (equivalent of 5–10 mg of fluoxetine) and increase every 2 weeks.
4. To monitor closely for worsening depression, worsening or new suicidal ideation or behaviours, and other behavioural side effects. These are most likely to occur in the first four to 6 weeks.
5. The FDA therefore suggests weekly monitoring at least for the first 4 weeks after the introduction of antidepressant therapy.

4.4.3 Pediatric Bipolar Disorder

Prepubertal bipolar disorder had been found to have a more malignant course (Geller et al. 2004). Greater baseline severity, comorbid attention deficit hyperactivity disorder and conduct disorder was noted to predict poorer treatment response (Masi et al. 2003, 2006). Comorbid ADHD had also been associated with poor long-term recovery (Biederman et al. 2004). A retrospective application of criteria for the subjects of some of these studies may indicate that they would fulfil criteria for DMDD rather than bipolar type I.

Valproate, Lithium, Risperidone, Olanzapine, Aripiprazole and Quetiapine remained first line treatments for acute manic or mixed episodes. The lack of medium to long-term studies to ratify this is astonishing and subsequently, their efficacy in maintenance treatment remains unclear (Jairam et al. 2012). Long-term prophylaxis may be indicated in children with family history of affective disorders, multiple bipolar episodes, when multiple medications were needed to treat the index episode or if subsyndromal symptoms were present (Jairam et al. 2004). We could not find more recent studies which gave direction on prophylaxis.

A recent review of acute treatment for mania in children and adolescents found consistent evidence favouring the use of second-generation antipsychotics (SGAs), limited evidence favouring the use of combinations of SGA with a mood stabilizer (MS), and no evidence supporting the use of MS monotherapy in this context. Various SGAs are not clearly separated in terms of efficacy, but differ in their side effect profiles. There are insufficient data to comment on the benefit of alternative treatments, psychological treatments and electroconvulsive therapy. Gaps remain about expected time to recovery, and when to augment or change treatment when there is lack of effect (Hazell and Jairam 2012).

In a retrospective chart review, 96 % recovered from the index episode and 90 % were either on lithium or valproate (Rajeev et al. 2003, 2004). The relapse rate was 35 and 89 % of the relapses occurred in the first 2 years following the index episode, 28 % of whom relapsed despite being on adequate therapeutic doses of lithium. This raised doubts about the efficacy of this drug in relapse prevention (Rajeev et al. 2004, Pravin et al. 2005). However, earlier studies have reported a threefold higher relapse rate in those who discontinued medications and that early relapse predicted a higher risk of later relapse (Strober et al. 1990).

Based on the evidence and current understanding, the recommendation is for an acute episode of mania or mixed affective state in an adolescent be treated with SGA with lithium/valproate/lamotrigine added for prophylaxis. The decision about prophylaxis including choice of agent is based on several factors including the type and duration of episode, the number of episodes, comorbidities, family history, response to treatment and functional impairment. At all times, the need to include the family in the discussion regarding treatment must be remembered. The efficacy of specific psychotherapeutic treatments in mania is unclear, but they may have a role in prophylaxis and enhancing the quality of life (Hazell and Jairam 2012).

4.4.4 Biomarkers of Treatment Response

Recent studies have focused on the identification of biomarkers related to the pathophysiological mechanisms underlying the development, clinical presentation, course and treatment response of bipolar disorder. The importance of clinically applicable biomarkers has been pursued and reviews have shown promising evidence for brain-derived neurotrophic factor and pro-inflammatory markers as clinically relevant biomarkers in Bipolar disorder. The adolescent population has been of particular focus in identifying biomarkers before onset of comorbid medical conditions and to enable early intervention (Goldstein and Young 2013). Sleep changes as a biomarker of bipolar disorder to predict the occurrence of an episode has also been examined (Lopes 2013). Identifying dysfunctional biochemical processes and neuronal circuits in mood disorders can help plan effective treatment strategies (Bredt et al. 2015).

Meta-analysis of amygdala volumes in children and adolescents with bipolar disorder has concluded that structural, functional and neurochemical amygdala differences may be useful as age-specific biomarkers of illness and treatment response (Pfeifer et al. 2008).

4.5 Course and Outcome

4.5.1 Depressive Disorder

Mean length of a depressive episode is around 7–9 months, with 90 % remission rates at the end of 2 years. Risk of Recurrence is about 40 % by 2 years and 70 % by 5 years. 5–10 % may have a protracted episode, lasting longer than 2 years. It is also found to be persistent into adulthood with a recurrence rate of 70 % (Lewinsohn et al. 1994; Kovacs et al. 1997; Rao and Chen 2009).

20–40 % of children and adolescents with MDD develop bipolar disorder within 5 years (Rao and Chen 2009). Predictors of bipolarity in depressed children include: rapid onset, presence of psychotic symptoms, psychomotor retardation, family history of affective disorders and drug induced hypomanic symptoms (Strober et al. 1993; Akiskal et al. 1995).

Suicide attempts and completion is one of the most significant sequelae of MDD. 60 % report having thought about suicide and 30 % attempt suicide. The risk of suicidal behaviour increases if there is a history of suicide attempts, comorbid disruptive disorders, substance abuse, impulsivity and aggression, availability of lethal agents, exposure to negative events and a family history of suicidal behaviour (AACAP 2007).

4.5.2 *Pediatric Bipolar Disorder*

With the introduction of DMDD, there is a need to review the literature to tease out those studies whose finding may have been 'contaminated' by the addition of those children who would now be diagnosed as DMDD. This leaves those studies that had applied the DSM criteria strictly in order to generate either a bipolar type I or type II disorder. A review of the available literature on the course and outcome of pediatric bipolar disorder revealed 12 outcome studies. Six were retrospectively designed, while six were prospective studies. In essence, with treatment, the mean index manic/mixed episode length was 10–14 weeks; 81–100 % showed episodic recovery with 50–80 % of them experiencing one or more recurrences over a 5-year period. Majority of recurrences occurred in the first 2 years following the index episode (Srinath et al. 1998; Jairam et al. 2004). The retrospective studies demonstrated that the majority of bipolar disorder (BD) in the adult population had its onset in adolescence. There is some preliminary evidence to indicate that the phenotype of BD becomes more classical as the person becomes older and additionally, that adolescent onset BD may have a poorer prognosis than adult onset BD. A number of predictors of both negative and positive outcomes were identified in prospective studies. Living with an intact biological family was positively associated with a faster time to recovery whereas the presence of previous affective episodes, comorbid ADHD, low SES and poor treatment adherence predicted a longer duration of index episode. In Strober et al.'s (1995) study those who had a mixed affective state were more likely to have relapses of their BD. Other factors associated with relapse were low maternal warmth, alcohol use, antidepressant treatment, no psychotherapeutic intervention post hospitalization and longer duration of index episode. These adolescents had high rates of hospitalization and health service utilization, high unemployment, legal problems and poor academic and psychosocial functioning (Geller et al. 2008; Jairam et al. 2008).

4.6 Conclusion

The developmental differences in the presentation of affective disorders in children and adolescents has received a greater focus over the years and the introduction of DMDD as a new diagnostic category in DSM 5 is indicative of the same. Using developmentally appropriate assessments has helped address some of the controversies centred around diagnosis of depression in the young. Research has provided insights into the course and outcome of affective disorders; however, controversies exists regarding their effective management in bringing about a more favourable outcome.

The current research is moving towards identifying reliable and clinically relevant biomarkers. This will inform clinical practice by providing a better understanding and predictability of treatment responses and thereby address some of the current unaddressed concerns related to management of affective disorders.

References

Akiskal, H. S., Maser, J. D., Zeller, P. J., et al. (1995). Switching from 'unipolar' to bipolar II. A 11-year prospective study of clinical and temperamental predictors in 559 patients. *Archives of General Psychiatry, 52*, 114–123.

American Academy of Child and Adolescent Psychiatry. (2004). Practice parameter for the use of electroconvulsive therapy with adolescents. *Journal of American Academy of Child and Adolescent Psychiatry, 43*, 1521–1539.

American Psychiatric Association. (2013). Diagnostic and statistical manual of mental disorders (5th ed., DSM-5). Washington, D.C.: American Psychiatric Association.

Angold, A., & Costello, E. J. (1993). Depressive comorbidity in children and adolescents: Empirical, theoretical, methodological issues. *American Journal of Psychiatry, 150*(12), 1779–1791.

Angold, A., Costello, E. J., & Erkanli, A. (1999). Comorbidity. *Journal of Child Psychology and Psychiatry, 40*, 57–87.

Axelson, D., Birmaher, B., Strober, M., Gill, M. K., et al. (2006). Phenomenology of children and adolescents with bipolar spectrum disorders. *Archives of General Psychiatry, 63*(10), 1139–1148.

Bhargava Raman, R. P., Seshadri, S. P., Janardhan Reddy, Y. C., Girimaji, S. C., et al. (2007). Is bipolar II disorder misdiagnosed as major depressive disorder in children? *Journal of Affective Disorders, 98*, 263–266.

Biederman, J., Mick, E., Faraone, S. V., Van Patten, S., Burback, M., & Wozniak, J. (2004). A prospective follow-up study of pediatric bipolar disorder in boys with attention-deficit/hyperactivity disorder. *Journal of Affective Disorders, 82*(1), S17–S23.

Birmaher, B., Brent, D., & AACAP Work Group on Quality Issues. (2007). Practice parameters for the assessment and treatment of children and adolescents with depressive disorders. *Journal of the American Academy of Child and Adolescent Psychiatry, 46*(11), 1503–1526.

Bredt, D. S., Furey, M. L., Chen, G., Lovenberg, T., et al. (2015). Translating depression biomarkers for improved targeted therapies. *Neuroscience and Biobehavioral Reviews, 59*, 1–15.

Cheung, A. H., Emslie, G. J., & Mayers, T. L. (2006). The use of antidepressants to treat depression in children and adolescents. *Canadian Medical Association Journal, 174*, 193–200.

Copeland, W. E., Shanahan, L., Egger, H., Angold, A., & Costello, E. J. (2014). Adult diagnostic and functional outcomes of DSM-5 disruptive mood dysregulation disorder. *American Journal of Psychiatry, 171*, 668–674.

Demeter, C. A., Youngstrom, E. A., Carlson, G. A., Frazier, T. W., et al. (2013). Age differences in the phenomenology of pediatric bipolar disorder. *Journal of Affective Disorders, 147*(1–3), 295–303.

Diamond, G. S., Reis, B. F., Diamond, G. M., Siqueland, L., & Isaacs, L. (2002). Attachment based family therapy for adolescents—a treatment development study. *Journal of the American Academy of Child and Adolescent Psychiatry, 41*(10), 1190–1196.

Dougherty, L. R., Smith, V. C., Bufferd, S. J., et al. (2014). DSM 5 disruptive mood dysregulation disorder: Correlates and predictors in young children. *Psychological Medicine, 21*, 1–12.

Emslie, G. J., Mayes, T., Porta, G., Vitiello, B., et al. (2010). Treatment of resistant depression in adolescents (TORDIA): Week 24 outcomes. *American Journal of Psychiatry, 167*(7), 782–791.

Essau, C. A. (2008). Comorbidity of depressive disorders among adolescents in community and clinical settings. *Psychiatry Research, 158*, 35–42.

Geller, B., Tillman, R., Bolhofner, K., & Zimerman, B. (2008). Child bipolar I disorder: Prospective continuity with adult bipolar I disorder; characteristics of second and third episodes; predictors of 8-year outcome. *Archives of General Psychiatry, 65*, 1125–1133.

Geller, B., Tillman, R., Craney, J. L., & Bolhofner, K. (2004). Four-year prospective outcome and natural history of mania in children with a prepubertal and early adolescent bipolar disorder phenotype. *Archives of General Psychiatry, 61*, 459–467.

Goldstein, B. I., & Young, L. T. (2013). Toward clinically applicable biomarkers in bipolar disorder: Focus on BDNF, inflammatory markers and endothelial function. *Current Psychiatry Reports, 15*(12), 425.
Hazell, P., & Jairam, R. (2012). Acute treatment of mania in children and adolescents. *Current Opinion in Psychiatry, 25*(4), 265–270.
Jairam, R., Hanstock, T., Cahill, C., Hazell, P., Walter, G., & Malhi, G. (2008). The changing face of bipolar disorder: Adolescence to adulthood. *Minerva Pediatrica, 60*(1), 59–68.
Jairam, R., Srinath, S., Girimaji, S. C., & Seshadri, S. P. (2004). A prospective 4–5 year follow-up of juvenile onset bipolar disorder. *Bipolar Disorders, 6*(5), 386–394.
Jairam, R., Prabhuswamy, M., & Dullur, P. (2012). Do We Really Know How to Treat a Child with Bipolar Disorder or One with Severe Mood Dysregulation? Is There a Magic Bullet? Depression Research and Treatment, 2012, 967302.
Kovacs, M., Lopez-Duran, N. L. (2012). Contextual emotion regulation therapy: A developmentally based intervention for pediatric depression. *Child and Adolescent Psychiatric Clinics of North America, 21*(2), 327–343.
Kovacs, M., Obrosky, D. S., Gatsonis, C., & Richards, C. (1997). First-episode major depressive and dysthymic disorder in childhood: Clinical and sociodemographic factors in recovery. *Journal of the American Academy of Child and Adolescent Psychiatry, 36*, 777–784.
Krishnakumar, P., & Geetha, M. G. (2006). Clinical profile of depressive disorder in children. *Indian Paediatrics, 43*, 521–526.
Lewinsohn, P. M., Clarke, G. N., Seeley, J. R., & Rohde, P. (1994). Major depression in community adolescents: Age at onset, episode duration, and time to recurrence. *Journal of the American Academy of Child and Adolescent Psychiatry, 33*, 809–818.
Lopes, M. (2013). Sleep complaint as a biomarker of bipolar disorder in children and adolescent. *Sleep Medicine, 14*, s1, e185–e186.
Luby, J. L. (2010). Preschool depression: The importance of identifying depression early in development. *Current Directions in Psychological Science, 19*(2), 91–95.
Luby, J. L., Gaffrey, M. S., Tillman, R., et al. (2014). Trajectories of preschool disorders to full DSM depression at school age and early adolescence: Continuity of preschool depression. *American Journal of Psychiatry, 171*(7), 768–776.
March, J. S., Silva, S., Petriycki, S., Curry, J., et al. (2007). Treatment for adolescents with depression study (TADS): Long-term effectiveness and safety outcomes. *Archives of General Psychiatry, 64*(10), 1132–1143.
McCain, J. A. (2009). Antidepressants and suicide in adolescents and adults: A public health experiment with unintended consequences? *Pharmacy and Therapeutics, 34*(7), 355–378.
Masi, G., Toni, C., Perugi, G., Travierso, M. C. et al. (2003). Externalizing disorders in consecutively referred children and adolescents with bipolar disorder. *Compr Psychiatry, 44*(3), 184–189.
Masi, G., Perugi, G., Toni, C., Millepiedi, S., et al. (2006). Attention-deficit hyperactivity disorder—bipolar comorbidity in children and adolescents. *Bipolar Disord, 8*(4), 373–381.
Narayan, Cl, & Shekhar, S. (2015). The mental Health Care Bill 2013: A critical appraisal. *Indian Journal of Psychological Medicine, 37*(2), 215–219.
National Institute for Clinical Excellence (NICE). (2005). Depression in children and young people: Identification and management in primary, community and secondary care. National Clinical Practice Guideline No., 28.
Pfeifer, J. C., Welge, J., Strakowski, S. M., Adler, C. M., & DelBello, M. P. (2008). Meta-analysis of amygdala volumes in children and adolescents with bipolar disorder. *Journal of the American Academy of Child and Adolescent Psychiatry, 47*(11), 1289–1298.
Pravin, D., Rajkumar, R. P., Prabhuswamy, M. Y., Srinath, S., Girimaji, S., & Seshadri, S. P. (2005). Course and outcome of bipolar affective disorder in children. *Journal of Indian Association for Child and Adolescent Mental Health, 1*(2), 5.

Rajeev, J., Srinath, S., Girimaji, S., Seshadri, S. P., & Singh, P. A. (2004). Systematic chart review of the naturalistic course and treatment of early-onset bipolar disorder in a child and adolescent psychiatry center. *Comprehensive Psychiatry, 45*, 148–154.

Rajeev, J., Srinath, S., Reddy, Y. C. J., Shashikiran, M. G., Girimaji, S. C., Seshadri, S. P., et al. (2003). The index manic episode in juvenile-onset bipolar disorder: The pattern of recovery. *Canadian Journal of Psychiatry, 48*, 52–55.

Rao, U., & Chen, L. A. (2009). Characteristics, correlates, and outcomes of childhood and adolescent depressive disorders. *Dialogues in Clinical Neuroscience, 11*, 45–62.

Roy, A. M., Lopes, V., & Klein, R. G. (2014). Disruptive mood dysregulation disorder: A new diagnostic approach to chronic irritability in youth. *American Journal of Psychiatry, 171*, 918–924.

Srinath, S., Prabhuswamy, M., Reddy, Y. C. J., Girimaji, S. R., Seshadri, S. P. (2008). Clinical practice guidelines for the treatment of children and adolescents with affective disorders. *Indian Journal of Psychiatry*, 238–248.

Srinath, S., Reddy, Y. C. J., Girimaji, S. C., Seshadri, S. P., & Subbakrishna, D. K. (1998). A prospective study of bipolar disorder in children and adolescents from India. *Acta Psychiatrica Scandinavica, 98*, 437–442.

Stalets, M. M., & Luby, J. L. (2006). Preschool Depression. *Child and Adolescent Psychiatric Clinics of North America, 15*(4), 899–917.

Strober, M., Lampert, C., Schmidt, S., & Morrell, W. (1993). The course of major depressive disorder in adolescents: I. Recovery and risk of manic switching in a follow-up of psychotic and nonpsychotic subtypes. *Journal of the American Academy of Child and Adolescent Psychiatry, 32*, 34–42.

Strober, M., Morrell, W., Lampert, C., & Burroughs, J. (1990). Relapse following discontinuation of lithium maintenance therapy in adolescents with bipolar I illness: A naturalistic study. *American Journal of Psychiatry, 147*, 457–461.

Strober, M., Schmidt-Lackner, S., Freeman, R., Bower, S., Lampert, C., & DeAntonio, M. (1995). Recovery and relapse in adolescents with bipolar affective illness: A five-year naturalistic, prospective follow-up. *Journal of the American Academy of Child and Adolescent Psychiatry, 34*, 724–731.

Tourian, L., LeBoeuf, A., Breton, J. J., et al. (2015). Treatment options for the cardinal symptoms of disruptive mood dysregulation disorder. *Journal of Canadian Academy of Child and Adolescent Psychiatry, 24*(1), 41–54.

Weisz, J. R., McCarty, C. A., & Valeri, S. M. (2006). Effects of psychotherapy for depression in children and adolescents: A meta-analysis. *Psychological Bulletin, 132*, 132–149.

Yen, S., Stout, R., Hower, H., Killam, M. A., et al. (2015). The influence of comorbid disorders on the episodicity of bipolar disorder in youth. *Acta Psychiatrica Scandinavica, 17*.

Chapter 5
Reflections on Suicide in Children and Adolescents

Alan Apter and Yari Gvion

Abstract Suicide attempts are the most common reason for seeking psychiatric care in the mid-teens. In the West, females predominantly attempt suicide while males usually commit suicide. In India, deaths in women occurred between 15 and 29 years and youth suicide is especially common. There are many risk factors to suicide behaviour in the young. Access to means is one of the most preventable of such factors. Psychiatric illness is one of the major risk factors in the young. Those include depression, conduct disorder, dissociative disorders and borderline personality disorder, anorexia and bulimia nervosa, and schizophrenia. When there is more than one disorder, then risks are multiplied. Three personality constellations are also evident in youngsters at risk for suicide attempts. Those include narcissism, perfectionism and the inability to tolerate failure; impulsive and aggressive characteristics combined with oversensitivity to life stress and hopelessness are often related to underlying depression and mental illness. Other risk factors are psychological. Suicidal adolescents should undergo a comprehensive clinical evaluation. It is important to emphasize seriousness of the problem to the child and the family and to ensure evaluation, since lack of compliance with treatment is characteristic of suicidal adolescents who are brought to emergency room. The chapter reviews some of the assessment measures that exist. Suicide prevention in youth includes primary, secondary and tertiary prevention strategies. Primary and secondary prevention programmes are often used at schools. The goal of tertiary prevention is to reduce the rate of relapse in adolescents with known suicidal ideation and attempts. Finally, the chapter reviews some of the interventions used in suicide behaviour.

A. Apter (✉) · Y. Gvion
Department of Psychology, Schneider's Children's Medical Center of Israel,
Bar Ilan University, Ramat Gan, Israel
e-mail: asapter@gmail.com

Y. Gvion
e-mail: yari@kadi.co.il

S. Malhotra and P. Santosh (eds.), *Child and Adolescent Psychiatry*,
DOI 10.1007/978-81-322-3619-1_5

Keywords Adolescent · Risk factors · Assessment · Prevention · Therapy · Suicidal behaviour

5.1 Introduction

Suicide is a leading cause of death in young people. In the USA, it is the third leading cause of death after car accidents and homicide. In India, it is the second most common cause of death in both boys and girls. Moreover, suicide attempts are the most common reason for seeking psychiatric care in the mid-teens and although attempts rarely predict a later suicide at this age they are nearly always associated with an impairing disorder (WHO 2014).

5.2 Terminology

Non-fatal suicidal behaviours include a heterogeneous spectrum of behaviours such as suicidal ideation, suicidal threats, suicidal gestures, suicide attempts, serious suicide attempts and interrupted attempts. Another related form of behaviour is self-cutting, which consists of repetitive and stereotypical cutting, the objective of which is to relieve distress/anger, pain and loneliness rather than to die. This often co-occurs with suicidal behaviour and is often termed "non-suicidal self-injury" (NSSI). NSSI was proposed for inclusion in the DSM 5 as a separate entity but this was not accepted and the decision was to await further evidence before making a final conclusion about the entity's final status.

5.3 Epidemiology

Suicide in the young is most common in Eastern Europe particularly in the countries of the former Soviet Union. The twentieth century showed huge increases in male youth suicides in the West except for the periods of both World Wars (WHO 2014). The explanation for the decrease is the camaraderie of soldiers giving each other support and also the effects of prohibition in the US. Just before the turn of the century, a gradual decrease in suicide rates occurred in young males, perhaps due to the increased use of specific serotonin uptake inhibitors (SSRI) for the treatment of adolescent depression. When the use of SSRI was suddenly decreased owing to the introduction of the black box label after a scare that SSRI agents could actually induce suicide, peaks of suicide in adolescent males reappeared. Indeed Gibbons et al. (2007) showed that between 2003 and 2005 youth suicide in the Netherlands increased by 49 % and in the USA by 14 %, while SSRI prescriptions for adolescents declined by approximately 22 % in both the USA and the Netherlands. Attempted suicide is less common in males than in females. The highest rate for females is in the age range of 15–19 years (Nock et al. 2008). Social class and suicide attempts are inversely related (Nock et al. 2008). In high income countries, suicide rates increase with increasing age but in India young women have the highest suicide rates of all ages and to a lesser extent this is also true of young males. Interestingly, higher educational status and marriage which are protective factors are actually risk factors in India (Patel et al. 2012). In India 40 % of suicide deaths in men and 56 % of suicide deaths in women occurred between 15 and 29 years and youth suicide is especially common in South India due to a combination of social problems and mental illness. The high suicide rates in South India might also be attributable to the social acceptance of suicide as a method to deal with difficulties as well as ready access to highly lethal pesticides (Patel et al. 2012).

Suicide attempts tend to cluster in the younger age groups especially in the mid- and late teens. They occur predominantly in females during the teenage years. In the West, the discrepancy between the facts that females predominantly attempt suicide while males usually commit suicide is known as the "Gender Paradox" (Nock et al. 2008).

5.4 Risk Factors

There are many and varied risk factors for youth suicide. "Access to means" is one of the most preventable of such factors. Thus, reducing the access to firearms has achieved consistently good results especially in Israel and in Switzerland where young soldiers had been encouraged to keep their rifles at home. When these policies were changed, suicide rates dropped significantly. The introduction of pesticide control significantly reduced the rates of suicide in young women in Sri Lanka. Social fragmentation also is a potent risk factor for the 15–44-year-old age group.

Psychiatric illness is a well-known risk factor at all ages. Some conditions are more specifically pertinent to the young. Apart from depression, these include conduct disorder, dissociative disorders and borderline personality disorder, anorexia and bulimia nervosa, and schizophrenia. When there is more than one disorder then risks are multiplied. In our experience, the following comorbid constellations are especially dangerous: schizophrenia, depression and substance abuse; substance abuse, conduct disorder and depression; affective disorder, eating disorder and anxiety disorders; affective disorder, personality disorder and dissociate disorder.

Schizophrenia in the young is paradoxically most dangerous in the better prognosis cases where insight is maintained. As the young person, especially male, realizes that he has an incurable mental illness which is destroying his identity, depression sets in. This can lead to self-medication often with alcohol or other psychoactive substances, which in turn makes for impulsive and faulty decision-making and then subsequent suicide. There is now considerable evidence to show that aggression turned outward does not reduce aggression turned inward but in fact can potentiate inward aggression. Thus, aggressive young people are very prone to suicide and detention centres and juvenile prisons have accordingly high rates of self-harm. When the adolescent with conduct disorder is incarcerated and depressed and when he is using alcohol and drugs his situation becomes all the more dangerous for suicide (Galaif et al. 2007).

Eating disorders are associated with high rates of suicide. Since anorexia nervosa is a disorder of females, this is surprising given the "gender paradox". However, this disease has the highest standard mortality rate of all psychiatric conditions. Bulimia nervosa is also associated with all forms of suicidal behaviour both fatal and non-fatal. The term multi-impulsive bulimia was coined by Lacey (1993) to describe the combination of impulsive suicidal, sexual and eating behaviour seen in these young women.

Borderline personality disorder is also prominently a condition found in young adolescent women. The hallmark of this disorder is non-fatal suicidal behaviour, however completed suicide is not rare in these patients. These girls are often prone to dissociative states, commonly related to childhood sexual trauma. These dissociative states are often potent proximal risk factors for suicide in young women (Stanley and Jones 2009).

5.5 Personality Constellations

Suicidal behaviour in adolescence is very heterogeneous and can occur within the context of a variety of personality constellations. Three such sets are narcissism, perfectionism and the inability to tolerate failure; impulsive and aggressive characteristics combined with over sensitivity to life stress and hopelessness are often related to underlying depression and mental illness.

The narcissistic and perfectionist constellation was very evident in a group of soldiers who committed suicide and who were investigated as part of a psychological autopsy study (Apter et al. 1993, 2008). These soldiers showed strong narcissistic and perfectionist patterns, schizoid traits in their personality, a strong need to prove their worth, high self-expectations and hopes and were termed by those who knew them as being private and isolated people. The following is a **fictitious conglomerate** picture of a subset of cases—it does **not** refer to any particular individual.

Daniel was a 20-year-old officer when he killed himself. His family was achievement oriented and had high moral standards Their ideals stressed controlling one's emotions and living up to high standards. Daniel was a natural leader and popular with his teachers and peers. In the army he excelled and was selected as an instructor for new recruits. His superiors commended him for his ability to perform under stress. He became totally involved in his new duties. He vowed that his platoon would win the prize for the best performance but although they did rather well, their overall performance rating was only average. Following the course graduation ceremony Daniel went to his room and shot himself.

Levi et al. (2008) have formulated a model to explain these types of suicide as follows: severe mental pain along with communication difficulty and the inability to ask for help lead to a high risk for suicide. As men in general have more difficulty in asking for help, this model might even explain why men are at higher risk for suicide than women.

The impulsive aggressive personality constellation is seen frequently in adolescents, in emergency rooms and adolescent inpatient units. The dynamics behind this type of suicidal behaviour can be described in terms of Menninger's famous triad: the wish to die, the wish to kill and the wish to be killed (Freud's "death instinct"). In these cases, the latter two wishes predominate (Menninger 1933).

The following is a **fictitious conglomerate** picture of a subset of cases—it does **not** refer to any particular individual. *Deborah had always been impulsive and oppositional from an early age. At about the age of 11 she developed anorexia nervosa probably because of her being an accomplished dancer in a ballet troop. With the onset of adolescence, she developed very severe bulimia. Her first admission to a psychiatric unit was occasioned by a suicide note, which she wrote to her teacher at school. In the unit, she was "an impossible patient". By the time, she was 22 she had made over 100 suicide attempts. She received all kinds of psychosocial and biological therapies but of no avail, although with age (now 25) there is some tempering of her emotional instability.*

These impulsive aggressive cases appear to be related to the concept of the "Serotonin-related anxiety/aggression stressor precipitated depression" (Apter et al. 1990). According to this concept, certain individuals faced with relatively minor life stressors react with anger and anxiety and develop a secondary depression often accompanied by suicidal behaviour. Interestingly, these kinds of suicidal behaviour appear to be under specific genetic control where as in older suicides the genetic of suicide are more related to the underlying psychiatric illness.

The final constellation is that of the demoralization—hopelessness constellation. In these cases the adolescent is usually suffering from an underlying mental illness more often depression. An example is a classic case from the literature, the case of Ellen West who was treated by the famous Swiss psychiatrist, Leon Binswanger.

She was the daughter of wealthy Jewish parents who had great control over her. Her father interfered twice when she became engaged and when she finally married it was to a cousin. From age 19 she developed the fear of becoming fat and by 21 had developed anorexia nervosa. She was hospitalized but this only increased her suicidal thoughts. She was discharged from the sanatorium at the request of her family. On the third day after returning home, she appeared to be a changed person. She ate and enjoyed a walk with her husband. That evening, she took a lethal dose of poison. In her diary published posthumously she described the tyranny of her thoughts about weight and food which could escape only by killing herself.

5.6 Psychological Risk Factors

There are of course a myriad of psychological risk factors for adolescent suicidal behaviour and there is only space here to highlight a few of special interests which may have a value for understanding adolescent suicidal behaviour.

Dysfunctional Attitudes are the corner stones of the learning theory approach to depression and suicide and form the central fulcrum for the cognitive behaviour approaches to depression and suicide developed by Brown et al. (2005) and adapted for adolescents by David Brent. They are the results of false beliefs that can be attacked by logical reasoning and Socratic argumentation.

Rumination/Distraction Rumination is the compulsively focused attention on the symptoms of one's distress, and on its possible causes and consequences, as opposed to its solutions. It is similar to worry except rumination focuses on bad feelings and experiences from the past, whereas worry is concerned with potential bad events in the future. Rumination has been widely studied as a cognitive vulnerability factor to depression; however its measures have not been unified in the Response Styles Theory proposed by Nolen-Hoeksema (2000). Distraction is the healthy alternative to rumination, where focus is directed to positive stimuli instead of distress. Rumination is believed to predict the duration of depressive symptoms.

In other words, ruminating about problems was presumed to be a form of memory rehearsal which was believed to actually lengthen the experience of depression. Many of the modern mindfulness therapeutic strategies for suicidal behaviour in adolescence are based on the notion that mindfulness combats rumination.

Autobiographical Memory There has been a suggestion that in the presence of early childhood adversity repression occurs. This leads to the production of overgeneralized autobiographical memories. The lack of specific autobiographical memories is associated with paucity of interpersonal problem-solving strategies which are in turn associated with the use of suicidal behaviours to solve such problems. This too can often be counteracted by mindfulness techniques (Arie et al. 2008).

Appraisal/Reappraisal (Carthy et al. 2010) **Cognitive reappraisal** is an emotion regulation strategy that involves changing the trajectory of an emotional response by reinterpreting the meaning of the emotional stimulus. For example, a person may fail a series of tests and think negatively about his or her performance upon first receiving the results. The person revisits his or her emotional response to the situation and later views the results as a way to challenge and better him or herself. This process involves two parts: (a) recognition of one's negative response and (b) reinterpretation of the situation to either reduce the severity of the negative response or exchange the negative attitude for a more positive attitude. This strategy is one of the three broad categories of coping which include appraisal-focused behaviour, problem-focused behaviour and emotion-focused behaviour. It differs from the other two methods of coping because it primarily addresses an individual's perception of a situation, rather than directly altering environmental stressors or emotional responses to those stressors.

Emotional Regulation Generally speaking, emotional dysregulation has been defined as difficulties in controlling the influence of emotional arousal on the organization and quality of thoughts, actions and interactions. Individuals who are emotionally dysregulated exhibit patterns of responding in which there is a mismatch between their goals, responses and/or modes of expression, and the demands of the **social environment** (Linehan et al. 1991). For example, there is a significant association between emotion dysregulation and symptoms of depression, anxiety, eating pathology and suicidal behaviour in adolescents. Dialectic behaviour therapy (DBT) probably the most effective form of therapy for suicidal adolescents is heavily focused on this psychological process.

5.7 Assessment

Suicidal adolescents should undergo a comprehensive clinical evaluation. It is important to emphasize seriousness of the problem to the child and the family and to ensure evaluation, since lack of compliance with treatment is characteristic of suicidal adolescents who are brought to emergency rooms.

Clinicians' ability to undertake accurate assessment of suicidality among adolescents has been compromised by a lack of well-defined terminology and understanding as to what constitutes suicidal behaviour (Posner et al. 2007). One important publication to deal with this problem is a study by Posner et al. (2007) describing the Columbia Classification Algorithm for Suicide Assessment (C-CASA), which is a standardized suicidal rating system providing data for the pediatric suicidal risk analysis of antidepressants conducted by the FDA.

Following the development of the C-CASA, a low-burden measure of the spectrum of suicidal ideation and behaviour, the Columbia-Suicide Severity Rating Scale (C-SSRS), was developed in the NIMH Treatment of Adolescent Suicide Attempters Study (TASA) to assess severity and track suicidal events through treatment. This clinical interview focuses on both ideation and behaviour. It can be administered during evaluation or risk assessment to identify the level and type of suicidality present. It can also be used during treatment to monitor clinical deterioration or improvement (Posner et al. 2007).

In young people, in whom assessment takes time, emergency room personnel tend to take a rapid history of present circumstances and briefly assess for depression, and the mistaken diagnosis of adjustment disorder is often made. In adolescents who are identified as being school dropouts, truants or unemployed, it is important to take a careful history of impulsive behaviour and conduct problems as well as history of drug and alcohol use. In adolescents, questions of identity and sexual orientation (Garofalo et al. 1999) must be sought in all patients (Eskin 2012).

5.8 Suicide Prevention in Youth

Suicide prevention in youth includes primary, secondary and tertiary prevention strategies. Current efforts to establish better empirical evidence for suicide prevention include the National Registry of Evidence-Based Programmes and Practices (NREPP), a federal registry of effective prevention programmes in the USA (Rodgers et al. 2007). Examples of successful primary prevention strategies are involvement of the media in responsible reporting of suicides (Pirkis et al. 2009; Niederkrotenthaler and Sonneck 2007) and limiting the access to commonly used and potentially lethal methods of suicide, such as guns, pesticides, pills, etc. (Biddle et al. 2008; Gunnell et al. 2007).

Secondary prevention strategies address individuals at risk, such as those with mental disorder, and aim to provide early treatment (Anderson and Jenkins 2006). An example of secondary prevention in youth is gatekeeper training in schools, community or health care settings. The idea is to train school staff and health care professionals to recognize youths at risk and refer them to appropriate treatment facilities/services.

Another secondary prevention strategy is screening of the general adolescent population for individuals with suicidal ideation and previous attempts, as well as depression and other suicide risk factors (Gould et al. 2005). The recent studies on the relation between bullying and suicidality suggest that early school years suicide prevention and active screening strategies should also focus on those who are frequently bullied and victimized.

Primary and secondary prevention programmes are often used at schools. They have become a significant feature of most national suicide prevention strategies (Gould et al. 2009). In school, children and adolescents can easily be reached, although dropouts comprise a definite risk group which is often missed. Some of those programmes are aimed at case finding using suicide awareness educational curricula, gatekeeper training or screening, while others aim at risk reduction through skills training or a combination of skills training and suicide awareness educational curricula. Thus far, signs of suicide (SOS) is one of the best empirically supported school-based prevention programme and is listed as such in the National Registry of Evidence-based Programmes and Practices (NREPP). SOS is a two-day programme for adolescents ages 13–18 years, combining a curriculum component (a video and teacher-led class discussion) aimed at raising awareness, with a screening component to identify students with depression and at risk of suicide. An evaluation in more than 6000 students in five high schools showed a 40 % short-term decrease in self-reported suicide attempts and modest changes in knowledge and attitudes. Yet, no changes were found in suicide ideation and help-seeking behaviours (Aseltine and DeMartino 2004). The most recent replication study of SOS (Aseltine et al. 2007) involved over 4000 adolescents from diverse ethnic/racial background in nine different high schools across three states in the USA. Results confirmed earlier findings and showed significantly lower rates of suicide attempts, greater knowledge about, and more adaptive attitudes towards, depression, independent of race/ethnicity, grade and gender. However, no effect was found for help-seeking behaviours. Both studies lack follow-up data beyond 3 months and baseline pretest data.

Another school-based strategy is skills training, with a specific focus on improving problem-solving and coping skills, thereby aiming to "immunize" youths against suicidal behaviour. These programmes also intend to reduce suicide risk factors, such as depression, hopelessness and drug abuse. Orbach and Bar-Joseph (1993) assessed a group-based prevention programme in Israeli schools and found that a gradual, controlled exploration of inner experiences and life difficulties related to suicidal behaviour, while teaching coping strategies, can immunize adolescents against self-destructive feelings.

The Awareness programme of primary intervention targets adolescents between 14 and 26 years old and increases pupils' awareness of mental health, healthy/unhealthy behaviour (Wasserman et al. 2012).

Question, persuade and refer (QPR) (http://www.hopes-wi.org/gpr.htm) is a gate keeping programme, designed to educate teachers and other school-based adults in identifying at-risk adolescents and referring them to mental health facilities (Wasserman et al. 2012).

Research on gatekeeper training has shown significant improvement in knowledge, attitudes, intervention skills and willingness to cope with a crisis, as well as referral practices among school personnel (King and Smith 2000; Wyman et al. 2008). Three gatekeeper programmes in particular have been widely used: Living Works' applied suicide intervention skills training (ASIST) (www.livingworks.net) and question persuade and refer (QPR) (Wasserman et al. 2012) (www.qprinstitue.com).

The goal of tertiary prevention is to reduce the rate of relapse in adolescents with known suicidal ideation and attempts. This requires multidisciplinary services with easy access, continuity of care and rehabilitation, as well as inclusion of the family in the process (Wasserman and Durkee 2009). The aim of post-intervention programmes is to assist survivors in their grief process, in addition to identifying and referring those who may be at risk of developing morbidity and mortality related to pathological bereavement. However, although the value of suicide post intervention is increasingly recognized, there is insufficient research on the efficacy of programmes targeting youths in general and school-based programmes in particular.

5.9 Psychosocial Therapies

Adolescent attempters often fail to attend and complete treatment. As a matter of fact, it has been suggested that about half of the adolescent suicide attempters do not receive adequate psychotherapy after their attempt. Parental denial and psychopathology may interfere with treatment planning. This poses a major problem in the management of adolescent suicide attempters (Rotheram-Borus et al. 1996).

The same problem occurs in family therapy, because of the high rejection rate by parents, as reflected by high levels of non-attendance at treatment sessions.

Little research is available on treatment targeting suicidal adolescents and, until recently, suicidal adolescents were excluded from clinical trials. Currently, there are only two psychotherapies that have been found to be effective in reducing suicide attempts among adults: CBT (Brown et al. 2005) and dialectical behaviour therapy (DBT) (Linehan et al. 1991). These have been adapted to adolescents and appear to be promising, as described below.

DBT has been adapted for adolescents with borderline features (DBT-A). DBT-A is based on a dialectical perspective and a mindfulness orientation (based on Eastern Zen Buddhist principles). The dialectic of the treatment is the emphasis on balancing change and acceptance. Identity problems, impulsivity, emotional instability and interpersonal problems are targeted by teaching mindfulness, distress tolerance, emotion regulation and interpersonal effectiveness. This is a 16-week treatment that includes individual psychotherapy, multifamily skills training group (a didactic framework in which the patients and parent/family members are taught four sets of skills and practice with one another) and the therapist's consultation team. Parents are an integral part of DBT-A and participate in the skills training group and in the individual sessions, as needed, to address familial issues. Behaviour change in DBT-A is facilitated by a combination of direct instruction about the skills to be learned, modelling of the behaviour, repeated practice by the patient and positive reinforcements offered by the therapist (Brunstein Klomek and Stanley 2007).

Mehlum et al. (2014) examined whether a shortened form of dialectical behaviour therapy, dialectical behaviour therapy for adolescents (DBT-A) is more effective than enhanced usual care to reduce self-harm in adolescents. They studied 77 out-patients adolescents with recent and repetitive self-harm who were randomly allocated to either DBT-A or enhanced usual care. Treatment retention was generally good in both treatment conditions, and the use of emergency services was low. DBT-A was superior to EUC in reducing self-harm, suicidal ideation, and depressive symptoms. Effect sizes were large for treatment outcomes in patients who received DBT-A, whereas effect sizes were small for outcomes in patients receiving enhanced usual care.

Another therapy for suicidal behaviour is the TASA therapy. It combines cognitive behavioural techniques based on Beck's model (Brown et al. 2005), skills enhancement based on DBT and family therapy. The family is encouraged to support; to improve the family's problem-solving skills, and modify the family's communication patterns (Brunstein Klomek and Stanley 2007). Results show positive outcome for adolescents vigorously treated with a combination of medication and psychotherapy. Adolescents with depression who have recently attempted suicide showed rates of improvement and remission of depression that seem comparable to those observed in no suicidal adolescents with depression (Vitiello et al. 2009).

Other psychotherapies include multisystemic therapy (MST) (Huey et al. 2004), psychoeducation and cognitive behavioural family therapy (Rotheram-Borus et al. 1996), home-based family therapy (Harrington et al. 1998), developmental group therapy (Wood et al. 1996) and Youth-Nominated Support Team (YST-1) (King et al. 2006). A recent study in Australia failed to replicate the benefits of the developmental group therapy (Hazell et al. 2009). As far as we are aware, none of the other studies has been replicated, so these therapies remain unproven.

5.10 Hospitalization

Some suicide attempters need hospitalization. Those include youngsters who express a persistent wish to die or who are psychiatrically ill (Brent 1997). In order for hospitalization to benefit the patient, a relationship with the suicidal adolescent and his family should be established in the emergency room and the importance of treatment should be stressed. An appointment and a follow-up plan should be scheduled before discharge. A "no-suicide contract", in which the child or adolescent agrees not to engage in self-harming behaviour and to tell an adult if he or she is having suicidal urges, may be useful but should not be relied on. The contract should never decrease a clinician's vigilance or curtail monitoring of the child or adolescent. Clinicians should also be aware of suicide contagion in the case of exposure to suicidal behaviour on a ward.

Suicidal adolescents should only be discharged home if adequate supervision and support will be available over the next few days and if a responsible adult has agreed to dispose of potentially lethal medications and firearms. Warning the child or adolescent and family about the dangerous disinhibiting effects of alcohol and other drugs is important. The first days after an attempt pose danger for repeated ideation and attempt, thus the clinician treating the suicidal child or adolescent should be available to the patient and family.

Once a therapeutic alliance is established and the child or adolescent has attended the first treatment sessions, the child or adolescent is more likely to continue treatment. Length of the treatment is individual, but 3–6 months should be a rule, with successively fewer contacts up to 1 or 2 years, sometimes longer (Harrington et al. 1998).

5.10.1 Psychopharmacology

Any medication prescribed to the suicidal child or adolescent must be carefully monitored by a third party and any change of behaviour or side effects should be reported immediately.

Only one medication, lithium, has been shown to have a potential anti-suicide effect (Cipriani et al. 2005). Apart from one report describing the preventive effects of lithium on suicidal thoughts and behaviours in adolescents (Masters 2008), there have been no studies on the effects of this treatment on adolescent suicidal behaviour (Bursztein and Apter 2009). Tricyclic antidepressants should not be prescribed for the suicidal child or adolescent as a first line of treatment. They are potentially lethal, because of the small difference between therapeutic and toxic levels of the drug, and they have not been proved effective in children or adolescents.

Selective serotonin reuptake inhibitors (SSRIs) reduce suicidal ideation and suicide attempts in non-depressed adults with cluster-B (borderline, antisocial, histrionic, narcissistic) personality disorders. They are safe in children and adolescents, have low lethality and are effective in treating depression in non-suicidal adolescents. Further research is needed to determine whether SSRIs influence suicidal behaviour or ideation in children and adolescents. Finally, it should be noted that the recent decrease in youth suicide rates may parallel the increased use of SSRI medications in this age group.

Other medications that may increase disinhibition or impulsivity, such as the benzodiazepines and phenobarbital, should be prescribed with caution in children and adolescent.

5.11 Conclusions

Adolescent suicide remains a cause of death in young people and a major health problem. Non-fatal suicidal behaviour causes also a great deal of morbidity and suffering. In order to improve the prediction of suicidality, to enhance assessment process, and find more effective treatment and more targeted prevention programmes, the identification of more specific risk factors is prerequisite. The presence of mental illness, alcohol and drug abuse, conduct disorder, poor communication within the family, personality disorder and lack of compliance with therapy make cases of suicide attempts difficult to treat.

References

Anderson, M., & Jenkins, R. (2006). The national suicide prevention strategy for England: The reality of a national strategy for the nursing profession. *Journal of Psychiatric and Mental Health Nursing, 13*(6), 641–650.

Apter, A., Bleich, A., King, R. A., Kron, S., Fluch, A., Kotler, M., et al. (1993). Death without warning? A clinical postmortem study of suicide in 43 Israeli adolescent males. *Archives of General Psychiatry, 2*, 138–142.

Apter, A., King, R. A., Bleich, A., Fluck, A., Kotler, M., & Kron, S. (2008). Fatal and non-fatal suicidal behaviour in Israeli adolescent males. *Archives of Suicide Research, 12*, 20–29.

Apter, A., van Praag, H. M., Plutchik, R., et al. (1990). Interrelationship among anxiety, aggression, impulsivity, and mood: A serotonergicaly linked cluster? *Psychiatry Research, 32*(2), 191–199.

Arie, M., Apter, A., Orbach, I., Yefet, Y., & Zalzman, G. (2008). Autobiographical memory, interpersonal problem solving, and suicidal behaviour in adolescent inpatients. *Comprehensive Psychiatry, 49*, 22–29.

Aseltine, R. H., & DeMartino, R. (2004). An outcome evaluation of the SOS suicide prevention program. *American Journal of Public Health, 94*(3), 446–451.

Aseltine, R., James, A., Schilling, E., & Glanovsky, J. (2007). Evaluating the SOS suicide prevention program: A replication and extension. *BMC Public Health, 7*, 161.
Biddle, L., Donovan, J., Hawton, K., Kapur, N., & Gunnell, D. (2008). Suicide and the internet. *BMJ, 336*(7648), 800–802.
Brent, D. A. (1997). The aftercare of adolescents with deliberate self-harm. *Journal of Child Psychology and Psychiatry, 38*, 277–286.
Brown, G. K., Have, T. T., Henriques, G. R., Xie, S. X., Hollander, J. E., & Beck, A. T. (2005). Cognitive therapy for the prevention of suicide attempts: A randomized controlled Trial. *JAMA, 294*(5), 563–570.
Brunstein Klomek, A., & Stanley, B. (2007). Psychosocial treatment of depression and suicidality in adolescents. *CNS Spectrums, 12*(2), 135–144.
Bursztein, C., & Apter, A. (2009). Adolescent suicide. *Current Opinion Psychiatry, 22*(1), 1–6.
Carthy, T., Horesh, N., Apter, A., Edge, M. D., & Gross, J. (2010). Emotional reactivity and cognitive regulation in anxious children. *Behaviour Research and Therapy, 48*, 384–393.
Cipriani, A., Pretty, H., Hawton, K., & Geddes, J. R. (2005). Lithium in the prevention of suicidal behaviour and all-cause mortality in patients with mood disorders: A systematic review of randomized trials. *American Journal of Psychiatry, 162*, 1805–1819.
Eskin, M. (2012). Problem solving therapy in the clinical practice. *Newnes*.
Galaif, E., Sussman, S., Newcomb, M., & Locke, T. (2007). Suicidality, depression, and alcohol use among adolescents: A review of empirical findings. *International Journal of Adolescent Medicine and Health, 19*(1), 27–36.
Garofalo, R., Wol, R. C., Wissow, L. S., et al. (1999). Sexual orientation and risk of suicide attempts among a representative sample of youth. *Archives of Pediatrics and Adolescent Medicine, 153*, 487–493.
Gibbons, R. D., Brown, C. H., Hur, K., et al. (2007). Early evidence on the effects of regulators' suicidality warning on SSRI prescriptions and suicide in children and adolescents. *American Journal of Psychiatry, 164*, 1356–1363.
Gould, M., Brunstein Klomek, A., & Batejan, K. (2009). The role of schools, colleges and universities in suicide prevention. In D. Wasserman & C. Wasserman (Eds.), *The Oxford textbook of suicidology and suicide prevention—A global perspective* (pp. 551–560). New York: Oxford University Press.
Gould, M. S., Marrocco, F. A., Kleinman, M., Thomas, J. G., Mostkoff, K., Cote, J., et al. (2005). Evaluating iatrogenic risk of youth suicide screening programs: A randomized controlled trial. *JAMA, 293*(13), 1635–1643.
Gunnell, D., Fernando, R., Hewagama, M., Priyangika, W. D., Konradsen, F., & Eddleston, M. (2007). The impact of pesticide regulations on suicide in Sri Lanka. *International Journal of Epidemiology, 36*(6), 1235–1242.
Harrington, R., Kerfoot, M., Dye, E., et al. (1998). Randomized trial of a home-based family intervention for children who have deliberately poisoned themselves. *Journal of the American Academy of Child and Adolescent Psychiatry, 8*(37), 512–518.
Hazell, P. L., Martin, G., McGill, K., Kay, T., Wood, A., Trainor, G., et al. (2009). Group therapy for repeated deliberate self-harm in adolescents: Failure of replication of a randomized trial. *Journal of the American Academy of Child and Adolescent Psychiatry, 48*(6), 662–670.
Huey, S. J., Henggeler, S. W., Rowland, M. D., Halliday-Boykins, C. A., Cunningham, P. B., Pickrel, S. G., et al. (2004). Multisystemic therapy effects on attempted suicide by youths presenting psychiatric emergencies. *Journal of the American Academy of Child and Adolescent Psychiatry, 43*, 183–190.
King, C. A., Kramer, A., Preuss, L., Kerr, D. C., Weisse, L., & Venkataraman, S. (2006). Youth-nominated support team for suicidal adolescents (Version 1): A randomized controlled trial. *Journal of Consulting and Clinical Psychology, 74*(1), 199–206.
King, K. A., & Smith, J. (2000). Project SOAR: A training program to increase school counselors' knowledge and confidence regarding suicide prevention and intervention. *Journal of School Health, 70*(10), 402–407.

Lacey, J. H. (1993). Self-damaging and addictive behaviour in bulimia nervosa. A catchment area study. *British Journal of Psychiatry, 162*, 190–194.

Levi, Y., Horesh, N., Fischel, T., et al. (2008). Mental pain and its communication in medically serious suicide attempts: An “impossible situation”. *Journal of Affective Disorders, 111*(2), 244–250.

Linehan, M. M., Armstrong, H. E., Suarez, A., Allmon, D., & Heard, H. L. (1991). Cognitive-behavioural treatment of chronically parasuicidal borderline patients. *Archives of General Psychiatry, 48*(12), 1060–1064.

Masters, K. J. (2008). Anti-suicidal and self-harm properties of lithium carbonate. *CNS Spectrums, 13*(2), 109–110.

Mehlum, L., Tørmoen, A. J., Ramberg, M., Haga, E., Diep, L. M., Laberg, S., et al. (2014, July). Dialectical behaviour therapy for adolescents with repeated suicidal and self-harming behaviour—A randomized trial. *Journal of the American Academy of Child & Adolescent Psychiatry, 53*(10), 1082–1091.

Menninger, K. A. (1933). Psychoanalytic aspects of suicide. *International Journal of Psychoanalysis, 14*, 376–390.

Niederkrotenthaler, T., & Sonneck, G. (2007). Assessing the impact of media guidelines for reporting on suicides in Austria: Interrupted time series analysis. *Australian and New Zealand Journal of Psychiatry, 41*(5), 419–428.

Nock, M. K., Borges, G., Bromet, E., Cha, C. B., Kessler, R. C., & Lee, S. (2008). Suicide and suicide behaviour. *Epidemiological Review, 30*, 133–154.

Nolen-Hoeksema, S. (2000). The role of rumination in depressive disorders and mixed anxiety/depressive symptoms. *Journal of Abnormal Psychology, 109*(3), 504–511.

Orbach, I., & Bar-Joseph, H. (1993). The impact of a suicide prevention program for adolescents on suicidal tendencies, hopelessness, ego identity, and coping. *Suicide and Life Threatening Behavior, 23*(2), 120–129.

Patel, V., Ramasundarahettige, C., Vijayakumar, L., Thakur, J. S., Gajalakshmi, V., Gururaj, G., et al. (2012). Suicide mortality in India: A nationally representative survey. *Lancet, 379*(9834), 2343–2351.

Pirkis, J., Dare, A., Blood, R. W., Rankin, B., Williamson, M., Burgess, P., et al. (2009). Changes in media reporting of suicide in Australia between 2000/01 and 2006/07. *Crisis, 30*(1), 25–33.

Posner, K., Oquendo, M. A., Gould, M., Stanley, B., & Davies, M. (2007). Columbia Classification Algorithm of Suicide Assessment (C-CASA): Classification of suicidal events in the FDA’s pediatric suicidal risk analysis of antidepressants. *American Journal of Psychiatry, 164*(7), 1035–1043.

Rodgers, P. L., Sudak, H. S., Silverman, M. M., & Litts, D. A. (2007). Evidence-based practices project for suicide prevention. *Suicide and Life Threatening Behaviour, 37*(2), 154–164.

Rotheram-Borus, M. J., Piacentini, J., Van Rossem, R., et al. (1996). Enhancing treatment adherence with a specialized emergency room program for adolescent suicide attempters. *Journal of the American Academy of Child and Adolescent Psychiatry, 35*, 654–663.

Stanley, B., & Jones, B. (2009). Risk for suicidal behaviour in personality disorders. In D. Wasserman & C. Wasserman (Eds.) *Oxford textbook of suicide prevention a global perspective* (pp. 287–292). Oxford: Oxford University Press.

Vitiello, B., Brent, D., Greenhill, L. L., Emslie, G., Wells, K., Walkup, J. T., et al. (2009, August 21). Depressive symptoms and clinical status during the treatment of adolescent suicide attempters study. *Journal of the American Academy of Child & Adolescent Psychiatry, 48*, 997–1004.

Wasserman, D., & Durkee, T. (2009). Strategies in suicide prevention. In D. Wasserman & C. Wasserman (Eds.), *The Oxford textbook of suicidology and suicide prevention—A global perspective* (pp. 381–386). New York: Oxford University Press.

Wasserman, C., Hoven, C. W., Wasserman, D., Carli, V., Sarchiapone, M., Al-Halabí, S., et al. (2012). Suicide prevention for youth—A mental health awareness program: Lessons learned from the saving and empowering young Lives in Europe (SEYLE) intervention study. *BMC Public Health, 12*, 77.

Wood, A., Harrington, R., & Moore, A. (1996). Controlled trial of a brief cognitive-behavioural intervention in adolescent patients with depressive disorders. *Journal of Child Psychology and Psychiatry, 37*(6), 737–746.

World Health Organization (WHO). (2014). *Preventing suicide: A global imperative*. Geneva: WHO.

Wyman, P. A., Brown, C., & Hendricks, I. (2008). Randomized trial of a gatekeeper program for suicide prevention: 1-year impact on secondary school staff. *Journal of Consulting and Clinical Psychology, 76*(1), 104–115.

Part II
Substance Use

Chapter 6
From Nihilism to Hope: Reframing the Concept of Addiction

Vivek Benegal and Deepak Jayarajan

Abstract The treatment of substance use disorders (SUDs) has been characterised by a focus on the goal of abstinence, fostering a sense of therapeutic nihilism when relapse occurs. This chapter will focus on an overview of the factors that determine individuals' vulnerability to SUDs, and how it differs between those at high risk and those at lower risk for an SUD. It will also discuss how this conceptual understanding can be used by clinicians to reframe the focus from an abstinence only model (focused solely on halting drug use) to a more nuanced interventional model that combines harm reduction along with interventions that target the underlying risk factors for addictive disorders, with a longer term focus on recovery.

Keywords Addiction · Externalising spectrum disorders · Dependence · High risk · Intervention · Model · Low risk · Substance use disorder · Vulnerability

Abbreviations

ADHD	Attention deficit hyperactivity disorder
ATOD	Alcohol, tobacco and/or other drugs
CNS	Central nervous system
ERP	Event-related potential
fMRI	Functional magnetic resonance imaging

V. Benegal (✉)
Centre for Addiction Medicine, Department of Psychiatry, National Institute of Mental Health and Neurosciences, Bangalore, India
e-mail: vbenegal@gmail.com

D. Jayarajan
Psychiatric Rehabilitation Services, Department of Psychiatry, National Institute of Mental Health and Neurosciences, Bangalore, India
e-mail: deepak.jayarajan@gmail.com

S. Malhotra and P. Santosh (eds.), *Child and Adolescent Psychiatry*,
DOI 10.1007/978-81-322-3619-1_6

HR	High-risk children, i.e. children of persons with dependence as well as two first-degree family members who also have substance dependence
LR	Low-risk children, i.e. children with no family history of substance dependence in their first- and second-degree relatives
TMS	Transcranial magnetic stimulation
VTA	Ventral tegmental area
SUD	Substance use disorder

6.1 Introduction

The treatment of addiction has been an activity in which its practitioners often feel dwarfed by a visceral perception of inevitable failure. The revolving doorway of sobriety and relapse, through which 'addicts' seem to pass so very frequently, has stymied client, therapist and concerned caregiver alike, albeit in different ways. When a client is working toward a goal of abstinence, that terminus can seem like a mirage, more illusion than reality. Even when abstinence is achieved, it can seem like a reward forever perched on the edge of an abyss, waiting for something as yet unseen or unheard to come and push it over into the depths of regret and despair. To understand why this process carries such an aura of nihilism, it is worthwhile to understand how the concept of addiction itself has evolved. The earliest treatment models of addiction were based on the conceptualisations of substance use prevalent in the era they arose in, from the moral model with the concept of demon rum to the temperance movement and prohibition. These models brooked no solution less than a complete cessation of consumption. The Alcoholics Anonymous concept of addiction as a lifelong disease, for which there is no cure with the only treatments available to reduce or suppress the urge to use drugs, has the potential to suggest that the disorder is deterministic with limited ability for the user to change other than to adopt faith in a higher power. The conceptualisation of addiction as a chronic relapsing disorder, which has its roots in individual vulnerability and which behaves similarly to other chronic disease processes (McLellan et al. 2000), has begun to suggest paradigm shifts in the approach to, and the treatment of addiction. This biopsychosocial understanding has helped us understand that while addiction (in the early onset subset of those who develop substance use disorders or SUDs) occupies the extreme end of a spectrum of substance use behaviours, harmful use and hazardous use, especially in young users, also require early intervention. Hence, while achieving abstinence from substance use can be a final goal for treatment providers to aspire to, the harm reduction has been found to be a developmentally congruent approach to the primary and secondary prevention of risky behaviour adolescents (Canadian Paediatric Society 2008). This chapter will focus on the theoretical framework for a change in approach, along with its implications in the management of substance use, and particularly substance use in adolescents.

6.2 Vulnerability to Addictive Disorders

While assessing adolescent substance users, it is important to evaluate certain key factors that underlie their vulnerability to develop a more severe or chronic SUD. These factors can be summarised as follows:

- Family history of substance use disorders: A high number of first-degree relatives who have substance use disorders can be understood to convey a higher potential to carry genetic markers of risk. However, it is important to keep in mind that this set of risk factors, that is shared by family members, do not reflect a risk to develop substance use disorders alone, but a wider spectrum of risky behaviours. In addition, when there are family members who use alcohol, tobacco or other drugs (ATOD), factors such as easier access to ATOD as well as modelling can also affect attitudes towards substance use and experimentation (social learning theory). Offspring of parents with alcohol-dependent parents also have an earlier onset of use of substances (Obot et al. 2001). For example, a study done in Thrissur, Kerala, by Chopra et al. showed that the prevalence of alcohol use among offspring of alcohol users (10 %) was significantly higher than in the offspring of non-users (3 %) (Chopra et al. 2008).
- Externalising spectrum disorders, including attention deficit hyperactivity disorder (ADHD): ADHD, both during childhood as well as adulthood, serves as a significant risk factor to develop more severe SUDs (Ohlmeier et al. 2008). However, it is important to note that the externalising group of disorders include constructs such as antisocial personality disorder, oppositional defiant disorder and conduct disorders, all of which share in common certain endophenotypes underlying this risk but to differing extents. One such externalising trait is sensation-seeking, which can predispose not only to substance use but to risky sexual behaviour as well (Chandra et al. 2003). In addition, the reward pathway (involving the ventral tegmental area (VTA), the nucleus accumbens and the prefrontal cortex) has been noted to show hypofunctioning in externalising spectrum disorders (Volkow et al. 2011).
- Chronic stress: Chronic stress is often conceptualised to mean psychosocial stress that persists for an extended period and is severe (e.g., sexual abuse, physical abuse, homelessness, extreme poverty and negative life events such as parental losses, parental conflict, parental separation, etc.). Sufferers tend to have higher rates of initiation of drug use as well as an increased incidence of other psychiatric disorders too (Sinha 2008; Burt et al. 2003; Kessler 2004; Clark et al. 1997). Other types of biological stressors, including poor nutrition and exposure to environmental pollutants such as lead, can also adversely increase the risk of developing future developmental and psychiatric disorders, thereby enhancing the risk for future substance use as well.
- Co-occurring mental illnesses: Anxiety disorders (Hulvershorn et al. 2015), mood disorders as well as schizophrenia all serve as diatheses which increase the likelihood of developing or exacerbating a substance use disorder.
- Easy availability of substances.

- Early use: The earlier in life, the substance of abuse are used, the more the chance of altered neuro-development and allostatic load (state of chronic reward dysregulation, wherein a substance user's drug-seeking behaviour becomes driven by a need to chase or recapture the initial rewarding effects of the drug) (Wand 2008). Drugs of abuse serve as pharmacological stressors in terms of brain development, altering developmental trajectories at critical periods of brain development, thereby augmenting the risk of a more severe course of substance use.

6.3 Do High-Risk Children and Adolescents Differ from Their 'Lower Risk' Counterparts?

Studies comparing high-risk children (HR—children of persons with dependence as well as two first-degree family members who also have substance dependence) with low-risk children (LR—children with no family history of substance dependence in their first- and second-degree relatives) have shown a number of differences which could mediate future risk for SUDs, even before either group have had their first substance use experience! Some of these differences are

- Structural differences in brain regions: HR subjects not only have significantly smaller volumes of their superior frontal, cingulate and parahippocampal gyri, amygdala, thalamus and cerebellum, but these reduced grey matter volumes correlated negatively with their externalising symptom scores. Trends toward a reduction of these differences with increasing age suggest a neuro-developmental lag in HR subjects (Benegal et al. 2007). Adolescents with SUDs show significantly greater psychological dysregulation along with prefrontal and parietal white matter disorganisation when compared to controls (Chung et al. 2013; Clark et al. 2012). *In addition, one imaging study done as part of a thesis in NIMHANS has revealed differences in the pattern of white matter tract myelination between HR and LR subjects* (Subbu et al. 2010).
- Electrophysiological differences: In terms of the externalising syndrome, a heritable disinhibitory complex, characterised by generalised increased brain hyperexcitability, is thought to underlie the disorder (Begleiter and Porjesz 1999). In a comparison done by Benegal et al. and Silva et al. between HR and LR children, the P300 component of event-related potential (ERP), a measure of the way the brain pays attention and discriminates between potentially important and non-important stimuli, shows reduced amplitude and this is associated with externalising psychopathology (Benegal et al. 1995; Silva et al. 2007). A difference in terms of the absence of the cortical silent period immediately following transcranial magnetic stimulation (TMS) of the brain, in HR subjects, which indicated inefficient inhibitory capacities of the brain resulting in a state of central nervous system (CNS) hyperexcitability (which strongly predict externalising symptoms) were found by Muralidharan et al. (2013) Hence, a

large number of brain endophenotypes/markers of brain development appear to indicate the presence of a brain development delay—associated with the manifestation of a spectrum of externalising behaviours: Poor attention allocation, impulsivity, difficulty in learning from mistakes, novelty seeking, oppositionality and conduct symptoms.
- Cerebral Activation patterns: Functional magnetic resonance imaging (fMRI) has shown altered patterns of brain activation to go/no-go tasks, though there are contrasting results in terms of whether there is increased or decreased activation in the frontal cortex and other cortical areas (Clark et al. 2013). On the anti-saccade task, a behavioural inhibition task that may be presented during fMRI, HR children made more anti-saccade task errors than did controls; and in the group of HR children, those with ADHD made more errors than those without ADHD (Habeych et al. 2006). On affect-laden tasks, HR children had greater amygdalar activation in response to seeing affect-laden faces than controls, indicating greater frontolimbic network hyper responsiveness to such stimuli (Thatcher et al. 2014).
- Altered CNS responsiveness to substance use: While HR subjects, after ingestion of alcohol, show greater CNS stimulation (a faster onset and longer duration of a switch from beta to alpha activity) and a greater reinforcing effect of alcohol (Jagadeesh et al. 1999), they can have low subjective awareness of intoxicating effects. Moreover, this is a genetically influenced characteristic that impacts on the alcoholism risk of HR subjects (Schuckit 2009).

This difference in the maturity, and hence the functioning, of brain circuits which mediate top-down patterns of information processing versus those that mediate the salience incentive and emotions (Casey et al. 2008). A confluence of mutually interacting environmental influences and genetic factors modulates this risk over time, resulting in a delay in brain maturation. Once again, it is important to understand that HR children carry a greater risk or propensity for certain behavioural characteristics when compared to LR children, and that these characteristics can predispose them to many types of risky behaviours, one of which is substance use and/or abuse.

6.4 What Does This Mean for Clinical Practice?

For illustration, let us take the case of Ms. X, 16-year girl, who was brought straight from a rehab centre (from where she has been going her class X exams) directly to the outpatient department (OPD), with her parents being very concerned about safety and escape from custody. X was being treated for multiple substance use disorders fulfilling criteria for dependence (Inhalants, cannabis, tobacco and alcohol) and severe emotional reactivity, with violence to self and others. She had been diagnosed as Borderline PD and had already had multiple admissions in rehabilitation and psychiatric nursing homes. X has also had early sexual experimentation with multiple medical terminations of pregnancies. She is currently on a combination of two antipsychotics with Carbamazepine and has been on long-term psychotherapy. The dominant theme X brings up during interviews is her reaction to her father's affair and his temporary abandonment of the family, and she does not see herself stopping alcohol and cannabis use at present. Her parents are seeking long-term confinement and care, as they believe that this is the only possible solution, while X is adamant that she 'will not go to rehab'. All3 of them are tired of the way things have been going...

It is obvious that HR children would seem to require a set of interventions, of which those directed specifically towards substance abuse would form a subset. The other components include interventions targeted at

- the early identification of both substance use disorders as well as comorbidities
- the amelioration of externalising disorders (with an armoury of both pharmacological and psychosocial methods)
- treating psychiatric comorbidities (such as anxiety, schizophrenia and mood disorders)
- life skills training
- stress management
- family interventions
- facilitating access to resources that further education and facilitate vocational skill building
- promoting healthy behaviours and/or positive addictions such as exercise and hobbies
- Parent Management Training
- making contingency plans and learning how to deal with lapse and/or relapse of substance use
- maintaining follow-up and aftercare.

In essence, adolescents with substance use who have been brought to treatment have a variety of needs that the clinician is able to help them with, many of which they may be more motivated to address than substance use. For example, a client is more likely to agree to help with an inability to finish projects or tasks because of ADHD, than address their use of cannabis which they perceive as normative. As we have seen that it has been suggested that ADHD shares underlying risk factors for SUD.

This refocusing from the initial problem on every caregiver's and therapist's mind, i.e. substance use, which the client may not be willing to address immediately or even acknowledge, to a vulnerability factor which the client acknowledges as problematic *in other dimensions of well-being* allows both the reluctant client and the eager therapist to set a common goal for treatment. Addressing the vulnerability factor helps to improve quality of life and drive change. It also facilitates a longer term engagement of the client in treatment, allowing time to build rapport and perhaps reconsider, eventually, their desire to continue substance use. While abstinence is a worthy final goal, this approach affords the therapist the ability to reduce ongoing harms from a number of risky behaviours and enhance quality of life. It allows clients to build the skills and the resilience factors which could help them reduce drug use as well as maintain this reduction or abstinence over time.

Hence, this approach of ***reframing*** the problem of substance use as a single aspect of a larger, overarching problem (i.e. vulnerability) can be a powerful way of engaging even reluctant clients and facilitating incremental change. In addition, it allows us to educate client and families about their vulnerability better. It allows parents and adolescents to set common goals for change, even if substance use is something they continue to disagree on. As a significant number of adolescents may not have developed a severe SUD but still have harmful or hazardous use, it allows a refocusing of priorities on underlying vulnerability factors and enhancing of the adolescent's quality of life. Let us see how this helped in Ms. X.

X is an overweight teenager with over-sexualised clothing and appearance. She is angry and blames her father and mother for escalating their interpersonal problems into a need for admission. She is tired of therapists and believes she knows exactly what every clinician is going to say. However, motivational interviewing, you are able to understand and reflect back to her that she truly feels sad about dreams and goals that now seem unrealizable to her. On the Adult ADHD self-rating scale (ASRS), she has high scores. When these concerns are amplified by questions about impulsivity and poor attention allocation, both she and her parents are concerned about her inability to achieve hopes and goals despite her high intelligence. She does not seem to have had a mood disorder.

Her difficulties in achieving her dreams and fulfilling her potential are what you reframe as the central tragedy of her story. This was something that she and her parents readily concur with and want to work on. You illustrate her ADHD's contribution to this by comparing her brain to a car, with her frontal cortex acting as the brakes (allowing her to regulate her behaviour) and her anterior cingulate acting as her gears (allowing her to change her behaviours in response to new situations). You describe her limbic system and the reward pathway in her brain as providing the drive to perform tasks that are important to her, or her engine. She is able to see that impulsivity and an impaired ability to finish tasks are barriers to her goals. Drug use has served as self-medication. X agrees to work on "tuning brakes and gears" while placing reduction of drug use as a "why use kerosene as fuel instead of petrol and ruin your car" argument.

Once agreement is achieved, treatment plans need to be made. Psychosocial interventions that could be used range from individual therapy to family therapy to community-based programmes. In terms of psychological programmes, in addition to CBT, dialectic behaviour therapy and interpersonal therapy have also been reported to show promising outcomes. Psychological interventions could have a range of components that target anxiety, mood disorders such as bipolar disorder and depression, eating disorders, disruptive and oppositional behaviours, self-harming or self-injurious behaviours, poor assertiveness, anger and aggressive behaviours, major psychiatric disorders such as schizophrenia along with substance use disorders (Ollendick and King 2004). Crucially, the intervention should focus on building confidence between adolescent and care-givers, planning for lapses/relapses and developing contingency plans, agreeing on follow-up in both routine and emergency situations and building positive hobbies and activities that are rewarding to the adolescent. These 'positive addictions' can help reduce the need to self-medicate with drugs and boost self-efficacy and esteem.

Comorbidities once identified need to be treated, both with psychosocial as well as pharmacological interventions based on need. One group that we have discussed is those who have externalising disorders. The pharmacological treatment for ADHD has been shown to not increase the risk for subsequent SUDs, as well as show protective effects from developing SUDs (Nigg 2013). While the literature has shown varying effects in terms of the effect of treating ADHD on comorbid SUD outcomes, a study by Benegal et al. in 262 males showed significant externalising symptom reduction, longer abstinence, shorter turnaround time and better quality of life while on atomoxetine (Benegal et al. 2013).

In terms of pharmacotherapy for severe substance use disorders in young adults, some promising new agents which can serve as agents that modify the allostasis, or altered hedonic tone caused by prolonged substance use are available. In terms of alcohol use, baclofen, topiramate and naltrexone have been used in early onset disorders. Case reports of baclofen in the treatment of solvent use have also been reported (Muralidharan et al. 2008). The glutamatergic agent, N-acetylcysteine, has been shown to increase the odds of reduction of cannabis use, as well as having some promise in other SUDs such as cocaine use and nicotine use (McClure et al. 2014). Opioid treatment guidelines now allow the use of opioid substitution therapy in adolescents when indicated. However, the use of these anti-craving agents as well as substitution therapy in adolescents needs to be evaluated much further. A proposed treatment paradigm is shown below in Fig. 6.1.

Ms. X is at first struck by the fact that she is not being labelled as a drug addict. She recognises that the formulation of persons with difficulties in sustaining interest and motivation—describes her well. She says that she also despairs of reaching her goals and fulfilling her desires, as she is never able to finish a task. Despite being clever and more creative, she lags behind her other friends and her repeated failures have made her despair of ever being good enough. And Yes! She would very much like to change that aspect of her if there is a solution. Perhaps even reduce her use of drugs! She is taken up by the concept of tuning her car/brain, now that she no longer has to defend herself of charges of being a drug addict and a bad person…

Ms. X was started on methylphenidate for the ADHD and initially baclofen for anti-craving. She received elements of Dialectical Behaviour Therapy and specific tips on handling problems with studying, emotional reactivity, craving and relapse. We intended to get the family into structured Family therapy but were never able to as they lived in another part of the country and could only come back for brief follow-up visits.

The girl went back to school and completed her class 10 and class 12 exams successfully. Briefly she was troubled by teachers who she felt, continued to scapegoat her, but subsequently she got into an undergraduate course in London, and is studying successfully, living alone. She continues to drink along with her friends at the pub on weekends, but has given up smoking cannabis. Importantly, she is happy on the whole and her parents are very proud of her achievements.

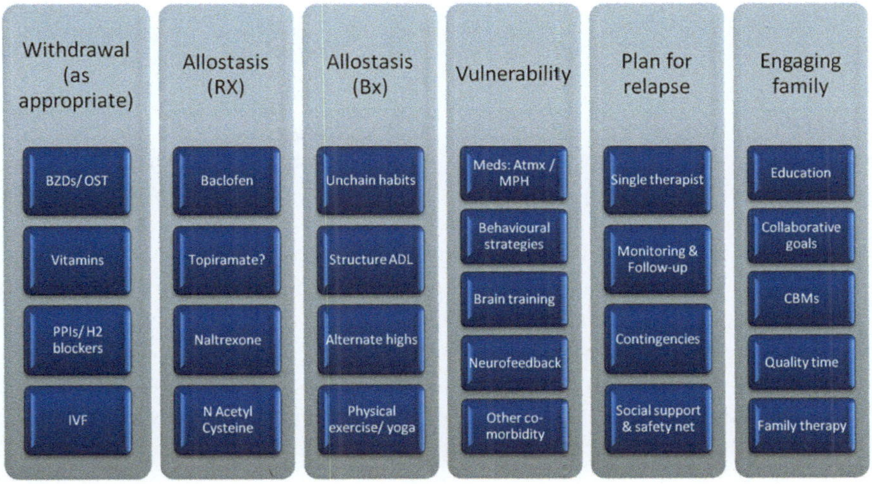

Fig. 6.1 Proposed treatment paradigm for early onset substance use disorders. *BZDs* Benzodiazepines; *OST* Opioid substitution therapy; *PPI* Proton pump inhibitors; *IVF* IV fluids; *ADL* Activities of daily living; *Atmx* Atomoxetine; *MPH* Methylphenidate; *CBM* Confidence building measures

In conclusion, we can see that a modified approach to substance use disorders in adolescents that focuses on addressing the vulnerability factors and comorbidities that have a direct bearing on SUDs has the potential to help clients with early substance use but not a disorder as well as clients with more severe SUDs. Therapists can use reframing to educate families as well as overcome resistance to therapeutic engagement. This approach allows the adolescent as well as her/his parents to set common goals and emphasise long-term and more holistic outcomes (e.g. quality of life) as their goals. It allows the therapist and the client to incorporate harm reduction measures and plan for contingencies, while not allowing relapses to derail treatment plans. Admissions should be considered when necessary, but long-term admissions which do not address the factors underlying substance use are unlikely to be effective.

It is important to understand that the risks that underlie addictions are also risk factors for other psychiatric disorders as well. Early identification, and interventions, for these very risks would allow us to help the young people who most need help, at the developmental period during which they need it most. Hence, a significant amount of research remains to be done on the factors, both environmental and individual, that crystallise the translation of these vulnerabilities into disorders. Some of these answers will come from cohort studies following children at risk. This long-term approach to addictive disorders as epiphenomena of underlying difficulties promises to be a more hopeful one to all stake-holders involved.

Learning outcomes
After reading this chapter, readers would understand that:

- Addictive disorders arise from a host of vulnerability factors, both individual and environmental.
- These vulnerability factors not only determine the risk for addiction, but to a significant number of psychiatric comorbidities, and can have a deleterious impact on an individual's quality of life.
- High-risk individuals show differences from those with low risk in various ways (including structural, electrophysiological and neurochemical alterations; cerebral activation patterns; altered CNS responsiveness to substance use, etc.), even before they develop an SUD.
- Treatment plans do need to incorporate harm reduction strategies for substance use, but they must target underlying risk factors with a combination of pharmacological and psychosocial interventions.
- Reframing the SUD as a problem arising from underlying factors which affect other aspects of a person's life helps generate shared treatment goals, and enhances the client's investment, as well as engagement, in treatment.
- Early identification of those young people at high risk, and the optimal timing of interventions that ameliorate the risk of developing SUDs, are important thrust areas for research.

References

Begleiter, H., & Porjesz, B. (1999). What is inherited in the predisposition toward alcoholism? A proposed model. *Alcoholism, Clinical and Experimental Research, 23*(7), 1125–1135.

Benegal, V., et al. (1995). P300 amplitudes vary inversely with continuum of risk in first degree male relatives of alcoholics. *Psychiatric Genetics, 5*(4), 149–156.

Benegal, V., et al. (2007). Gray matter volume abnormalities and externalizing symptoms in subjects at high risk for alcohol dependence. *Addiction Biology, 12*(1), 122–132. Available at: http://dx.doi.org/10.1111/j.1369-1600.2006.00043.x

Benegal, V., et al. (2013). The efficacy of atomoxetine as adjunctive treatment for co-morbid substance use disorders and externalizing symptoms. *Asian Journal of Psychiatry, 6*(6), 544–547. Available at: http://www.ncbi.nlm.nih.gov/pubmed/24309869

Burt, S. A., et al. (2003). Parent-child conflict and the comorbidity among childhood externalizing disorders. *Archives of General Psychiatry, 60*(5), 505–513. Available at: http://www.ncbi.nlm.nih.gov/entrez/query.fcgi?cmd=Retrieve&db=PubMed&dopt=Citation&list_uids=12742872

Canadian Paediatric Society. (2008). Harm reduction: An approach to reducing risky health behaviours in adolescents. *Paediatrics and Child Health, 13*(1), 53–60.

Casey, B. J., Jones, R. M., & Hare, T. A. (2008). The adolescent brain. *Annals of the New York Academy of Sciences, 1124*, 111–126. Available at: http://www.pubmedcentral.nih.gov/articlerender.fcgi?artid=2475802&tool=pmcentrez&rendertype=abstract

Chandra, P. S., et al. (2003). High-risk sexual behaviour and sensation seeking among heavy alcohol users. *Indian Journal of Medical Research, 117*, 88–92. Available at: http://www.nimhans.kar.nic.in/cam/CAM/Hi_risk_sex_behav_in_heavy_alc_users_IJMR_03.PDF

Chopra, A., et al. (2008). Association between parental and offspring's alcohol use—Population data from India. *Journal of Indian Association for Child and Adolescent Mental Health, 4*(2), 38–43.

Chung, T., Pajtek, S., & Clark, D. B. (2013). White matter integrity as a link in the association between motivation to abstain and treatment outcome in adolescent substance users. *Psychology of Addictive Behaviors : Journal of the Society of Psychologists in Addictive Behaviors*, *27*(2), 533–542. Available at: http://www.ncbi.nlm.nih.gov/pubmed/22369222

Clark, D. B. et al. (2012). Psychological dysregulation, white matter disorganization and substance use disorders in adolescence. *Addiction (Abingdon, England)*, *107*(1), 206–214. Available at: http://www.ncbi.nlm.nih.gov/pubmed/21752141

Clark, D. B. et al. (2013). Neuroimaging methods for adolescent substance use disorder prevention science. *Prevention Science: The Official Journal of the Society for Prevention Research*, *14*(3), 300–309. Available at: http://www.pubmedcentral.nih.gov/articlerender.fcgi?artid=3640678&tool=pmcentrez&rendertype=abstract

Clark, D. B., Lesnick, L., & Hegedus, A. M. (1997). Traumas and other adverse life events in adolescents with alcohol abuse and dependence. *Journal of the American Academy of Child and Adolescent Psychiatry*, *36*(12), 1744–1751. Available at: http://www.ncbi.nlm.nih.gov/entrez/query.fcgi?cmd=Retrieve&db=PubMed&dopt=Citation&list_uids=9401336

Habeych, M. E., et al. (2006). Impaired oculomotor response inhibition in children of alcoholics: The role of attention deficit hyperactivity disorder. *Drug and Alcohol Dependence, 82*(1), 11–17.

Hulvershorn, L. A., Quinn, P. D., & Scott, E. L. (2015). Treatment of adolescent substance use disorders and co-occurring internalizing disorders : A critical review and proposed model. *Current Drug Abuse Reviews*, 41–49.

Jagadeesh, A., et al. (1999). Differential EEG response to ethanol across subtypes of alcoholics. *Molecular Psychiatry*, *4*(S45).

Kessler, R. C. (2004). The epidemiology of dual diagnosis. *Biological Psychiatry*, *56*(10), 730–737. Available at: http://www.ncbi.nlm.nih.gov/entrez/query.fcgi?cmd=Retrieve&db=PubMed&dopt=Citation&list_uids=15556117

McClure, E. A., et al. (2014). Potential role of N-acetylcysteine in the management of substance use disorders. *CNS drugs*, *28*(2), 95–106. Available at: http://www.pubmedcentral.nih.gov/articlerender.fcgi?artid=4009342&tool=pmcentrez&rendertype=abstract

McLellan, A. T., et al. (2000). Drug dependence, a chronic medical illness. *Jama*, *284*(13), 1689. Available at: http://www.ncbi.nlm.nih.gov/pubmed/11015800. Accessed November 26, 2015.

Muralidharan, K., et al. (2008). Baclofen in the management of inhalant withdrawal: A case series. *Primary Care Companion to the Journal of Clinical Psychiatry*, *10*(1), 48–51. Available at: http://www.ncbi.nlm.nih.gov/pubmed/18311421

Muralidharan, K., et al. (2013). Relationship between motor threshold and externalizing symptoms in subjects at high risk for alcohol dependence: A TMS study. *American Journal on Addictions, 22*(1), 84–85.

Nigg, J. T. (2013). Attention-deficit/hyperactivity disorder and adverse health outcomes. *Clinical Psychology Review*, *33*(2), 215–228. Available at: http://www.ncbi.nlm.nih.gov/pubmed/23298633

Obot, I. S., Wagner, F. A., & Anthony, J. C. (2001). Early onset and recent drug use among children of parents with alcohol problems: Data from a national epidemiologic survey. *Drug and Alcohol Dependence*, *65*(1), 1–8. Available at: http://www.ncbi.nlm.nih.gov/pubmed/11714584

Ohlmeier, M. D., et al. (2008). Comorbidity of alcohol and substance dependence with attention-deficit/hyperactivity disorder (ADHD). *Alcohol and Alcoholism*, *43*(3), 300–304. Available at: http://www.ncbi.nlm.nih.gov/pubmed/18326548

Ollendick, T. H., & King, N. J. (2004). Empirically supported treatments for children and adolescents: advances toward evidence-based practice. In P. M. Barrett & T. H. Ollendick (Eds.), *Handbook of interventions that work with children and adolescents: Prevention and treatment.* London: Wiley.

Schuckit, M. A. (2009). An overview of genetic influences in alcoholism. *Journal of Substance Abuse Treatment, 36*(1), S5–14.

Silva, M. C., et al. (2007). Cognitive deficits in children of alcoholics: At risk before the first sip! *Indian Journal of Psychiatry, 49*(3), 182–188.

Sinha, R. (2008). Chronic stress, drug use, and vulnerability to addiction. *Annals of the New York Academy of Sciences, 1141*, 105–130. Available at: http://www.ncbi.nlm.nih.gov/pubmed/18991954

Subbu, S. S., et al. (2010). *An exploration of differences in brain white matter between subjects at high and low risk for alcohol dependence: A diffusion tensor imaging study.* Unpublished MD Thesis, National Institute of Mental Health and Neurosciences.

Thatcher, D. L., et al. (2014). Amygdala activation and emotional processing in adolescents at risk for substance use disorders. *Journal of Child and Adolescent Substance Abuse, 23*(3), 200–204.

Volkow, N. D., et al. (2011). Motivation deficit in ADHD is associated with dysfunction of the dopamine reward pathway. *Molecular Psychiatry, 16*(11), 1147–1154. Available at: http://www.ncbi.nlm.nih.gov/pubmed/20856250

Wand, G. (2008). The influence of stress on the transition from drug use to addiction. *Alcohol Research and Health, 31*(2), 119–136. Available at: http://www.ncbi.nlm.nih.gov/pubmed/23584814

Chapter 7
Tobacco Use and Its Developmental Effects in Children and Adolescents

Pratima Murthy, Aniruddha Basu and Prabhat Kumar Chand

Abstract Tobacco use often starts in adolescence. Early initiation of tobacco use contributes to significant health morbidity and mortality attributable to tobacco use. The Global Youth Tobacco Survey (GYTS) reports that one among five school-going boys and one in ten girls currently uses tobacco. Developmental animal studies point to the role of nicotine as a gateway drug and its priming effect on future drug use. Psychological factors associated with early use of tobacco include a vulnerable temperament, lower self-efficacy, peer influence, role modelling, and other factors. Social factors include norms and social acceptance. Interview and physical examination for tobacco use should be an integral part of the assessment of adolescents. Specific assessment scales help in determining the severity of nicotine addiction. Preventive approaches, i.e. tobacco-free laws, effective health warnings, restricting access to minors form the mainstay of intervention. Studies on the effectiveness of pharmacological interventions do not suggest significantly positive tobacco cessation outcomes for children and adolescents, except perhaps for the selective use of nicotine replacement for the heavy tobacco using adolescent.

Keywords Tobacco · Children · Adolescents · Smoking · Smokeless · Intervention · Prevention

---

P. Murthy (✉) · A. Basu · P.K. Chand
Department of Psychiatry, Centre for Addiction Medicine, NIMHANS, Bangalore, India
e-mail: pratimamurthy@gmail.com

A. Basu
e-mail: draniruddhabasu@gmail.com

P.K. Chand
e-mail: prabhatkumarchand@gmail.com

S. Malhotra and P. Santosh (eds.), *Child and Adolescent Psychiatry*,
DOI 10.1007/978-81-322-3619-1_7

Abbreviation List

WHO	World Health Organization
SEARO	South East Asia Regional Office
NFHS	National Family Health Survey
GYTS	Global Youth Tobacco Survey
GATS	Global Adult Tobacco Survey
DAMS	Drug Abuse Monitoring System
NCPCR	National Commission for Protection of Child Rights
MYTRI	Mobilizing Youth for Tobacco-Related Initiatives
HRIDAY	Health-Related Information Dissemination Among Youth
DANDY	Development and Assessment of Nicotine Dependence in Youth
SECASPS	Social and Emotional Contexts of Adolescents Smoking Patterns Study
NDSS	Nicotine Dependence Syndrome Scale
HONC	Hooked on Nicotine Questionnaire
mFTQ	Modified Fagerstrom Tolerance Questionnaire
FTND	Fagerstrom Test for Nicotine Dependence
IMPACT	Interventional Model for Prevention of Adolescent and Children against Tobacco
SHS	Second-Hand Smoke
THS	Third-Hand Smoke
NoT	Not on Tobacco
NRT	Nicotine Replacement Therapy
ENDS	Electronic Nicotine Delivery Systems
COTPA	The Cigarettes and Other Tobacco Products Act, 2003
NNS	Nicotine Nasal Spray

7.1 Introduction

> A custom loathsome to the eye,
> hateful to the nose, harmful to the brain,
> dangerous to the lungs, and in the black stinking
> fume thereof nearest resembling the horrible
> stygian smoke of the pit that is bottomless.
> 'Counterblast to Tobacco', 1604.

Tobacco use is one of the most important preventable causes of mortality worldwide. It kills nearly 6 million people each year and is projected to kill more than 8 million persons globally by 2030 (WHO 2015a) Epidemiological studies show that 90 % of the adult smokers begin smoking before 20 years of age—hence it is aptly called a 'pediatric disease' (Torres et al. 2008). Early initiation makes the adolescent smoker at even higher risk for different medical complications and early mortality (Peto 1994). Tobacco-related harm is aptly illustrated in the opening lines from the historic Counterblast to Tobacco attributed to James I (Goldsmid 2007).

7.2 Epidemiology

Among all WHO regions, boys aged 13–15 years from the South-East Asia Region and Eastern Mediterranean Region have the highest rate of tobacco use (over 20 %) (WHO 2015a). The rates at which adolescent girls aged 13–15 use tobacco average around 8 % globally. This average does not include the WHO European Region or the WHO African Region due to unavailability of comparable data. In India, given that 35 % of the population consists of young people below 19 years of age, tobacco use among adolescents is undoubtedly a serious public health problem. Tobacco in its diverse forms has been integral and widely prevalent as illustrated by epidemiological studies since the 1970s.

7.2.1 School-Based Surveys

The earliest school-based study done in 1979 (Mohan et al. 1979) was followed by a multitude of such studies. A systematic review of Indian studies on high school students (sixth to twelfth standard) between 1991 and 2007, shows a 18 % median prevalence of ever use of tobacco (Tsering et al. 2008). The prevalence of tobacco use in the 13–15 year age group was 14 % for boys and 6.34 % for girls. Other recent school-based surveys (Table 7.1) show a variation in the prevalence (Ravishankar and Nagarajappa 2009; Tsering et al. 2010; Narain et al. 2011; Muttappallymyalil et al. 2012). The Global Youth Tobacco Survey (GYTS) was undertaken in India in 2009 on 10,112 students studying in eighth, ninth and tenth standards (WHO 2009) A two-stage cluster sample design was selected to screen the population, collect data on the prevalence of cigarette and other tobacco use and data on five determinants of tobacco use—availability and accessibility of tobacco, exposure to second-hand smoke, smoking cessation, media, advertising, and school curriculum regarding tobacco.

Important findings of Global Youth Tobacco Survey (GYTS India 2009)

14.6 % used* one or other form of tobacco (Boys = 19.0 %, Girls = 8.3 %).
4.4 % smoked* cigarettes (Boys = 5.8 %, Girls = 2.4 %).
12.5 % used* other tobacco products (Boys = 16.2 %, Girls = 7.2 %).
Two-thirds of the students thought smoke from others was harmful to them.
Over 6 in 10 students thought smoking in public places should be banned.
*current use

Table 7.1 Recent school-based surveys of adolescent tobacco use from different parts of India

Author, place, year	Methodology	Findings
Awasthi et al., Haldwani (Uttarakhand), 2010	Randomly selected 594 students of grades eighth, ninth and tenth selected by a stratified random sample design	About 21.2 % of the students were found as current tobacco users; tenth and ninth standard students used tobacco more often than eighth standard students
Tsering et al., Kolkata (West Bengal), 2010	Cross-sectional study in two high schools; 416 students, in classes VIII, IX and X by a pretested questionnaire	The prevalence of ever use/lifetime use was 8.60 % (rural) and 11.04 % (urban) students
Rajnarain et al., Noida (Delhi), 2011	A cluster sample design was used to produce a representative sample of schools; students of class VII (age: 11–19 year) and XII were tested through a pretested, anonymous, closed and open-ended self-administered questionnaire	Lifetime users—11.2 %; 8.8 %—'ever smokers'; 4.6%—'ever chewers'; the mean age of initiation 12.4 year; 70 % of boys and 80 % of girls $\leq$ 15 year initiated the habit of tobacco before 11 years; significant early initiation of tobacco chewing reported from private compared to government school students
Sashidhar et al., Bangalore, 2011	Cross-sectional study in 2 randomly selected schools (age group-12–17 years). Pretested anonymous self-administered questionnaires	Prevalence of current smoking—6.8 %; half occasional smokers (once in 3 months); Initiation—at mean age of 13 years; half had a smoker in the house and about 40 % had no idea about dangers of smoking; majority of participants had never been taught about smoking either in school or at homes and more than half obtained information about smoking from television
Gunjal Sandeep et al., Nagpur, 2012	Cross-sectional study at purposively selected residential tribal schools. Predesigned and pretested pro forma was used	41.74 %—smokeless form, 2.86 % smoker (4.10 % boys—smokers, 1.57 % girls)
Jayakumari et al., Kannur (Kerala), 2013	All 3000 school students (14–18 years) both genders from ten randomly selected schools. A self-administered, pretested, structured, close-ended questionnaire was used for data collection	Overall prevalence of 5.5 % for users. Associations between father's and friend's tobacco habits were observed
Vidhubala et al., Chennai, 2014	School children ($n = 15{,}186$, 45 % boys and 55 % girls) between 10 and 15 years of age from 42 randomly chosen schools completed a seven item pretested structured questionnaire	Ever use of tobacco was 3.2 % (boys 2.6 %; girls 3.7 %) and 1.6 % reported intention to use tobacco in future; pre-teen 11 (5.8 %) and 12 (3.7 %) and 15 years (3.6 %) appear to be vulnerable to tobacco use; 56.3 % were exposed to passive smoking at home

Thus, although the awareness of harm and negative perceptions of tobacco has increased, the prevalence, accessibility and use is also higher as compared to earlier studies.

7.2.2 Community-Based Epidemiological Studies

School-based surveys are not representative of the population. However, community-based surveys on children and adolescents are scarce. A community-based study in rural Wardha revealed that 68.3 % boys and 12.4 % girls had consumed one or other tobacco products in the past 30 days (Dongre et al. 2008). Among the main forms of tobacco, 79.2 % consumed *kharra* and 46.4 % consumed *gutka*. Another community-based study from rural Jamnagar (Gujarat) found that 33.1 % of the adolescents (mostly in the age group 17–19 years) were addicted to tobacco chewing (Makwana et al. 2007). The limitation of these studies is that they are regional and not nationally representative. The National Family Health Survey 2005–2006 (NFHS-3) was carried out on a representative household sample across the country (NFHS 2007). Among 15–19-year-old boys ($n = 13{,}009$), 28.6 % reported tobacco use and among girls ($n = 24,\ 811$), 3.5 % reported tobacco use. This appears to show an upward trend from the previous round of the survey (NFHS-2; 1998–1999). However, the latest round of NFHS-4 (2015–16) showed optimistic trends of decreasing prevalence of tobacco use at least in the above 15 years age group. As per the latest round of GATS, 9.6 % of minors (15–17 years) consumed tobacco in some or other form whereas in the age group of 15–24 years, 27.4 % (23.1 %-smokeless, 9.7 %-smoking) of males and 8.4 % (smokeless-8.2 %, smoking-0.3 %) of females reported current use of tobacco (Ram and Lahiri 2010). A more recent study by the National Commission for Protection of Child Rights reached out to a total of 4024 school-going children (selected by convenience sampling and two-stage randomized clustered sampling) with 78 % living at home while the rest about 22 % lived in streets (Tikoo et al. 2013). Among children using other drugs, who formed the primary respondents of this study, 82 % were lifetime users of tobacco and 79 % were current users. Prevalence of past one month of tobacco use among adolescent drug using girls was 72 %. The overall average age of initiation of tobacco irrespective of gender was 12 years.

7.2.3 Studies Among Street Children and in Marginalized Populations

An estimated 18 million children in India live on the streets. They comprise a highly vulnerable population and about 50–75 % of this population uses tobacco in some form or the other. The average age of initiation of tobacco use in this group is 9–10 years. Children as early as 5 years of age have been reported to use tobacco. Community-based studies conducted in urban slums in India reported significantly high rates of adolescent substance use—for e.g. one study in Bangalore reported a prevalence of 70.1 % and another in urban Orissa in 2008 a prevalence of 43.4 %. Tobacco use constituted 90 % of all substance use (Sarangi et al. 2008). Among other marginalized populations, for e.g. among under-trial adolescents in observation homes in juvenile justice boards, tobacco use, particularly of the smokeless variety is very common (Malhotra et al. 2007). Other populations where tobacco use is more common are youth engaged in manual labour. A study of adolescent tea plantation labourers in Assam showed that about 58 % consume some form of tobacco.

Overall, it can be concluded that SEARO and India has a high prevalence of adolescent tobacco use. Studies in India have shown that an adolescent tobacco user is typically an older adolescent male (15–19 years of age), from a lower socio-economic status, mostly working. If from a rural area, he is likely to be a smokeless tobacco user and if from an urban area, likely to be a smoker (Narain et al. 2011) (for recent studies in India see Table 7.1).

7.3 Variation in Prevalence and Changing Pattern

From all these epidemiological studies, it is evident that there are considerable variations in prevalence with respect to the age group (younger versus older adolescents), gender, socio-economic status and place of residence (rural versus urban). Other attributable causes for such differences may be study methodology (the definition used for 'current smokers' may be variable, there may be a recall bias or low self-reporting). Although older studies have shown that men are four times more likely than women to smoke, GYTS data shows that boys aged 13–15 years were only 2–3 times more likely to smoke than girls. In many countries, there are no differences by gender in onset of cigarette smoking and other tobacco use. This has an important implication for gender-based interventions (Sagarkar et al. 2013). There are also regional variations in India, with prevalence varying from 1.9 % (Delhi) to 75.3 % (Mizoram) (Sinha et al. 2003). Sinha et al. (2003) has shown that children in some parts of the country are given tobacco as a dentifrice as part of traditional use. This practice ranges from 6 % in Goa to 68 % in Bihar. Overall, cigarette smoking among youth is high in the central, southern, and northeastern regions of India.

7.3.1 Age of Initiation

The average age of initiation of tobacco use in most Indian studies is between 8 and 15 years, similar to data from other countries (Narain et al. 2011). Lower age of initiation has been reported from the northeastern States of India, Uttar Pradesh and from rural areas of Gujarat, Tamil Nadu, Karnataka, Kerala and Goa where a large percentage of children under the age of 10 years experimented with smoking or smokeless tobacco in some form (Sinha et al. 2003; Gajalakshmi et al. 2004). Lower age of initiation is also associated with significant psychosocial risk factors. In a school-based study in India under project MYTRI, by comparing the psychosocial risk factors between the sixth grade cohort and the eighth grade cohort it has been found that the former had greater intentions and susceptibility to use tobacco than the latter and had significantly smaller scores on the scales for knowledge and self-efficacy related to tobacco control. Thus, the students in lower grades were more socially susceptible to tobacco use compared to those in higher grades (Dhavan et al. 2009). However, most of these studies are cross-sectional and are prevalence studies. For a better understanding of the tobacco epidemiology in the young, there is a need for longitudinal studies studying tobacco use from a lifespan perspective.

7.3.2 *Hospital Audits*

Though 70–80 % of the adults start smoking during adolescence, as per the Drug Abuse Monitoring System (DAMS), persons seeking treatment for tobacco dependence constitute only around 5 % of this population. Reasons for such low levels of treatment seeking may include low acknowledgment of use, low motivation to quit and lack of specialized services for tobacco cessation among youth.

In a tobacco cessation clinic at a tertiary care centre in north India, a majority (83 %) were in the age group of 15–19 years. Smokers constituted the single major group (60 %), out of whom 38 % additionally used smokeless tobacco (Malhotra et al. 2009). Tobacco users reported peer pressure as the single most important cause for initiation; however after a period of use, nicotine withdrawal maintained their habit. A majority (75 %) had made no earlier attempt to quit.

7.4 Etiopathogenesis of Tobacco Use in the Younger Population

Research in the past five decades has shown that the development of addiction is a complex process. Its initiation and maintenance is mediated by biological, psychological and sociocultural factors (Fig. 7.1).

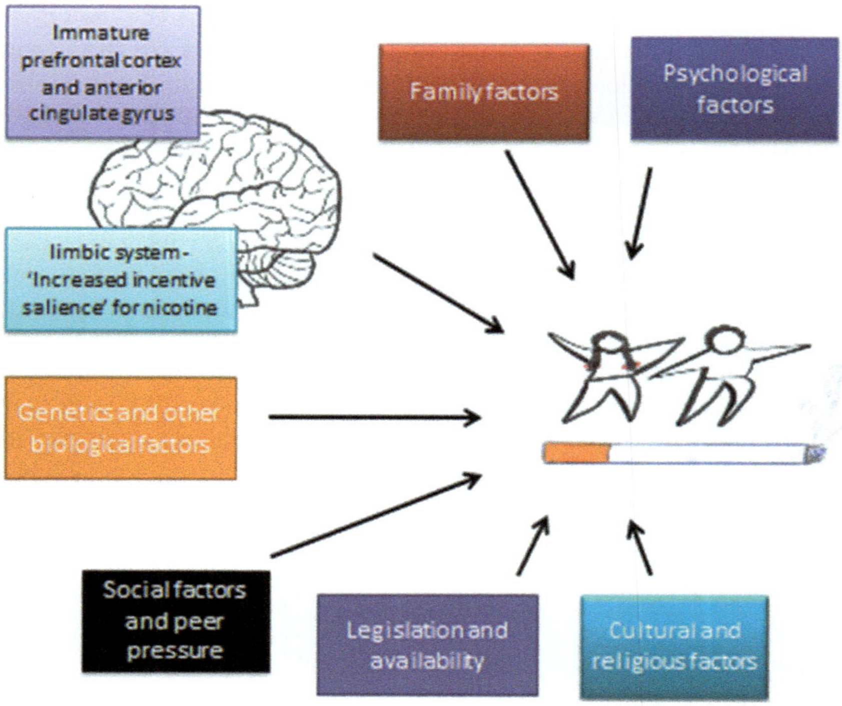

Fig. 7.1 Different factors leading to nicotine use in adolescents

7.4.1 Biological Mechanisms

Neuro-biologically, adolescence is one of the most active phases in one's life. A large percentage of pruning and myelination occurs during this phase, predominantly in the human prefrontal cortex. Synaptic density in major axonal reception zones increases between the ages of 1 and 5 and decreases by late adolescence (Huttenlocher 1979). Structural imaging studies show a dynamic alteration in white and grey matter, and different rates of maturation of the subcortical limbic structures maturation and cortical structures that are responsible for executive function and impulse control (Lydon et al. 2014). This leads to an overall increase in novelty seeking and risk-taking behaviour. It is also seen that firing of limbic dopamine cells is higher in adolescents than adults. D2 receptor mediated GABA mediated inhibitory control to the prefrontal cortex is also impaired (Yuan et al. 2015). Adolescents also have functional immaturity of nicotinic brain receptors which leads to increased binding potential of $\alpha4\beta2$ and $\alpha7$ receptors and altered expression of the respective genes (Schepis et al. 2008).

These alterations have been demonstrated in animal studies which show that adolescent rats are more vulnerable to nicotine. They are more sensitive and more susceptible to alterations in nicotine receptors and nicotine-induced neurotoxicity and to the experience of reward, (Bang and Commons 2011). In addition, adolescent rats exposed to nicotine for the first time have a greater likelihood of its self-administration, both in rate and amount. They also have greater chances of developing dependence compared to first exposure in adulthood. Mice initially primed with nicotine show increased place preference with cocaine and not when the two substances are used in the reverse order. This suggests that nicotine acts as a gateway drug and exerts a priming effect on cocaine in the sequence of drug use through global acetylation in the striatum and other epigenetic mechanisms, creating an environment primed for the induction of gene expression for addiction through Fos B (Kandel and Kandel 2014). Studies show that even a single day of nicotine exposure in adolescent rats can enhance sensitivity to aversive stimuli later in life (Iñiguez et al. 2009). Among humans, the majority of cocaine users smoke during the month they began using cocaine. Furthermore, in a large, longitudinal national study it was found that the rate of cocaine dependence (addiction as measured in the population) was highest (20.2 %) among users who started using cocaine after having smoked cigarettes. Dependence was much lower among persons who had begun using cocaine before they started smoking and among those who had never smoked more than 100 cigarettes (Kandel and Kandel 2014). This and other similar studies emphasize the importance of nicotine as a gateway drug.

7.4.2 Psychological Factors

Temperamental factors that may lead to early onset of tobacco use are increased impulsivity, novelty, sensation seeking and decreased harm avoidance. Among cognitive biases important in shaping the expectancies and incentive salience related to tobacco use in adolescents, attention, approach and memory biases are prominent. Different school-based studies indicate that the psychological factors important during this period are lower general self-efficacy, and maladjustment in school and with peers (Kumar et al. 2014). Tobacco use by boys may also be a part of their self-esteem and psychosexual development—the desire to be 'man-like' and impress the opposite sex (Dongre et al. 2008). Adolescent girls, on the other hand, may use tobacco as a stress reliever. In some cultures, girls use tobacco to allay menstrual pain. These reasons apart, childhood psychosocial adversity, particularly child physical and sexual abuse have also been shown to have an association with early onset tobacco use among adolescents (Kristman-Valente et al. 2013). Though the psychosocial correlates of early tobacco use among adolescents are more or less well established, those for avoiding tobacco are less well understood. However, focused group discussions in qualitative studies show that fear about habit forming, cancer, heart diseases, giddiness and nausea after using tobacco, poor oral hygiene may be deterring factors for tobacco use (Dongre et al. 2008).

7.4.3 Temperament and Psychiatric Co-morbidity

Tobacco use is more prevalent among children and adolescents with behavioural problems and psychiatric co-morbidity. Thus, smoking is more prevalent among children with externalizing traits, particularly those with attention deficit hyperactivity disorder, oppositional defiant and conduct disorder. The opposite temperament, i.e. the internalizing disorders like depression or emotional dysregulation disorders are also associated with higher tobacco use (Hockenberry et al. 2011). Not only is tobacco use co-morbid but it also a risk factor for the future development of mood and anxiety disorder—for example prospective studies have shown that smoking at an early age leads to the development of anxiety disorder in adulthood(Moylan et al. 2013).

7.4.4 Sociocultural Factors

Local custom, social norms and belief systems influence tobacco use in both rural and urban areas. In some rural areas, tobacco is believed to protect against scorpion and snake bites as well as pneumonia and mothers apply tobacco leaf soaked in castor oil over the rapidly breathing infant's chest (Dongre et al. 2008). Urban teenagers are influenced by media, advertisements and the commercial promotion of tobacco. Such factors and peer influence has made tobacco attractive and led to newer modalities of tobacco use including e-cigarettes and renewed hookah use.

There are also other factors that may prevent or promote tobacco use. These include parental influence, family structure, peer influence, as well as the ease of availability and accessibility of tobacco. In marginalized populations like street children, victims of exploitation or trafficking, those living in abject poverty, tobacco use may become a form of coping with hunger, frustration and sadness.

Thus, a variety of sociocultural influences determine the initiation and progression of tobacco use among children and adolescents.

While sociocultural factors including availability and access may influence initiation, psychological and biological factors may influence both initiation and maintenance of the habit, as well as consequent harm from the use of tobacco.

7.4.5 Clinical Features

While the initiation of tobacco use among adolescents is common, progression to dependence occurs in less than a third of users. Progression to daily smoking has been correlated with a variety of factors, including gender, sociocultural and socio-economic characteristics (including parental and peer use of tobacco, early dating), religiosity, legal restrictions, personality variables (including self-efficacy, disorderly conduct) academic achievement, ethnicity, mental health status, use of other drugs and experience with the first smoke (Hu et al. 2008; Nonnemaker et al. 2006). Leventhal and Leary suggested initiation of smoking is followed by a complex ontogeny. The developmental history of a smoker moves through several stages (Leventhal and Cleary 1980). Some authors have argued about the continuous nature of the developmental stages rather than discrete categorical stages. However, empirical evidence in this regard is equivocal (Mayhew et al. 2000).

Adolescent smoking topography (patterns by which the individuals regulate and keep the nicotine extraction constant like the puff volume, number, duration and inter-puff interval) is similar to that of adults. It therefore appears that the adult smoking topography develops very early during dependence. A more fundamental question is when 'dependence' sets in. The Development and Assessment of Nicotine Dependence in Youth (DANDY) study concluded that the first symptoms of nicotine dependence can appear within days to weeks of the onset of occasional use, often before the onset of daily smoking' (DiFranza et al. 2002). The proponents of "hooked on nicotine" programme have gone a step further and proposed that adolescents can lose autonomy over smoking after smoking the very first puff in their lifetime and even when they have only been exposed to second-hand smoke (Gervais et al. 2006). One radical proposition suggests that all symptoms can be reduced to 'craving' which does not depend on tobacco consumption or other behaviours (Dar and Frenk 2010). However, such a radical view has not been supported by empirical research. Longitudinal follow-up studies like the Social and Emotional Contexts of Adolescents Smoking Patterns (SECASP) report that development of even a few dependence symptoms predict later daily smoking (Dierker et al. 2015). Unlike its previous versions, the latest edition of the Diagnostic and Statistical Manual has also made significant changes—taken a dimensional approach and included all the entities under one rubric 'Tobacco Use Disorders' (Black and Grant 2014).

7.4.5.1 Physical Consequences of Adolescent Tobacco Use

Apart from mental health consequences, early tobacco exposure to tobacco is associated with adverse physical consequences. In a tobacco cessation clinic at a tertiary care centre in north India, 31 % of all treatment seeking adolescent tobacco users had symptoms of cardiovascular/respiratory system, which included breathlessness, chest pain, dry cough and cough with sputum. More than one in ten users (12 %) reported oral lesions e.g. white patches in oral cavity, ulcerations, red patches, etc. Of those with identified physical co-morbidities, only 5 % were under treatment for these symptoms and had been told by their treating physicians that these were tobacco-related (Malhotra et al. 2009).

7.4.5.2 Tobacco: Developmental Impact

The effects of tobacco on children start at the foetal stage, with maternal exposure to tobacco. According to the GATS, 39 % of women in India are exposed to SHS at home even though they do not use tobacco in any form. Pregnant smokers are at greater risk of ectopic pregnancy, spontaneous abortion, placenta previa, placental abruption, intra-uterine growth restriction, premature rupture of membranes, preterm birth and still birth (Cnattingius 2004). Many adverse pregnancy outcomes such as decreased gestational age and low birth-weight have also been reported among pregnant women chewing tobacco (Gupta and Sreevidya 2004). The effects of prenatal exposure of nicotine on smoking mothers, teratogenic effects and developmental effects on children are shown in Fig. 7.2 (Galanter et al. 2014). Prenatally exposed infants demonstrate problems in attention, inhibitory gating, cognitive, intellectual development and mood regulation often culminating in disruptive behaviour disorders in childhood and later development of mood disorders including bipolarity (Barros et al. 2011). Finally, as offspring pass through adolescence, higher rates of substance use and antisocial traits are reported. Apart from prenatal exposure children and adolescents may also be exposed to second-hand smoke (SHS). The GYTS data suggests that one in five students live in homes where others smoke and are exposed to SHS. More than one-third of the students are exposed to smoke outside of the home; one-quarter of the students have at least one parent who smokes (WHO 2009). Like prenatal tobacco exposure, SHS also increases the risk of bronchial asthma, future heart ailments and

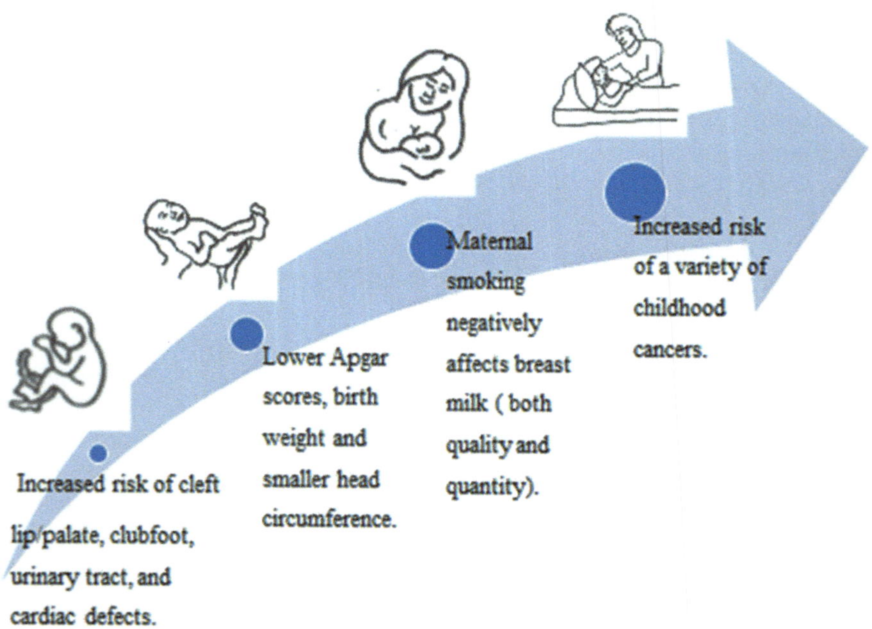

Fig. 7.2 Effect of smoking on foetus, infant and child

produce adverse effects on cognitive, intellectual development and mood (Yolton et al. 2005). Exposure to third-hand smoke (pollutants that remain on surfaces and in dust after tobacco has been smoked are re-emitted into the gas-phase, or react with other compounds in the environment to form secondary pollutants) can also produce detrimental effects on the child's health. Indoor surfaces can represent a hidden reservoir of THS constituents that could be re-emitted long after the cessation of active smoking (Ferrante et al. 2013).

7.5 Management

Two important goals for tobacco use among adolescents include:

(a) Preventing initiation of tobacco use
(b) Helping current tobacco users to quit.

7.5.1 Assessment

All adolescents, particularly in societies where tobacco use is highly prevalent should be screened for tobacco use. Apart from detailed history, the tobacco user should be examined for stigmata of tobacco use like nicotine stains on the oral mucosa, teeth and fingers. Breath carbon monoxide measures, biochemical monitoring with nicotine or cotinine levels may be used to corroborate clinical findings. Tobacco use can be assessed with the help of the Fagerstorm Test of nicotine dependence (FTND: a 6 item scale) for smokers, modified for smokeless tobacco use. FTND has been validated for the adolescent population (Colby et al. 2000). There is also a seven item modified Fagerstrom Tolerance Questionnaire (mFTQ) (Prokhorov et al. 1998) recommended for use among adolescent smokers. Like FTND, mFTQ has a linear method of scoring, i.e. higher the score, more likely the physical dependence to nicotine. Other recent instruments include the Nicotine Dependence Syndrome Scale (NDSS) (SAMHSA 2002; Shiffman et al. 2004), the Hooked on Nicotine Checklist (HONC) (DiFranza et al. 2000; O'Loughlin et al. 2003), and the Wisconsin Inventory of Smoking Dependence Motives (WISDM-68) (Piper et al. 2002). All these assessments except FTND are recent and "tolerance" is the common measure across all these scales. Questions have often been raised about the validity of self-report among adolescents regarding tobacco. However, studies suggest that self-report can be useful when confidentiality is ensured.

The GYTS 2009 suggests that two-thirds of current smokers want to stop smoking. However, only 4–6 % can quit unassisted. This indicates the need for effective interventions.

Interventions for this group can be either family-based, community-based, school-based or individual-level interventions where the person is treated with pharmacotherapy, individual psychotherapy or counselling sessions (WHO 2009). Comprehensive interventions involving the community and family are required to decrease environmental tobacco exposure.

7.5.2 Preventive Interventions

Though treatment is desirable, preventive approaches are a priority, particularly for adolescents. Three types of preventive approaches have been described in tobacco prevention interventions for children and adolescents. The first is the IMPACT intervention framework which includes policy-level approaches (increased taxation on tobacco products, smoke-free laws in public places and work places, effective health warnings, prohibiting tobacco advertising, promotions and sponsorships, and restricting access to minors); community-level approaches (school health programmes, mass media campaigns, community-based interventions, promoting tobacco free norms) and individual approaches (Arora et al. 2013). Among preventive interventions in the United States, one of the most prominent interventions for adolescents aged 14–19 years had been the American Lung Association's Not on Tobacco (NoT) intervention (Dino et al. 2001). It consists of ten 50-min, gender-specific group sessions usually held in schools during school hours and led by trained facilitators. NoT has also been used in community settings. The sessions are developmentally appropriate, expressed in teen-friendly language, and conducted in small groups (no more than 10–12 teenagers). Topics include motivation, stress management, the effects of smoking, preparation to quit, relapse prevention, dealing with peer pressure, media awareness, support networks and healthy lifestyles. The NoT program has been found to be more effective than brief intervention; the former had a quit rate of 15 % whereas for the latter it was 8 %. In a school-based short-term tobacco prevention programme in India, it has been shown that there is improvement in students' knowledge of smoking and its harmful effects, and elicit better anti-smoking attitudes (Verma et al. 2015). In a community-based intervention study among urban slums in Delhi in India by HRIDAY, a significant difference in current use of tobacco was observed in the intervention group (exposed to interactive activities, pretested posters, audio and video films, lectures and street plays). The intervention group showed a reduction in new users as compared to an increase in new users among the control group. However, no significant differences in the quit rate were shown in the two groups (Arora et al. 2010). An SMS text-based messaging system for school students in Switzerland was compared to an assessment-only control group. While there were no statistically different differences between the two groups on smoking cessation, there was significantly reduced consumption of cigarettes and significantly more attempts to quit in the intervention group (Haug et al. 2013; Zin et al. 2013). In a rural community-based intervention, it has been shown that a smoke-free initiative may be helpful in reducing second-hand smoking among children and adolescents (Nichter et al. 2015). The smoke-free homes initiative is based on the principle of collective efficacy. Recognizing the difficulty for individual women to effect change in their household, the movement establishes a smoke-free community mandate.

Legislature is also of paramount importance in preventing smoking. The Cigarettes and Other Tobacco Products Act, 2003 (COTPA) bans the sale of tobacco to minors as well as sale of tobacco within 100 yards of schools (Kaur and Jain 2011). Recently, there has been a ban on sale of loose cigarettes which may reduce tobacco use among youth (Shrivastav et al. 2012). Community-based interventions for tobacco prevention are usually complex multi-component interventions with coordinated activities and support from multiple pre-existing social structures within the community.

7.5.3 Psychosocial Interventions

Among adolescent tobacco users, psychosocial intervention is advocated as the primary treatment modality. Given that many adolescents are in the "honeymoon phase" of their nicotine addiction, recognition of the "slippery slope" of the addiction trajectory and its consequences is an approach worth exploring. Thus, psychosocial interventions in this age group can use motivational interviewing approaches, focusing on behaviour change. Brief personalized counselling focussing on adolescent issues, fixing a quit date and physician support has been found to be effective. However, studies show that motivational interviewing and brief intervention always do not translate to greater smoking abstinence particularly in adolescents with different psychosocial challenges. Such interventions may hold more promise as a prelude to more intensive smoking interventions with adolescents than as stand-alone interventions (Simon et al. 2015). Therefore, more rigorous relapse prevention sessions to identify exact triggers of relapse (both external and internal cues) are often necessary. An important innovation in this regard has been the web-based intervention. Strategies vary from listing websites on smoking cessation, e-mail reminders, short messaging services to interactive voice response. A recent study among high school students utilized an internet-based virtual reality world intervention and compared it with motivational intervention by a counsellor (Woodruff et al. 2007). Results showed significant abstinence rates in the short term. Given the popularity of technology among young population as well their cost—effectiveness, such interventions hold promise for the future.

7.5.4 Pharmacotherapy

1. **Nicotine Replacement Therapy (NRT)**: The different NRTs that have been used in adolescents include nicotine gums, patches and nicotine nasal spray (NNS). Given the small number of trials, it is difficult to ascertain whether NRT is an effective aid in smoking cessation. The scarce data that is available

suggest that nicotine patch is more efficacious than other nicotine replacement products. Higher abstinence rates with patches could be due to lower medication compliance rates with gums and NNS among adolescents (Moolchan et al. 2005; Rubinstein et al. 2008).

However, a long-term RCT using NRT did not yield any significant differences. Thus, it is still unclear whether it is useful to prescribe nicotine replacement to adolescents. There are also safety concerns, as there is some evidence of toxicity from nicotine to the developing brain. Nicotine replacement may also prime the developing brain for further substance use (Slotkin 2008). In the absence, however, of definite evidence for toxicity of NRT and the risks of smoking, current approaches tend to follow a harm minimization approach and consider NRT as less toxic compared to smoking (Bailey et al. 2012). NRT among adolescents is otherwise well tolerated without any severe or life-threatening adverse effects. Adolescents, however, report more adverse effects with nicotine nasal spray-like nasal irritation/burning and complaints of taste and smell dysfunction.

A study among pediatricians from US, showed that less that a fifth (17 %) are prescribing NRT to adolescent smokers and a majority of the pediatricians did not feel confident to prescribe NRT (Price et al. 2007).

2. **Non-Nicotine Medication**: At present, no smoking cessation medications are approved for children and adolescents below 18 years of age.

   Bupropion: This norepinephrine dopamine reuptake inhibitor is a standard treatment for nicotine dependence in adults. The end of treatment efficacy of bupropion in adolescent tobacco users at a dose of 150 mg sustained release was variable, ranging from 10 to 55 %. Only a few studies have reported significant improvement (Karpinski et al. 2010). There is an interest in using bupropion for adolescents with nicotine dependence and co-morbid attention deficient hyperactivity disorder (ADHD). One important methodological issue in studies involving bupropion is the dosage. It is unclear whether to use the conventional adult dosage of 300 mg or use 150 mg as some of the studies have done (Muramoto et al. 2007). Given the caution raised about treatment-emergent suicidal ideation, it is prudent to be careful in using bupropion. This combined with the lack of consistent efficacy, there has been no recommendation for its use in standard clinical practice guidelines for treatment of tobacco dependence among adolescents (Bailey et al. 2012).

   Varenicline: This drug is a partial agonist at $\alpha4\beta2$ receptor thereby reducing the reinforcing effects of nicotine. Precautions are advised for young people under the age of 18 years in view of the black box warning of increased suicidality. In a recent pilot study where varenicline was compared with bupropion-sustained release, it was seen that both medications were well tolerated and hence their effectiveness need to be evaluated in further studies in older adolescents (Gray et al. 2012).

In summary, the currently available evidence for pharmacotherapy is modest. The overall treatment efficacy is reported to be 30 % with a concern about side effect particularly for bupropion and varenicline. Erratic tobacco use patterns among adolescents also leads to the problem of the use of biochemical validation. A recent Cochrane review has shown scant evidence in favour of existing pharmacotherapies for adolescents (Stanton and Grimshaw 2013). Hence hopes are pinned on other α4 β 2 partial agonists like cytisine and nicotine vaccines, which are still in the experimental stages.

E-cigarettes: These are battery-operated electronic nicotine delivery systems (ENDS) which were introduced for the safe delivery of nicotine. However, they have been found to contain toxins like heavy metals and silicate particles. For these reasons, the World Health Organization has issued a warning against their use as there is no adequate evidence currently of their efficacy. On the contrary, it is suggested that their use may be detrimental to health (WHO 2015b). It has even been suggested that for adolescents, such devices may act as a gateway to other drugs of abuse (Wasowicz et al. 2015). Adolescents view e-cigarettes as a safer option—hence peer pressure and aggressive marketing of the so-called innocuous e-cigarettes may lead to the development of dependence in future.

Standard practice guidelines for tobacco cessation among children and adolescents include the National Institute of Clinical Excellence (NICE) guidelines and American Academy of Pediatrics (AAP) committee on substance abuse guidelines. In view of the scanty evidence for pharmacotherapy in adolescents, these guidelines are in favour of psychosocial interventions, and suggest the use of pharmacotherapy particularly nicotine gums only when needed (Simon et al. 2015).

7.6 Conclusion

Although the just released NHFS 4 survey (National Family Health Survey NFHS4 2015) findings suggest a welcome reduction in smoking in the population, tobacco use among children and adolescents is a growing problem, with young children initiating tobacco use. A variety of factors influence the initiation and maintenance of tobacco use in this population. Early age of exposure to tobacco is associated with greater physical as well as psychiatric problems in later life. Psychological interventions such as life skill education, increasing awareness, counselling, school-based program, etc. are preferred. Established pharmacological treatments for adults hold less promise for children and adolescents, for whom prevention and psychosocial interventions form the main intervention. Tobacco use as a gateway to other drug abuse is another important concern highlighting the need for its prevention. Newer devices like e-cigarettes pose newer challenges to children and adolescents.

7.7 Learning Points

- Tobacco use among adolescents is a growing public health problem.
- Younger adolescents are particularly vulnerable to tobacco initiation
- Initiation is multifactorial—reasons include a combination of biological, social and psychological factors.
- Tobacco use in pregnancy is associated with developmental impact on the newborn and has long-term consequences in terms of future emotional and behavioural problems.
- Exposure to second-hand smoke poses particular danger to children and adolescents and this should be countered on a priority basis.
- Proper assessment should be done emphasizing the psychosocial risk factors, psychiatric co-morbidity and medical complications in all adolescents who use tobacco in one or other form.
- Management is mostly by non-pharmacological means with both community-based and school-based psychosocial interventions.
- Nicotine Replacement may be used cautiously and currently there is no recommendation to use any of the electronic nicotine delivery systems.

Acknowledgments Ms Sharanya Mohan for the illustrations.

References

Arora, M., Mathur, M. R., & Singh, N. (2013). A framework to prevent and control tobacco among adolescents and children: introducing the IMPACT model. *Indian Journal of Pediatrics, 80*(Suppl 1), S55–S62.

Arora, M., Tewari, A., Tripathy, V., Nazar, G. P., Juneja, N. S., Ramakrishnan, L., et al. (2010). Community-based model for preventing tobacco use among disadvantaged adolescents in urban slums of India. *Health Promotion International, 25*(2), 143–152.

Awasthi, S., Jha, S. K., Rawat, C. M. S., Pandey, S., & Swami, S. S. (2010). Correlates of tobacco use among male adolescents in schools of Haldwani, Nainital. *Health and Population: Perspectives and Issues, 33*(1), 42–49.

Bailey, S. R., Crew, E. E., Riske, E. C., Ammerman, S., Robinson, T. N., & Killen, J. D. (2012). Efficacy and tolerability of pharmacotherapies to aid smoking cessation in adolescents. *Paediatric Drugs, 14*(2), 91–108.

Bang, S. J., & Commons, K. G. (2011). Age-dependent effects of initial exposure to nicotine on serotonin neurons. *Neuroscience, 179*, 1–8.

Barros, M. C. M., Mitsuhiro, S. S., Chalem, E., Laranjeira, R. R., & Guinsburg, R. (2011). Prenatal tobacco exposure is related to neurobehavioral modifications in infants of adolescent mothers. *Clinics (São Paulo, Brazil), 66*(9), 1597–1603.

Black, D. W., & Grant, J. E. (2014). DSM-5 guidebook: The essential companion to the diagnostic and statistical manual of mental disorders. American Psychiatric Pub.

Cnattingius, S. (2004). The epidemiology of smoking during pregnancy: Smoking prevalence, maternal characteristics, and pregnancy outcomes. *Nicotine & Tobacco Research: Official Journal of the Society for Research on Nicotine and Tobacco, 6*(Suppl 2), S125–S140.

Colby, S. M., Tiffany, S. T., Shiffman, S., & Niaura, R. S. (2000). Measuring nicotine dependence among youth: A review of available approaches and instruments. *Drug and Alcohol Dependence, 59*(Suppl 1), S23–S39.

Dar, R., & Frenk, H. (2010). Can one puff really make an adolescent addicted to nicotine? A critical review of the literature. *Harm Reduction Journal, 7*, 28.

Dhavan, P., Stigler, M. H., Perry, C. L., Arora, M., & Reddy, K. S. (2009). Patterns of tobacco use and psychosocial risk factors among students in 6th through 10th grades in India: 2004–2006. *Asian Pacific Journal of Cancer Prevention, 10*(5), 807–813.

Dierker, L., Hedeker, D., Rose, J., Selya, A., & Mermelstein, R. (2015). Early emerging nicotine dependence symptoms in adolescence predict daily smoking in young adulthood. *Drug and Alcohol Dependence, 151*, 267–271.

DiFranza, J. R., Rigotti, N. A., McNeill, A. D., Ockene, J. K., Savageau, J. A., St Cyr, D., et al. (2000). Initial symptoms of nicotine dependence in adolescents. *Tobacco Control, 9*(3), 313–319.

DiFranza, J. R., Savageau, J. A., Fletcher, K., Ockene, J. K., Rigotti, N. A., McNeill, A. D., et al. (2002). Measuring the loss of autonomy over nicotine use in adolescents: the DANDY (Development and Assessment of Nicotine Dependence in Youths) study. *Archives of Pediatrics and Adolescent Medicine, 156*(4), 397–403.

Dino, G., Horn, K., Goldcamp, J., Fernandes, A., Kalsekar, I., & Massey, C. (2001). A 2-year efficacy study of Not On Tobacco in Florida: An overview of program successes in changing teen smoking behavior. *Preventive Medicine, 33*(6), 600–605.

Dongre, A., Deshmukh, P., Murali, N., & Garg, B. (2008). Tobacco consumption among adolescents in rural Wardha: Where and how tobacco control should focus its attention? *Indian Journal of Cancer, 45*(3), 100–106.

Ferrante, G., Simoni, M., Cibella, F., Ferrara, F., Liotta, G., Malizia, V., et al. (2013). Third-hand smoke exposure and health hazards in children. *Monaldi Archives for Chest Disease, 79*(1), 38–43.

Gajalakshmi, V., Asma, S., & Warren, C. W. (2004). Tobacco survey among youth in South India. *Asian Pacific Journal of Cancer Prevention: APJCP, 5*(3), 273–278.

Galanter, M., Kleber, H. D., & Brady, K. (2014). The American psychiatric publishing textbook of substance abuse treatment. American Psychiatric Pub.

Gervais, A., O'Loughlin, J., Meshefedjian, G., Bancej, C., & Tremblay, M. (2006). Milestones in the natural course of onset of cigarette use among adolescents. *CMAJ: Canadian Medical Association Journal = Journal de l'Association Medicale Canadienne, 175*(3), 255–261.

Goldsmid, E. (2007). A CounterBlaste to Tobacco. By King of England James I. Dodo Press.

Gray, K. M., Carpenter, M. J., Lewis, A. L., Klintworth, E. M., & Upadhyaya, H. P. (2012). Varenicline versus bupropion XL for smoking cessation in older adolescents: a randomized, double-blind pilot trial. *Nicotine & Tobacco Research: Official Journal of the Society for Research on Nicotine and Tobacco, 14*(2), 234–239.

Gunjal Sandeep, S., Borle Amod, L., Narlawar Uday, W., Ughade Suresh, N., Chaudhari Vijaya, L., & Humne Arun, Y. (2012). Tobacco and alcohol use in tribal school students from Central India.

Gupta, P. C., & Sreevidya, S. (2004). Smokeless tobacco use, birth weight, and gestational age: Population based, prospective cohort study of 1217 women in Mumbai, India. *BMJ, 328*(7455), 1538.

Haug, S., Schaub, M. P., Venzin, V., Meyer, C., & John, U. (2013). Efficacy of a text message-based smoking cessation intervention for young people: A cluster randomized controlled trial. Journal of Medical Internet Research, *15*(8).

Hockenberry, J. M., Timmons, E. J., & Weg, M. W. V. (2011). Adolescent mental health as a risk factor for adolescent smoking onset. *Adolescent Health, Medicine and Therapeutics, 2*, 27–35.

Hu, M.-C., Muthén, B., Schaffran, C., Griesler, P. C., & Kandel, D. B. (2008). Developmental trajectories of criteria of nicotine dependence in adolescence. *Drug and Alcohol Dependence, 98*(1–2), 94–104.

Huttenlocher, P. R. (1979). Synaptic density in human frontal cortex—developmental changes and effects of aging. *Brain Research, 163*(2), 195–205.

Iñiguez, S. D., Warren, B. L., Parise, E. M., Alcantara, L. F., Schuh, B., Maffeo, M. L., Bolaños-Guzmán, C. A. (2009). Nicotine exposure during adolescence induces a depression-like state in adulthood. *Neuropsychopharmacology: Official Publication of the American College of Neuropsychopharmacology, 34*(6), 1609–1624.

Kandel, D. B., & Kandel, E. R. (2014). A molecular basis for nicotine as a gateway drug. *The New England Journal of Medicine, 371*(21), 2038–2039.

Karpinski, J. P., Timpe, E. M., & Lubsch, L. (2010). Smoking cessation treatment for adolescents. *The Journal of Pediatric Pharmacology and Therapeutics, 15*(4), 249–263.

Kaur, J., & Jain, D. C. (2011). Tobacco control policies in India: implementation and challenges. *Indian Journal of Public Health, 55*(3), 220–227.

Kristman-Valente, A. N., Brown, E. C., & Herrenkohl, T. I. (2013). Child physical and sexual abuse and cigarette smoking in adolescence and adulthood. *The Journal of Adolescent Health: Official Publication of the Society for Adolescent Medicine, 53*(4), 533–538.

Kumar, V., Talwar, R., Roy, N., Raut, D., & Singh, S. (2014). Psychosocial determinants of tobacco use among school going adolescents in Delhi, India. *Journal of Addiction, 2014*, 170941.

Leventhal, H., & Cleary, P. D. (1980). The smoking problem: A review of the research and theory in behavioral risk modification. *Psychological Bulletin, 88*(2), 370–405.

Lydon, D. M., Wilson, S. J., Child, A., & Geier, C. F. (2014). Adolescent brain maturation and smoking: what we know and where we're headed. *Neuroscience and Biobehavioral Reviews, 45*, 323–342.

Makwana, N. R., Shah, V. R., & Yadav, S. (2007). A study on prevalence of smoking and tobacco chewing among adolescents in rural areas of Jamnagar district, Gujarat state. *JMSR, 1*(1), 1–13.

Malhotra, C., Sharma, N., Saxena, R., & Ingle, G. K. (2007). Drug use among juveniles in conflict with the law. *Indian Journal of Pediatrics, 74*(4), 353–356.

Malhotra, S., Malhotra, A., Kakkar, N., Das, P. P., & Singh, J. (2009). The clinical and demographic profile of Nicotine users among Children and Adolescents. *German Journal of Psychiatry, 54*, 31-2.

Mayhew, K. P., Flay, B. R., & Mott, J. A. (2000). Stages in the development of adolescent smoking. *Drug and Alcohol Dependence, 59*(Suppl 1), S61–s81.

Mohan, D., Thomas, M. G., Sethi, H. S., & Prabhu, G. G. (1979). Prevalence and patterns of drug use among high-school students: A replicated study. *Bulletin on Narcotics, 31*(3–4), 77–86.

Moolchan, E. T., Robinson, M. L., Ernst, M., Cadet, J. L., Pickworth, W. B., Heishman, S. J., et al. (2005). Safety and efficacy of the nicotine patch and gum for the treatment of adolescent tobacco addiction. *Pediatrics, 115*(4), e407–e414.

Moylan, S., Jacka, F. N., Pasco, J. A., & Berk, M. (2013). How cigarette smoking may increase the risk of anxiety symptoms and anxiety disorders: a critical review of biological pathways. *Brain and Behavior, 3*(3), 302–326.

Muramoto, M. L., Leischow, S. J., Sherrill, D., Matthews, E., & Strayer, L. J. (2007). Randomized, double-blind, placebo-controlled trial of 2 dosages of sustained-release bupropion for adolescent smoking cessation. *Archives of Pediatrics and Adolescent Medicine, 161*(11), 1068–1074.

Muttappallymyalil, J., Divakaran, B., Thomas, T., Sreedharan, J., Haran, J. C., & Thanzeel, M. (2012). Prevalence of tobacco use among adolescents in north Kerala, India. *Asian Pacific Journal of Cancer Prevention: APJCP, 13*(11), 5371–5374.

Narain, R., Sardana, S., Gupta, S., & Sehgal, A. (2011). Age at initiation & prevalence of tobacco use among school children in Noida, India: A cross-sectional questionnaire based survey. *The Indian Journal of Medical Research, 133*, 300–307.

National Family Health Survey 2015-16 (NFHS4): States fact sheets. Retrieved August 27, 2016 from http://www.indiaenvironmentportal.org.in/content/424110/nationalfamilyhealthsurvey201516nfhs4statesfactsheets/

Nichter, M., Padmajam, S., Nichter, M., Sairu, P., Aswathy, S., Mini, G. K., et al. (2015). Developing a smoke free homes initiative in Kerala, India. *BMC Public Health, 15*, 480.

Nonnemaker, J., McNeely, C. A., & Blum, R. W. (2006). Public and private domains of religiosity and adolescent smoking transitions. *Social Science & Medicine (1982), 62*(12), 3084–3095.

O'Loughlin, J., DiFranza, J., Tyndale, R. F., Meshefedjian, G., McMillan-Davey, E., Clarke, P. B., et al. (2003). Nicotine-dependence symptoms are associated with smoking frequency in adolescents. *American Journal of Preventive Medicine, 25*(3), 219–225.

Peto, R. (1994). Smoking and death: the past 40 years and the next 40. *British Medical Journal, 309*(6959), 937–939.

Piper, M. E., Federman, E. B., Piasecki, T. M., Bolt, D. M., Fiore, M. C., & Baker, T. B. (2002, February). The Wisconsin dependence motives questionnaire: A new measure of tobacco dependence. Paper presented at the 8th annual meeting of the Society for Research on Nicotine and Tobacco, Savannah, GA

Price, J. H., Jordan, T. R., & Dake, J. A. (2007). Pediatricians' use of the 5 A's and nicotine replacement therapy with adolescent smokers. *Journal of Community Health, 32*(2), 85–101.

Prokhorov, A. V., Koehly, L. M., Pallonen, U. E., & Hudmon, K. S. (1998). Adolescent nicotine dependence measured by the modified Fagerström Tolerance Questionnaire at two time points. *Journal of Child & Adolescent Substance Abuse, 7*(4), 35–47.

Ram, F., Lahiri, S., et al. (2010). *Global adult tobacco survey 2009–2010*, New Delhi.

Ravishankar, T. L., & Nagarajappa, R. (2009). Factors attributing to initiation of tobacco use in adolescent students of Moradabad, (UP) India. *Indian Journal of Dental Research: Official Publication of Indian Society for Dental Research, 20*(3), 346–349.

Reddy, S. (2007) Advancing cessation of tobacco in vulnerable Indian tobacco consuming Youth. *Grantome*. Retrieved from http://grantome.com/grant/NIH/R01-TW007933-03

Rubinstein, M. L., Benowitz, N. L., Auerback, G. M., & Moscicki, A.-B. (2008). A randomized trial of nicotine nasal spray in adolescent smokers. *Pediatrics, 122*(3), e595–e600.

Sagarkar, A. R., Sagarkar, R. M., Arabbi, K. C., & Shivamallappa, S. M. (2013). A substantive review on tobacco use among school-going adolescents in India. *Journal of International Society of Preventive & Community Dentistry, 3*(1), 7–11.

SAMHSA [Substance Abuse and Mental Health Services Administration]. (2002). *Results from the 2001 National Household Survey on Drug Abuse: Volume I. Summary of national findings* (Office of Applied Studies, NHSDA Series H-17, DHHS Publication No. SMA 02–3758). Rockville, MD: Author.

Sarangi, L., Acharya, H. P., & Panigrahi, O. P. (2008). Substance abuse among adolescents in urban slums of sambalpur. *Indian Journal of Community Medicine: Official Publication of Indian Association of Preventive & Social Medicine, 33*(4), 265–267.

Schepis, T. S., Adinoff, B., & Rao, U. (2008). Neurobiological processes in adolescent addictive disorders. *The American Journal on Addictions/American Academy of Psychiatrists in Alcoholism and Addictions, 17*(1), 6–23.

Shiffman, S., Waters, A., & Hickcox, M. (2004). The nicotine dependence syndrome scale: a multidimensional measure of nicotine dependence. *Nicotine & Tobacco Research, 6*(2), 327–348.

Sinha, D. N., Gupta, P. C., & Pednekar, M. S. (2003). Tobacco use among students in the eight North-eastern states of India. *Indian Journal of Cancer, 40*(2), 43–59.

Shrivastav, R., Nazar, G. P., Stigler, M. H., & Arora, M. (2012). Health promotion for primordial prevention of tobacco use. *Global Heart, 7*(2), 143–150.

Simon, P., Kong, G., Cavallo, D. A., & Krishnan-Sarin, S. (2015). Update of adolescent smoking cessation interventions: 2009–2014. *Current Addiction Reports, 2*(1), 15–23.

Slotkin, T. A. (2008). If nicotine is a developmental neurotoxicant in animal studies, dare we recommend nicotine replacement therapy in pregnant women and adolescents? *Neurotoxicology and Teratology, 30*(1), 1–19.

Stanton, A., & Grimshaw, G. (2013). Tobacco cessation interventions for young people. *The Cochrane Database of Systematic Reviews, 8*, CD003289.

Tikoo, V. K., Dhawan, A., Pattanayak, R. D., Chopra, A. (2013). Assessment and pattern, profiles and correlates of substance use among children in India. National Commission on Protection of Child Rights (NCPCR), New Delhi

Torres, O. V., Tejeda, H. A., Natividad, L. A., & O'Dell, L. E. (2008). Enhanced vulnerability to the rewarding effects of nicotine during the adolescent period of development. *Pharmacology, Biochemistry and Behavior, 90*(4), 658–663.

Tsering, D., Pal, R., & Dasgupta, A. (2008). Tobacco use among high school students of West Bengal, India. *Indian Journal of Community Medicine: Official Publication of Indian Association of Preventive & Social Medicine, 33*(3), 207–208.

Tsering, D., Pal, R., & Dasgupta, A. (2010). Licit and illicit substance use by adolescent students in Eastern India: Prevalence and associated risk factors. *Journal of Neurosciences in Rural Practice, 1*(2), 76–81.

Verma, A., Muddaiah, P., Krishna Murthy, A., & Sanga, R. (2015). Exploring an effective tobacco prevention programme for Indian adolescents. *Public Health, 129*, 23–28.

Vidhubala, E., Sahaya, G., Vijayalakshmi, S., Bharathi, P., & Quarishy, Z. B. (2014). Prevalence of tobacco use among school children, exposure to passive smoking and their knowledge level about tobacco control in Chennai city, Tamil Nadu-A School Based Survey. *Journal of Indian Association for Child & Adolescent Mental Health, 10*(2).

Wasowicz, A., Feleszko, W., & Goniewicz, M. L. (2015). E-Cigarette use among children and young people: the need for regulation. *Expert Review of Respiratory Medicine, 1–3.*

World Health Organization. (2009). Tobacco use among students and teachers. Findings from the Global Youth Tobacco Survey (GYTS) and the Global School Personnel Survey (GSPS) 2003–2009. World Health Organization, Centre for Diseases Control, Ministry of Health and Family Welfare, Government of India.

World Health Organization. (2015b). Electronic cigarettes (e-cigarettes) or electronic nicotine delivery systems. *Statement March 2015*. Retrieved August 31, 2015 from http://www.who.int/tobacco/communications/statements/eletronic_cigarettes/en/

World Health Organization Tobacco. (2015a). Tobacco Fact Sheet July. Retrieved August 27, 2015 from http://www.who.int/mediacentre/factsheets/fs339/en/

Woodruff, S. I., Conway, T. L., Edwards, C. C., Elliott, S. P., & Crittenden, J. (2007). Evaluation of an Internet virtual world chat room for adolescent smoking cessation. *Addictive Behaviors, 32*(9), 1769–1786.

Yolton, K., Dietrich, K., Auinger, P., Lanphear, B. P., & Hornung, R. (2005). Exposure to environmental tobacco smoke and cognitive abilities among U.S. children and adolescents. *Environmental Health Perspectives, 113*(1), 98–103.

Yuan, M., Cross, S. J., Loughlin, S. E., & Leslie, F. M. (2015). Nicotine and the adolescent brain. *The Journal of Physiology, 593*(16), 3397–3412.

Zin, V., Meyer, C., John, U. (2013) Efficacy of a text message-based smoking cessation intervention for young people: A cluster randomized controlled trial. *Journal of Medical Internet Research, 2, 15*(8), e171.

Part III
Environment and Cultural Influences

Chapter 8
Rapid Sociocultural Change, Child-Rearing Crisis, and Children's Mental Health

Kang-E. Michael Hong

Abstract This article presents clinical observations and epidemiological empirical studies on the impacts of rapid sociocultural change on children's mental health in developing Asian countries. In addition, psychopathogenic mechanisms and processes and implications on the mental health of children are formulated and discussed from developmental, psychopathological, ecological, and ethological perspectives. Rapid modernization and "Westernization" have occurred in many Asian societies and brought about many benefits; however, this has been accompanied by large increases of mental health problems. The author suggests that one of the most critical pathogenic factors could be the rapidity and extensiveness of change rather than the change itself. This compressed form of modernization occurred within the span of only 40–50 years in most Asian countries, while it was accomplished gradually over 200–300 years in Western countries. The important mediating pathogenic processes are the breakdown of the traditional value orientation, a marked change of the family system from extended to nuclear, a weakening of major emotional support networks, and serious problems and crises in child-rearing practices. The new tides of globalization and the coexistence of multi-culturalism in most Asian countries will increase these risks. The critical importance of proper early child rearing and the quality of mother–infant attachment are emphasized for the future mental health of children in globalized world. The author advocates the need for new guidelines and paradigms to bring up mentally healthy children in this complex, ever changing world. A solution may be found in integrating the old and the new as well as integrating the East and the West.

Keywords Rapid social changes · Children's mental health · Child-rearing crisis · Developing countries in Asia

---

K.-E.M. Hong (✉)
Professor Emeritus, Department of Neuropsychiatry, Seoul National University Bundang Hospital, 300 Gumi-dong, Bundang-gu, Seongnam-si, Gyeongi-do, Korea
e-mail: kmhong@snu.ac.kr

S. Malhotra and P. Santosh (eds.), *Child and Adolescent Psychiatry*,
DOI 10.1007/978-81-322-3619-1_8

8.1 Introduction

During the latter half of the twentieth century, almost all the countries in Asia went through their own forms of "modernization" in which drastic economic, political, and social changes occurred to various extents and at varying speeds. This modernization involved industrialization, urbanization, family system changes from the extended to the nuclear, and "Westernization" through which a Western ideology and value orientation including democracy, capitalism, individualism, human rights, gender equality, and freedom of choice issues were introduced.

While these changes certainly brought about improvements in many areas of Asian life, such as standards of living, sanitation, nutrition, education, and physical health, they seem to have been accompanied by a disconcerting increase in the number of mental health problems in children and adolescents. These mental health problems include developmental, emotional, and behavioral disorders, child abuse and neglect, school violence, delinquency, suicide, and many other forms of social deviance. This is a paradox. Material wealth does not seem to guarantee psychological well-being.

The author has witnessed dramatic sociocultural changes and their salutary as well as pernicious consequences in South Korea for the past 70 years and has accumulated clinical observations and research data while establishing child psychiatry services in South Korea over the past 40 years. This article is to share the author's worries and concerns about the status of mental health of children in relation to social and family changes in Asian countries. Initially, the author wanted to cover all Asian countries but found it too difficult to gather the necessary information and data from all Asian countries. Therefore, the article focuses mostly on the South Korean case and extends to Japan and China as much as possible. Despite this limitation in scope, the author has found that the more information he assembles, the more convinced he becomes that situations are quite similar in most Asian countries with regards to these matters. The author does not want to claim that this article is rigorously scientific or that it presents a thorough review of the relevant literature. Instead, it is first a presentation of clinical observations and research on children's mental health during the period of compressed modernization in South Korea, and second a plea for the public and professionals of any countries undergoing rapid sociocultural changes to recognize the serious child mental health consequences and the importance of child rearing as a major mediating variable determining the effects of sociocultural changes on mental health.

8.2 Social Changes in South Korea Over the Past 50 Years

Modernization in Korea began 120 years ago during the last period of the Chosun dynasty. However, a truly substantial form of modernization did not begin until the end of World War II in 1945. In 1945, Korea was divided into North and South

Table 8.1 Indices of social changes in Korea

	1960s	2000s
GNI	<$100	$20,000
Urban population	<10 %	>90 %
Women working	25 %	50.6 %
Longevity	52.4 year	80.2 year
Senile population	3.0 %	10.7 %
Birth rate	4.1	1.19
# of children/family	4–5	1–2
Nuclear family	46 %	82 %
Crude divorce rate	0.4	3.4/1000
Suicide rate	<10	31/100,000
Internet user	0	>70 %

Korea. North Korea took a communist route and South Korea began to establish itself as a democratic, capitalistic, industrial country under U.S. influence. The American influence became stronger with the outbreak of the Korean War in 1950. Over the following five decades, South Korean society underwent rapid, massive, dramatic modernization, including industrialization, urbanization, and the introduction of democracy and a capitalistic economic system. Several important indices of social changes associated with these industrial revolutions are presented in Table 8.1. Gross annual income per capita (GDP) in Korea increased from $69 dollars/year right after the Korean War (1955) to about $10,000 in 1997, $20,000 in 2005, and near $30,000 in recent years. Major occupations changed from being agriculture-related (63 %) to being industry-related (33.1 %) and service and sales-related (40.5 %). Females now represent over 50 % of the work force, compared with 25 % in the 1960s. Over 90 % of the total population reside in either metropolitan area or in small- and medium-sized cities and less than 10 % live in rural areas. South Korea started with its manufacturing and petroleum "chimney" industries and it has now become the fifth largest automobile producing and largest ship building country in the world.

South Korea is now one of the leading countries in the IT industry. The changes have been sweeping, massive, drastic, and almost "miraculous," considering that these accomplishments took only 50 years since the 1960s.

The characteristics of Korean modernization are summarized as the following: First, modernization in Korea involved a very abrupt transformation from a closed totalitarian monarchy to a democratic, capitalistic, individualistic Western style. Korea imported not only the technology but also the ideology of the West, including democracy, human rights, freedom of choice, gender equality, and individualism. Therefore, modernization in Korea can almost be equated with Westernization. Second, modernization in Korea has involved rapid and massive industrialization accompanied by urbanization and rushing migration into metropolitan cities, such as Seoul, which has a population over 12 million. This has resulted in a sudden shift in major occupations, from agriculture-related jobs to either sales/service or industry-related jobs. However, the most important associated change might be the introduction of the nuclear family system as opposed to the extended family system, which constituted the backbone of the agrarian Korean society for 1000 years. Third, a prominent characteristic of Korean modernization is the speed and length of time required to achieve the current state of modernization, which took only 50 years, while modernization in the Western world took approximately 2–300 years. This rapidity and the extensiveness of change seem to be responsible for the confusion and problems in social norms, authority hierarchy, social orders and cultural values, moralities, and interpersonal relationships.

8.3 Family System Changes

The most significant changes associated with the modernization processes in South Korea are the changes of structure, functions, and roles of the family system. According to the 2003 Korean government report, 19.1 % of the Korean families are one generation families, 52 % are two generation families, and 15.5 % are one person families. Three or more generations are living together in only 13.5 %. This indicates that more than 80 % of the families are "nuclear." It appears that indeed Korean families changed sweepingly from the extended to the "nuclear" family. However, there are many types of "nuclear" families, in addition to the typical "nuclear" family consisting of a couple and their children and these include one person family of unmarried persons or aged persons, one-parent family, grandparents–grandchildren family, atypical family of children without adult and the global split family. Thus, it is not a simple nuclear family system; instead, the diversification and coexistence of different family structures characterize the family system in modern Korean society.

8.4 Changes of Sociocultural Values

This "compressed modernization" in South Korea inevitably brought about marked changes in the life goals and cultural values of Korean people. Koreans have made dramatic improvements in their standards of living and they no longer worry about the shortage of food, shelter, or clothing. As they became more profitable in their capitalistic adventures, achievement and competitiveness, material success, and social status have become dominant values in Korea. Unfortunately, the pursuits of certain higher virtues such as integrity of personality, humanism, harmony, good interpersonal skills, and a control of emotions (which was cherished so much in the past) have gone astray, becoming regarded as somewhat unnecessary. Traditional values based on Confucianism, Buddhism, and Taoism have been denied, and they are now considered obsolete (Choi 1988). Christianity

Table 8.2 Comparison of the Eastern and the Western cultures sociocultural values

Eastern/'traditional'	Western/'modern'
Relationship orientation	Achievement orientation
Suppression of emotion	Self-assertiveness
Integrity, holism	Self-actualization
Humanism, inner life	Rationalism, materialism
Collectivism, interdependence	Individualism, independence
Social control of behavior	Self-control of behavior
Harmony	Equality, human right
Authority, seniority	Democracy, freedom of choice
Male dominance	Gender equality
Confucianism, Buddhism	Christianity
"Shame culture"	"Guilt culture"

Coexist with conflicts and confusions in Korea

is now the most popular and active religion (50 %). Because individualism overshadows collectivism and people invest so much emotional energy into themselves, there is very little left to spare for child rearing and caring for other people. Koreans today rarely talk in public about Confucian teachings such as filial piety (孝). If they do, they are regarded as obsolete or extremely conservative. People have become preoccupied with importing and emulating the Western way of thinking and behaving. Many Koreans seem to care only for the materialistic and social achievements, and they show very little concern for others and the future. Korean people in general, particularly parents, have decided that the most important survival tool in this modern society is to invest all their energy into educating their children. A good education, scholastic achievement, and admission to a top-rated college would guarantee the advancement of their social status and lead to material success. Scholastic achievement has emerged as the most important competition method in the newly transformed country (Table 8.2).

Cultural standards are suffering from duality and confusion due to the coexistence of two contrasting value systems: traditional versus modern and Korean versus Western. People recognize the importance of family cohesion, "me as a member of a family," but they cannot help pursuing "me as an individual," "me," and "we" are in conflict, without hope of resolution. The authority of an adult over the next generation has been lost, and seniority is no longer respected. Instead, the younger generation is revered for their aggressiveness, assertiveness, and vitality.

Most South Korean people today may believe that there is nothing wrong with these changes because they are living well, and they do not have to worry about clothes, food, and shelter as they did in the past. Such opinions might be correct if we disregarded the phenomenal increases in the numbers of children's emotional and conduct disorders, violence and sex-related crimes, drug abuse cases, divorce, and broken families.

8.4.1 Children's Mental Health Problems and Issues in Korea

The author's clinical experience with child psychiatry in South Korea has demonstrated the existence of all disorders classified in the Diagnostic and Statistical Manual of Mental Disorders-IV (DSM-IV) and the International Classification of Diseases-10 (ICD-10). In the early years of child psychiatry development in Korea, several prevalence studies were carried out on several different disorders, with reported prevalence rates of 7.6 % for ADHD, 3.8 % for conduct disorder, 4.2 % for oppositional defiant disorder 4.2 % (Cho and Shin 1994), 9.2/10,000 for autism (Hong 1999), and 2.4 % for dyslexia among third and fourth graders (Lee and Hong 1985). Overall, the prevalence of psychiatric morbidity among Korean school adolescents was 31 % (Kim et al. 1983). Most recently, a school-based epidemiological study in Seoul (Park et al. 2015) demonstrated prevalence of ADHD at 13 %, ODD at 12 %, specific phobia at 15.6 %, anxiety disorder at 8 %, mood disorder at 2 %, and tic disorder at 3.9 %.

What was most notable in clinical child psychiatry practice in Korea was that there were many "reactive," "transient," and "mild" forms of emotional–behavioral–developmental problems which mimic classical psychopathology, but they cannot be definitely diagnosed according to DSM or ICD manuals. For example, transient tic, test anxiety, separation anxiety, and various forms of psychosomatic symptoms are noted very frequently and they seem to be related to many types of stress due to life changes and parental pressure on scholastic achievement. In lay terms, "senior high disease" indicates that senior high students are victims of the endless pressure to study to get high grades in order to enter a top-ranked college. Mild forms of conduct problems and extremely spoiled behaviors are frequently observed in public and school and many children behave like "a little tyrant" as described in China and they tend to have poor social skills and poor peer relationships. This seems to relate to being an only child, parental overprotection, and permissive child-rearing practices.

Another disconcerting problem observed in the early developmental years is a sharp increase in the number of autism-like children referred to child psychiatric clinics for diagnosis. Many meet the diagnostic criteria for reactive attachment disorders or PDD NOS (Hong et al. 1992; Hong and Youn 1996; Shin et al. 1999). There are also sharply increasing incidences of child abuse and neglect. They are related to a variety of adverse environmental factors and a lack of appropriate parental care and stimulations in their development.

The incidence of school bullying, including "wang-ta," which is a kind of rejection and isolation of an individual student by peers (similar to "Ijime" in Japan), is very high (48 %) and the rate of extreme school violence is 3 % (Kim 2001). There are also rapidly growing numbers of school refusal. Another intriguing form of adolescent violence is parent abuse, the prevalence of which is 2.8 % (Lee et al. 1997). Some of these adolescents do not have any other problems except that they are socially isolated, secluded, and withdrawn; a condition similar to "hikkigomori" in Japan and the violent behaviors are directed only at their own parents.

Most recently, a new form of behavioral addiction has emerged. More than 90 % of South Korean adolescents are using the Internet and the prevalence of internet addiction is reportedly 3.5 % among Internet users (Whang et al. 2003). Internet use seems to serve various functions, such as experimenting with relationships, searching for an identity, providing a sexual outlet, and seeking help for depression and social isolation. Severe forms of game addiction seem to accompany frequently serious comorbidities such as ADHD and depression. Another very serious psychosocial problem among adolescents is the high suicide rate (28/100,000) and 4.4 % of adolescents have a history of attempting suicide (Juon et al. 1994).

8.4.2 Crisis and Problems of Child Rearing in South Korea

Some clinical observations and research data from sociological and education fields suggest a crisis in parenting and child rearing in Korea. These are described and presented as potential causative and mediating factors explaining the relationship between sociocultural changes and increasing children's mental health problems in Korea.

1. Increased unwanted pregnancies and unwanted children: The major causes of unwanted pregnancies are marital conflicts, divorce, economic hardship, both parents working, unwanted sex, and teenage pregnancy which could be considered consequences of modernization. Recently, some married couples have questioned whether they should have a child. They often feel that having a child will disturb their couple-centered life, the advancement of their career, and "self-actualization." Unwanted pregnancies are often terminated by illegal abortions. An informal statistic claims that about 1 million illegal abortions occur each year, which is more than the number of live births (around 600,000 per year).

2. Avoidance and refusal of child rearing and custody: Many parents avoid or refuse their parental roles after their children are born. Each year, 13,000 infants and children are abandoned on the street or in infant care facilities. It is surprising to see that recently older children have been abandoned during divorce processes. Both mother and father refuse to take custody of their children. There has been a sharp increase in the divorce rate during the 1990s in Korea. The crude divorce rate rose from 0.4 in the early 1970s to 3.2 in 2003. This is a drastic change from the past, when a child was treasured and considered an important linkage of family tree. Now children are often regarded as obstacles to remarriages and career advancements after divorce.

3. Confusion and inappropriateness in infant-rearing practice: Many young couples lack sufficient knowledge and skills to raise their children well. They are often confused, frustrated, and filled with misunderstandings about child rearing. Young parents are embarrassed because they do not know how to handle or feed

an infant or how to soothe the infant when cries. Young parents today are unsure about the purposes and proper methods of discipline, and they use corporal punishment more often (even during early infancy) and are more punitive than previous generations. This situation seems to be a cause for the alarming increases in infant–child maltreatment, neglect and abuse (Lee et al. 2000; Ahn and Hong 1987). It has been noted that there are two peaks of prevalence of child abuse: one occurs around one to two years of age and the other at 6–7 years of age. The abuse of one or two year olds seems to be related to the failure of attachment on the mother's part and their lack of sensitivity, empathy, and responsibility toward the infant. The mothers are so self-centered that they feel bothered and irritated by the baby's usual cries or demands. Abuses around the second peak seem to be related to discipline.

Hong et al. (1992), Hong and Youn (1996), and Shin et al. (1999) reported a significant increase in the number of infants and preschoolers with autism-like features, yet different from typical autism. Some of these children could be diagnosed as "PDD NOS," "maternal deprivation," or "reactive attachment disorder." One common feature among these children is adverse environmental factors, either inadequacy or inappropriateness of mothering and child-rearing practices. They were not grossly neglected or abused but were emotionally neglected. Environmental adversity includes the following four factors: (1) mother's post-partum depression, marital conflicts, and conflicts with in-laws; (2) mother's working without provision of appropriate substitute care; (3) a child being born abroad and a mother's inability to care for the baby due to her social isolation, depression, and failure to culturally adapt; and (4) mother's inability to provide sensitive, appropriate emotional care, or the mother's use of grossly inappropriate caring methods, such as letting the baby watch TV or videos all day. Similar clinical syndromes of serious attachment disturbance were reported by Rutter (1999) and Mukkades et al. (2000).

4. Inappropriate or inadequate discipline: Overprotection and over-control.

Many young couples simply have the wrong ideas about discipline and they do not know the real purpose and function of discipline. This is due to mother's self-centeredness, a lack of experience and education, and a lack of empathetic understanding of an infant's behaviors and needs. The drastic decline in the number of children in the family, from 4 or 5 to 1 or 2 per family, has significantly changed the dynamics between the baby and the parents. There is an increased risk of either overprotection or over-control. Overprotection comes from the belief that a baby's demand should be met immediately and generously to increase self-confidence and self-esteem in the child. Often the child is an only child or a sickly child or a "special" child. Many children have the "prince syndrome" or "princess syndrome." These children are spoiled, egocentric, and lacking self-control. They cannot get along with their peers and they have difficulty adjusting to school life. Over-control is motivated by various factors. It can arise from a parental need to possess a child and a parent's projected wish of social achievement. These, "tiger moms," think they can mold the child as they want and "early education" in infancy has been a recent fad in Korea. Many young mothers try hard to stimulate cognitive development and special talents. They try to make their children smart and competitive, and they often disregard the child's emotional needs.

5. Changes in sexual roles and attitudes, and sex stereotypes: Recently Korea has witnessed a dramatic change in family relationships and sex roles due to the nuclear family system, the women's equal rights movement, and an increase in the number of working mothers. The traditional, dominant-male/submissive-female relationship has been weakened and the roles that were previously clearly prescribed as either male or female are no longer taken for granted. This has resulted in an increase in competition and struggle between male and female partners. Being raised in a nuclear family and living in separate dwellings from grandparents has resulted in negligible supervision from elders and an increase in power of the mother within the family. The younger generations tend to have more spousal conflicts and quarrels, and they easily resort to divorce.

6. Prime emphasis and endless pressure on scholastic achievement: Perhaps one of the most serious problems in Korea is that intellectual ability and scholastic achievement are regarded as the most important asset parents must cultivate for their children to be successful in this competitive society. Parents encourage competition and push children to reach the highest rank in school, instead of cultivating harmony and caring for other people and suppressing emotions, as in the past. A syndrome known as "senior disease" involved a complex combination of anxiety, depression, and stress experienced while preparing the college admission. This test anxiety is now so pervasive and universal that even primary school pupils experience test anxiety. It is shocking to see many parents hiring special tutors to stimulate the intelligence and cognition of their one or two year olds.

8.5 Immediate Causes of Crisis and Problems of Child Rearing

The author suggests the following findings as immediate causes of confusion, problems, and crisis of child rearing in Korea.

1. Predominant nuclear families and reduced number of children in a family: The successful Family Plan Project of the Korean Government, the high economic burden of living and education, and delayed marriage have brought about drastic reductions in the number of children in a family from the previous average 3.6 to the recent 1.1. The birth rate has steadily declined for the last three decades; it hit a low point of 1.17 in the 2010s. A small nuclear family has both pros and cons from a child rearing and child developmental point of view. The advantages are that the parents can provide full attention and adequate care for an individual child and they can foster intellectual development and self-assertiveness in this competitive, achievement-oriented society. On the other hand, relationships between the parents and the child may become so intense that a slight trauma or changes in the relationship could result in serious disturbances. The reduced number of children

in a nuclear family also increases parental expectations regarding each child's scholastic and occupational achievements and increases the risks of over-control and overprotection. Moreover, the absence of grandparents deprives the family of constructive supervision for the parents and compensatory care for the child which could alleviate the possible emotional neglect and trauma inflicted by their immediate parents. Children in modern Korea no longer experience their grandparents' overindulgence and unconditional affections. In addition, the reduction or absence of siblings eliminates such valuable experiences as sibling rivalry, competition, and cooperation. This will be a contributing factor to peer relation difficulties later.

2. Rising number of working mothers: Women made up 50 % of the workforce in Korea in the 2000s. The real problem is not the increase in working mothers per se, but rather the lack of appropriate substitute childcare while mothers work. In the past, mothers did most of the child rearing. Women in modern Korea tend to look at full-time housewives as being undesirable; they may shame these women. Who cares for the children while they work? Grandparents are not willing to offer substitute care and there are not enough quality daycare facilities or other infant care facilities. The result is the increased risk that the infant's care will be unsatisfactory. This increases the risk of insecure attachment or other relationship problems between the mother and infant. When the risk becomes a reality, we see many disturbed mother–child relationships, attachment disturbances, child neglect and abuse, and many other early developmental problems.

3. Active women's equal rights movement: The women's equal rights movement and feminist movement have been very active in the past 30 years in Korea. They have challenged traditional gender stereotypes, such as automatic male dominance and female submission, and they have been successful in reducing prejudices against women. They have also improved women's rights and their status in society in general. Husband and wives have become more equal than ever. Many women now have good occupations and have become economically independent. They demand equal rights and self-actualization. These changes have made males unsure of their masculinity and their roles. This has resulted in an increased power struggle between the two sexes. On top of these changes, Korea is in the process of a sexual revolution and women have become more liberal and active in their sexual relationships. These dynamic changes in sexual relationships cannot be dismissed as non-significant cause of the increased divorce rate and problems associated with sex role and sexual identity in Korean adolescents today.

4. Few opportunities to learn how to raise a child and to be a parent.

In contemporary Korean society, it is shocking to find that young parents have very few opportunities to observe, experience, and participate in raising a child while growing up, mainly because they grew up in a nuclear family and they were often only child and did not have more than one sibling. This situation is in a stark contrast to the traditional extended family, in which older siblings can observe and help mother or aunt raise a younger sibling or cousin. They also are deprived of receiving assistance, supervision, and advice from experienced grandparents and other adult relatives.

On top of this lack of informal learning experience, there is no formal course to teach child development and child rearing in secondary schools and college. Both at home and at school, children are busy learning mathematics, science, and English. A short lecture series on "how to raise a child" is offered to parents-to-be during pregnancy but only a few take it.

Young parents are confused about the goals of child rearing and are opinionated regarding certain methods. These confusions and biases come from the coexistence of information on child rearing in the traditional and Western styles. Overall, most young couples are not prepared to provide a good-enough parenting.

5. Confusing and often contradictory advice by "professionals" on child rearing: Besides being uneducated on child rearing and parenting, young parents are often confused and have difficulties choosing what and whose advice to follow. The number of "child specialists" is mushrooming in South Korea. The books that parents resort offer quite varied orientations and emphases, and "experts" on television, radio, and daily newspapers prescribe rules for how to raise children according to their different theoretical orientations. Most child experts are educated abroad, mostly in the United States and some in Europe. They have different educations; therefore, their theoretical backgrounds are quite diverse. Unfortunately, most of them have not paid any attention to traditional child-rearing practices and they lack the knowledge and appreciation of early infancy. Their advice and teachings are often downward extensions of what they know about older children or adults; therefore, they emphasize the intellectual development, learning, scholastic achievement, and peer socialization.

Many books on child rearing and child development are available although they are mostly translations of foreign books. It is a shame that few studies and books are available regarding traditional child-rearing practices in Korea. Further, it is unfortunate that few Korean scholars and professionals have really studied and learned about traditional child-rearing practices; instead, they are busy with deciphering a Western way of child rearing and trying to apply it in Korea. In addition, parents themselves seem to prefer the "new Western style" of child rearing, believing that it will guarantee success in a modern society. Parents tend to think that Western ways are always better and they are always ready to follow the Western-oriented professionals' advice.

The author proposes that the child-rearing and parenting problems described above are the most important intermediating mechanisms explaining how rapid social and family changes bring about mental health problems in children.

8.5.1 Traditional and Modern Child-Rearing Practices in Korea

Many current child-rearing practices in South Korea appear to be imitations of Western style child rearing. However, it is likely that the majority of Korean

Table 8.3 Comparison of the Eastern and the Western culture child-rearing style and attitude

The Eastern	The Western
Interdependence	Independence
Infants sleep with mother	Sleep in separate bed and room
Skinship; extensive, prolonged	Talking, stimulating, minimal contact
Surrounded by many caretakers	Mother, father
Parents make a choice for them	Encourage the child to make a choice
Plays with them	Let them play by themselves
A few toys	A number of toys
Highest motivation to explore when with mother	Highest motivation to explore when allowed to make his own decision
Encourages a concern with others' feeling	Ask questions about objects and supply information about them

mothers might have maintained the essence of traditional child rearing without recognizing it. Thus, it is very difficult to tease out what is Western and what is traditional. It is most likely that both methods coexist (Table 8.3).

One of the most important underlying dynamics of child rearing in traditional Korean culture is that the mother's mode of existence and the meaning of her life were derived through child rearing and child education, and ultimately her offspring becoming successful social members (Kim 1974). In other words, mothers used to achieve self-actualization through their children and their husbands. Therefore, they willingly sacrificed themselves to take care of their children and they attempt to achieve happiness by raising their children well. Koreans believe in fetal education. Pregnant mothers try to keep their minds clean and peaceful during pregnancy, and they are cautious about what they say and what they eat, because they believe that their fetuses can be educated through their appropriate and proper attitudes and minds.

The most salient point in Korean child-rearing practice in the past was that an infant was provided with almost constant physical contact. This contact was mostly with the mother and when she worked, the baby was handed to a grandmother or sometimes to the oldest daughter. Babies slept with the mother and they were breast-fed and carried around on their mothers' back wrapped in "podaegi" (carrying blanket), even when the mothers worked. They were rarely separated from the mother. This plentiful supply of physical contact and affection enable infants to feel content and sensually gratified and to establish a sense of basic security, trust, and belongingness. Some people call Korean society a "Jeong (情) society." Jeong can be defined as the attachment and affection through which a mother's care, contact, comforts, and sense of worthiness can be transmitted, and play an important role in adult interpersonal relationships.

Toilet training was not harsh. It was carried out by a benevolent grandmother who gently pushed the child in a rather loose, permissive way. In contemporary Korea, the majority of Korean children are bottle-fed and the parents are very rigid and harsh about toilet training.

During their preschool years, children experienced diverse relationships with multiple adults in their extended family. There were many children of differing ages in the extended family. They had plenty opportunities to observe different relationships between the two sexes, not only mother and father, but also grandma and grandpa, and uncle and aunt. Therefore, they did not have an intense triangular relationship with only their mother and father. They could diffuse the acuteness of the "Oedipal strivings" with multiple grown-ups in the family.

It appears that most contemporary Koreans prefer child-rearing practices in Western style. However, traditional child rearing might be more suitable to meet the basic instinctual needs of a child, while modern child rearing might be necessary to adapt to modern, individualistic, highly technical society. The coexistence of these two contrasting child-rearing orientations and subsequent confusions and conflicts might be responsible for the increased children's mental health disturbances.

8.6 Relationship Between Modernization and Mental Health—A Selective Literature Review for Discussion

It could be readily accepted that modernization usually promotes physical health, improves standards of living, increases job opportunities, and improves socio-economic status. However, modernization seems to have both positive and negative results in relation to the effects on mental health.

Early studies such as Mussen and Beytagh (1969) and Inkeles and Smith (1970, 1974) did not support the assertion that modernization is regularly associated with increased emotional or behavioral disorders in a developing country.

However, a growing number of empirical studies indicate at least an increased risk of psychopathology in relation to modernization. Almeida-Filho (1998) reviewed literature on social and mental health changes in Latin America and challenged the conclusions of Inkeles and Smith. He suggested that mental health in this region worsened during the 1980s and that urban social mobility, the class formation process, and capitalistic modes of production are the main factors involved in increased emotional disturbances. He claimed that the new type of economy and the phenomenon of "hypertrading" on a global scale has produced social inequalities and has created a new poverty.

Rhaim and Cederblad compared two epidemiological studies of Sudanese children. The original study was done in 1965 (Cederblad 1968) and it was replicated in 1980 (Rahim and Cederblad 1984). During the 15-year interval, significant urbanization occurred in Sudan. Tribal distribution changed from comprising 90 % of nomadic tribes in 1965 to only 38 % in 1980, and the number of fathers holding a job in agriculture reduced from 17 to 4 %. The average overall income increased 2.5-fold, and sanitary conditions improved dramatically. School attendance rose from 30 to 90 %. The most interesting finding was that while older children had better physical health status in 1980 compared with 1965, younger children were in a significantly worse state of health; only 45 % being healthy in 1980, compared to 62 % in 1965. Regarding mental health, significantly more behavioral symptoms were reported in 1980 than in 1965. The frequency of psychosomatic headaches and stuttering tripled while hyperactivity doubled in children of 7 years of age. The gender differences were very striking; boys had more symptoms in general. They speculated that certain factors in Sudanese culture seem to protect the mental health of Sudanese children in times of rapid social change, such as the tendency of a whole extended family settling in the same area of the city and the low divorce rate, and these factors result in a low crime rate and less problems of disorientation, alienation, broken homes, and alcohol abuse. The urbanization and socio-economic changes did not alter the basic features of community life in this area.

Harpham (1994) strongly suggested that changes in social support and life events due to urbanization and industrialization in developing countries affect mental health, mainly causing depression and anxiety in general populations. Marsella (1992) and Kleinman et al. (1999) proposed that rapid social changes are associated with social problems, such as street violence, alcoholism, illicit drug abuse, domestic abuse, and other mental and behavioral health problems. Conger (1987) commented on a paradox in which the same social changes that promote individual health and achievement work against the maintenance of social support systems and a sense of community. Therefore, it seems that the consequences of modernization can be both pernicious and salutary.

The negative effects of modernization on mental health seem to be mediated by increased acculturation stress, social class changes, and reduced social support, particularly, the breakdown of the family system. Kleinman and Kleinman (1999) suggested that improved material prosperity and worsening mental and social health outcomes can occur together and that they may be produced by social inequality. Minde (1988) reviewed the evidence linking social change to psychological problems in school age children and their families.

The fact that not all individuals suffer from psychological problems when exposed to the same kinds of social change suggests that social change per se is not the cause of social or psychological disorders; instead, the cause is the failure of individuals or groups to adapt to social change which can create symptoms of social and psychological distress. Mediating variables are cultural proximity, gender differences, cognitive factors, contact experiences and social support systems, social economic class, and patterns of upbringing (Marsella 1992). Hong (1995, 2006) asserted that problems of child rearing and parenting associated with social changes are the most important mediating variables. Other important variables are the speed of change, the presence or absence of preceding ideological/philosophical changes, and the role of traditionalism.

We should also consider mental health factors that protect against the negative effects of social changes. These positive factors include regular, stable, formal employment (Rahim and Cederblad 1984); the maintenance of a good relationship with the parents (Brody 1973); the existence of an extended family (Cederblad

1968); and a sense of coherence and preservation of the traditional culture and literacy (Brody 1973).

Western countries do not seem to be immune to these processes and the effects of social change on mental health. Conger (1981) commented on the effects of the social changes in the USA from "freedom to be me, to do one's own thing" in the 1960s to the "me and its new narcissism" decade of the 1970s (Lasch 1979). In the 1980s, preoccupation with oneself and a diminished concern for the needs of others emerged. One of the most important recent social changes is the decline in respect for authority, for authority's sake. There has been a loss of the unquestioning faith in social institutions and an increase in skepticism regarding the infallibility of scientists and health professionals. All these changes of attitudes tend to increase the relative isolation of individuals and families. An atmosphere of shared responsibility has become rare. On a more personal level, Americans have become more interested in their own physical and psychological well-being which has led to a diminished concern for the needs of others. The great preoccupations with self-realization, self-expression, and freedom to be me are associated with a feeling of a diminished ability to establish intimate and lasting relationships with others (Lasch 1979).

8.6.1 Modernization, Mental Health, and Child Rearing

The author proposes that both positive and negative effects of modernization on child development and mental health can be decisively mediated through child-rearing practices, especially in early infancy. Child-rearing practices depend on how adults in a modernizing, developing country view the nature of children. It also depends on what kind of child-rearing knowledge and experience parents have. It has been suggested that all too often, many non-Western developing countries have idealized and emulated the West without realizing how natural and culturally relevant their traditional child-rearing practices are. Many parents in non-Western developing countries are confused by the coexistence of Western and traditional child-rearing methods, and they often do not recognize that differences exist. Child rearing is the most important influential factor through which the processes of modernization exert their deleterious or beneficial effects on child development and its deviations; in the form of various reactive, developmental, emotional, and behavioral disturbances. Notable progresses in developmental psychology and infant psychiatry have repeatedly confirmed the importance of infant development in personality formation and psychopathology (Sameroff and Emde 1989; Bowlby 1969; Rutter 1997). However, child psychiatrists and mental health workers have not paid enough attention to the significance of early child-rearing experiences in their diagnostic formulation and intervention planning (Fig. 8.1).

Major problems in child rearing and parenting in contemporary globalizing world cannot be dismissed as unrelated to psychopathology, simply because associated problems do not meet formal diagnostic criteria. Many developmental and

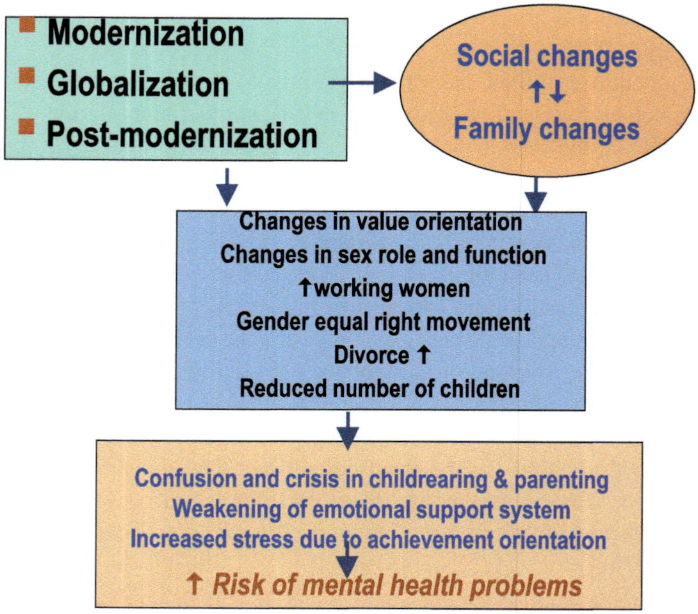

Fig. 8.1 Modernization and mental health

emotional–behavioral problems occur in association with rapid environmental changes and they are often transient, reactive, and temporary. However, they can be forerunners of psychiatric disorders. They also may mimic major psychopathology. These pose significant clinical implications. Certain disorders, such as autistic spectrum disorder (ASD) and ADHD, are mistakenly diagnosed or over-diagnosed if transient and reactive emotional–behavioral problems are not recognized properly. The dramatic increase of child abuse and neglect, ASD, school violence, conduct disorder, ADHD, and Internet addiction cannot be explained as true increases in the incidences of these disorders and a significant portion of them could be the result of including these reactive and transient developmental, emotional, and behavioral problems. Thus, the children's mental health professionals should be aware of this phenomenon in their clinical practice.

8.7 Meaning of Cross-Cultural Differences of Child Rearing

Swanwick (1996) recently reviewed child rearing across cultures and identified three themes as major functions of child rearing in most cultures: survival, family cohesion, and transmission of cultural values. Harkness (1992) commented that traditional ways of life are being modified by increased interethnic contact and social pressure from peers, family, and, in some instances, health care professionals, and they may disturb the security of early caregiver–infant relationships. Stopes Roe and Cochrane (1989) studied family traditionalism in Asian and British populations and found that the British population was the least traditional in attitude and the Asian population the most traditional. Asians valued conformity more and self-direction less than the British group. Caudhill and Frost (1973) also noted that Japanese mothers spent a long time soothing and lulling their infants rather than stimulating them with active chatting, as American mothers did. Ekblad (1988) studied Chinese primary school children and compared them with Scandinavian children. Chinese mothers seem to be more in control of their children and Ekblad concluded that parents' belief about the basic nature of children and theories of how one molds a child into their ideas makes a cross-cultural difference. Similarly, Weisz et al. (1989) proposed a higher rate of over-control problems for Thai children than American children because Thai adults are unusually intolerant of under-controlled behaviors such as aggression, disobedience, and disrespect. Thais believe children should be peaceful, polite, and deferent and that they should inhibit and control the expression of anger and other strong emotions.

Harkness (1992) saw cultural differences in child rearing resulting from adult beliefs about the nature of children. A mother's innate sensitivity to respond to infant signals for nurturance and the cultural perspective that guides parents are shaped by a culture-specific model of interpersonal relationships; child-rearing practices have evolved based on these two dynamic factors over the past 1000 years. For example, an independence model of child rearing for middle-class Americans is appropriate in individualistic cultures and an interdependence model of child rearing for middle-class Japanese parents is appropriate in collectivistic cultures.

8.8 Child Rearing and Mental Health from an Ecological and Ethological Perspective

Why do non-Western parents seem to engage in more Western child-rearing practices as opposed to traditional ones? While it cannot be denied that many parents in non-Western cultures imitate the Western style vigorously on the surface, the phenomenon is more likely to be the result of dynamic forces in their new modern environments. In other words, it may be an adaptation to a drastically changing ecological niche, created by industrialization, urbanization, improved living conditions, reductions in the number of children, nuclear family systems, and others (Bronfenbrenner 1979).

A broader perspective might be that similar phenomena might have occurred several times during the 100,000 year history of human existence. Homo sapiens evolved over millions of years before they appeared only 100,000 years ago as modern humans. They lived in hunting–gathering society for the first 90 % of human history. Therefore, the evolutionary adaptiveness of the human being, such as physiological structures and behaviors, was suited to a hunting–gathering society where they had close contact and integration with nature (Swanwick 1996). However, this evolutionary adaptiveness of human beings had to change when societies began to become agrarian around 10,000 years ago. This was followed by yet another major revision of their lives when their societies became industrialized around 200–300 years ago. Now, we are in the midst of another evolutionary adaptation process due to unprecedented advances in the fields of science and technology, Information Technology and Biotechnology. Therefore, we might be near another quantum jump in evolution (Teihard de Chardin 1959).

Newborn infants have to learn more as civilization progresses. Parents have to put force a great deal of energy to raise their children to utilize all the conveniences and benefits of their advanced civilization. However, it has become difficult to meet evolutionary-based social, instinctual and emotional needs, as society progresses further away from nature and becomes more sophisticated and complicated. From the ethological perspective, modern humans in highly technological societies with all the conveniences and benefits of civilization may have no problem in finding food, clothes, or shelter. Questions of self-actualization, the meaning of existence, and other uniquely human achievements may have no direct relevance to mental health. Instead, the basic biological and instinctual behavioral systems, such as attachment, aggression, and sexuality, are problematic in terms of regulation, gratification, and renunciation. Skills to meet and regulate these evolutionary-based instinctual, emotional, and behavioral demands should be established and taught during early infancy through proper child-rearing practices. A lack of appreciation for these basic instincts neglects and inappropriate child rearing might be the most damaging etiological factors causing the psychopathologies of human beings in modern society. Individualism, materialism, hedonism, and achievement orientation, which are the predominant currencies around the world, produce plenty of "marketing personalities" with diminished humanism and humanity, and make it difficult to maintain a sense of belonging and integrity with family and other human beings. The exclusiveness of a couple-oriented life style and a barely sustained nuclear family will produce modern humans who possess much of what they want, yet feel empty inside and pessimistic about their whole lives. Difficulties maintaining the balance between "me as a true autonomous independent self" and "me as a part of family and society" will be a perennial problem for all human beings to overcome.

The young generation spends much of their time with computers. They can chat, play, and have cyber sex with characters in cyberspace. They are trying to meet their emotional needs through cyberspace and they might form a "cyber identities." They spend hours on the computers and becoming addicted to them. They utilize all the conveniences of an advanced, post-industrial society. The critical problem is that they are moving further away from evolutionary adaptiveness as they accommodate new, advanced, technical society. The more they adapt to the new environment, the greater the risk that they will have unmet human emotional and instinctual needs such as attachment, aggression, and sexuality. This is the very reason why emotional and behavioral problems increase as a civilization progresses further away from the natural environment to which human beings had originally adapted so well.

8.9 Globalization: A New Challenge and a New Demand

The current trends of changes and transformations in social structures, cultural values, and behavioral patterns will continue in the twenty-first century, because the world is compressed in time and space and has become one "nation." People will move around the world, migrate and return, live abroad, and raise children abroad. They are bound to live together with other ethnic and cultural groups and to get in touch with different cultural orientations and values. "Cultural invasions," cultural pluralism, and cultural clashes among people are inevitable. New crises or the intensification of existing child rearing and mental health crises should be expected. In addition, the recent resurgence of religion, anti-Western sentiment, the rediscovery of traditional values and indigenous cultures, the transformation of traditions in global and universal perspectives, and the search for a new world order (Huntington 1993) are bound to bring about conflicts, confusion, and disorientation in the field of child rearing.

Conflicts between cultures and the clashes between civilizations (Lee 1998) may occur not only on an international level but also within a country, even within an individual, because the majority of countries in the world are modernizing and globalizing. During the past era of modernization, Western values, institutions, and culture have dominated the world as the highest, most liberal, most enlightened, most rational, most advanced, and most civilized forms of thinking in humankind. However, Huntington (Lee 1998) predicted that as globalization progresses further, Western influence will decline and other civilizations, such as East Asian civilization, will raise leading to a shift in the direction of influence. Asia might "transmit to the rest of the world their Asian values" and Confucian virtues, such as self-discipline, diligence, family cohesion, and the primacy of the social group's interest over the individual need (Huntington 1993; Lock 1983). Globalizations in economics, politics, and cultures, and the consequential clashes of civilizations demand a global ethics and a new way to coexist.

We are now forced to think of the implications of globalization on mental health and the need to develop effective, preventive, therapeutic interventions on a global scale. Perhaps, international organizations such as International Association of Child and Adolescent Psychiatry and Allied Professions (IACAPAP), World Association of Infant Mental Health (WAIMH), International Society of Adolescent Psychiatry (ISAP), regional organizations such as Asian Society of Child, and Adolescent Psychiatry and Allied Profession (ASCAPAP) should begin to pay attention to these issues and make an appropriate action plan. Minde (1988) has suggested that any preventive interventions to reduce the risk for children and families due to social change should be based on the following three principles:

① maintain traditional family ties and support structures, ② preserve a high level of personal autonomy in the involved population group, and ③ provide support structures for existing cultural practices, instead of replacing them with new ones.

8.10 Conclusions: A Plea for an Integration of the East and the West, the Past and the Present in Child rearing

The author is not simply insisting that we should go back to the "good old days" and resort to traditional child-rearing practices. There is no tradition that does not accommodate new cultural values and new human achievements. Instead, the author strongly suggests that we, particularly non-western people, should study and learn more about traditional ways of child rearing as well as the purposes of and underlying reasons for those old ways. They must have some relevance and applicability in raising the children of today because all human beings have had and will continue to have common, basic, social instincts, such as love, attachment, control and sublimation of aggression, and proper gratification for and renunciation of sexuality. These instinctual needs and other basic human needs will exert their power as long as the human race exists. Basic instincts are the main forces of human existence. We must learn how to fulfill those instincts and how to compromise when they are in conflicts with social restrictions. These biological instinctual behavioral systems will not change even though society and the environment might change a lot. What should be changed is not human needs per se, but rather the ways in which we fulfill the needs. Therefore, the function of child rearing is to promote infants' abilities to regulate and fulfill their needs while meeting societal demands.

This can be achieved only through a satisfactory mother–infant relationship and appropriate child-rearing practices. We want our children to be competent, adaptive, and happy. People say we need a new morality and "global ethics." However, the author proposes that this kind of universal and global ethical standards cannot be established without an appropriate and "good-enough" child rearing. The experiences and skills obtained through "good-enough" child rearing will be the main force in meeting the challenges and solving various emotional–behavioral problems in this ever-growing technological society. We should put our children at the center stage again and provide them with sufficient and good child-rearing experiences through which their basic skills to survive can develop in this rapidly changing world.

At this point, the author suggests that there should be no differences between the East and the West in the purposes of child rearing which helps develop basic survival skills and basic human relationship skills. Differences might exist in external "ways of life" and "ways of thinking" in adults. However, there is no need for any major differences how we raise our children because we all are human and our basic biological and social needs are not different. Therefore, parents in non-Western countries should not merely imitate the exterior of Western child rearing, but should try to understand the philosophy and functions in their own right; further, they should study and learn traditional and indigenous child-rearing practices in their own right as well. It is the author's contention that parental roles are similar in the East and the West. Even if there are some differences, they might be complementary rather than contradictory.

It is strongly suggested that all children's mental health professionals examine themselves, ask what the main sources of their expertise and theoretical background are, and reflect on whether they are trying to apply what they learned from a different culture, directly to their culture. We, children's mental health professionals, regardless whether we live in the East or the West, must learn the essential functions of child-rearing practices and their implications on children's mental health. As globalization progresses further, the East and the West will continue to meet and clash with each other. We have an obligation to find out what to cherish, what to preserve, what to give up, what to import and export, and how to integrate them into the soundest child-rearing practices for our time. We also have an obligation to carry out cross-cultural examinations on different child-rearing practices and different cultural values from different civilizations, so we can learn from each other and become better parents. We must formulate the best child-rearing methods for our time and the future.

Our forefathers in Korea tried to do this a long time ago. "Cherish the old and appreciate the new (溫故知新)," "Study the old and create the new (法古創新)," and "Integration of the East and the West" (東西統合) were three proverbs from Korean tradition. We have failed in accomplishing these goals, mainly because we have not attempted to put them into practice. Therefore, we should study our old ways of life and dig out hidden jewels which we can pass on to the new generations in the East and the West.

References

Ahn, D. H., & Hong, K. M. (1987). A survey of child abuse by physicians' reports. *Mental Health Research, 6*, 53–65.

Almeida-Filho, N. (1998). Becoming modern after all these years: Social change and mental health in Latin America. *Culture, Medicine and Psychiatry, 22*, 285–316.

Bowlby, J. (1969). *Attachment and Loss* (Vol. I. Attachment). London: Basic Books.

Brody, E. B. (1973). Psychiatric implications of industrialization and rapid social change. *The Journal of nervous and mental disease*, *156*(5), 300–305.

Bronfenbrenner, U. (1979). *The ecology of human development*. Cambridge: Harvard University Press.

Caudhill, W., & Frost, I. A. (1973). Comparison of maternal care and infant behavior in Japanese-American, American and Japanese families. In W. Lebra (Ed.), *Youth socialization and mental health*. Honolulu: University of Hawaii.

Cederblad, M. (1968). A child psychiatric study of Sudanese Arab children. *Acta Psychiatrica Scandinavica*, Suppl 200.

Cho, S. C., & Shin, Y. O. (1994). Prevalence of disruptive behavior disorders. *Journal of the Korean Academy of Child and Adolescent Psychiatry, 5*, 141–149.

Choi, B. Y. (1988). *Korean culture and Korean people*. Seoul: SaGaeJul Press.

Conger, J. J. (1981). Freedom and commitment: Families, youth and social change. *American Psychologist, 36*, 1475–1484.

Conger, J. J. (1987). Behavioral medicine and health psychology in a changing world. *Child Abuse and Neglect, 11*, 443–453.

Ekblad, S. (1988). Influence of child-rearing on aggressive behavior in a transcultural perspective. *Acta Psychiatrica Scandinavica, 78*(Suppl 34), 133–139.

Harkness, S. (1992). Cross-cultural research in child development: A sample of the state of the art. *Development Psychology, 28*(4), 625–662.

Harpham, T. (1994). Urbanization and mental health in developing countries: A research role for social scientists, public health professionals and social psychiatrists. *Social Science and Medicine, 39*(2), 233–245.

Hong, K. M. (1995). Crisis in child rearing and parenting in Korea. *Psychotherapy, 9*(1), 43–55.

Hong, K. M. (1999). Prevalence of autistic disorder in a medium size city of Korea: A total population study. *Journal of Autism Spectrum Disorder, 1*(1), 1–25.

Hong, K. M. (2006). Impacts of rapid social and family changes on the mental health of children in Korea. *Psychiatry Investigation, 3*(1), 6–25.

Hong, K. M., & Youn, H. S. (1996). A follow-up study of 30 children with reactive attachment disorder. Paper presented at the 1st Congress of Asian Society of Child and Adolescent Psychiatry.

Hong, K. M., Youn, H. S., & Shin, M. S. (1992). Comparison of developmental and psychopathological characteristics of RAD and PDD children. *Journal of the Korean Academy of Child and Adolescent Psychiatry, 3*(1), 3–13.

Huntington, S. P. (1993). The clash of civilization. *Foreign Affairs*, 72(3).

Inkeles, A., & Smith, D. (1970). The fate of personal adjustment in the process of modernization. *International Journal of Comparative Sociology, 2*(1), 81–113.

Inkeles, A., & Smith, D. (1974). *Becoming modern: Individual changes in six developing countries*. Boston: Harvard University Press.

Juon, H. S., Nam, J. J., & Ensminger, M. E. (1994). Epidemiology of suicidal behavior among Korean adolescents. *Journal of Child Psychology and Psychiatry, 35*(4), 663–676.

Kim, J. E. (1974). *The psychology of Korean family*. Seoul: Ewha Women's University Press.

Kim, K. I., et al. (1983). Mental health survey of high school students. *Mental Health Research, 1*, 1–50.

Kim, Y. S. (2001). School bullying and related psychopathology in elementary school students. *Journal of Korean Neuropsychiatric Association, 40*(5), 876–906.

Kleinman, A., & Kleinman, J. (1999). The transformation of everyday social experience: What a mental and social health perspective reveals about Chinese communities under global and local change. *Culture Medicine and Psychiatry, 23*, 7–24.

Kleinman, A., Kleinman, J., & Lee, S. (1999). Introduction to the transformation of social experience in Chinese society: Anthropological, psychiatric and social medicine perspectives.

Lasch, C. (1979). *The culture of narcissism: American life in an age of diminishing expectations*. New York: Norton.

Lee, K. Y. (1998). In the defense of Asian value. *Time*.

Lee, H., Chun, R., Min, S., Oh, K., & Lee, S. (1997). Adolescent violence toward parents. *Journal of the Korean Academy of Child and Adolescent Psychiatry, 8*, 199–206.

Lee, Y. S., & Hong, K. M. (1985). Specific reading disorder in Korean Elementary School children-A pilot study. *Journal of Korean Neuropsychiatry Association, 24*, 103–110.

Lee, J. Y., Hong, K. E., Cho, H. S., Lee, Y. H., Ahn, D. H., Kwak, Y. S., et al. (2000). The National Survey of Child Abuse. *Journal of Korean Council for Children's Rights, 4*(2), 97–112.

Lock, M. (1983). Japanese response to social change-making the strange familiar. *Western Journal of Medicine, 139*(6), 829–834.

Marsella, A. J. (1992). *Urbanization and mental disorders: An overview of theory and research, and recommendations for interventions and research*. Mental Health Division: WHO.

Minde, K. K. (1988). Effect of social change on the behavior of school-age children, preventive services for school-age children. *Pediatrics, 15*, 170–175.
Mukaddes, N. M., Bilge, S., Alyanak, B., & Kora, M. E. (2000). Clinical characteristics and treatment responses in cases diagnosed as reactive attachment disorder. *Child Psychiatry Human Development, 30*(4), 273–287.
Mussen, P., & Beytagh, L. A. M. (1969). Industrialization, child-rearing practices, and children's personality. *The Journal of Genetic Psychology, 115*, 195–216.
Park, S., & Kim, B. N. et al. (2015). Prevalence, correlates, and comorbidities of DSM-IV psychiatric disorders in children in Seoul, Korea. *Asia-Pacific Journal of Public Health, 27*(2), NP1941-NP1942.
Rahim, S. I. A., & Cederblad, M. (1984). Effects of rapid urbanization on child behavior and health in part of Khartoum, Sudan. *Journal of Child Psychology and Psychiatry, 25*(4), 629–641.
Rutter, M. (1997). Clinical implications of attachment concepts; retrospect and prospect. In L. Atkinson & K. J. Zucker (Eds.), *Attachment and psychopathology* (pp. 17–461). New York: Gilford Press.
Rutter, M. (1999). Quasi-autistic patterns following severe early global privation. *Journal of Child Psychology and Psychiatry, 40*(4), 537–549.
Sameroff, A. J., & Emde, R. N. (1989). *Relationship disturbances in early childhood; a developmental approach*. New York: Basic Books.
Shin, Y., Lee, K., Min, S., & Emde, R. N. (1999). A Korean syndrome of attachment disturbance mimicking symptoms of pervasive developmental disorder. *Infant Mental Health Journal, 20*(1), 60–76.
Stopes Roe, M., & Cochrane, R. (1989). Traditionalism in the family: A comparison between Asian and British cultures, and between generations. *Journal of Comparative Family Studies, 20*(2), 141–158.
Swanwick, M. (1996). Child rearing across cultures. *Paediatric Nursing, 8*(7), 13–17.
Teihard de Chardin, P. (1959). *The phenomenon of man*. New York: Harper & Row Pub.
Weisz, J. R., Suwanlert, S., Chaiyasit, W., Weiss, B., Achenbach, T. M., & Trevathan, D. (1989). Epidemiology of behavioral and emotional problems among Thai and American children: Teacher reports for ages 6–11. *Journal of Child Psychology and Psychiatry, 30*(3), 471–484.
Whang, L. S., Lee, S., & Chang, G. (2003). Internet over-users' psychological profile: A behavior sampling analysis on internet addiction. *CyberPsychology and Behavior, 6*, 143–150.

Chapter 9
Street Children: Stories of Adversity and Resilience

Cornelio G. Banaag Jr.

Abstract The concept of resilience has initiated a paradigm shift in the fields of child development and prevention. This shift has focused on the innate capacity of individuals to face up to adverse events, withstand considerable hardships, and be made stronger by these events. There are few conditions in life that can be more adverse than to be young and live in the streets of major cities of the world. This chapter involves a study of a group of street children and youth in Manila who had shown evidence of resilience in the face of adversity. A search was made for the factors that made for their resilience, with the hope that these factors can be enhanced and be made useful in the battle against the dangers in the streets, particularly the danger of substance abuse.

Keywords Resilience · Adversity · Street children · Resilience factors

9.1 The Meaning of Resilience

Resilience is the capacity of individuals to face up to an adverse event, withstand considerable hardship, not only overcome it but also be made stronger by it. The concept of resilience has been discussed in the past studies as involving both the idea of stressor and an innate capacity of children to respond, endure, and develop normally in spite of the presence of stressors (Richmond and Beardslee 1988). The concept offers a comforting device because the consequences of childhood adversity can be potentially devastating. There is rich evidence in the research literature linking adverse life events and psychiatric disorders in adult and children (Freidrich et al. 1982), substance abuse (Biafora et al. 1994; Duncan 1977), and suicidal behavior (de Wilde et al. 1992). Wolff (1995) underscores the

C.G. Banaag Jr. (✉)
University of the Philippines, Quezon City, Philippines
e-mail: cgbanaag@yahoo.com

S. Malhotra and P. Santosh (eds.), *Child and Adolescent Psychiatry*,
DOI 10.1007/978-81-322-3619-1_9

usefulness of the concept of resilience for research and practice in at least three ways: First, the notion of resilience and vulnerability, of risk and protective factors, highlights the complexity of psychiatric disorders and their causes. It stresses the need to go beyond simple associations between antecedents and consequences, and to look at exceptions rather than the expected outcome. Second, the discovery of why some children caught up in adversity nevertheless do well helps us to identify previously undetected possibilities for preventive action. Finally, the idea of resilience keeps hope alive in clinical practice; however much the odds against good outcome, we know that many children escape their expected fate. This is illustrated by one of the earliest longitudinal studies on high risk children in the Hawaiian island of Kauai exposed to both biologic and psychosocial risk factors (Werner 1994). In her study which began in 1955, Werner identified 201 high risk newborns whose lives she followed from the perinatal period to the age of 32. Of these 201 subjects, 72 grew into competent, confident, and caring adults. The results of the study showed that the effects of reproductive stress decreased with time and that the developmental outcome of practically every biological risk factor was dependent on the quality of the rearing environment. All the studies cited involved populations other than street children. This chapter focuses on street children in response to the growing number of these children found living and working in the streets of major cities all over the world. Furthermore, many of these children get involved in the trafficking and use of psychoactive substances, licit and illicit. Understanding the resilience of many of these children may help organizations working with them develop more appropriate intervention programs.

9.1.1 Resilience and Development

Resilience is best understood from the perspective of developmental process and transactional models (Sameroff and Mckenzie 2003). Individuals pass through the various stages of development continually interacting with other social and physical systems. "Individual adaptation arises from many dynamic processes *within* the individual at the biological (e.g., genetics, hormonal) and behavioral (e.g., attention, capacity for learning) levels as well as between the individual and the different systems in which the individual is embedded [close relationship with caregivers and peers, influence from school and community (Masten and Powell 2003)]". This complex network of interacting systems can influence the impact of adverse events on the individual, either increasing or decreasing the individual's capacity to successfully adapt.

The concept of resilience initiated a paradigm shift in the fields of child development and *prevention*. This shift has moved from focusing on decreasing the environmental risk factors that make individuals susceptible to the development of maladaptive behavior and psychiatric disorders to the highlighting of resilience and its promotion. In this paradigm, it is essential to identify environmental and individual protective factors that can serve as a buffer against the detrimental effects of risk factors, as well as the individual's vulnerabilities that can pose as a threat to resilient outcome. Resilience, therefore, is viewed as a product of interaction between individual and environmental factors, something that can be fostered through the developmental years of childhood and adolescence. It can be developed by strengthening the protective elements in a child's environment while simultaneously promoting the child's life and other personal strengths.

9.1.2 Resilience Factors

Many studies have identified critical factors associated with the resilience of some children. These factors include external supports and resources available to a child (for example, family, school, and community institutions), personal strengths that the child develops (like self-esteem, a capacity for self-monitoring, spirituality and altruism), and social skills the child acquires (such as conflict resolution and communication skills). Werner's 1955 study specifically indentified individual and environmental factors that were linked to successful adaptation in high risk situations. Among these were: (1) temperamental characteristics that allowed the subjects to elicit positive reactions from others, thus facilitating positive relationships, (2) skills and values that allowed efficient use of their abilities and talents, (3) care-giving skills of the parents that fostered competence and self-esteem in the children, (4) adult support, and (5) opportunities for major life transitions.

The study of O'Sullivan (1991) showed that the presence of an adult who takes interest in a child can have a clear positive effect on the child's later life as an adult, even in the presence of a dysfunctional parent. It is obvious that resilience does not develop in a vacuum but grows within the context of the family and the community. As children become older, they assume increasing responsibility for their resilience. The challenge is how to help the children be more capable in promoting resilience in themselves and how to help adults contribute to this resilience more effectively. Findings related to different cultures and different age groups indicate that all cultures draw from the same pool of resilience factors but in different combination and dynamics. The age of the child has been found to play a critical role. There is a notable change from dependence on external supports and services on the part of younger children to a greater reliance on social and interpersonal skills on the part of older children, looking up to adults as models (Grothberg 1995). The data suggest that inner, personal strengths continue to build over the years.

As Wolff points out, resilience is an enduring aspect of a person. Genetic and constitutionally based qualities both determine and are in turn modified by life experiences. Good intelligence, easy adaptability, social temperament, and an appealing appearance attract positive responses in others, which in turn contribute to an inner sense of self-worth, competence, and sense of self-efficacy that have been consistently related to resilience. The importance of the macro environment in fostering resilience cannot be overstressed. The adversities associated with poverty are great and quite susceptible to intergenerational transmission. These adversities contribute to domestic violence, maternal depression, parental discord, coercive and non-vigilant parenting, and child abuse. On the other hand, some studies suggest that these same adversities may serve to strengthen the resilience of children. Turner et al. (1993) synthesized various studies on resilience factors that serve to promote positive psychological growth and development. Turner et al. classified these factors into individual and environmental factors that decrease individual vulnerability and increase individual resilience. They include factors such as an easy temperament, intellectual capacity, self-efficacy, a realistic appraisal of one's environment, social problem-solving skills, a sense of direction or mission, a capacity for empathy, a sense of humor, a capacity for adaptive distancing, and gender. For environmental factors, they included family, school, and community protective elements such as early parental care, enduring warm and positive relationships with at least one adult, a positive family environment and bonding, high parental expectations, family responsibilities, positive modeling, good parenting skills and supervision, family and rituals, support for the youth's competencies and life goals, extended family support, opportunities for students involvement in various school activities, a caring, supportive school climate, and positive community norms.

9.2 Resilience in Special Population

The Philippine government has increasingly focused on children in need of special protection. These children are seen as a special population in need of attention and special interventions. This population of children includes those who are neglected, abandoned, physically and/or sexually abused; those who are in conflict with the law or caught in armed conflicts; victims of child labor; victims of substance abuse; and those who live and work in the streets (street children).

Many of the studies on resilience had been done with children and youth living with families under various circumstances of adversity. There are very limited studies done on the resilience of special populations like the street children. In a critical review of resilience literature and its relevance to homeless children, Neiman (1988) identified certain factors associated with resilience among street children. She grouped these factors into individual (constitutional factors, gender, temperament) and environmental factors (positive mother–child relationship, protective family relationships, extrafamilial factors).

9.2.1 The Street Children

There are very few conditions in life that can be more adverse than to be young and live in the streets of major cities in the world. Estimates reported by the WHO

Project on Street Children and Substance Abuse put the number of the street children between 10 and 100 million worldwide. The criterion for defining street children varies from country to country and with time, making it difficult to arrive at any precise global estimates. In the Philippines, there are 1.5 million street children nationwide. About 75,000 of them are found in Metro Manila alone (DSWD 1988). In more recent report, the estimate number is 220,000 nationwide (CWL 2006).

Why are these children and youth on the streets? The interweaving political, economic, and psychological conditions that have driven children to the streets are too complex to give a simple explanation for this worldwide phenomenon. Poverty, like the kind spawned by the political and socioeconomic conditions in many developing countries, is the most commonly cited leading cause. Most children of poor families are forced to stop going to school and instead go to the streets to earn. However, beyond poverty, one suspects that the breakdown of traditional family and community values and structures serves as a major factor in the increase of children on the streets. Symptoms of such breakdown include the neglect and abuse of children, dysfunctional parents who could not adequately care for their children, lack of support from the traditional extended family system, abuse of psychoactive substances by the parents or by other members of the family, domestic violence, lack of employment opportunities, lack of access to basic community services, congestion in slum areas, violence in the community, deterioration of values permitting exploitation of children, and finally breakup of families.

9.2.1.1 Street Children and Health Hazards

Children and youths on the streets experience serious health risks and physical danger. They are exposed to high levels of violence, victimization, sexual exploitation by pedophiles and pimps, and to the use of harmful substances. Many suffer from psychiatric symptoms and mental health problems.

The percentage of substance abusers among street children varies greatly. Studies in different parts of the world indicate that between 25 and 90 % of street children abuse psychoactive and harmful substances. In the Philippines, about 50 % of the street children abuse substances. The most common substances used include: alcohol, nicotine, inhalants, marijuana, and amphetamines (CWL 2006).

9.2.1.2 Street Children and Interventions

In the Philippines, a large number of governmental and nongovernmental organizations (often offered to as agencies by the street children) responded to the growing crisis of the street children. Community-based, center-based, and street-based programs of intervention were created to help these children and their families. These interventions primarily addressed the deficits in the environment of these children that pushed them to life in the streets. In the course of their work, people involved in helping street children were impressed with remarkable capacity of some of these children to survive adversities of life in the streets. Not only do they overcome these adversities, but are also made stronger by their encounter with adversities. Though confronted everyday with the multiple risk factors in their environment, they had been able to avoid substance abuse, prostitution, teenage pregnancy, and other major pitfalls in living on the streets. These children were later identified as resilient.

9.3 The Study

Supported by the UNICEF Philippines and the National Project on Street Children of the Philippine government, a descriptive study in the resilience of street children and youth in Manila was conducted. The study was, in part, motivated by the concern over the highly prevalent use of harmful substances among street children. The objective of the study was to identify individual, family, and environmental factors that made for the resilience of the subjects in the study, with hope that, once identified, these factors can be enhanced and made useful in the battle against substance abuse. A modified social stress model, derived from the original work of Rhodes and Jason (1990) and modified for use in the WHO Programme on Street Children and Substance Abuse, was used as the framework for identifying the children's resilience traits as well as the risk and protective factors in their environment. This model views the risk of substance abuse as directly proportional to risk factors (which include stress, mechanisms by which use of harmful substance is "normalized," and the desired experience with substance) and inversely related to protective factors (positive attachments, coping skills, and available resources).

This study is descriptive and qualitative in nature, based on a case study method. The objective is to identify individual, familial, and community factors that contribute to the resilience of a group of street children. While large sample sizes strengthen the quantitative design of a study, case study and other qualitative methods can provide deeper insights into the complex dynamics of the subjects' interactions and life experiences. Twenty-five (25) street children (17 males and 8 females) were interviewed for the study. The age range of the subjects was 12–20 for the males and 14.5–19 for the females.

These children were selected from various nongovernmental organizations or agencies linked with the UNICEF Program on Psychosocial Intervention. The children included in the study came from a pool of 50 names submitted by the different organizations who, at the time of the study, had demonstrated at least 2 years of steady, even though at times shaky, positive psychological development.

Based on the modified social stress model, the investigator developed a questionnaire for use in the evaluation of the subjects. The questionnaire was designed to assess individual, familial, and environmental factors that make for resilience. A series of in-depth interviews was done with each subject. A detailed mental status examination was done on each subject. Personal and family histories were gathered from direct interviews of the subjects as well as from the existing records. Whenever possible, interviews were also made with peers, staff members, and family members with the consent of the subjects involved. Home visits were also done by a social worker when applicable. In some cases the subject was the only source of information, limiting the data gathered to the subject's memory and view of his word.

9.3.1 Individual Resilience Traits

As previous studies show, a cluster of personality traits enable high stressed children to overcome their stresses and develop a sense of competence and control in their lives. These traits enhance their resilience.

In this study, a sense of direction or mission and self-efficacy are the two most common individual traits identified by the street children. The positive effects of a sense of direction or mission can be attributed to the relative stability that a goal offers as opposed to the drifting nature of a directionless life. Many of the children affirmed that a sense of direction gave them a purpose or a life task that guided the decisions they made. One of the subjects, Ronnel, was guided by his self-chosen mission to save his younger siblings as well as other children from experiencing the life he had on the streets. His dream of becoming a policeman someday can be seen as an extension of a sense of mission to save other children who go astray.

> At 17, Ronnel is one of the older boys at KAIBIGAN (FRIEND), a non-governmental community based center for street children. He felt responsible for the younger boys and tried to act like a role model by actively participating in the center's activities such as sports like swimming and basketball, as well as handicraft making. During his extra time he worked as a "car wash boy" outside the center. Having known the damaging effects of abusing substances, he felt he had a responsibility to save other street children from drug abuse. When he met children in the streets using drugs, instead of joining or ignoring them as he might once have done, Ronnel would talk to them to warn them of the dangers in abusing harmful substances. Specifically, Ronnel wanted to make sure that his younger siblings would not have to go through what he had undergone. In his words "I didn't' take good care of myself back then, so now I intend to guide and care for my younger siblings"

The importance of a sense of direction can be seen in the case of Joel, an 18-year-old high school senior. His desire to go to school goaded him to continue studying despite the many upheavals and changes in his life.

> Joel remembered that his family was too poor to send the children to school regularly. After his father left them, his family moved in with some friends in another section of the city. Subsequently, he and his mother moved to the reclamation area by the Manila Bay. Joel never gave up on his school. He completed grade 6 while living in the reclamation area and subsequently went to high school with the help of a street children organization. According to Joel, he wanted to finish his schooling because he believed he could get a better job than what he did in the streets and a better chance to help his family.

Closely related to the sense of direction or mission is the sense of *self-efficacy.* Self-efficacy has been defined as a "positive perception of one's competence to perform certain tasks" (Bandura 1977). It includes the faith of an individual in his ability to control his or her life and environment in positive ways. Seen in this light, self-efficacy gives an individual a feeling of self-empowerment and self-worth that is needed to attain one's goal. Almost all the children interviewed constantly demonstrated their sense of self-efficacy through repeated and effective daily behavior aimed at gaining a livelihood in the streets. Rafael, for example, believed in his abilities to change his future. He approached the staff of KANLUNGAN (SHELTHER) seeking help to enroll in a vocational course; he eventually learned refrigerator and air condition repair. This sense of self-efficacy could be seen even earlier in his life.

> At 17, Ronnel is one of the older boys at KAIBIGAN (FRIEND), a non-governmental community based center for street children. He felt responsible for the younger boys and tried to act like a role model by actively participating in the center's activities such as sports like swimming and basketball, as well as handicraft making. During his extra time he worked as a "car wash boy" outside the center. Having known the damaging effects of abusing substances, he felt he had a responsibility to save other street children from drug abuse when he met children in the streets using drugs, instead of joining or ignoring them as he might once have done, Ronnel would talk to them to warn them of the dangers in abusing harmful substances. Specifically, Ronnel wanted to make sure that his younger siblings would have not to go through what he had undergone. In his words "I didn't' take good care of myself back then, so now I intend to guide and care for my younger siblings"

The importance of a sense of direction can be seen in the case of Joel, an 18-year-old high school senior. His desire to go to school goaded him to continue studying despite the many upheavals and changes in his life.

> Joel remembered that his family was too poor to send the children to school regularly. After his father left them, his family moved in with some friends in another section of the city. Subsequently, he and his mother moved to the reclamation area by the Manila Bay. Joel never gave up on his school. He completed grade 6 while living in the reclamation area and subsequently went to high school with the help of a street children organization. According to Joel, he wanted to finish his schooling because he believed he could get a better job than what he did in the streets and better chance to help his family.

Many of the street children who shared their life stories demonstrated *social problem-solving skills* and street *survival skills* as important factors in their survival. Both sets of skills are important in that they allow the street children to live in the streets and survive. Maximiano, 14 years old, illustrated good social problem-solving skills. When he left home, his immediate concern was where to eat and sleep in the streets. He quickly asked around at nearby stores, offering to work for food and shelter. He was eventually hired by a canteen owner to help out in the kitchen, and learned how to cook in the process.

> Jerry and the other boys quickly found out that much to their dislike, they had to resort to begging, occasionally stealing and handbag snatching in order to survive. They felt they had no choice because they were hungry and had no money. They slept in different places such as sidewalks and under the Light Rail Transit (LRT) station. All of them learned to

> do drugs, two of them even engaged in prostitution for some time. But each of them made a turn around when they faced up to their mistakes and corrected them.

Problem-solving skills reinforce one's sense of competence and self-esteem. Street survival skills, on the other hand, often involve self-damaging behavior that heightens the risk of failure in a street child who is not resilient. Whereas the case of Jerry and the other boys focused more on survival skills, the case of Marlon M. is an example of social problem-solving skills:

> When Marlon went to Cubao, a busy commercial district, he continued to earn by begging and watching cars. From his earning, he bought food and clothing. He slept almost always alongside a particular bank. When he needed to go to a restroom, he would go to restaurants. His friends also brought him to homes where street children would be allowed to use the toilet and bathroom for a fee.

Adaptive distancing, seen in most of the children, is an important trait that helped the street children in the study effect healthy separation from the immediate problems in their lives. The children with this trait managed to separate themselves physically and/or psychologically from the risk factors in their environment. Many street children interviewed, did not identify with dysfunctional patents and found healthy role model elsewhere. They did not feel responsible for their parents' problem. Some even felt compassion but detached toward their parents. Such is the case of Susan who, although disappointed with her mother continued to love her and exerted efforts to save her from abusive boyfriend. She preferred to live in a residential center that helped her go to school. In her words:

> My problem has to do with my mother and her live-in partner. I cannot do anything to separate them. That is why I believe this problem will never be solved. I love my mother, and I will try to help her whenever I can.

Jerry also exhibited his capacity for adaptive distancing.

> He would leave the house when his foster parents fought. Although he wished to stop the fight, he knew there was nothing to do. Mr. D (Jerry's foster father) was alcoholic. When drunk he would become violent, provoke fights, would shout a lot, and sometimes would physically abuse his wife. Whenever the couple fought, Jerry would just leave the house. He wanted to stop the fights but was afraid to do so.

Having a hobby or a creative talent as sport, singing, dancing, writing, and painting serves a s coping mechanism through which children can distance themselves from problems and at the same time foster in them feelings of competence, self-worth, identity, and a feeling of worth in the community. In some instances, in fact, the creative talents have served a purpose of "therapy" or self-healing because these activities allowed expression of conflicted feelings. A good example is the case of Rommel who had sublimated his conflicts into theater arts. Through his work in the street theater he also realized that he could be useful to the community.

> Supported by Maryville Foundation, a community-based center, Rommel joined workshops in theatre arts. He took a 10-day live-in course in script writing. He discovered his great love for the performing arts, especially drama, acting, directing and script writing. He also realized that he could make himself useful to the community by directing plays,

acting, and writing drama with lesson for the audience to learn. His involvement in theatre arts meant a deeper involvement with his own self.

Marlon P., who represented his school in karate tournaments and at the same time taught it in his school, demonstrated the importance of a special talent.

In order to act effectively for themselves or for others, the street children need a *realistic view of their environment.* Most children showed a good capacity for appraising their situation realistically. These children seemed to know what was possible and attainable in their situations, allowing them to act on opportunities that could their long term goals. They also knew what they could and could not change in their life situations. Many of the children have learned to accept their dysfunctional parents for what they were. Others have accepted the limitations that their environments placed on their dreams.

Joel B. dreamed of becoming a computer scientist someday or a pilot "so I can visit other countries". But he was aware these dreams were not readily within his reach. So he planned "to be an electrician after high school, then work, save money, and take up computer engineering."

Self-monitoring skills and self-control are regarded by more than half the children as important factors in their lives. Self-monitoring, the ability to regularly assess one's self and situations, makes for resilience through constant awareness of where one stands in his or her life. By monitoring the events in his life and the effects of these on the self, the street child is able to appraise his or her environment realistically. He or she is able to make good choices, and able to avoid options that can bring harm to him or her, like substance abuse. Self-control refers to the ability of individuals to control impulses and disengage from temptations and pressures. It involves an internal focus of control, thereby reinforcing their sense of self-efficacy. Obviously, the youngsters in this study who had been able to say "no" to drugs, street brawls, and early risky sexual experimentation and exploitation have illustrated adequate self-control; an illustrative case is Michael:

At 12 years old Michael was introduced to the use of marijuana and other substances like cough syrup and "shabu" (amphetamine) by the people he worked with at the market place. When told by a concerned adult of the harmful effects of the substances, Michael decided to stop using them. He left his work in order to get away from the temptations and company of the addicts. He figured that he could get another job by asking his friends in the streets.

Intellectual capacity was roughly gauged through academic achievement and responses shown by the street children during interviews. Very few of them had psychological tests. More than half of the children interviewed showed a notable degree of intelligence reflected particularly in their achievements in school. The street children who showed comparatively higher intelligence also placed a high premium on the importance of schooling. They saw formal education as a means of improving their situation in life. Nina, for example, viewed the completion of her education as the most important goal in life. Another street child, Eric had just graduated from high school and was employed as a décor painter in the furniture factory. Aside from the relative advantage that intelligence gives a person in order to survive., the belief in the value of education as a possible means of improving one's condition had given the street children a firm anchor that kept them from engaging in self-destructive behavior. Joel is a good example of one who valued education

> Joel never gave up on school. He wanted to complete his high school education because he planned to work and help his family. He admired a cousin who received academic honours in his school, and hoped to be like his cousins. He knew his classmates and friends had high expectation of him, and wanted to remain a good role model for other children.

There were six subjects who, prior to their inclusion in the study, had formal psychological assessments. It is interesting to note that these subjects had I.Q. measurements that were much lower than what one would expect, given their adaptive capacities. This raises the question whether the standard instruments used to measure intelligence are appropriate for special populations like the street children.

Ten of the subjects appeared to possess an *easy temperament and disposition,* allowing them to maintain positive relationships especially with people in a position to help them. They gravitated easily toward good connections. As cited in the earlier studies, an easy temperament aids in fostering good interpersonal relationships thus allowing other people to treat them in more positive manners. These relationships reinforce the children's sense of self-worth and at the same time open more opportunities for self-development. In Val's case, it was easier for him to empathize with friends who were in trouble. He tried to entertain them, to talk to them, or play with them. He considered himself to be humorous, "good at making people laugh and be happy."

Nine of the subjects showed the *capacity to recognize mistakes* they had made in the past and instead of succumbing to these or simply accepting them, they used the knowledge brought on by experience to create better, more positive lives. The subjects who had exhibited this trait were generally more *altruistic* and *emphatic*. They used their experiences to help younger children so that they could avoid making the same mistakes that they themselves had made in the past. Rommel, for example, having known the damaging effects of substance abuse now felt a responsibility to keep other children from committing the same mistakes he had made.

> Rommel, whose talent in the theatre arts had been cited earlier, had been involved in drugs, alcohol and gambling. He worked in a gambling house as an errand boy. It was an easier job than collecting garbage. He also earned much more. He had more than enough pocket money for school needs, clothes, shoes, and food for his family. He began to neglect his school responsibilities. With the help of a social worker, he got connected with the Maryville foundation. He decided to stop working at the gambling den, and proceeded to graduate from high school. This became the turning point in his life.

Another boy, Eric, gave up life in the streets and drugs, concentrated on his studies, and had been steadily self-employed. He still occasionally would go to his old neighborhood trying to help pull his friends away from the streets.

Many studies identify *a sense of humor* as an important element of resilience. These factors came out clearly in eight of the subjects. Humor allows an individual to cope with the situation that can threaten to overwhelm him or her. The ability to laugh at oneself, and see the lighter side of situations can open help in dealing with the stressful events in one's life. Humor reduces tensions and restores perspective. Rafael and Val, for example, attributed their ability to get along well with others to their sense of humor.

Leadership skills, altruism and empathy are attributes that are "others-oriented" allowing the individual to actively help other people. Seventeen of the subjects showed leadership skills and altruism. These attributes gave them a sense of purpose, worth, and self-empowerment, and allowed them to go beyond themselves in trying to achieve goals that would benefit others, Empathy, shown by 15 of the subjects, allowed the subjects to feel for others. Through their actions, the subjects in the study were recognized in their various communities. In some cases they acted as *"kuyas"* (older brothers) and "*ates*" (older sisters) for those younger than they. They became role models for the younger ones, using their knowledge and experience to help just as they themselves were helped in the past by others. Marissa was recognized and awarded by the Philippine National Red Cross as among the most outstanding junior health workers the year prior to the study. She had shown leadership skills by organizing seminars on health care for street children in KANLUNGAN (SHELTER), a community-based center for street children.

> In her first year with KANLUNGAN, Marissa finished a three-week dressmaking course and became involved in helping the staff work with the children on the streets. Her work involved talking to street children and educating them about the dangers of harmful substances. At the age of 15, she was selected by the KANULUNGAN staff to represent the center at a training seminar for junior health workers sponsored by the Manila chapter of the Philippine National Red Cross. After her training, she organized seminars for street children at KANLUNGAN on health promotion. She assisted the staff in first aid, and helped bring the children to the hospital for emergency and out-patient treatment. A staff worker commented, "after the training, Marissa immersed herself in health work, showing efficiency and effectiveness in performing her duties. She knew more about hospital procedures than I did." That year she was voted as the *"Bantog na Junior Health Worker"* (Outstanding Junior Health Worker). A recognition given by the National Red Cross, Manila Chapter. She was cited for her organizational skills and leadership qualities.

Another subject, Teresa, showed similar traits:

> Teresa demonstrated her leadership skills and altruism as a student leader. In grade school, she was always voted as class president. She had a soft heart for children like her, poor but deeply committed to studying. Her capacity for empathy had led her sometimes to make mistakes in the past. In grade school, she remembered feeling sorry for a friend who had lost a book. She took a book from the library to replace the one her friend had lost. She was caught and was heavily reprimanded. She never forgot the mistake she made.

Eleven of the 25 subjects took special note of how a *sense of morality* guided their actions and choices in daily life. They attributed to their sense of right and wrong their capacity to avoid the use of illegal drugs and the use of sex for money. A sense of morality reinforces self-control, and contributes to feeling of efficacy.

> Marissa claimed her friends in the streets engaged in sex for money. She refused to engage in such activity because she thought of it as morally wrong. She would rather beg.

Religion or *faith in God* was regarded to be very important by 10 of the subjects.

They cited prayers and going to church as sources of support that helped them through difficulties. All ten had expressed the belief that the power of faith had helped them stay away from trouble. Some of these children admitted that they did not go to church regularly. Nevertheless their behavior showed that they had a personal relationship with God. Marlon had a good relationship with God and would go to church frequently when feeling troubled; he also prayed before each meal. Marissa claimed that she generally turned to God first whenever she encountered problems or felt downhearted.

Ronnel, though young in age, had developed a philosophical attitude about life. He believed that given the right time, things would fall into their proper places. He felt a personal relationship with God. Though he did not attend church regularly, he believed that God had a special mission for him.

The last resilience factor identified among street children is *"pakikisama."* This is a very common Filipino trait that can be loosely defined as "going along with a group to avoid confrontations." It may also be seen as an individual's attempt to seek attachment or to belong to a group. This trait can have either positive or negative effects depending on the kind of group that the individual attaches himself to. Therefore, it is important for the street children to connect to a good group that can offer them access to positive involvement. Michael, after he left his work in the market to avoid the "addicts" was able to connect himself to the "Scout Ranger Brotherhood," a fraternity that he described as "a group of upright, stable, and supportive young men who avoided violence." Here he felt a sense of brotherhood and belonging that strengthened his own sense of self-worth.

Joel B. showed this trait when he joined a residential center for street children and readily became part of it. When admitted to MASIGLA, Joel had scabies all over his body. He was very thin and evidently malnourished. He adjusted quickly to life in the center. He related easily to the staff and other residents.

The individual resilience traits identified in this study, and demonstrated in the vignettes, are not mutually exclusive. Many of the traits, in fact, are closely related to each other and were clustered accordingly. The subjects in the study registered an average of eleven individual resilience traits. Some showed a minimum of seven traits while others showed considerably more. These traits appear to have interplayed with one another in each child in a manner that is empowering.

9.3.2 Individual Traits and Environmental Factors

Individual traits, while very important, are not always sufficient for the development of resilience. Resilience involves interaction between the individual and environmental factors, not just fixed attributes or traits within the individual. This observation is especially true among children and adolescents. Young people need elements in their environment that will not only reinforce but also protect the individual traits which help them become resilient. In the study, a search for family, community, and peer protective factors, was made in order to show the dynamic interaction of individual resilience traits with protective factors in the individual's environment resulting in positive adaptive outcomes.

9.3.2.1 Family Protective Factors

The family is the single institution that can respond to the basic needs of children on a long term basis. It exerts the most powerful influence over the child's emotional, social, psychological, and physical development. Whether it is a two-parent, single-parent, adoptive or foster family, it normally provides significant protective factors that help build resilience in the individual. In some instances, as in a dysfunctional family, it may be a source of significant risk.

In the study, the most commonly cited protective factor was that of *having family responsibilities.* Twenty-three of the twenty-five subjects mentioned this factor as being important. This factor included not only household chores and taking care of younger siblings, but also earning extra income for the impoverished family. In many instances, this sense of responsibility implied firm and clear parental discipline and supervision. Bleuler (1978) has a partial explanation for the effect of this factor on the individual. Bleur found that "youth whose families need them to do tasks will feel that they have something to contribute and will feel valued and empowered." This empowerment can be seen in the life of Teresa.

Teresa learned to do her chores at home such as cleaning washing dishes, and throwing the garbage without question or resistance. To help earn for the family, she began working in the streets when she was 8 years old. She learned how to be resourceful in the streets. After school, she sold barbeque and "kakanin" (rice cake) in the streets. She usually came home from school at 2:00 p.m. and during *merienda (snack)* time she would make her rounds at the Pandacan market. On a fine day, her goods would be sold out. At times, she would have some left over that she took home for the family. She would earn enough for the day which augmented the family income and her school expenses.

Family traditions and rituals cited by the subjects in the study included the celebrations of recognition days or achievements, social and family gatherings, meals together, and most commonly going to church together. Rituals and traditions serve as powerful protective factors, even in the face of family dysfunction and chaos. The family can begin to see itself as somehow enduring even if it is not always cohesive. Traditions and rituals often act as recognition of one's place or position in the world and enhance a sese of belonging to a group. No matter what else is going on, if the family could eat together on special days or hear Mass together on Sunday, the children will internalize a routine around which they can build their identity. The family praying together also enhances the child's religious feeling and faith in God, which as shown earlier, many of the street children interviewed regarded as important in facing up to adversity.

Susan, for example, related how much she appreciated her mother's efforts to keep family rituals despite their poverty. When she was much younger, her mother would prepare a modest meal to celebrate her birthday with the family and friends.

Among the street children interviewed, eight mentioned having *positive family environments and bondings*. This relatively low item was not surprising when one considers that the very reason many street children are out in the streets is their desire to escape their dysfunctional families. Many of the children interviewed experienced positive family environments with substitute families that had adopted them. Jerry, for example, found a home in Mr. D's family who accepted him as one of their own. Marlon P. continued to live with his foster family. Moreover, most of the eight subjects who mentioned having positive family environments no longer had such families at the time of the interview. The subjects were actually looking back at their lives when their families were still intact and deriving strength from these memories.

> The family of Norma, while unusual in its extremely positive nature showed the importance of a positive family environment. Her parents raised their children sharing the household chores that included dish washing, laundry, and cleaning. Despite their poverty, they always emphasized the importance of education. No matter how little they had in life. Norma's parents always made sure that all their children went to school. Norma described her family as being close-knit. They always celebrated special days like Christmas and other holidays at home. During birthdays her mother would fix something special for the family. When the children were much younger, the family always attended Mass together.

Another highly expressed protective factor was that of *a warm, positive relationship with a parent.* Considering the frequent observation that many street children fail to establish close and effective bonds with their parents, the scope of this definition was made to include various adults in the street child's life such as foster parents, relatives, and other adults who show interest and concern for the street children.

> Rommel, known for his stage work described his father as a "family man" working hard all day and going straight home on time for supper. The father had no vices and was close to the children. Rommel strongly identified with him in his disposition, especially in his father's love for the arts. His father wrote plays and poems and influenced Rommel towards this inclination.

Some of the street children related how having a warm bond with a sibling was important to them. It is not uncommon for the sibling of street children to be street children themselves and the shared experiences of living in the streets often cause siblings to turn to one another. Such bonding obviously provides a protective element for each of the siblings.

Among his siblings, Antonio was closest to the eldest, Mary Anne, who used to take him along to the market. He also looked up to his brother, Anmar, with whom he identified in terms of work and study.

A warm, positive relationship with an adult fosters feeling of importance in street children, making them feel that someone does care for them. An older person to whom they can run for support or advice serves as a positive adult model.

Positive adult models acted as guide in life for many of the street children. Early parental modeling was expressed by 15 of the 25 respondents as a guiding factor even if the parent was no longer involved with them in some instances. This can be seen in the case of Jerry. Although his father had died when he was five years old, Jerry wished to complete his education because he believed his father had wanted that of him. According to Jerry, he had taken after his father both in personality traits and physical attribute. He wished to become a soldier, as his father had been. Many of the subjects mentioned foster parents as their role models. Such parent substitutes were common in the lives of the streets children studied. Jennifer, for example developed a strong bond with her caregiver (Ate Glo) in the center where she stayed. Jennifer described Ate Glo as being patient and caring and a source of inspiration for her.

Twelve of the subjects felt special affection from the members of their extended families. In some cases, an aunt or an uncle had cared for the children in lieu of a mother or father. In other instances, a grandparent had taken over parenting even for only a brief period in the child's life, an experience that the child could remember for years to come. A member of the extended family toward whom the subject felt particularly close became role model. The extended support system provided the protective factor at critical points in the child's life. In a number of cases, the affectionate bond was established with a sibling rather than with the parents.

Although many of the street children interviewed did not maintain frequent contact or involvement with their families, nine respondents said that their *families were morally supportive of them* in their struggle to attain their goals. Some mentioned that their parents had high expectations of them. Supportiveness of the child's ability and high parental expectations enhance a child's resilience. The child enhances his belief in his abilities when he knows his parents have faith in him and have high expectations of him. Parents who expect a child not to take drugs and make that expectation known have tremendous influence in the child's decisions not to abuse substances. Similarly, parents who have high but realistic expectations of their child's performance in school can inspire their children to strive well. For example, Antonio's father stressed the need for him to finish college in order to liberate himself from their poverty. This has sustained Antonio's efforts in his studies. Support and belief in the children appear to be positive protective factors only as long as these are realistic. Parents who have high expectations beyond the children's abilities may instill feelings of inadequacy and failure in their children.

9.3.2.2 Resilience and Community Factors

The protective elements identified in the peer group, school, and community at large, like individual and family resilience factors are not exclusive of one another. There is a constant interplay among different categories of resilience factors. For example, leadership skills are fostered and bolstered by family support but need a community that allows positive involvement that can sustain these skills. A community where there is a sense of caring, mutual protection, and nondrug use norms is likely to foster resilience in the young people.

Together with the protective factors in the family, community protective factors had been identified to be critical in the lives of street children in the study. Among these community factors, *agency intervention* or the help provided by street children organizations was the single factor consistently mentioned by all subjects as having positive effects in their lives. A certain bias toward this finding, however, is to be expected because all the respondents interviewed were accessed through various nongovernment organizations (NGO) that had identified them as being resilient. All these organizations, except two, are community based. They supported the children while they lived in their families and worked and go to school. Two of the NGOs are center-based, i.e., the children lived in the centers. According to the street children, the agencies acted as foster families from whom they could receive the warmth, care, and support that their own families were unable to provide effectively and continuously. These agencies facilitated opportunities for schooling, involvement with peers, and basically functioned as surrogate families to which street children could turn in time of need. All the 25 subjects in the study attributed the adaptive outcomes in their lives to the protective influence provided by the agencies.

An opportunity for involvement with the community was mentioned in 15 of the 25 cases. These opportunities—like street theater, working as junior health educators, teaching martial arts, participating in extracurricular activities—allowed positive personal growth and instilled feelings of adequacy and self-worth, as well as a sense of belonging to a community.

School experience was regarded by many of the subjects as a powerful element in the community. Thirteen of the subjects mentioned the importance of having a *caring and supportive school climate*. Seven mentioned that *high expectations from the school* with regard to their performance inspired them to work hard. The support and expectations generally came from a particular teacher or one's peers in the school setting with whom the bonds of friendship had been formed. These factors fostered in the street children feelings of self-efficacy, the belief that they themselves had some power over their circumstances and therefore could work toward attaining their dreams and aspirations. Being in school also lent a sense of purpose to these children, at the same time providing a structure and guidance in their lives. The effects of a supportive school climate can be seen in the example of Antonio.

> Antonio took more interest in subjects taught by teachers who were warm, concerned and supportive. He was nine years old and in fourth grade when one such teacher learned from his classmate that his father was an innocent stabbing-victim in a street brawl. She asked Antonio in class how his father was and he tearfully narrated what happened. Antonio was afraid that his father would die and he felt consoled by her concern and his classmates' silent support. It inspired him to carry on with his studies and his work in the midst of the family crisis.

9.4 Conclusion

The street children included in this study have been identified as resilient by NGO involved in helping them and their families. These are the children who have been able to maintain a steady and productive development despite the adversities of working in the streets. The search for what makes each one of them resilient shows a pool of traits universally shared by resilient people. In many cases, street children have dysfunctional families that, to begin with, push them to the adversities of life in the streets. Understanding the resilience of many of these children should help create interventions that should not only focus on supplying what is deficient in their lives but should equally emphasize efforts at enhancing their resilience. There is need for further studies on how helping agencies, the schools, the families and the rest of the street children's community could interact in a manner that can facilitate the development and strengthening of resilient traits among these children.

There is evidence in research literature that adverse life conditions breed a host of maladaptive behaviors among which is substance abuse. On the other hand, studies of resilient individuals demonstrate good adaptive outcomes in the face of adversities. Furthermore, there is evidence that resilience can be systematically enhanced and nurtured, especially during the developmental years of childhood and adolescence, through proactive interventions. Examples of such interventions include the life skills program and effective parenting training. Resilience—a product of dynamic interaction between individual vulnerabilities and positive traits, between risk and protective factors in the environment—empowers the individual to make sensible choices during critical moments in life. Such resilience may be the important element in changing the trajectory of the lives of street children.

References

Bandura, A. (1977). *Social learning theory*. Englewood Ciffs, NJ: Prentice Hall.

Biafora, F. A., Warheit, G. L., Vega, W. A., Gil, A. G. (1994). Stressful life events and changes in substance abuse among a multiracial/ethnic sample of adolescent boys.

Bleuler, M. (1978). *The Schizophrenic disorders*. New haven, CT: Yale University Pres.

de Wilde, E. J., Kienhorst, I. E. W. M., Diekstra, R. F. W., & Wolfers, W. G. G. (1992). The relationship between adolescent suicidal behavior and life events in childhood and adolescence. *American Journal of Psychiatry, 149*, 45–51.

Duncan, D. F. (1977). Life stress as a precursor to adolescent drug dependence. *International Journal of Addiction, 12*, 1047–1056.

Freidrich, W., Reams, R., & Jacobs, J. (1982). Depression and suicidal ideation in early adolescent. *Journal of Youth and Adolescence, 11*, 403–407.

Grothberg, E. (1995). *The international resilience project*. Resilience: Research, Application, and Policy, Civitan International Research Center, University of Alabama at Birmingham, Alabama, U.S.A. resilnet.uiuc.edu/library/grotb95a.html

Masten, A. S., & Powell, J. L. (2003). A resilience framework for research, policy, and practice. In S. S. Luthar (Ed.), *Resilience and vulnerability: Adaptation in the context of childhood adversities*. New York, NY: Cambridge University Press.

Neiman, L. (1988). A critical review of resilience literature and its relevance to homeless children. *Children's Environments Quarterly, 5*, 17–25.

O' Sullivan, C. M. (1991). The relationship between childhood mentors and resilience in adult children of alcoholics. *Family Dynamics of Addiction Quarterly, 1*(4), 49–49.

Rhodes, J. E. & Jason, L. A. (1990). A social stress model of substance abuse. *Journal of Consulting and Clinical Psychology, 58*(4), 395–401.

Richmond, J. B. & Beardslee, W. R. (1988). Resilience: Research and practical applications for pediatricians. *Journal of Developmental and Behavioral Pediatrics, 9*(3), 157–163.

Sameroff, A. J., & Mckenzie, M. (2003). Research strategies for capturing transactional models of development: The limit of the possible. *Development and Psychopathology, 15*, 613–640.

Department of Social Welfare and Development (DSWD), United Nations Children Fund (UNICEF). (1988). The Situation of Street Children in Ten Cities.

The Council of the Welfare of Children (CWL). (2006). The situation of Children in the Philippines.

Turner, S. Norman, E., & Zunz, S. (1993). From risk to resilience, a paradigm shift, a literature review and annotated bibiliography. Fordham University Graduate School of Social Sciences.

Werner, E. E. (1994). Overcoming the odds. *Journal of Developmental and Behavioral Pediatrics, 15*(2), 131–136.

Wolff, S. (1995). The concept of resilience. *Australian and New Zealand Journal of Psychiatry, 29*(4), 565–574.

Chapter 10
Cyberage and Child Mental Health

Jillian Sok Teng Boon and Daniel Shuen Sheng Fung

Abstract Most people will have no qualms about visiting a hospital for medical attention for a physical ailment but may have concerns about visiting a hospital for mental health issues. The stigma in mental health is prevalent despite improved healthcare services and efforts to educate the public. Due to the prevalence of mental health disorders, they should be targeted by population-based interventions. In Singapore, a national program was developed to address mental health issues by working across the health and education sectors. This was done using a community team called Response, Early Assessment and Intervention in Community Mental Health (REACH), which was regionally deployed. REACH provided early identification of emotional and behavioral difficulties through assessment, intervention, and training to school counselors and relevant community agencies. Leveraging on the network that REACH developed, technology has created novel and exciting alternative approaches to traditional heathcare delivery models. Serious games, a classification of video games with objectives other than entertainment, such as learning and performing desirable behaviors and skills have been increasingly explored. Recent studies have shown some of the benefits of serious games and their abilities for building positive therapeutic relationships. Essentially, game technology holds potential promise in delivering skills and knowledge to children using interactive features, simulations, and immersive

J.S.T. Boon · D.S.S. Fung
Department of Child and Adolescent Psychiatry, Institute of Mental Health, Singapore, Singapore
e-mail: jillian_st_boon@imh.com.sg

D.S.S. Fung (✉)
Yong Loo Lin School of Medicine, Singapore, Singapore
e-mail: Daniel_fung@imh.com.sg

D.S.S. Fung
Duke-NUS Graduate Medical School, Singapore, Singapore

D.S.S. Fung
Lee Kong Chian School of Medicine, Nanyang Technological University, Singapore, Singapore

S. Malhotra and P. Santosh (eds.), *Child and Adolescent Psychiatry*,
DOI 10.1007/978-81-322-3619-1_10

environments. This means that the power of treatment can be readily accessed through downloading applications onto any mobile device. Efforts to modify traditional face-to-face psychological interventions by leveraging on game-based environments can enhance existing mental health services.

Keywords Community mental health · Games · Children · Adolescents · Population mental health · Serious games · Gamification

10.1 Introduction

The term cyberage refers to the high technology era that modern living is now part of. It refers to the regular use of computers in all its forms, from the desktop personal computers that function as work and home tools to the mobile and other portable devices that assist us in daily living. We hope to describe the impact of this technologically advanced world on the practice of mental healthcare and in particular how we evaluate and treat mental health disorders in children. We will provide a brief history of the development of population mental health and the use of computers as enablers in this process. We will explain the concept of serious games and its use in mental health and we will provide a brief description of examples in Singapore.

10.2 The Mental Health Label

Stigma is described by the Webster Merriam dictionary as "a mark of shame or discredit." Research has suggested that the stigma of mental health disorders can significantly impact on treatment and individual engagement (Mueller et al. 2012). Perceived dangerousness of individuals with mental health disorders and skepticism toward medication are likely to influence an individual's decision to seek help. Although information can now be easily accessed and readily available, the public opinion of mental health disorders is still poor due to the lack of scientific information published by the media (Barkley et al. 2002). The importance of properly curated medical information that is accurate, up to date and evidence based is necessary to overcome misinformation that leads to stigma.

10.3 Mental Health Prevalence and the Treatment Gap

The prevalence of mental health disorders has been estimated to be as high as 20 % (Steel et al. 2014; SAMHSA 2013). Emotional disorders, such as anxiety and depression, are probably the most common. However, more serious disorders such as schizophrenia and bipolar disorder can affect up to 1 % of the population (Perälä et al. 2007). These numbers are consistent across many countries and give rise to a treatment gap between identifiable problems and the access to help. Treatment gaps can be very large and represent a public health challenge for both developed and developing countries. The World Health Organisation (2011) has indicated that the Mental Health Gap as a critical issue for health authorities to address.

In order to bridge the treatment gap, there is a need to take a different approach to managing disorders. Traditional mental health approaches focus on developing clinical services based in hospitals with a high concentration of specialist clinicians (physicians, psychologists, nurse, and other professional staff) operating in a face-to-face consultation approach. These approaches cannot meet the treatment gap which will require a systems-based population approach. Population health approaches focus on the health of entire populations and the strategies for improving health outcomes (Kindig and Stoddart 2003). Ultimately, the goal of population health is to target the determinants of health via government policies and strategies, some of which are not within the traditional mandate of health (Kindig et al. 2008). Traditional systems focus on illness and episodic care but do not consider the needs of entire populations. This results in uneven eventual care and difficulties in preventing serious illness from occurring (Lynn et al. 2007). The importance of national strategies to improve population outcomes cannot be underestimated.

10.4 Community Mental Health

Recognizing the importance of population-based approaches, governments have been developing community-based services that bring healthcare within easy reach of individuals and families. This includes making people more aware of common disorders. Health promotion has replaced approaches that focus predominantly on prevention of illnesses. Many of such approaches focus on developing healthy lifestyles such as improving nutrition, regular exercise for physical fitness, reducing smoking in the population and managing stress by improving emotional resilience (Prochaska and DiClemente 1983). Many countries also organized community mental health efforts by upskilling primary care physicians and family practitioners to be able to identify and treat common high prevalence mental health disorders, such as anxiety and depression. Use of technology to supplement these systems is rapidly increasing. For public education, web portals, social media, and mobile applications have grown exponentially. Many of these educational portals (and books) are now available online and often in the public domain. Assessments in mental health practice often include a technological element. Standard assessment batteries have online or standalone versions which allow self-assessment and preclinical self-evaluations. Intelligence testing and other psychoeduational and cognitive batteries have all gone into electronic versions. Interventions are also taking on electronic significance. Electronic cognitive behavior therapy (eCBT) is one common example of such enablers to illness prevention and treatment (Cavanagh and Shapiro 2004). Mobile applications on the ubiquitous cellular phone (which today are more like high powered computers on the go) have taken treatment into the realm of smart monitoring with wearable sensors either connected to the phone or as an accessory device (like a smart watch or band).

10.5 Community Mental Health Programme in Singapore

Singapore developed a healthy lifestyle approach to health promotion in 1992 and set up the Health Promotion Board in 1996 to drive this effort. Mental health promotion was targeted as an arm of this healthy lifestyle campaign and for several years focused on knowledge awareness and the risk reduction of high burden mental health disorders such as schizophrenia and depression (Toh et al. 2002). These efforts were jointly developed by the Health Promotion Board and the Institute of Mental Health, the national center for the treatment of mental health disorders. The National Committee for Mental Health was coordinated in 2005 that lead to the formation of a National Mental Health Blueprint in 2007. It was recognized that a national strategy was necessary to maintain good mental health, identify mental health disorders early and establish a comprehensive intervention program in both educational and healthcare settings. The initial focus of the Blueprint for children and adolescents was in the school system, as education is compulsory and schools form an obvious base for preventative as well as early intervention efforts. This was provided through a community team called Response, Early Assessment and Intervention in Community Mental Health (REACH), which was regionally deployed (Fung et al. 2013).

The partnership between the Ministries of Health and Education is school-centered and progressively implemented in 360 mainstream and 20 special schools throughout Singapore over 5 years. The REACH teams form the framework for early identification of emotional and behavioral difficulties. The REACH team has trained 386 school counselors in child mental health topics, thus increasing the counselors' capability in detecting, assessing, and managing affected students. With training, the counselors were also able to identify students requiring tertiary care. Similarly, school staff were taught to identify and manage problems by the counselor. Primary care physicians and social service agencies within the school's vicinity were similarly engaged to form a network of community support for students and families. Parent support groups from schools as well as national disease support groups were included in to improve understanding and knowledge transfer.

The REACH program showed that a national preventative and early intervention system could be implemented. The initial implementation showed that a number of clinically relevant questions have emerged; an almost equal number of behavioral and emotional disorders were assessed suggesting that anxiety and depression were clearly underdiagnosed. This potential treatment gap between what was being seen and what was prevalent in the population suggested the need for some form of screening at school entry. Similiarly, a need for research informing on how health screening could be conducted in schools. However, as in other areas of the world, there is a pressing need for early prevention programs even before school entry. The empirical base for Singaporean mental health services is drawn largely from Western studies and there is a need to examine the determinants of risk and resilience within this unique Asian setting. The presence of a strong extended Singaporean family, with culturally distinct family practices, such as a "confinement period" for 30 days following the birth of a child, and an emphasis on academic success are a few examples of the influences facing Singaporean children. Singapore is one of several East Asian countries that represent the most technologically advanced societies with high penetration of smart technology in daily use and high gaming amongst the young. Singapore is therefore an ideal site for development of technology enabled population mental health.

10.6 E-Interventions in Population Mental Health

Computers, the Internet and mobile communication devices now permeate every aspect of our lives. In 2012, there are nearly 2.1 billion Internet users (or approximately 30.2 %) of the world's population around the globe (Fung and Lim-Ashworth 2012). In Singapore, the number of Internet users doubled from 35 to 71.1 % of the population over a 10 year period between 2000 and 2010. (World Bank 2010). Mobile phones are used by nearly 80 % of the world's population and out of these a quarter of them are smart phone users. The development of technology has impacted various industries in different ways. Some industries like retail and banking have become completely technology-driven allowing improved accessibility, rapid information exchange, and better efficiency and increasing value for customers. Other industries like healthcare and education continue to view technology with some concern and teachers and doctors continue to operate within traditional boundaries of the classroom and hospitals. But this is changing.

The mental healthcare industry is traditionally focused on a relationship between a clinical specialists armed with knowledge with his patient who does not have that knowledge base. This one to one relational treatment puts a heavy burden on specialized resources that can only attend to a limited number of patients a day. The use of technology to improve this process is relatively unknown. The concern that clinicians have is that technology can only hinder this relationship and reduce the recovery process. Most psychological therapies do not follow a stringent therapeutic plan but require dynamic face to face interactions between clinicians and patients on a regular basis (Wahle and Kowatsch 2014). In essence, technology appears to dehumanize the clinical process yet recent studies have suggested that technology can treat some pervasive mental disorders, such as depression, as effectively as traditional face-to-face therapy (Wagner et al. 2014).

In addition, the use of technology is able to lower individual's reservation toward mental health treatment and the social stigma attached to it (Clement et al. 2014).

Telemedicine, a term used interchangeable with Telehealth, is an example of the use of teleconferencing through the internet (Nelson et al. 2013). This enables patients who are unable to access specialists in the community due to various physical, socioeconomic, linguistic, and cultural backgrounds. Telehealth encompasses a wide range tools to compliment the patient's needs (US Department of Health and Human Services 2015). These tools include—online therapy, e-health resources, mobile applications, health forums, and online support groups. Studies have shown that videoconferencing provided effective in-person care that extends beyond age, outcomes, satisfaction for single consultation, assessment, or follow ups (Nelson et al. 2013).

Within the healthcare industry, mobile devices are used for treatment monitoring, appointment reminders, health promotion, health surveys, patient record keeping and, delivery of patient services via video or audio systems (WHO 2011). Software applications are constantly being developed for providing mental healthcare globally (Ly et al. 2014). The cost of mobile devices are inexpensive compared to that of a whole computer system and allows greater portability with less power requirements. This would be advantageous to communities from lower socioeconomic backgrounds. In addition, development of mobile applications is cheaper than that of computer systems and programs (Hilty et al. 2013).

When reaching out to the young who are at risk of mental health disorders, we need to identify how they connect with others and get information. Today's children enjoy interactive ways of learning and are often exposed to some form of technological device at a young age (e.g., learning new words, picture books, nursery rhyme songs with accompanied animations). They learn to seek out information and knowledge through the Internet and mobile devices (Ellis et al. 2012). This changes the way information is being accessed from young. Traditionally, individuals go to the doctor when they are unwell. The new generation will be able to look online for help, discuss in online forums to identify common symptoms and difficulties, look up medication side effects, all without having to step into the doctor's office. The Pew Research Center (Raine et al. 2012) report found that over 31 % of mobile phone users have used their devices to access health related information through their smartphones. This was also observed with caregivers who are critical elements in the support network of patients. Due to the stigma of mental healthcare, and the reluctance to see mental health professionals, this easy accessibility allows more rapid help seeking behaviors through the Internet or via mobile applications. This is an opportunity to allow for self-education, early identification, and early intervention. The main caveat is that the information is well curated and able to outreach the population easily.

10.7 Games and Their Purposes

Gamification is the concept of applying game design thinking to nongame applications to make them fun and engaging (Derryberry 2007). A core gamification strategy is to reward players who accomplish the desired task. Rewards, points, achievement badges, or levels are some of the motivation techniques used in gamification. Making tangible rewards for the accomplishment of tasks are ways of motivating players. Allowing meaningful choices, increasing challenges, and adding narratives are some other techniques used in this approach.

Gamification is an emerging form of 'purposeful' gaming sometimes being called serious games, in which games are being utilized beyond entertainment functions. McCallum defined serious games as "a term used to describe the development of games specifically designed to achieve some change in the player" (McCallum 2012). This change could be in knowledge, attitude, physical ability, cognitive ability, health, or mental wellbeing. This distinguishes them from games that have been designed for entertainment, where changes in the player are merely side effects.

Serious games can be pleasurable and entertaining but their primary purpose is often to train, investigate or educate, often through problem solving. Serious games can be classified into different types (Noor et al. 2012). These terms are often used loosely in combination with an underlying learning objective. Typically, video game genres are classified according to the type of gameplay, such as sports, shooters, etc. In contrast, serious games are often categorized by their purpose. Edutainment is a blend of education and entertainment. Games-based learning or game learning has distinct learning objectives which balance the subject matter with the gameplay and the ability of the player to retain and apply this to the real world (Alvarez and Rampnoux 2007). Simulation games are used for the practice and acquisition of various skills such as simulation for driving different vehicles (cars, trains, airplanes; e.g., FlightGear); simulation of managing of businesses or industries (e.g., Transport Tycoon). Games for Health refers to games for psychological and rehabilitation purposes (Putnam and Chong 2008). In this category, therapy is made accessible to patients without actually seeing a therapist. This can apply to physical rehabilitation as well as psychosocial training. Exergaming are games that incorporate elements of exercise (Alvarez and Rampnoux 2007) and incorporate new ways of playing and recreate movements in sports, leisure, and healthy exercises. Art Games are games used to express artistic ideas or art. Productivity gaming are games which award points for accomplished real-world organizational/ planning related tasks, e.g., to-do lists (Alvarez and Rampnoux 2007). Advergames uses games for advertising and include numerous different ways such as interactive video games that enable the user to be constantly exposed to the advertised brand or product as well as product placement or banners in-game (Alvarez and Rampnoux 2007).

With the array of serious games possibilities, the technology can provide a platform for various industries to reach the population.

10.8 Serious Games in Mental Health

The application of serious games to mental health would allow users to use knowledge, intervention, or have assessments done regardless of time and settings. Additionally, these are inexpensive as compared to the traditional desktop or laptop. A good proportion of patients with mental illness own mobile devices. A recent survey conducted in a Chicago outpatient psychiatry clinic suggested that 70 % of 100 patients owned a smart phone, of these, 50 % were willing to download mobile applications to monitor their mental health status (Torous et al. 2014). There are a large number of applications which look into mood tracking and variations of CBT in both the Apple app store (for Apple devices) and Google play (for Android devices). Chan et al. (2014) ran a basic search of the number of available applications for specific disorders. Table 10.1 presents the number of available mobile applications in Apple and Android devices.

With these statistics in mind, mobile applications can be used as an extension of psychotherapy to help patients to monitor their own mental health status—such as mood, medication adherence, addictions, activity, and movement tracking (Harrison et al. 2011). In the United States, the use of mobile applications for mental health is widely seen in the Veterans Administration, one of the largest providers of healthcare services for the country (US Department of Veterans Affairs 2015a, b). The National Center for Telehealth and technology have piloted and released applications to empower caregivers, health providers, and patients. These include treatment of posttraumatic stress disorder (PTSD) symptom tracking with direct integration into their own electronic medical records. There are also applications that help with prolonged exposure tasks in treatment for PTSD.CBT applications, such as CBT-I Coach which allows individuals to document an electronic diary of their sleep, activity coupled with CBT techniques and psychoeducation (US Department of Veterans Affairs 2015a, b). Researchers in Sweden have also

Table 10.1 Available mobile applications for specific mental health disorders (As of January 2014), Chan et al. (2014) (Adapted)

Search terms	Google Play	iOS Apple Store	Examples
Depression	1615	586	Sleep Cycle—helps improve your sleep cycle
Anxiety	1296	775	Health through Breath—teaches breathing techniques
Schizophrenia	67	20	Big White Wall—app for communal sharing to reduce stigma
Bipolar	151	90	Optimism—app for tracking moods and trggers
Psychiatry	168	149	PTSD Coach—app for self-assessment and tracking of symptoms
Alcoholism	1911	146	12 Steps AA Companion—Alcoholics Anonymous a helpful app developed by AA

included behavioral activation and mindfulness techniques in smartphone applications for patients with depression (Ly et al. 2014).

10.9 Serious Games in Population Mental Health

The concerted use of serious games as part of a national strategy for population mental health will now be described. Singapore has developed a national strategy for providing mental health support for schools through the REACH program. This program provides a network of support for school counselors to identify and intervene for those at risk of and suffering mental health disorders early. The development of technology to support the program is needed for widespread adoption and implementation. The basis of this strategy is to adopt a disruptive and innovative process in three main areas: (1) Creating a curated resource for mental health disorders typically occurring in school children that targets school personnel, parents, and children themselves; (2) Self-education and treatment resources that target entire student populations with surreptitious aid for those with significant mental health disorders and; (3) Technology enabled interventions that improve on traditional treatment methods and are engaging for children.

10.10 Reaching Out Beyond the Clinic: (Roc-N-Ash) Web Portal

Attention deficit hyperactivity disorder (ADHD) and Anxiety disorders are two of the most common mental health disorders seen at our child guidance clinics (CGC). However, due to limited professional manpower resources, there is often a long wait time before children with these disorders receive treatment at a specialist clinic. Hence, ROC-N-ASH, (http://www.roc-n-ash.com) was developed as part of the solution to provide early intervention to children with ADHD and Anxiety disorders.

ROC-N-ASH involved a tripartite collaboration between mental health professionals, infocomm experts, and e-Learning/gaming professionals. It was developed as an innovative and holistic IT system to manage the mental wellness of the child and adolescent. ROC-N-ASH enables healthcare professionals to leverage on the system to promote mental wellness and facilitate early detection and intervention for children and adolescents at risk of mental health disorders. This also encouraged the involvement of schools and caregivers with greater empowerment of knowledge of mental disorders and treatment strategies.

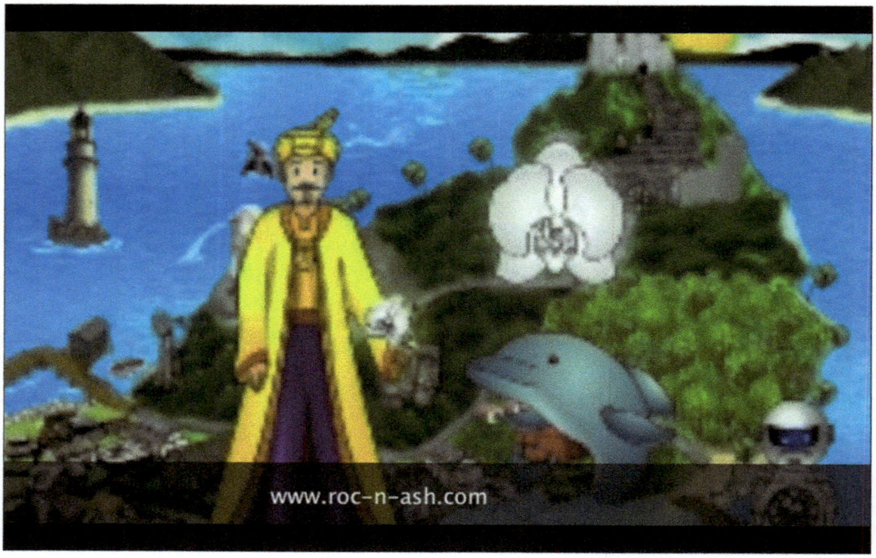

The ROC-N-ASH portal is an interactive system with information courseware on ADHD and childhood anxiety, books for purchase, events announcements, and therapeutic games. The information courseware was publically accessible online, aimed to increase knowledge of ADHD and anxiety disorders and strategies on managing child and adolescent with such disorders were provided at no cost. Specifically, the ADHD module comprises of a screening tool that helps parents and school personnel to screen for the risk of inattention and/or hyperactivity-impulsivity symptoms and its severity. The public can also purchase mental health related books, be informed of upcoming mental health public forums and workshops and register online through the portal. The therapeutic games immerse the child and adolescent in the role of an avatar, earning gold coins, and completing missions of various stages. One such example is a game called 'Saving Loumba' which is a literacy software designed to help ADHD child and adolescent with literacy difficulties learn ways to concentrate better and be less impulsive while engaged in reading and spelling activities. Computer Assisted Strategies To Lessen Excessive Anxiety in Children (CASTLE-AC) teaches child and adolescent skills in managing their anxiety through missions and quests to defeat anxiety monsters. Schools can subscribe to the games and can be trained on the use of the program. The development of ROC-N-ASH also serves to be a resource to the REACH community teams as part of a population-based approach. The website was active for 7 years and has been retired as use of web portal is increasingly being replaced by mobile applications. The information section of the portal had been ported onto the REACH portal (www.reachforstudents.com).

10.11 Specific Population-Based Game for Managing Anger: RegnaTales

Social and problem-solving skills training (SPSST) was developed as part of the treatment available for children with ADHD and anger (Ooi et al. 2007). A computer-based game was developed as part of an ongoing PhD student dissertation using SPSST concepts. The software prototype has undergone preliminary evaluation. The first part of the study involved 12 students (6 boys and 6 girls) of a primary school (aged 10 years) and the goal was to obtain the students' views on the usability and playability of the prototype. The students felt that the prototype was enjoyable and they could learn useful concepts for anger management (Tan et al. 2010). In April 2011, the study team obtained funding to further develop the mobile application version of the SPSST. The team partnered a local gaming company to develop the mobile application game, "RegnaTales." The main objective of this game is for the player to learn social responsibility in an entertaining environment with specific skills training in anger management and social communication. Through the use of role playing game (RPG) environments, the player is encouraged to learn skills for identification of feelings, perspective taking, coping skills, empathy, pro-social skills, and problem solving. These skills form the underlying goals of each mission. The missions have been designed to test and reinforce relevant skills on managing anger serendipitously through game play.

RegnaTales is set in a fantasy world with both modern and medieval influences. The balance between the good (Flame) and bad (Shadow) energy is managed by a special machine which is being targeted by the villain on the piece, a dark lord named Abaddon. The protagonist, a young boy/girl depending on the avatar the player chooses, must encounter a series of challenges and skills training in order to save the machine, his/her parents and ultimately the world. The player is supported by various characters in the game who act as guides and helpers to manage his/her emotions as he/she develops increasingly sophisticated anger management skills to battle Abaddon and his minions.

To motivate the player, audio and visual animations are common features throughout the game. Positive or negative game consequences will be awarded when the player manages to fulfill tasks or fail tasks, respectively. Incorporation of skills within the game and assessment of application of these skills are done at every level. These skills include deep breathing (use of the 'wind box'), visualization and, cognitive restructuring (e.g., positive self-talk). To reinforce and encourage the use of these skills, the player has to maintain a reasonable amount of flame energy which is in the toolbar at the bottom of the screen. When the flame energy gets low, the player is prompted to exercise self-care by doing visualization exercises. Flame energy is reduced with concomitant increase in shadow energy when the player exhibits socially inappropriate, aggressive, and impulsive behavior in the game. Reducing flame energy and increasing shadow energy would either slow down or completely interrupt game play. The player has full control of his/her avatar as well as customizations, such as dressing and weapons by earning points within the game.

The goal of developing RegnaTales is to understand how children respond to games, and how games can teach skills without making them overtly educational. This area of research is limited and there is a need for evidence to show its applicability and effectiveness in improving emotional regulation.

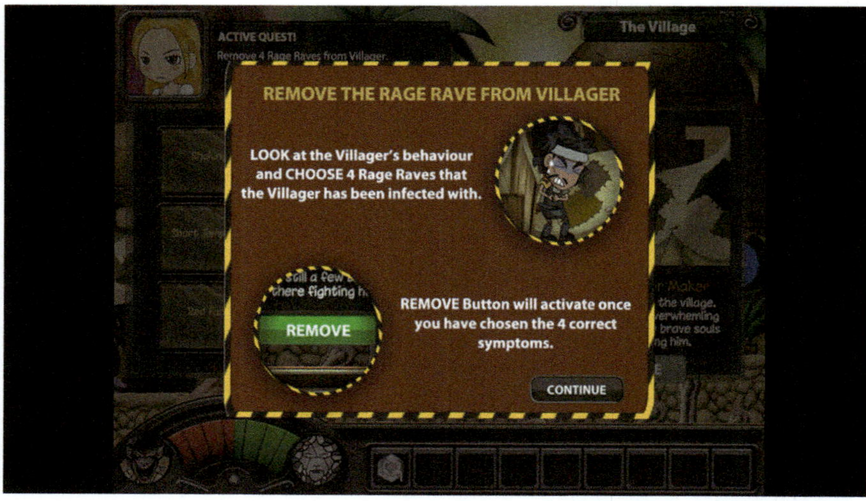
ACTIVE QUEST!
Remove 4 Rage Raves from Villager.
The Village
REMOVE THE RAGE RAVE FROM VILLAGER
LOOK at the Villager's behaviour and CHOOSE 4 Rage Raves that the Villager has been infected with.
REMOVE
REMOVE Button will activate once you have chosen the 4 correct symptoms.
CONTINUE

The next phase of the game development would include pilot testing of the playability of the game applications where children are selected at random to play the game. The app is available in the Apple App Store.

10.12 Technology-Enabled Interventions: BCI and VRET

We describe two examples of using technology to enhance the traditional mental health treatments. The Brain-computer interface (BCI) is the science and technology of devices and systems which directly respond to neural and cognitive processes (Monastra et al. 2005). A development team at the Agency for Science and Technology Research, NUS-Duke Graduate Medical School and the Institute of Mental Health have developed a progressive series of training games using electroencephalogram (EEG)-based BCI. Three-channel EEG signals are recorded from the frontal and parietal positions. These EEG signals first pass through a filter bank to be broken down into various frequency subbands covering the theta, alpha, beta 1, and beta 2 waves. The filtered signals are then sent to the respective spatial filters corresponding to each frequency band, which enhance the detection of information from the brain's electrical rhythm. A parametric model derived through machine learning from the multi-band EEG signals will divide the EEG signals into either attention or inattention states. These states are translated into a score which represents the attention level of the subject (Lim et al. 2012). This is set up in a calibration task in which the subjects have to perform attention and relaxation activities in which their EEG signals are collected. This allows the results to be individualized and personal. As the system makes use of a subject's direct attention to control a game, it works on a feedforward mechanism. Results of a pilot study of 20 subjects with this BCI game demonstrated an improved attention score over 10 weeks rated by both parents and teachers although these scores were not statistically significant when compared with the control group (Lim et al. 2012). A large-scale randomized control trial is currently underway to further investigate this game-based intervention.

Virtual reality exposure therapy (VRET) is an increasingly common treatment for anxiety and specific phobias (Wiederhold and Wiederhold 2000). The emergent use of virtual reality exposure therapy (VRET) has been used to treat anxiety disorders where graduated exposure is required. (Roy et al. 2003). Graduated exposure requires individuals with anxiety to be exposed to anxiety provoking situations in a systematic manner. VRET immerses users in a computer-generated simulation or virtual environment (VE). The program responds to the individual's body gestures through the use of in-built motion sensors. Computer-generated stimulation and VE provides the opportunity for users to be systematically exposed to specific anxiety provoking situations (Pull 2005). These exposure experiences allow the rehearsal of skills learnt during therapy to be applied to the scenario. According to Wilhelm et al. (2005), "VRET compliments the emotion-processing model, which holds that the fear network must be activated through confrontation with threatening stimuli and that new, incompatible information must be added into the emotional network."

Our clinic developed a prototype VRET system and exposure protocol for children with selective mutism. Selective mutism (SM) is a rare condition characterized by a child's anxiety, fear or phobia of having to speak at school or in other social settings. A review of 23 studies on the treatment of SM including psychodynamic, behavioral, and cognitive-behavioral approaches suggested that behavioral and cognitive-behavioral techniques appeared most effective for SM (Cohan et al. 2006). There remains a need for research on treatment models for children with SM. The use of virtual reality exposure therapy (VRET) has increasingly becoming a well-supported alternative to exposure in-vivo in the treatment of anxiety disorders, and is regarded as an extension of the exposure component of behavioral therapy (Powers and Emmelkamp 2007; Morina et al. 2014). Six children, with a clinical diagnosis of SM, were recruited from the outpatient clinic of a psychiatric hospital. They were referred into the study by their attending clinician after completing at least 8 anxiety management psychotherapy sessions. The system consists of a novel interactive subsystem, a large LED display, and a 3D environment rendering computer. The exposure-based protocol required participants to complete five different scenarios in a virtual local-classroom environment. Participants had to interact with the scenarios via gestures or speech which are positively reinforced during the scenarios. All six parents reported a decrease in overall anxiety and more than 60 % of the parents reported a decrease in symptoms related to social phobia across participants. This is consistent with clinical trials, uncontrolled designs, qualitative reviews (Botella et al. 2004; Hoffman et al. 2003; Pull 2005) that suggest VRET as a good treatment option for anxiety.

10.13 Challenges Ahead

One of the most difficult challenges in developing a serious game is the balancing of what is a mental health intervention with what gamers like. Games traditionally leverage on four factors for player engagement, amusement for relaxation and entertainment, curiosity in discovering something new, challenges with a sense of accomplishment and socializing during play. In a serious game, we need to introduce a form factor that fits the four factors but also incorporate the serious objective for the game.

Translating the skills from the manualized social problem-solving skills training program into a game was an uphill task. A lot of the strategies and ideas that were possible translations into a game were hindered by budget or the lack of resources/manpower to work on designing or engineering such missions for children to work on. At the same time, as computer engineers have no training in mental healthcare, their perception of the skills that were to be translated in the games was superficial. This required a lot of supervision and revision in developing the skills training within the game.

Despite the heavy use of smartphones amongst the young, health applications are prevalently accessed and used less. The Pew reported that less than one in five smartphone users had an application to track mood or sleep and only 2 % used applications for tracking use of medication, and treatment management. The low and slow absorption of healthcare mobile applications exemplify the need for change in treatment and management means for patients and by providers.

Socioeconomic status and technology literacy also hinder other groups from using mobile applications and devices. Some of these are age related—elderly where a large proportion of their lives were without the use of the internet (Parish and Yellowlees 2014). Thus, penetration of mobile application with certain populations may not be as effective and widespread.

In the research field, a lot of the studies focused on older technologies. These included the use of telephones, text messaging and video recorders (Free et al. 2013). Fewer clinical trials published on smartphone applications. This has resulted in lesser reliability on smartphone applications and greater difficulty in securing funding or requesting for funding due to the small pool of available evidence-based serious games.

It is agreed by many that game technology holds potential promise in delivering skills and knowledge to children as children find the interactive features, simulations, and immersive environments in games both enticing and engaging (Gunter et al. 2008). Indeed the growth in gaming technology has created novel and exciting alternative approaches to traditional delivery methods to meet needs of a newer generation of children with their preference for emerging game technologies (Shaffer et al. 2005). The game world is known to provide the player with a relatively "safe" environment to practice behaviors in role-play situations, rule learning, and repetition of tasks (Parsons and Mitchell 2002). Given the potential advantages and benefits that can be gained in using games for addressing the social and emotional problems encountered by children, it is worthwhile to modify traditional face-to-face psychological interventions by leveraging on opportunities available in the game-based environment.

10.14 Moving Forward—Future of Mental Health in the Cyberage

The future for technology in mental health lies in three main areas: The first is its application in self-care. Technology can enable a lay person to have clinical decision support in terms of education, identification of risk, and personalized self-monitoring of healthcare indices. The second is in supporting healthcare professionals in the evaluation of a patient. Instead of traditional evaluations often done in combination with patient and caregiver providing information in the form of interviews and rating scales, such evaluations can be either done remotely or obtained surreptitiously through the activities of daily living. The third area is the inclusion of treatment into mainstream activities in which serious games are fast becoming a useful platform. Mental health treatments could be administered into (as far as possible) everyday life. These three developmental areas are an increasing reality in a future cyberage which we believe is less science fiction and more science fact, provided that resources are given in this direction.

References

Alvarez, J., & Rampnoux, O. (2007, April). Serious game: Just a question of posture? *Conference in Artificial & Ambient Intelligence, AISB'07* (p. 420–423), Newcastle, UK.

Barkley, R. A., Fischer, M., Smallish, L., & Fletcher, K. (2002). The persistence of attention deficit hyperactivity disorder into young adulthood as a function of reporting source ad definition of disorder. *Journal of Abnormal Psychology, 111*(2), 279.

Botella, C., Quero, S., Banos, R. M., Perpina, C., Garcia Palacios, A., & Riva, G. (2004). Virtual reality and psychotherapy. *Studies in Health Technology and Informatics, 99*, 37–54.

Cavanagh, K., & Shapiro, D. A. (2004). Computer treatment for common mental health problems. *Journal of Clinical Psychology, 60*(3), 239–251.

Chan, S. R., Torous, J., Hinton, L., & Yellowlees, P. (2014). Mobile tele-mental health: Increasing applications and a move to hybrid models of care. *Healthcare, 2*, 220–233.

Clement, S. Schauman, O., Graham, T., Maggioni, F., Evans-Lacko, S., Bezborodovs, N., et al. (2014). What is the impact of mental health-related stigma on help-seeking? A systemic review of quantitative and qualitative studies, *Psychological Medicine (FirstView)* (pp. 1–17).

Cohan, S. L., Chavira, D. A., & Stein, M. B. (2006). Psychosocial treatments for children with selective mutism: A critical evaluation of the literature from 1990–2005. *Journal of Child Psychology and Psychiatry, 47*(11), 1085–1097.

Derryberry, A. (2007). Serious games: Online games for learning. http://www.imserious.net. Accessed May 15, 2015.

Ellis, L. A., Collin, P., Davenport, T. A., Hurley, P. J., Burns, J. M., & Hickie, I. B. (2012). Young men, mentalhealth, and technology: Implications for service design and delivery in the digital age. *Journal of Medical Internet Research, 14*, e160.

Evans, R., & Stoddart, G. C. (1990). Producing health, consuming health care. *Social Science and Medicine, 33*, 1347–1363.

Free, C., Phillips, G., Watson, L., Galli, L., Felix, L., Edwards, P., et al. (2013). The effectiveness of mobile-health technologies to improve health care service delivery processes: A systematic review and meta-analysis. *PLOS Medicine, 10*, e1001363.

Fung, D. S. S., & Lim-Ashworth, S. J. N. (2012). Opening minds: The use of technology to provide a personalized population based mental health programme. *Asia Pacific Biotech News, 16*(2), 35–37.

Fung, D., Ong, L. P., Tay, S. L., & Sim, W. H. (2013). *REACH Chronicles, a community mental health model for children and adolescents in Singapore*. Singapore: World Scientific.

Gamification. [Online]. Available: http://gamification.org/wiki/Gamification. Accessed Wednesday 19, 2015.

Gunter, G., Kenny, R., & Vick, E. (2008). Taking educational games seriously: Using the retain model to design endogenous fantasy into standalone educational games. *Educational Technology Research and Development, 56*, 511–537.

Harrison, V., Proudfoot, J., Wee, P. P., Parker, G., Pavlovic, D. H., & Manicavasagar, V. (2011). Mobilemental health: Review of the emerging field and proof of concept study. *Journal of Mental Health, 20*, 509–524.

Hilty, D. M., Ferrer, D. C., Parish, M. B., Johnston, B., Callahan, E. J., & Yellowlees, P. M. (2013). The effectiveness of telemental health: A 2013 review. *Telemedicine and e-Health, 19*, 444–454.

Hoffman, H., Garcia-Palacios, A., Carlin, A., Furness, T., & Botella-Arbona, C. (2003). Interfaces that heal: Coupling real and virtual objects to treat spider phobia. *International Journal of Human– Computer Interaction, 16*, 283–300.

Kindig, D., Asada, Y., & Booske, B. (2008). A population health framework for setting national and state health goals. *JAMA, 299*, 2081–2083.

Kindig, D. A., & Stoddart, G. (2003). What is population health? *American Journal of Public Health, 93*, 366–369.

Lee, J. J., & Hammer, J. (2011). Gamification in education: What, how, why bother? *Academic Exchange Quarterly, 15*(2), [Online]. Available: http://www.gamifyingeducation.org/files/Lee-Hammer-AEQ-2011.pdf. Accessed: Tuesday 21, 2013.

Lim, C. G., Lee, T. S., Guan, C., Fung, D. S. S., Zhao, Y., Teng, S. S. W., et al. (2012). A brain-computer interface based attention training program for treating attention deficit hyperactivity disorder. *PLoS ONE, 7*(10), e46692.

Ly, K. H., Trüschel, A., Jarl, L., Magnusson, S., Windahl, T., Johansson, R., et al. (2014). Behavioural activation versus mindfulness-based guided self-help treatment administered through a smartphone application: A randomised controlled trial. *BMJ Open, 4*, p. e003440.

Lynn, J., Straube, B. M., Bell, K. M., Jencks, S. F., & Kambic, R. T. (2007). Using population segmentation to provide better health care for all: The "bridges to health" model. *The Milbank Quarterly, 85*(2), 185–208. doi:10.1111/j.1468-0009.2007.00483.x.

McCallum, S. (2012). Gamification and serious games for personalized health. *Student Health Technology Information, 177*, 85–96.

Monastra, V. J., Lynn, S., Linden, M., Lubar, J. F., Gruzelier, J., & LaVaque, T. J., (2005). Electroencephalographic biofeedback in the treatment of attention-deficit/hyperactivity disorder. *Applied Psychophysiology and Biofeedback, 30*(2), June, 2005.

Morina, N., Brinkman, W.-P., Hawtanto, D., & Emmelkamp, P. M. G. (2014). Sense of presence and anxiety during virtual social interactions between a human and virtual humans. *Peer Journal, 2*, e337. doi:10.7717/peerj.

Mueller, A. K., Fuermaier, A. B., Koerts, J., & Tucha, L. (2012). Stigma in attention deficit hyperactivity disorder. *ADHD Attention Deficit and Hyperactivity Disorders, 4*(3), 101–114.

Nelson, E.-L., Davis, K., & Velasquez, S. E. (2013). Ethical considerations in providing mental health services over video teleconferencing. In C. Turvey, & K. M. Myers, (Eds.) *Telemental health: Clinical, technical, and administrative foundations for evidence-based practice* (pp. 47–62), London, UK: Elsevier. Patrick Stack. History of Video Game Consoles. Time Magazine website 2005.

Noor, H. A. M., Shahbodin, F., & Naim, C. P. (2012). Serious game for autism children: Review of literature. *World Academy of Science, Engineering and Technology, 64*, 647–652.

Parish, M. B., & Yellowlees, P. (2014). The rise of person-centered healthcare and the influence of health informatics and social network applications on mental health care. In M. Lech, I. Song, P. Yellowlees, & J. Diederich (Eds.), *Mental health informatics* (Vol. 491) Berlin, Heidelberg: Springer.

Ooi, Y. P., Ang, R. P., Fung, D. S. S., Wong, G., & Cai, Y. (2007). Effects of CBT on children with disruptive behavior disorders: Findings from a Singapore study. *ASEAN Journal of Psychiatry, 8*, 71–81.

Parsons, S., & Mitchell, P. (2002). The potential of virtual reality in social skills training for people with autistic spectrum disorders. *Journal of Intellectual Disability Research, 46*, 430–443.

Perälä, J., Suvisaari, J., Saarni, S. I., Kuoppasalmi, K., Isometsä, E., & Pirkola, S. (2007). Lifetime prevalence of psychotic and bipolar I disorders in a general population. *Archives of General Psychiatry, 64*(1), 19–28.

Powers, M. B., & Emmelkamp, P. M. G. (2007). Virtual reality exposure therapy for anxiety disorders: A meta-analysis. *Journal of Anxiety Disorders, 22*(3), 561–569.

Raine, L., Zuckuhr, K., & Duggan, M. (2012). Mobile connections to libraries. Pew Research Center US Department of Health and Human Services. Telehealth. Available online: http://libraries.pewinternet.org/2012/12/31/mobile-connections-to-libraries/. Accessed on June 23, 2015.

Prochaska, J. O., & DiClemente, C. C. (1983). Stages and processes of self-change of smoking: Toward an integrative model of change. *Journal of Consulting and Clinical Psychology, 51*, 390–395.

Pull, C. B. (Ed.). (2005). Current status of virtual reality exposure therapy in anxiety disorders: Editorial review. *Current Opinion in Psychiatry, 18*, 7–14.

Putnam, C., & Chong, L. (2008). Software and technologies designed for people with autism: What do users want? *ASSETS'08: Proceedings of the 10th International ACM SIGACCESS Conference on Computers and Accessibility* (pp. 3–10). New York, USA: ACM.

Roy, S., Klinger, E., Legeron, P., Lauer, F., Chemin, I., & Nugues, P. (2003). Definition of a vr-based protocol to treat social phobia. *Cyberpsychology and Behavior, 6*, 411–420.

Shaffer, D. W., Squire, K., Halverson, R., & Gee, J. P. (2005). Video games and the future of learning. *Phi Delta Kappan, 87*, 104–111.

Steel, Z., Marnane, C., Iranpour, C., Chey, T., Jackson, J. W, Patel, V. et al. (2014). The global prevalence of common mental disorders: A systematic review and meta-analysis 1980–2013. *International Journal of Epidemiology, 43*(2), 476–493. doi: 10.1093/ije/dyu038. Epub 19 March, 2014.

Substance Abuse and Mental Health Services Administration. (2013). Results from the 2012 National Survey on Drug Use and Health: Mental Health Findings, NSDUH Series H-47, HHS Publication No. (SMA) 13–4805. Rockville, MD: Substance Abuse and Mental Health Services Administration.

Tan, J. L., Goh H. L., Ang, R. P. & Huan, V. (2010). Child-centered interaction in the design of a game for social skills intervention. *Proceedings of the ACM CiE 7th International Conference on Advances in Computer Entertainment Technology*. Taipei, Taiwan.

Torous, J., Friedman, R., & Keshvan, M. (2014). Smartphone ownership and interest in mobile applications to monitor symptoms of mental health conditions. *JMIR mHealth and uHealth, 2*, e2.

Toh, C. M., Chew, S. K., & Tan, C. C. (2002). Prevention and control of non-communicable diseases in Singapore: A review of national health promotion programmes. *Singapore Medical Journal, 43*(7), 333–339.

US Department of Health and Human Services. (2015). Telehealth. Available online: http://www.hrsa.gov/ruralhealth/about/telehealth/. Accessed on 13 May, 2015.

US Department of Veterans Affairs. (2015a). Department of Veterans Affairs (VA). Mobile Health Fact Sheet Final, 2013. Available online: https://mobilehealth.va.gov/sites/default/files/files/VAMobileHealthFactSheet.pdf. Accessed on 13 May, 2015.

US Department of Veterans Affairs. (2015b). Mobile App: CBT-i Coach. Available online: http://www.ptsd.va.gov/public/pages/cbti-coach-app.asp/. Accessed on 13 May, 2015.

Wahle, F., & Kowatsch, T. (2014). Towards the design of evidence-based mental health information systems: A preliminary literature review, *35th International Conference on Information Systems*, Auckland, New Zealand.

Wagner, B., Horn, A. B., & Maercker, A. (2014). Internet-based versus face to face cognitive-behavioral intervention for depression: A randomized controlled trial. *PLoS ONE 8*(7), e62873.

WHO Global Observatory for eHealth. (2011). *mHealth new horizons for health through mobile technologies*. Geneva, Switzerland: World Health Organization.

Wiederhold, B. K., & Wiederhold, M. D. (2000). Lessons learned from 600 virtual reality sessions. *Cyberpsychology and Behavior, 3*, 393–400.

Wilhelm, F. H., Pfaltz, M. C., Gross, J. J., Mauss, I. B., Kim, S. I., & Wiederhold, B. K. (2005). Mechanisms of virtual reality exposure therapy: The role of the behavioral activation and behavioral inhibition systems. *Applied Psychophysiology Biofeedback, 30*, 271–284.

Chapter 11
Childhood Sexual Abuse: Lifting the Veil of Denial

Ruchita Shah and Aakanksha Singh

Abstract The reality and enormity of child and adolescent sexual abuse, especially in the Asian subcontinent had been until recently shrouded by *collective denial* and *a conspiracy of silence*. Child sexual abuse (CSA) in its various forms is alarmingly common. In a 2007 large-scale study undertaken by the Government of India, as many as 53 % of children reported being subjected to one or more forms of sexual abuse, several fold higher than that reflected in legal statistics. In a large number of these cases, the perpetrator is someone in the family or someone responsible for the child's care like a school teacher. Risk factors involved in occurrence of CSA include lower socio-economic status, single parenthood, parental substance use amongst others. The response of the family and community is often that of disbelief, blaming the child and holding her/him responsible, and fear of and actual stigma and ostracism. Such a response coupled with insensitivity towards, anticipated harassment and inadequate protection of victims by concerned agencies and authorities increases the woes of the child. This also often results in under-reporting and 'out of court settlements'. Unfortunately, the psychological impact of sexual abuse on children though unequivocally clear and well documented in the literature, is completely neglected in the aftermath. This is partly due to efforts of the family in protecting itself from social ostracism at the cost of protection and psychological health of the child—*hushing rather than discussing*. Partly, it is due to lack of defined governmental policies and guidelines or its implementation and of trained mental health professionals working in this area. Thus, occurrence of CSA and its consequences are enmeshed in a complex web of many aspects of the child's life and circumstances, societal attitudes, attitude of the government and its agencies, and attitude and commitment of professionals.

R. Shah (✉) · A. Singh
Department of Psychiatry, Post Graduate Institute of Medical Education and Research, Chandigarh, India
e-mail: drruchitashah@gmail.com

A. Singh
e-mail: aakankshapgi@gmail.com

S. Malhotra and P. Santosh (eds.), *Child and Adolescent Psychiatry*,
DOI 10.1007/978-81-322-3619-1_11

In this chapter, epidemiological, clinical and policy-related matters shall be discussed to understand this complex web, particularly in Asian context.

Keywords Asian · Child sexual abuse · Culture · Epidemiology · Laws · Policies · Sociocultural context

11.1 Introduction

Child sexual abuse (CSA) is neither a recent phenomenon nor a rare occurrence. Rather CSA has always existed behind closed doors, "below the surface" (Martin and Silverstone 2013), and at times even socially sanctioned as in the 'Devadasi' system and child marriages in India (Singh et al. 2014) and the 'Deuki' system in Nepal (UNICEF 2001). Till recently, the complex problem of CSA was never discussed in the public domain, but remained a concern of a few professionals and activists. In 2007, the Department of Women and Child Welfare, Government of India undertook a nation-level study (Ministry of Women and Child Development, Government of India [MoWCD, GOI] 2007) on child abuse where more than 12,447 children and adolescents aged 5–18 years were surveyed. Despite certain methodological issues, the study revealed some eye-opening statistics—more than half of the children had faced one or more forms of sexual abuse, with 22 % reporting severe forms of sexual abuse. These findings led the then Hon. Union Minister for Women and Child development to name this phenomenon as a "conspiracy of silence" (MoWCD, GOI 2007). It has been well recognized that CSA bears serious consequences for the health and wellbeing of the individual not only in the immediate aftermath of its occurrence, but also through adulthood. Additionally, it has wider implications for family and society as a whole. Despite this, research suggests that in over 95 % of cases the CSA is never disclosed to authorities (Martin and Silverstone 2013). To understand this phenomenon, it is important to reflect on the contextual factors. Contextual factors are those that work not just at the individual level of victim and perpetrator, but also at the level of family and society in general. Acceptance of and tolerance for violence and abuse towards women and children, shaming of the victim and sexuality as a tabooed subject, are some of these contextual factors. These factors may potentially affect perpetration and disclosure of CSA as well as the response to CSA from various quarters, including health professionals, police and judiciary, who are also part of the larger society. Moreover, the quality and magnitude of response from the professionals and lawmakers and preventive measures through the policymakers may further affect the prevalence and facilitation of disclosure. In other words, CSA needs to be understood in the complex sociocultural context in which it occurs. In this chapter, epidemiological, clinical and policy-related matters shall be discussed with an emphasis on these factors, especially in the Asian context. Needless to say, role of these factors cannot be neatly divided as relevant to prevalence, clinical aspects or law and policy making. Rather, most of these can be expected to be over-arching. Also, role of many of these factors may be hypothetical rather than evidence based. Towards the end of the chapter, it has been discussed how this knowledge can be utilized for prevention of and response to CSA.

11.2 Definition

The World Health Organization (World Health Organization [WHO] 2003) defines CSA as "the involvement of a child in sexual activity that he or she does not fully comprehend, is unable to give informed consent to, or for which the child is not developmentally prepared and cannot give consent, or that violates the laws or social taboos of society. CSA is evidenced by this activity between a child and an adult or another child who by age or development is in a relationship of responsibility, trust or power, the activity being intended to gratify or satisfy the needs of the other person" (p. 75) (WHO 2003). In another definition given by WHO, CSA is defined as 'inappropriate sexual behaviour with a child, acts being committed by a person responsible for the care of a child (for example a baby-sitter, a parent, or a day care provider), or related to the child' (WHO, Updated 2003). Recent understanding of CSA has been more inclusive. Sexual abuse extends to both contact and non-contact activities that result in the sexual gratification of an adult or a significantly older or more mature child/adolescent. Activities that fall under the spectrum of child sexual abuse include penetrative and non-penetrative assault including touching or fondling of genitals, oral acts involving genitalia, sexual exploitation of the child for material gain (prostitution, child pornography), voyeurism, exhibitionism, exposure to sexually explicit talk or material (Protection of Children from Sexual Offences Act [POCSO] 2012) and cybercrimes. Any act that involves coercion, force or the threat of force is also categorized as child sexual abuse. Further, the POCSO Act (2012) labels sexual assault as 'aggravated' if the child is less than 12 years or physically or mentally disabled or if assault is committed more than once or if the perpetrator is someone responsible for the protection of the child including police, hospital staff and relatives. The Criminal Law (Amendment) Act [CLA] (2013) of India has replaced the word rape with 'sexual assault' and includes penetrative as well as non-penetrative sexual activities. Also, the age of consent for consensual sexual activity has been increased to 18 years, and hence any sexual activity involving a woman aged less than 18 (other than in a marital situation) is punishable.

Much disparity exists regarding the age for sexual consent or sexual maturity across countries ranging from 12 or 13 (e.g. Tonga, Spain) to 17 or 18 years (e.g. in many Asian countries, US, Australia) (Graupner 2000) highlighting the sociocultural norms and context of CSA. Despite this, conceptually, when one child is older or developmentally more mature than the other child participating in sexual activity, one child is physically bigger or in a higher social position, or controls resources to which a younger child wants access, threat and coercion are at work (Goodyear-Brown et al. 2012) that may result in CSA.

11.3 Epidemiology—Prevalence, Reporting and Non-disclosure

It is difficult to determine how frequently CSA occurs because of gross under-reporting, methodological differences between studies (Gilbert et al. 2009a, b), and varying definitions of CSA and different populations studied (based on age, e.g. children, adolescents or adults, vulnerability, e.g. street children, in juvenile homes, etc.). Globally, CSA affects more than one out of five females and one in 10 males (Collin-Vézina et al. 2013). In the recent World Mental Health Surveys, sexual abuse was reported to be around 1.6 % (Kessler et al. 2010). A meta-analysis conducted in the year 2009 analyzed 65 studies in 22 countries and estimated an "overall international figure" of sexual abuse in 7.9 % of males and 19.7 % of females before the age of 18 years (Wihbey 2009). According to this meta-analysis, the highest prevalence rate of CSA was seen in Africa (34.4 %), closely followed by that in Asia (23.9 %).

In Asia, studies have been conducted across the continent. The prevalence has varied from 6 % in Hong Kong (Tang 2002) to 41 % for girls and 29.5 % for boys in China (Luo et al. 2008; Song et al. 2014) in individual studies. The United Nations International Children Education Fund (UNICEF) study on Child maltreatment in East Asia and the Pacific (2012) reported that physical contact sexual abuse ranged from 1.7 % in Hong Kong to 11.6 % in the Pacific Islands. In a landmark study from Nepal, trafficking and sexual abuse among street children in Kathmandu were studied. The respondents reported a significantly high frequency (80 %) of sexual exploitation among their friends. The most important forms of sexual abuse faced included masturbation, oral and anal sex. Foreigners/tourists were the prime sexual abusers (66.7 %), followed by the leader of street children (23.8 %) (Subedi 2002). It has been suggested that the growing tourism industry in Asia puts the vulnerable children at risk of CSA perpetrated by the tourists (O'Briain 2008).

Indian studies in this context are especially important because India is home to 19 % of the world's children. In the nation-wide study (MoWCD, GOI 2007) more than 12,447 children aged 5–18 years were surveyed. It was found that about 53 % of these children had faced one or more forms of sexual abuse, with around 22 % being victims of severe forms of sexual abuse. On the other hand, children on street, children at work and children in institutional care reported the highest incidence of sexual assault. Around 17 % of children who had been sexually assaulted fell in the age range of 6–10 years. In half of the cases, abuser was a person known to the child or in a position of trust and responsibility, mainly an uncle or a male cousin (MoWCD, GOI 2007). Similar findings had been reported earlier by the NGO RAHI in 1998 (RAHI 1998). A UNICEF survey from 2005 to 2013 reported that 10 % of Indian girls might have experienced sexual violence when they were 10–14 years of age and 30 % during 15–19 years of age (Ray 2014). In a recent study from Kerala amongst 1614 adolescents (15–19 years) found that 36 % of boys and 35 % of girls had experienced sexual abuse at some point in their lives. Most of the incidents had occurred while using public transport (Krishnakumar et al. 2014). Two other school-based studies in older children and adolescents with sample sizes of 320 and 1060 revealed that the perpetrators were usually relatives, elder siblings and teachers (Deb and Modak 2010; Daral et al. 2016). In another study done among college students, 10 % reported that someone exposed his/her private parts to them, while in 6.4 % of the cases, the perpetrator forced the study participants to expose their private parts (Bhilwar et al. 2015). Around 40 % of Indian children are susceptible to threats like being homeless, trafficking, drug abuse, forced labour and crime (Human Rights Watch 2013); every second child is being exposed to some form of sexual abuse and every fifth child faces critical forms of it (Behere et al. 2013).

On the other hand, the legal statistics might reflect major barriers to disclosure. For example, in India, the number of cases registered under POCSO Act, 2012 from 2012 till 2015 were a little more than 45,000. In other words, CSA cases are either not recognized or reported. This could be because of various reasons. The studies from India lend some information regarding the factors related to non-disclosure of CSA. The MoWCD, GOI (2007) study revealed that across various forms of sexual abuse, more than 70 % of children did not report to anyone and preferred to keep quiet about their vicitmisation. In case of sexual assault, amongst those who reported, the majority of children shared the incident with their parents followed by a sibling (6.7 %), and only 3.4 % children reported the matter to police. Amongst young adults, only 17.24 % were in favour of harsh punishment to the abuser, while the majority, i.e. 51.31 % of felt that the matter should remain within the family or household and only family members should handle the problem. In another study (Bhilwar et al. 2015), a majority informed parents, siblings, friends or teachers. Amongst those who did not inform, around 32 % gave the reason that they were afraid that their parents would be angry, 28 % cited feeling of shame as the main reason for not disclosing. Another 12 % passed off the incident as being unimportant. Since the abuser is usually a person known or even related to the child, the matter is suppressed by the family for fear of disintegration of the family. Further, inadequate communication skills of young or disabled children to report such events, and lack of judgment of a child to recognize the action as improper worsens this problem (Kaufman et al. 1995; Kelly et al. 2002). In majority of cases, CSA continues for a long period of time. It has been suggested that children progressively adjust to sexual abuse by a trusted person, by accommodating psychologically to the inherent contradictions, confusions and enforced secrecy accompanying the experience (Summit 1983). It may constitute a coping strategy which enables some children to remain asymptomatic during the abuse and leaving the abuse undiscovered. The abuser's own pattern of denial of the abuse through cognitive distortions lessens his potential discomfort and enables him to continue the abuse. Therefore, by the time sexual abuse is discovered in childhood, it has usually occurred many times (Johnson 2004). Besides these factors that apply globally, importantly in our context, the idea that such matters are to be kept within family (apparently irrespective of the perpetrator) seems deep rooted as reflected in the findings of various studies (MoWCD GOI 2007; Bhilwar et al. 2015). The characteristics of inter-dependence and loyalty to the group in collectivistic societies may be playing a major role. Similar observations regarding cultural differences in response to sexual harassment in Asian women have been made earlier (Zimbroff 2007). Even when the child discloses to the family, disbelief, anger towards and shaming of the victim, fear of social ostracism, inadequate or discouraging response from legal quarters and coercion or threat on part of the perpetrator may also result in under-reporting. Some of these factors have been referred to earlier by Fontes and Plummer (2010) and Gilligan and Akhtar (2006).

11.4 Vulnerability to Child Sexual Abuse

Sexual abuse is construed as abuse of power of the more powerful onto the weaker or vulnerable individuals. This is particularly true for children. The child's vulnerability by virtue of age, female gender, being an unwanted baby, mental or physical disability, neglect or social isolation, poverty, being in foster care or adopted, war/armed conflict, parents with mental illness or substance abuse, single parent, dysfunctional families increases the likelihood of sexual abuse (WHO Report 2006). Street children and children who are employed are much more vulnerable (MoWCD GOI 2007). Adolescents with poor social bonding and poor coping are also vulnerable. In case of younger children, they may not even understand what is being done to them and the wrongfulness of the same. Also, if they understand, they may not be in a position to resist. Witnessing or being a victim of sexual abuse and domestic violence during childhood or substance use may increase the likelihood of becoming a perpetrator. Perpetrators may prefer seduction and gaining trust over coercion, by becoming the child's friend, playing games with them, and offering them gifts ranging from money and toys to beer and cigarettes. Beyond these individual and familial factors, certain risk factors work at community and societal levels. These include tolerance of violence especially towards women and children, considering women and children traditionally as objects of honour, gender and social inequality, poverty, low levels of education and easy accessibility of substance.

11.5 Consequences of Child Sexual Abuse

CSA results in not only physical trauma, but grave emotional trauma with long-lasting effects. Rather, physical consequences are less likely in child sexual abuse. Non-contact abuse does not result in any physical findings. HIV and other sexually transmitted infections are seen in children with CSA. In addition, there are definite negative consequences for the child and her/his family.

CSA can have both immediate and long term adverse psychological effects that carry over into adulthood (Wyatt and Powell 1988). It has been suggested that CSA alters a child's cognitive and emotional orientation to the world and causes trauma by distorting their self-concept and affective capacities, issues of trust and intimacy (Finkelhor and Browne 1985). This can further lead to psychological and behavioural consequences which may extend to adulthood. The immediate psychological consequences include emotional disturbances in the form of fear, depression, anger, hostility and low self-esteem. Other initial effects of abuse are guilt, shame, sleep disturbances and eating disorders (Browne and Finkelhor 1996). These children also present with recent onset anxiety disorders (fearfulness, nightmares, phobias), post-traumatic stress disorder (PTSD), hysterical reactions, self-injurious and suicidal behaviour and substance abuse, aggressive and criminal behaviour, truancy and suicidal attempts (King et al. 2002; Garnefski and Arends 1998). Almost two-thirds of CSA victims develop some psychological problems with depression being the most common outcome (Patel et al. 1997) and 20–70 % of victims of CSA suffer from PTSD (McLeer et al. 1992). Other long-term effects include anxiety, negative self-concepts, interpersonal problems, conduct problems and self destructive behaviours (Kohli 2004). Adolescents sexually abused in childhood are more likely (five times) to report non-clinical psychotic experiences such as delusions and hallucinations than their non-abused counterparts (Lataster et al. 2006). Besides this child sexual abuse can also lead to 'reactive abuse (abuse of other children by a victim of abuse)'. The behavioural consequences of sexual abuse depend on the child's age, developmental level, physical acts performed, threats, fear of retribution, fear of culpability, chronicity of acts, child's resilience and relationship to the perpetrator and effective treatment (Haj-Yahi and Tamish 2001; Molnar et al. 2001). Behavioural changes include sexualized behaviours like genital manipulation, 'mummy/daddy' and 'nurses/doctors' related themes in their play (Browne and Finkelhor 1996), becoming withdrawn, behavioural/developmental regression, nightmares, sleep disturbance, frequent crying, clinginess/fears and refusal to stay alone or with a particular person, fear of males, enuresis and encopresis, headaches, stomach aches, unusual interest or curiosity about sexual matters, school disturbances including learning difficulties, poor concentration and declining grades (O'Keefe 2004; Browne and Finkelhor 1996).

Despite so many consequences reported in literature, it is important to note that around one-third of the abused children show no psychological symptoms or only non-specific symptoms and abuse goes on undetected (Kendall-Tackett et al. 1993). This can be explained by the extremely diverse characteristics of CSA which lead to a wide range of potential outcomes (Saywitz et al. 2000). Common reasons for asymptomatic survivors of sexual abuse include inability on part of treating team to detect the symptoms, insufficient severity of abuse, development of avoidant coping styles that mask victims' distress or having more resilience in such condition (Williams and Nelson-Gardell 2012). Studies suggest that various protective factors that influence resilience capacities of CSA victims are support from their non-offending parents, no past history of abuse (Hébert et al. 2006), less reliance on avoidant coping strategies to deal with the traumatic event (Bal et al. 2003), higher emotional self-control (Kassis et al. 2013), interpersonal trust and feelings of empowerment (Daigneault et al. 2007), less personal attributions of blame and of stigmatization (Feiring et al. 2007) and high family functioning and secure attachment relationships (Beaudoin et al. 2013).

11.6 Sociocultural Context of CSA

Sociocultural context was earlier referred to in some detail in the sections on Epidemiology—Prevalence, Reporting and Disclosure and Vulnerability to CSA (Sects. 11.3 and 11.4). Researchers have consistently recognized that cultural norms play a major role in defining sexual violence (Kalof 2000; Singleton 2004). Data suggest that child maltreatment is the product of a complex interaction of parental characteristics and the social and cultural conditions in which they exist (Agathonos-Georgopoulou 1992). The problem of CSA in Asia and particularly in India (Human Rights Watch 2013) has traditionally remained shrouded in a "conspiracy of silence" due to a multitude of familial, sociocultural and economic factors. Most of the times, community either blame victim for the abuse and their families are labelled. Besides contrary to the western population, Asian victims are often alienated and ostracised by their own families and by the whole community, if they go public with allegations of abuse. Usually, victims and their families face tremendous pressure to drop their cases. Such a problem is not about religion or race but about a culture where notions of shame result in the blaming of victims rather than perpetrators. Various untold stories explain how a culture of shame in Asia perpetuates abuse. Rao et al. (1992) investigated the types of sexual abuse encountered by the victims according to ethnicity and found that Asians are more likely to internalize their feelings rather than act out and approximately 60 % of Asian victims were abused by a male relative including the father.

A 16-year-old girl was brought by her maternal aunt as she was having severe anxiety and depressive symptoms for the past few months. The girl used to stay with this aunt and her family for undergoing some educational training locally. During the past few months of her stay, she was repeatedly being touched inappropriately by her aunt's husband. The girl did not tell it to anyone as she was afraid no one would believe her and at times, thought that she was simply mistaken. On some days, when she would be surer of herself, the idea of disclosing it would occur to her. But, she would think, "it would ruin my aunt's life...my cousins would hate me, they would never forgive me". One day, she spoke to her mother who was visiting her. Her mother advised her to keep quiet for her aunt's sake and it was "ghar ki baat" (a family matter). She better not tell it to her friends. Also, she asked her not to abruptly leave their house as it might seem suspicious. The girl was waiting for her academic year to end. (Maternal aunt was not aware of the abuse at that time; mother described the girl as 'samajhdar' (wise) for not having told anyone).

This case vignette (with some modifications) reflects the various contextual factors that are playing a role. The most prominent are the feelings of guilt and blame in the victim. Importantly, reaction of the mother points towards other factors such as loyalty to family and importance given to ties rather than individual suffering.

It has been emphasized earlier in literature that non-disclosure and non-reporting leaves the victim to suffer in silence without protective or therapeutic supports. Hence, it is extremely important to understand these factors from the standpoint of protection and prevention. Collectivistic values and tolerance and acceptance of violence against women and children have already been referred to earlier. Some other factors relevant to Asian culture are presented below.

11.6.1 Family Structure

In Asian culture, the roles of different family members are well defined. In almost whole of Asian culture elders and males are higher in the hierarchy (Ho 1990; Uba 1994). Father is the head of the family (Uba 1994). Mother is usually ranked lower in the family hierarchy when compared to her husband, in-laws and at times, her son. This patriarchal aspects of Asian cultures place children and adolescents at risk for sexual victimization (Lee 1996). Daughters tend to lack authority within the family. These decrease reporting of sexual abuse to authorities, particularly when the perpetrator is a man within the family (Hall et al. 1998).

11.6.2 Shame

CSA victims grow in environment of secrecy, guilt and shame (Damon et al. 1992). Children tend to blame themselves for the abuse due to egocentric thinking (Damon et al. 1992). In Asian culture parents instil guilt and shame to control the behaviour of children (Sue 1997). Feelings of guilt and shame prevent child from disclosing sexual abuse experiences to others. This, 'shame' and 'loss of face' are experienced by the individual and others associated with the individual (Lum 1998). Due to stigma attached to child sexual abuse victims and their family members have a tendency to move away from friends and relatives (Okamura et al. 1995). Victims engage in face-saving behaviours like denial or non-acceptance of blame (Rao et al. 1992). This serves as a coping for preserving the integrity of the ego/self (Thomas 1992). Several of the studies amongst Asians have been conducted in immigrant populations and therefore are not truly emic in nature. However, of recent there have been research, both case studies and larger studies from India and other Asian nations that refer to shame and loss of honour among victims and their families (MoWCD GOI 2007; Bhilwar et al. 2015; Chan 2009).

11.6.3 Honour

Traditionally, sexual abuse of girls and women has been a method to bring dishonour to that family or community. CSA then is taken as a personal humiliation ('murder of honour') and may invoke revenge (WHO 2006). Family honour is considered more important than the health and safety of the victim, which results in complete neglect of the victim. Also, family response that concentrates on restoring "lost" family honour puts the blame on the victim without punishing men (WHO 2006).

11.6.4 Attitudes Towards Sexuality

Sexuality is generally considered a taboo topic for discussion in Asian culture and discussion on this topic is avoided (Bhugra and Cordle 1988). The discussions of sexuality are usually limited to same-sex conversations. Due to lack of knowledge many Asian children are vulnerability of sexual abuse (Thomas 1992). This taboo of discussing sexual issues hinders child's ability to inform adults and adults' initiative to report to authorities (Wong and Wittet 1987).

There are other important societal factors that creates barrier for disclosure and indirectly perpetuate crime. The fears that the family shall be ridiculed by the police, the child would have to undergo interviews and interrogations, and might be blamed, humiliated and threatened in the fight for justice prevents many from seeking help. Human Rights Watch report (2013) has presented several case studies proving this point.

11.7 Clinical Aspects and Management

The focus of treatment is related to abuse on one hand and its causes and consequences on the other. Commonly encountered problems are confidentiality, secrecy and denial on part of the part of the family members, liaison with different agencies and working with the family according to their sociocultural background. Treatment is usually carried out in different settings, i.e. individual, group and family. Individual approach aims at enabling the children to describe their abuse and feelings.

11.7.1 Treatment

As CSA is under reported, children usually present with some other physical and psychological complaints to the clinician. These subtle signs are physical and psychological consequences of child sexual abuse and should be identified at earliest (MacMillan et al. 2013). As disclosure of abuse requires access to a trusted adult, specialized interviewing skill is required so that child feels protected and accepts treatment (Johnson 2004). Children usually do not disclose abuse until they feel much safer and protected. To facilitate this, a multidisciplinary team including pediatric services and mental health professionals as well as other social service agencies that can interface with law enforcers and take care of the safety of the child is needed. The abused child should be seen as soon as possible and at least within 72 h to detect injuries before they heal, to avoid further abuse and reduce chances of threats and bribery (Gosset and Hédouin 2002). Interview should be conducted step-wise including rapport building, asking open-ended questions, telling the truth, introducing the topic of concern, free narration, general questions and lastly specific questions. Repeated interviews should be avoided (Yuille et al. 1997). In addition, play observation may be a useful mode of examination. Associated psychological aids like drawings (Burgess and Hartman 1993), anatomically correct dolls, projective tests, behavioural checklists have been found to be useful (Chantler et al. 1993; Friedrich et al. 1991; Leifer et al. 1991). Any statement made by the child should be recorded in available formats as guided by the law and provisions of the State. Detailed physical examination including genital and rectal examination should be done at the earliest by pediatricians or gynaecologists or a trained medical officer.

The immediate focus of treatment should address the psychological distress, feelings of insecurity, lack of trust, self-blame and guilt. An attempt should be made to evaluate and address ideas of self-harm or suicide. It is equally important to address the psychological state of the parents or that of the non-offending parent. Studies have found that court appearances are the most stressful aspect of abuse assessments (Johnson 1999). Children and their families will need ongoing care from mental health professionals as well as social service agencies. Hence, a liaison between different professionals is of paramount importance. In the long-run, it is imperative to address issues of trust, self-esteem, self-image and sexuality, along with ongoing assessment of depression, anxiety disorders and PTSD. In cases of severe PTSD or depression or suicidality, inpatient management may be warranted. Anti-depressants may be used judiciously in severe cases, though psycho-therapeutic interventions remain the mainstay. Several psychotherapies have been studied in this population like psychodynamic abuse-focused therapy, CBT, Group therapy, Supportive psychotherapy, Dialectical Behavior Therapy, Play therapy and Art therapy. Trauma-Focused Cognitive Behavioural Therapy (TF-CBT) incorporates cognitive-behavioural, attachment, humanistic, empowerment and family therapy models (MacMillan et al. 2013). Studies suggest that sexual abuse-specific cognitive behavioural therapy is more effective than nondirective supportive therapy (Cohen and Mannarino 1998).

11.7.1.1 Working with Children and Their Families from Asian Continent

Many of the Asian traditional values mentioned previously may discourage victims and their families from seeking psychological support. The principles behind psychotherapy like individualism, self-determinism and self-fulfilment are in direct conflict with several traditional Asian cultural values of collectivism, interdependence and loyalty towards the family (Chan and Leong 1994). Stigma and shame attached with mental illness in the Asian community inhibits them from seeking psychological services (Rao et al. 1992). Asians tend to view mental illness as a personal weakness and lack of will power which conflicts with the valued Asian values of self-control, suffering, and persevering in the face of adversity (Ho 1990). Seeking psychological support for CSA is considered as a punishment for past wrongs of the family, poor guidance and discipline from the family elders (Chan and Leong 1994). Asians may be more likely to obtain treatment and follow through with treatment if it is recommended by a court of law. Asian patients are at special risk for premature termination of treatment. This may be due to unfamiliarity with the process of psychotherapy, conflict over the direction of psychotherapy and cultural values (Root 1985). In the therapy, Asian patients are likely to be reluctant to rely on the clinician as an authority figure. They expect the clinician to tell them what is wrong and solve their problems and mostly somaticize their symptoms (Chin 1998). The Asian values of hierarchy and respect for authority may be used by the therapist to work with the family (Ho 1990). Ho (1990) also suggests that community and family elders may be useful sources of support during the process of therapy.

Given the taboo of discussing sexual behaviours and issues in Asian culture, direct initial questions about the sexual abuse experience should be avoided. Child should be interviewed with the trusted adult to whom he or she initially disclosed the abuse who may or may not be the family member (Okamura et al. 1995).

Usual strategies described in different studies (Ho 1990; Sue and Sue 1999) for Asian clients and families are as under:

(a) Refrain from asking too many personal questions during the initial session
(b) Take an active and directive role
(c) Assess the problem from the client's perspective and culture
(d) Focus on the specific problem as identified by the client
(e) Assess current financial and social needs, as well as safety needs
(f) Time-limited therapy focused on resolution of problems

In the beginning phase of therapy, appropriate self-disclosure from the clinician is required to develop trust and confidence. There is a need to form a social and cultural connection with the family and appreciate client's cultural background. It is important to engage the family and to develop rapport with them. We should avoid direct confrontation or a discussion of cultural taboos (Lee 1996). Client should discuss who among family members should be included in therapy. While, western culture relies on verbal communication, Asian culture tends to emphasize non-verbal and indirect communication (Cheng 1997). Asians traditionally use indirect styles of communication and avoid confrontation (Lee 1996). In working with sexual abuse victims it is important that therapists notice non-verbal behaviour during the course of therapy. During the second, problem-solving phase, it is suggested to focus on the problems the family presents and a psycho-educational approach should be followed as education is highly valued in Asian cultures. Therapist should capitalize on family strength and community support. In the last, termination phase Asian client do not usually verbalize anger or separation anxiety. Asian clients usually view relationship with their clinician as that of a friend that will continue after termination and appreciate clinician's role by bringing a gift. However, these culturally appropriate gestures should not be interpreted as pathological.

Lastly, Asian community often consults herbalists, community elders, fortune tellers and priests in times of need. Given the community's preference for these resources, these groups of community professionals may benefit from education on child sexual abuse.

11.8 Legislation and Policies

In Asia, the policy and legislative framework for child protection have evolved over the past few decades. We have focused mainly on India, taking it a case study. Recent policies adopted in India include the Juvenile Justice (Care and Protection of Children) Act 2000 and Delhi Rules 2009 which have the provision of age appropriate segregation of children in residential facilities, standards of care for the physical infrastructure and training of staff (Delhi Juvenile Justice—Care and Protection of Children Rules 2009). A major breakthrough was achieved by the enactment of the POCSO Act (2012) (Sagar 2014). The POCSO has increased the quantum of punishment and provided for special courts. It also provides for relief and rehabilitation of the victims. Section 19 of POCSO provides for mandatory reporting of sexual offences by any person who has knowledge that a child has been sexually abused. Thus, this Act extends responsibility to the treating doctor to report the matter to the law enforcing agencies if it was not done by the patient or his/her family. Following POCSO, in 2013, the Indian government introduced the National Policy for Children. The NPC aims towards creating a caring, protective and safe environment for all children (MoWCD GOI 2013). The Delhi Commission for Protection of Child Rights (Guidelines for Prevention of Child Abuse 2014) recently introduced its guidelines based on the principle of '*zero tolerance*' for child abuse in any form. This involves set of procedures and processes for schools, residential facilities, and other institutions in form of recruitment processes, capacity building, child protection safeguards and transport-related guidelines. A national level plan of action also exists in several Asian nations such as India, Nepal and Sri Lanka for combatting trafficking and commercial exploitation of children and women. However, despite the strong provisions of the existing laws, the implementation and the outcome has been far less encouraging. Since its implementation, though 45,000 cases have been registered under the POCSO Act (2012), almost 40,000 cases were pending with the police or judiciary. The data from 2014 reveals a poor conviction rate of 24.6 % under the POCSO Act (MoWCD GOI 2016). Lack of proper collection and preservation of material evidence and inadequate medico-legal documentation are cited as major reasons for low conviction rates. The state of affairs is expected to be similar in other developing nations of Asia. Besides a culture of silence around the issue, lack of knowledge and understanding cause problems in implementation. In keeping with this, the Ministry of Women and Child Development, GOI along with the National Commission held a consultation with all stakeholders responsible for implementing the POCSO Act and emphasized that there is a need for dissemination of information, creation of awareness and registration of cases under POCSO Act. The Government of India has also begun a process of regional consultations with medical professionals with the aims to sensitize and train them to respond to CSA. Indian Medical Association along with UNICEF has come up with the initiative on CSA in form of training of the trainers (doctors with minimum 5 years' experience) through regional workshops and to train doctors of various medical colleges of the country. Overall, it is imperative that the doctors, police and judiciary be sensitized and trained regarding the practical aspects of dealing with CSA. It is also recommended that Child helpline number should be displayed in the clinics and hospitals for reporting any case of known or suspected child abuse or neglect (Sagar 2014).

11.9 Prevention of CSA

The approach to prevention of CSA has to be multi-pronged, working at different levels and on various contextual factors. According to WHO report (2013), childhood experience of sexual abuse and witnessing domestic violence as a child are the major predictors of perpetration of violence during adulthood. Hence, programs geared towards life skills and coping management for school children that are either universal or targeted, may play an important role. The second most frequent approach is that of primary prevention and involves universal educational programs generally delivered in schools and is aimed at potential victims. These universal programs intervene in the individual, family or societal preventive sphere (Finkelhor 2009). In a meta-analysis on the effectiveness of school-based child abuse prevention programs, the programs with four or more sessions produced the highest effect sizes (Davis and Gidycz 2000). In another review almost all studies found a small but significant average gain in self-protective knowledge by programs like modelling, group discussion and role play (Topping and Barron 2009). Also, a culture of 'zero tolerance' towards CSA needs to be developed. Gender equality, empowerment of women, non-tolerance towards violence of any form on children and women and sensitization of teachers and parents are some of the deeper changes at the societal level that have the potential to decrease the occurrence of CSA. Also, these same strategies can indirectly affect the cultural barriers to disclosure of CSA. For example, in the case vignette presented, the mother's advice and action would have been different if from a young age she would have been encouraged to stand against any form of abuse. Besides the skill training of professionals responsible for responding to CSA, it is important that they gradually adopt value systems that are based on equality and respect for the integrity of the other person (be it a boy or a girl). If the legal process becomes child friendly and efficient, it would become a deterrent for the perpetrators. These prevention strategies thus, operate on multiple levels, viz. level of minors; adults who live or work with children; societal and legislative level, and finally, on the level of conscious or "less than conscious" attitudes which protect the abuse perpetrators (Zollner et al. 2014). However, it is important that the prevention programs are suitably adapted to relevant specific cultural contexts and needs.

11.10 Conclusion

Child sexual abuse occurs in the context of a complex interplay of individual, familial and social factors. Further, socio-culture specific issues such as family structure and inter-dependence, and constructs of shame and dishonour influence prevalence, reporting, treatment seeking, available and accepted modes of treatment of sexual abuse. CSA is associated with a high degree of physical and psychological problems besides the legal and social issues. Despite this, the contextual factors may result in non-disclosure leaving the victim to suffer silently. Its alarming rate and long-lasting harmful consequences clearly calls for extensive and powerful policy and practice efforts. To effectively prevent CSA, universal preventive approaches, targeting personal, family and societal conditions should be developed to protect the next generations of children and youth from sexual victimization. It is absolutely essential that all those involved in responding to CSA victims should be sensitized and trained in performing their specific roles. An active effort is required for the development of strategies to address the barriers to disclosure and reporting. While treating the psychological consequences, it is imperative to consider the cultural differences. Although some advancement in the recent decade at policy and legislation level has been made, but more and sustained efforts are needed across disciplines and services to tackle this hidden menace.

References

Agathonos-Georgopoulou, H. (1992). Cross-cultural perspectives in child abuse and neglect. *Child Abuse Review, 1*(2), 80–88.

Bal, S., Van Oost, P., De Bourdeaudhuij, I., & Crombez, G. (2003). Avoidant coping as a mediator between self-reported sexual abuse and stress-related symptoms in adolescents. *Child Abuse and Neglect, 27*(8), 883–897.

Beaudoin, G., Hébert, M., & Bernier, A. (2013). Contribution of attachment security to the prediction of internalizing and externalizing behavior problems in preschoolers victims of sexual abuse. *Revue Europeenne de Psychologie Appliquee, 63*(3), 147–157.

Behere, P., Rao, T. S. S., & Mulmule, A. N. (2013). Sexual abuse in women with special reference to children: Barriers, boundaries and beyond. *Indian Journal of Psychiatry, 55*(4), 316–319.

Bhilwar, M., Upadhyay, R. P., Rajavel, S., Singh, S. K., Vasudevan, K., & Chinnakali, P. (2015). Childhood experiences of physical, emotional and sexual abuse among college students in South India. *Journal of Tropical Pediatrics, 61*(5), 329–338.

Bhugra, D., & Cordle, C. (1988). A case control study of sexual dysfunction in Asian and non-Asian couples 1981–1985. *Sexual and Marital Therapy, 3*, 71–76.

Browne, A., & Finkelhor, D. (1996). Impact of child sexual abuse: A review of the research. *Psychological Bulletin, 99*, 66–77.

Burgess, A. W., & Hartman, C. R. (1993). Children's drawings. *Child Abuse and Neglect, 17*(1), 161–168.

Chan, K. L. (2009). Sexual violence against women and children in Chinese societies. *Trauma, Violence, and Abuse, 10*, 69–85.

Chan, S., & Leong, C. W. (1994). Chinese families in transition: Cultural conflicts and adjustment problems. *Journal of Social Distress and the Homeless, 3*, 263–281.

Chantler, L., Pelco, L., & Mertin, P. (1993). The psychological evaluation of child sexual abuse using the Louisville behavior checklist and human figure drawing. *Child Abuse and Neglect, 17*(2), 271–279.

Chin, J. L. (1998). Mental health services and treatment. In L. C. Lee & N. W. S. Zane (Eds.), *Handbook of Asian American psychology* (pp. 485–504). Thousand Oaks, CA: Sage.

Cheng, B. K. (1997). Cultural clash between providers of majority culture and patients of Chinese culture. *Journal of Long-Term Home Health Care, 16*, 39–43.

Cohen, J. A., & Mannarino, A. P. (1998). Interventions for sexually abused children: Initial treatment outcome findings. *Child Maltreatment, 3*(1), 17–26.

Collin-Vézina, D., Daigneault, I., & Hébert, M. (2013). Lessons learned from child sexual abuse research: Prevalence, outcomes, and preventive strategies. *Child and Adolescent Psychiatry and Mental Health, 7*(1), 22.

Daigneault, I., Hébert, M., & Tourigny, M. (2007). Personal and interpersonal characteristics related to resilient developmental pathways of sexually abused adolescents. *Child and Adolescent Psychiatric Clinics of North America, 16*(2), 415–434.

Damon, L. L., Card, J. A., & Todd, J. (1992). Incest in young children. *Assessment of family violence: A clinical and legal sourcebook* (pp. 148–172). New York: Wiley.

Daral, S., Khokhar, A., & Pradhan, S. (2016). Prevalence and determinants of child maltreatment among school-going adolescent girls in a semi-urban area of Delhi, India. *Journal of Tropical Pediatrics,* doi:10.1093/tropej/fmv106

Davis, M. K., & Gidycz, C. A. (2000). Child sexual abuse prevention programs: A meta-analysis. *Journal of Clinical Child Psychology, 29*(2), 257–265.

Deb, S., & Modak, S. (2010). Prevalence of violence against children in families in Tripura and Its relationship with socio-economic factors. *Journal of Injury and Violence Research, 2*(1), 5–18.

Delhi Juvenile Justice (Care and Protection of Children) Rules. (2009). Govt of NCT of Delhi, India.

Feiring, C., Miller-Johnson, S., & Cleland, C. M. (2007). Potential pathways from stigmatization and internalizing symptoms to delinquency in sexually abused youth. *Child Maltreatment, 12*(3), 220–232.

Finkelhor, D. (2009). The prevention of childhood sexual abuse. *The Future of Children/Center for the Future of Children, the David and Lucile Packard Foundation, 19*(2), 169–194.

Finkelhor, D., & Browne, A. (1985). The traumatic impact of child sexual abuse: A conceptualization. *The American Journal of Orthopsychiatry, 55*(4), 530–541.

Fontes, L. A., & Plummer, A. (2010). Cultural issues in disclosures of child sexual abuse. *Journal of Child Sexual Abuse, 19*, 491–518.

Friedrich, W. N., Grambsch, P., Broughton, D., Kuiper, J., & Beilke, R. L. (1991). Normative sexual behavior in children. *Pediatrics, 88*(3), 456–464.

Garnefski, N., & Arends, E. (1998). Sexual abuse and adolescent maladjustment: differences between male and female victims. *Journal of Adolescence, 21*, 99–107.

Gilbert, R., Kemp, A., Thoburn, J., Sidebotham, P., Radford, L., Glaser, D., et al. (2009a). Recognising and responding to child maltreatment. *Lancet (London, England), 373*(9658), 167–180.

Gilbert, R., Widom, C. S., Browne, K., Fergusson, D., Webb, E., & Janson, S. (2009b). Burden and consequences of child maltreatment in high-income countries. *Lancet (London, England), 373*(9657), 68–81.

Gilligan, P. A., & Akhtar, S. (2006). Cultural barriers to the disclosure of child sexual abuse in Asian communities: Listening to what women say. *British Journal of Social Work, 36*, 1361–1377.

Goodyear-Brown, P., Fath, A., & Myers, L. (2012). Child sexual abuse: The scope of the problem. *Handbook of child sexual abuse* (pp. 1–5). New York: Wiley.

Gosset, D., & Hédouin, V. (2002). Sexual assaults. *La Revue Du Praticien, 52*(7), 734–738.

Graupner, H. (2000). Sexual consent: The criminal law in Europe and overseas. *Archives of Sexual Behavior, 29*(5), 415–461.

Guidelines for Prevention of Child Abuse. (2014). *Delhi commission for protection of child rights*. India: Govt of NCT of Delhi.

Haj-Yahi, M. M., & Tamish, S. (2001). The rates of child sexual abuse and its psychological consequences as revealed by a study among Palestinian university students. *Child Abuse and Neglect, 25*(10), 1303–1327.

Hall, G. C., Windover, A. K., & Maramba, G. G. (1998). Sexual aggression among Asian Americans: Risk and protective factors. *Cultural Diversity and Mental Health, 4*(4), 305–318.

Hébert, M., Collin-Vézina, D., Daigneault, I., Parent, N., & Tremblay, C. (2006). Factors linked to outcomes in sexually abused girls: A regression tree analysis. *Comprehensive Psychiatry, 47*(6), 443–455.

Ho, C. K. (1990). An analysis of domestic violence in Asian American communities: A multicultural approach to counseling. *Women & Therapy, 9*(1–2), 129–150.

Human Rights Watch. (2013). Breaking the silence: Child sexual abuse in India.

Johnson, C. F. (1999). The use of charts and models to facilitate a physician's testimony in court. *Child Maltreatment, 4*, 228–241.

Johnson, C. F. (2004). Child sexual abuse. *Lancet (London, England), 364*(9432), 462–470.

Kalof, L. (2000). Ethnic differences in female sexual victimization. *Sexuality and Culture, 4*, 75–97.

Kassis, W., Artz, S., Scambor, C., Scambor, E., & Moldenhauer, S. (2013). Finding the way out: A non-dichotomous understanding of violence and depression resilience of adolescents who are exposed to family violence. *Child Abuse and Neglect, 37*(2–3), 181–199.

Kaufman, K., Johnson, C. F., & Weller, A. M. (1995). The victims of female and male perpetrators of sexual abuse: A comparative study. *Journal of Interpersonal Violence, 3*, 322–333.

Kelly, R. J., Wood, J. J., Gonzalez, L. S., MacDonald, V., & Waterman, J. (2002). Effects of mother-son incest and positive perceptions of sexual abuse experiences on the psychosocial adjustment of clinic-referred men. *Child Abuse and Neglect, 26*(4), 425–441.

Kendall-Tackett, K. A., Williams, L. M., & Finkelhor, D. (1993). Impact of sexual abuse on children: A review and synthesis of recent empirical studies. *Psychological Bulletin, 113*(1), 164–180.

Kessler, R. C., McLaughlin, K. A., Green, J. G., Gruber, M. J., Sampson, N. A., Zaslavsky, A. M., et al. (2010). Childhood adversities and adult psychopathology in the WHO World Mental Health Surveys. *The British Journal of Psychiatry: The Journal of Mental Science, 197*(5), 378–385.

King, M., Coxell, A., & Mezey, G. (2002). Sexual molestation of males: Associations with psychological disturbance. *The British Journal of Psychiatry: The Journal of Mental Science, 181*, 153–157.

Kohli, A. (2004). Child sexual abuse. *Bulletin PGI, 38*, 152–159.

Krishnakumar, P., Satheesan, K., Geeta, M. G., & Sureshkumar, K. (2014). Prevalence and spectrum of sexual abuse among adolescents in Kerala, South India. *Indian Journal of Pediatrics, 81*(8), 770–774.

Lataster, T., van Os, J., Drukker, M., Henquet, C., Feron, F., Gunther, N., et al. (2006). Childhood victimisation and developmental expression of non-clinical delusional ideation and hallucinatory experiences: Victimisation and non-clinical psychotic experiences. *Social Psychiatry and Psychiatric Epidemiology, 41*(6), 423–428.

Lee, E. (1996). Asian American families: An overview. In *Ethnicity and family therapy* (2nd Ed., pp. 227–248). New York: The Guilford Press.

Leifer, M., Shapiro, J. P., Martone, M. W., & Kassem, L. (1991). Rorschach assessment of psychological functioning in sexually abused girls. *Journal of Personality Assessment, 56*(1), 14–28.

Lum, J. L. (1998). Family violence. *Handbook of Asian American psychology* (pp. 505–525). Thousand Oaks, CA: Sage.

Luo, Y., Parish, W. L., & Laumann, E. O. (2008). A population-based study of childhood sexual contact in China: Prevalence and long-term consequences. *Child Abuse and Neglect, 32*(7), 721–731.

MacMillan, H. L., Tanaka, M., Duku, E., Vaillancourt, T., & Boyle, M. H. (2013). Child physical and sexual abuse in a community sample of young adults: Results from the Ontario child health study. *Child Abuse and Neglect, 37*(1), 14–21.

Martin, E. K., & Silverstone, P. H. (2013). How much child sexual abuse is "below the surface", and can we help adults identify it early? *Frontiers in Psychiatry, 4*, 58.

McLeer, S. V., Deblinger, E., Henry, D., & Orvaschel, H. (1992). Sexually abused children at high risk for post-traumatic stress disorder. *Journal of the American Academy of Child and Adolescent Psychiatry, 31*(5), 875–879.

Ministry of Women and Child development. (2007). Study on child abuse: India. Government of India.

Ministry of Women and Child Development. (2013). National Policy for Children. Ministry of Women and Child Development, Government of India.

Ministry of Women and Child Development. (2016, March 3). Conviction under POCSO Act.

Ministry of Women and Child Development, Government of India. http://pib.nic.in/newsite/PrintRelease.aspx?relid=137261

Molnar, B. E., Buka, S. L., & Kessler, R. C. (2001). Child sexual abuse and subsequent psychopathology: Results from the National Comorbidity Survey. *American Journal of Public Health, 91*(5), 753–760.

O'Briain, M. (2008). Sexual exploitation of children and adolescents in tourism. A contribution of ECPAT International to the World Congress III against Sexual Exploitation of Children and Adolescents, Bangkok.

Okamura, A., Heras, P., & Wong-Kerberg, L. (1995). Asian, Pacific island, and Filipino Americans and sexual child abuse. *Sexual abuse in nine North American cultures: Treatment and prevention* (pp. 67–96). Thousand Oaks, CA: Sage.

O'Keefe, M. (2004). A case of suspected child sexual abuse. *Journal of Clinical Forensic Medicine, 11*(6), 316–320.

Patel, R. R., Methiwalla, S., Rane, A., & Gore, S. (1997). Child sexual abuse: Psychosocial aspects. *Indian Journal of Psychiatry, 39*(Suppl), 56.

Protection of Children from Sexual Offences (POCSO) Act. (2012). Government of India.

Rao, K., DiClemente, R. J., & Ponton, L. E. (1992). Child sexual abuse of Asians compared with other populations. *Journal of the American Academy of Child and Adolescent Psychiatry, 31*(5), 880–886.

Ray, A. (2014, September 12). 42 % of Indian girls are sexually abused before 19: UNICEF. The Times of India.

Root, M. P. (1985). Guidelines for facilitating therapy with Asian American clients. *Psychotherapy, 22*, 349–356.

Sagar, R. (2014). *Child sexual abuse: Need for a preventive framework in Indian context, 19*, 53–55.

Saywitz, K. J., Mannarino, A. P., Berliner, L., & Cohen, J. A. (2000). Treatment for sexually abused children and adolescents. *The American Psychologist, 55*(9), 1040–1049.

Singh, M. M., Parsekar, S. S., & Nair, S. N. (2014). An epidemiological overview of child sexual abuse. *Journal of Family Medicine and Primary Care, 3*(4), 430–435.

Singleton, K. W. (2004). Strategies of survival: Coping, characteristics of resiliency, and perceived impact of abuse in resilient black female survivors of sexual trauma. Dissertation abstracts international section B. *The Sciences & Engineering, 64*, 12–B.

Song, Y., Ji, C.-Y., & Agardh, A. (2014). Sexual coercion and health-risk behaviors among urban Chinese high school students. *Global Health Action, 7*, 24418.
Subedi, G. (2002). Trafficking and sexual abuse among street children in Kathmandu. International Programme on the Elimination of Child Labour. International Labour Organization, Kathmandu, Nepal.
Sue, D. (1997). The interplay of sociocultural factors on the psychological development of Asian in America. In *Counseling American minorities: A cross-cultural perspective* (5th Ed., pp. 205–213). Boston: McGraw-Hill.
Sue, D. W., & Sue, D. (1999). *Counseling the culturally different: Theory and practice* (3rd ed.). New York: Wiley.
Summit, R. C. (1983). The child sexual abuse accommodation syndrome. *Child Abuse and Neglect, 7*(2), 177–193.
Tang, C. S. (2002). Childhood experience of sexual abuse among Hong Kong Chinese college students. *Child Abuse and Neglect, 26*(1), 23–37.
The Criminal Law (Amendment) Act. (2013). Government of India.
Thomas, J. (1992). An interview with Amy Okamura. *The Advisor: American Professional Society on the Abuse of Children, 8*, 16–18.
Topping, K. J., & Barron, I. G. (2009). School-based child sexual abuse prevention programs: A review of effectiveness. *PubMed Health.*
Uba, L. (1994). *Asian Americans: Personality patterns, identity, and mental health.* New York: Guilford.
UNICEF. (2001, December). Commercial sexual exploitation and sexual abuse of children in South Asia. Kathmandu, Nepal. UNICEF.
UNICEF. (2012). Child maltreatment: Prevalence, incidence and consequences in the East Asia and Pacific Region: A systematic review of research strengthening child protection systems series: No 1. UNICEF.
Wihbey, J. (2009). Global prevalence of child sexual abuse. *Journalist Resource.*
Williams, J., & Nelson-Gardell, D. (2012). Predicting resilience in sexually abused adolescents. *Child Abuse and Neglect, 36*(1), 53–63.
Wong, D., & Wittet, S. (1987). *Be aware, be safe*. Renton, WA: King County Rape Relief.
World Health Organization. (2003). Guidelines for medico-legal care for victims of sexual violence, gender and women's Health, family and community health injuries and violence prevention, non-communicable diseases and mental health. Geneva, World Health Organization.
World Health Organization, Updated. (2003). Guidelines for medicolegal care for victims of sexual violence. *Child sexual abuse*. Geneva. World Health Organization, Updated.
World Health Organisation. (2006). Sexual violence. Geneva. World Health Organization http://www.who.int/violence_injury_prevention/violence/global_campaign/en/chap6.pdf
WHO report. (2013). Global and regional estimates of violence against women. Prevalence and health effects of intimate partner violence and non-partner sexual violence. Available from:http://apps.who.int/iris/bitstream/10665/85239/1/9789241564625_eng.pdf?ua=1. Accessed 4 Oct 2016.
Wyatt, G., & Powell, G. (1988). Identifying the lasting effects of child sexual abuse. In *The lasting effects of child sexual abuse* (pp. 15–17), CA: Sage.
Yuille, J. C., Hunter, J., Joffe, R., & Zaparnuik, J. (1997). Interviewing children in sexual abuse cases. In Child Victims (Ed.), *Child witnesses: Understanding and improving testimony*. New York: Illford.
Zimbroff, J. (2007). Cultural differences in perceptions of and responses to sexual harassment. *Duke Journal of Gender Law & Policy, 14*, 1311–1341.
Zollner, H., Fuchs, K. A., & Fegert, J. M. (2014). Prevention of sexual abuse: Improved information is crucial. *Child and Adolescent Psychiatry and Mental Health, 8*(1), 5.

Chapter 12
The Lifelong Impact of Childhood Parental Loss: Manifestations and Management

Salman Akhtar

Abstract This contribution deals with the lifelong emotional impact of childhood parental loss. It seeks to elucidate the struggles, vulnerabilities, and occasional triumphs, of individuals whose parents have died early on in their lives. Realms of aggression, narcissism, love, temporality, and feelings about one's own mortality are explored. Important caveats are entered to preclude superficial generalizations and to assure that the assessment of such individuals stays nuanced and specific to each particular situation. The contribution then extends to include guidelines for treating such patients in psychotherapy and psychoanalysis. It emphasizes the need to provide a greater than usual illusion of 'holding,' to validate the gravity of their loss, to unmask the defenses against the awareness of the pervasive impact of the loss and to interpret the patients' defensive uses of their status as an orphan. The chapter pays special attention to their difficulties with interruptions in the course of treatment and even more so in dealing with the termination of treatment.

Keywords Orphan · Loss · Narcissism · Validation

12.1 Introduction

Words matter. They help us express and convey or hide and camouflage our thoughts and inner experiences. For us psychoanalysts, this is an issue of paramount importance. We depend upon 'associations'—a river-like, undulating chain of words—to deduce the psychologically elusive layers of striving and fear in our patients. Words are our allies. We listen to them and use them with utmost care. As yet we remain vulnerable to collusion with the public at large in avoiding the use

S. Akhtar (✉)
Psychoanalytic Center of Philadelphia, 833 Chestnut East, Suite 210-C,
Philadelphia, PA 19107, USA
e-mail: Salman.Akhtar@jefferson.edu

S. Malhotra and P. Santosh (eds.), *Child and Adolescent Psychiatry*,
DOI 10.1007/978-81-322-3619-1_12

of words felt as too anxiety-provoking or deemed 'politically incorrect.' We refer to the external female genitalia as 'vagina' instead of the medically correct 'vulva,' lump all militant uprisings as 'terrorism,' and recoil from calling anyone 'mentally retarded' or 'handicapped.' Under the guise of updating our vocabulary, we renounce powerful and direct communication. We struggle to think and speak fearlessly but Freud's (1897) *matrem nudam*[1] is the outer wall of our lexical prison.

These introductory remarks, long-winded though they might seem, are intended to underscore the noticeable absence of the word 'orphan' from our literature. Indeed, the word 'orphan' does not appear in the index to the standard edition of *The Complete Psychological Works of Sigmund Freud* nor is it mentioned in any of the 27 glossaries published over the 120 years history of our profession (Akhtar 2009a). A quick search of Psychoanalytic Electronic Publishing (PEP)-Web, the computerized compendium of the contents of 29 psychoanalytic journals[2] reveals that although there is much written about those who have suffered parental loss during childhood, only 2 papers (Gordon and Sherr 1974; Carveth 1992) are with the word 'orphan' in their titles. This can be attributed to fashions of the times and to our well-intentioned desire to avoid hurtful labels. However, one wonders whether there is some anxiety resulting in such linguistic avoidance. An attempt to explore the origin of such unease might begin from examining the word itself.

The word 'orphan' has its roots in the Latin *orphanus* meaning destitute or without parents, and the Greek *orphanos* meaning bereaved, comfortless, and one who has lost parents during childhood. Somewhat greater latitude in the connotation of the word 'orphan' evolved over time (e.g., in its application to animals, unpopular technology, and a single line of a paragraph appearing at the end of the page) but the most prevalent meaning continued to be a child whose parents are dead. Two quibbles arise in this context. Does one have to lose both parents to qualify as an orphan? And, what is the cut-off point, age-wise, after which the death of a parent does not lead to one being considered an orphan?

A quick look at Spanish, Chinese, Hindi, and Arabic, the four languages that are collectively spoken by more than half of the world's population, reveals varying answers. Spanish and Chinese have only one word, *huerfano* and *gu'er*, respectively, for orphan, and restrict its use to children who have lost both parents to death. Hindi too has only one word, *anath*, for orphans, but its origins do not refer to the death of parents. The word actually means 'not protected by anyone,' or 'not belonging to anyone.' Moreover, the word is used only for those who have lost their fathers; there is no specific word for children who have lost their

[1]Freud's (Letter to Wilhelm Fleiss, October 3, 1897, cited in Masson 1985, p. 268) lapsing into Latin, *matrem nudam*, while describing, at age 41, the childhood memory of having seen his mother naked attests to the power of certain words and the strenuous efforts we make to avoid using them.

[2]The Web also contains the contents of 56 major psychoanalytic books and the entire 24 volume set of the Standard Edition of The Complete Psychological Works of Sigmund Freud.

mothers. In contrast, Arabic shows a remarkable latitude and sophistication. Not only does it have different words for those who have lost a father (*al yateem*), a mother (*al munqateh*), or both parents (*al la lateem*) during childhood, it implicitly suggests a continuum of the trauma's severity. *Al yateem* translates roughly into 'one has no identity or no self of his own,' *al munqateh* into 'one who has been severed and lacerated,' and *al la lateem* into 'one who is in utter despair.' Fascinatingly, the Arabic distinction between paternal and maternal loss centers upon conflicts of individuation versus the rupture of a fused self-object representation (see the section on mental pain below).

Linguistic and cultural variations aside, the common custom is to restrict the use of the word 'orphan' for those who have lost at least one parent before ceasing legally to be a minor. The word thus has inherently painful and helpless connotations. There is also an air of immutability associated with a designation of this sort and the nihilism that this can portend makes one recoil from it.[3]

At the same time, the background of deprivation and of being raised by people other than parents allows rich avenues for writers' imaginations. Orphans are therefore often chosen as protagonists of literary fiction. Gordon and Sherr (1974) provide a comprehensive list of novels and plays where the main character has lost one or both parents.[4] While familiarity with the fictional characters in their list can enhance empathy for such individuals, it is the step-by-step deconstruction of the intrapsychic vicissitudes of this trauma that truly enlightens the clinician.

12.2 The Lifelong Impact of Childhood Parental Loss

The impact of parental loss during childhood is lifelong. Its myriad manifestations can be broadly grouped under the following categories: (i) continued intrapsychic relationship with the dead parent(s), (ii) mental pain and defenses against it, (iii) narcissistic imbalance, (iv) disturbances in the development of aggressive drive, (v) problems in the realm of love and sexuality, (vi) disturbances in the subjective experience of time, and (vii) attitudes toward one's own mortality. In what follows, I will address the phenomenological and psychodynamic aspects of these areas in some detail.

---

[3]Paradoxically, the aversion is diminished if the broader context of parental loss is even more horrifying. A dramatic illustration of this is constituted by the nearly 4000 children orphaned as a result of the bombings of Hiroshima and Nagasaki toward the end of World War II. They continue to be called the 'A-bomb orphans.'

[4]Prominent among their list are *The Adventures of Augie March* (Bellow 1953), *Great Expectations* (Dickens 1860), *Tom Jones* (Fielding 1749), *The Vicar of Wakefield* (Goldsmith 1766), *Demian* (Hesse 1919), and *Of Human Bondage* (Maugham 1915).

12.2.1 Continued Intrapsychic Relationship with the Dead Parent(s)

In *Mourning and Melancholia*, his seminal contribution to the topic of loss and grief, Freud (1917) declared that

> Reality testing has shown that the loved object no longer exists, and it proceeds to demand that all libido shall be withdrawn from its attachments to that object. This demand arouses understandable opposition – it is a matter of general observation that people never willingly abandon a libidinal position …normally, respect for reality gains the day. Nevertheless, its orders can not be obeyed at once. They are carried out bit by bit, at great expense of time and cathectic energy, and in the meantime, the existence of the lost object is psychically prolonged. Each single one of the memories and expectations in which the libido is bound to the object is brought up and hyper-cathected, and detachment of the libido is accomplished in respect of it…. When the work of mourning is completed, the ego becomes free and uninhibited again (pp. 244–245).

This stance became the centerpiece of the psychoanalytic perspective on mourning and only recently has come under question (Meyers 2001; Masur 2001). Rather than undergoing decathexis, the lost object is now seen as getting psychically relocated. It continues to have an existence in the mind but the relationship between it and the self is altered and carries a lesser degree of affect. Freud, who had originated the decathexis idea, took this latter position elsewhere. In a 1929 letter to a friend whose son had died, Freud spoke of grief in the following terms:

> We know that the acute sorrow we feel after such a loss will run its course, but also that we will remain inconsolable, and will never find a substitute. No matter what may come to take its place, even should it fill that place completely, it yet remains something else. And that is how it should be. It is the only way of perpetuating a love that we do not want to abandon" (cited in Fichtner 2003, p. 196).

Such an outcome is even more marked in children. Though there are individual variations, generally the cathexis of primary love objects is maintained for years after loss and decathexis occurs slowly and painfully in toddlers (e.g. Spitz 1946, 1950, 1965; Bowlby 1960, 1963, 1969; Furman 1974). With somewhat older children, the opposite seems to be the case; there is an inability to decathect the object-representation of the deceased (Pollock 1961; Wolfenstein 1966; Nagera 1970). This is due to a developmental lack of tolerance of mental pain and the deeply disturbing threat of narcissistic imbalance; a parent has after all been a 'self object' (Kohut 1977) in addition to being a separately experienced object. Thus a split in the ego is established. One part knows that the parent is dead. The other part holds on to the internal representation of the parent, intrapsychically 'behaving' as if he or she were fully alive. Even when they know that the parent is dead, children often show intense distress and make all sorts of actual and imaginary efforts to bring the dead parent back to life.[5]

---

[5]The award-winning French movie, *Ponette* (Les Films Alain Sarde 1996) poignantly depicts a four-year old girl's anguish upon losing her mother as well as her desperate measures to bring her back to life.

Pollock (1961) observed approximately similar phenomena in three adult patients who had lost a parent before the age of six. He noted that:

> Throughout the years there had been a retention of the deceased parent in the form of a fantasy figure who was in heaven; to whom the patient could talk and tell whatever he or she wished; who never verbally or actively responded to the patient; and who was always all-seeing and omnipresent (p. 350).

Cournos (2001) comes very close to this in describing her lifelong reactions to the loss of her father at age three and mother, at age eleven. She notes that she "could certainly recite the fact that my mother was dead and never returning. This belief existed side by side with the fantasy of remaining in an on-going relationship with her" (p. 141). Echoing Furman (1974), she emphasizes that a child has limited choice in seeking a substitute parental figure and thus finds an adaptive value in maintaining a living image of the deceased parent.[6] The parent might appear to 'spiritually' accompany the child, and later, the adult, everywhere. Or, the belief in his or her being alive might be betrayed by a dream image.

Clinical Vignette: 1

During his late teens, Charles LeRoy[7] who had lost his mother at age seven, felt a sudden sense of discomfort while watching the scene where the protagonist's mother is hiding in the Valley of Lepers in the movie, *Ben Hur* (Metro-Goldwyn-Mayer 1959). Two days later, he woke up from sleep in an emotional turmoil that had elements of shock, regret, and sadness. He had dreamt that he was walking on a street and a construction worker invited him to see what was hidden under the ground. With great effort, the latter unscrewed the manhole and lifted it. When Charles looked inside, his found his mother fully alive. Apparently she had not died at all and had been living under ground for several years. Charles was shocked by the discovery and felt deeply regretful that he had not known this before.

Less dramatic evidences of a lifelong internal tie to the deceased parent come in myriad forms. Aimless wandering that is unconsciously intended as a search for the lost love object is another manifestation. 'Agoraphilia' (Glauber 1955), involving an inordinate fascination for outdoors, especially ruins and wilderness, is a specific variation of such aimless wandering. Here "the love of the dead mother and the need to master the fears of her, have become the love and mastery of, or triumph over, the petrified aspects of Mother Nature" (p. 703).

---

[6]The findings of the Harvard Childhood Bereavement Study (Silverman and Worden 1993) confirm this. The investigation was based upon contacting families seen by funeral directors in the Boston, MA, area where a parent had died leaving behind a child between the ages of 6 and 17. Approximately half of the eligible families agreed to participate in the study; this included 125 children whose average age was 12. When interviewed, 81 % felt that the deceased parent was watching over them and 57 % reported speaking to him or her.

[7]All names of patients in the clinical vignettes are fictitious.

12.2.2 Mental Pain and Defenses Against It

While they might not have consciously experienced or registered it as such during childhood, adults orphaned as children remain forever vulnerable to separation anxiety, or to use Pine's (1979) more evocative term, 'separateness anxiety'; this involves discomfort and disorientation over the sense of separateness from others. However, it is the emergence of mental pain, with its characteristic admixture of hurt, disbelief, bitterness, and anger that forms the greatest threat for their ego stability. The dysphoric experience can readily emerge at the slightest of betrayals.

Since the nature of this affect is elusive and literature assessing it is meager, it might not be out of place to elucidate the concept here at some length. Freud (1926) introduced the concept in psychoanalytic literature under the rubric of *Seelenshmerz* (literally, soul-pain). He acknowledged that he knew very little about this affect and fumbled in describing it. He referred to a child's crying for his mother and evoked analogies to bodily injury and loss of body parts. He also mentioned a sense of 'longing' and 'mental helplessness' (pp. 171–172) as being components of mental pain. In the *Project* he suggested that mental pain resulted from a marked increase in the quantity of stimuli impinging upon the mind. This caused "a breach in the continuity" (1895, p. 307) of the protective shield. Pain was a direct result of such shock trauma. In *Mourning and Melancholia*, Freud related pain to object loss and said that the complex of melancholia behaved like "an open wound" (1917, p. 253). It was, however, not until an addendum to *Inhibition, Symptoms and Anxiety* (1926, pp. 169–172) that Freud linked his economic explanations to his object-related hypothesis regarding the origins of mental pain. He suggested that where there is physical pain, in increase in narcissistic cathexis of the afflicted site occurs and the same is true of mental pain. In illustrating his ideas through the situation of an infant separated from his mother, Freud implied that the object loss leading to mental pain occurred at a psychic level of ego-object non-differentiation. Weiss (1934) made this explicit by stating that:

> Pain arises when an injury – a break, so to speak, in the continuity –occurs within the ego…Love objects become, as we know, libidinally bound to the ego, as if they were parts of it. If they are torn away from it, the ego reacts as though it had sustained mutilation. The open wound thus produced in it is just what comes to the expression as mental pain (p. 12).

Thus was born the notion that mental pain is not an accompaniment of any object loss by only of the object loss that leads to an ego rupture. It is perhaps in this spirit subsequent analysts used words such as "pining" (Klein 1940, p. 360) and "longing" (Joffee and Sandler 1965, p. 156) in association with mental pain. They also resorted to somatic analogies and metaphors. Indeed, in mapping out the affective world, Pontalis (1981) placed pain "at the frontiers and juncture of body and psyche, of death and life" (p. 131). In a recent effort at bringing these and other scattered writings (Khan 1979; Joseph 1981; Kogan 1990) on this subject together I stated:

> Mental pain consists of a wordless sense of self-rupture, longing, and psychic helplessness that is vague and difficult to convey to others. It usually follows the loss of a significant object or its abrupt refusal to meet one's anaclitic needs. This results in the laceration of an unconscious, fused self-object core of the self. Abruptly precipitated discrepancies between the actual and wished-for self-states add to the genesis of mental pain. Issues of hatred, guilt, moral masochism, as well as fantasies of being beaten can also be folded into the experience of mental pain. The feeling is highly disturbing and is warded off by psychic retreat, manic defense, induction of pain into others and changing the form and function of pain. Each of these can have a pathological or healthy outcome depending upon the intrapsychic and social context upon whether they ultimately permit mourning to take place of not (Akhtar 2000, p. 223).

Among the defenses mentioned above, 'manic defense,' with its trio of idealization, denial of dependence, and omnipotence (Klein 1935; Winnicott 1935), is especially suited for warding off mental pain. *Idealization* tenaciously retains an 'all good' view of the world and oneself which, in turn, defends against guilty recognition of having injured others in fact or fantasy. *Denial* is aimed at erasing the awareness of dependence upon others. *Omnipotence* is utilized to control and master objects, but without genuine concern for them. Excessive reliance upon 'manic defense' depletes the capacities for mature aloneness, self-reflection, and genuine attachment. Mild, transient, and focal (i.e., only in one or the other area of psychosocial functioning) deployment of manic defense, on the other hand, can safeguard mental stability, and, in a paradoxical fashion, permit gradual acceptance of current and childhood losses.

12.2.3 Narcissistic Imbalance

A frequent result of parental loss during childhood is lowering of self-esteem. Not having someone to belong to and nobody to call one's own result in a sense of existential shame. One feels different from others, sensing that something is missing that should have been there in one's environment (and in its internalized representative, one's psychic structure). This feeling of being different is more marked in association with preadolescent parental loss and tends to persist throughout the later course of life. Ameliorative impact of substitute caregivers (i.e., grandparents, stepparents) helps but does not wipe out this inner shame completely.

Such narcissistic imbalance has many consequences. Idealization of parents, parenthood, and parenting is common. Envy of friends and relatives who did not lose parents in childhood is often evident and so is the tendency to overprotect one's own offspring. Hunger for belonging and narcissistic demonstration of finally having someone to call one's own extends to the marital context, leading, at times, to behavior patterns that could be annoying to the spouse.

Clinical Vignette: **2**

> Sharmila Ghosh, a thirty-five year old school teacher, was in psychotherapy with me. Having married a somewhat older man who was an internist, she had expected to receive a

sense of protection and support besides financial security from him. He was known to be a generous man and, for all external appearances, lived an opulent life. Soon after marriage, Sharmila saw the real picture. Her husband chronically spent beyond his means and his indulgent attitude towards others had a driven quality. She and her husband began to argue about household expenses, among other things. This led to marital strife and, later, to her seeking my help.

As our work unfolded, an interesting detail of their interaction emerged. This involved her husband's handing over the telephone to her whenever a family member or a friend called him or even when he had initiated the call. He somehow appeared incapable of carrying out a phone conversation from the beginning to end on his own. I initially thought that Indian cultural emphasis upon communal togetherness (Roland 1988) was responsible for this behavior of his. However, when I learned that he had lost both his parents during early childhood, I surmised differently. His handing over the phone to her now appeared his way to tell others that he did have someone in his life, and that someone did belong to him. When I shared this insight with Sharmila, she instantly understood and experienced a sense of tenderness toward her husband. Her telling this experience to him led to a softening of the tension between them.

Narcissistic imbalance consequent upon early parental loss might not remain restricted to such 'minor' psychopathology, however. A tendency to view oneself as an 'exception' (Freud 1916) might also develop, leading to egregious violations of societal limits and taboos. Arrogance, promiscuity, stealing, embezzlement, and near-incestuous cross-generational sexual activity may all arise out of such an unduly entitled attitude.

12.2.4 Disturbances in the Development of Aggressive Drive

A frequent concomitant of early parental loss is the disturbed development of the aggressive drive. Three kinds of problems can occur. In the order of decreasing severity, these include the aggressive drive undergoing atrophy, splitting, and repression. In order to understand the first of these concepts, namely the atrophy of aggression, one has to revisit Freud's (1974) statement that a coherent aggressive drive can only evolve if there is certainty of a libidinal object being available. In simpler words, one can be meaningfully angry only if there is someone there to be angry with. This is precisely what is lacking in the life of orphans. Ever uncertain of their belonging to anyone, children without parents fail to develop the normal entitlement to be angry. They lack a 'healthy capacity for indignation' (Ambassador Nathaniel Howell, personal communication, April 4, 1996). As adults, they either do not adequately register conflict with others or readily withdraw inwards; instead of confrontation, there is mere resignation. Commonly seen in schizoid (Akhtar 1987, 2009c, d) and 'as if' (Deutsch 1942) personalities, such striking absence of reactive aggression is not based upon repression. No displaced and disguised forms of resentment and anger can be found. This distinguishes atrophy of aggression from repression of aggression since the latter is inevitably accompanied with derivative (e.g., via dreams and parapraxes) or displaced expressions.

The second type of disturbance in the metabolism of aggression involves its splitting-off from the libidinal and affectively neutral sections of personality. This results in a personality organization that is essentially 'borderline' (Kernberg 1975) in structure. Self-and object-constancy do not develop if the parental loss has occurred during the first two years of life or are retrospectively weakened if the parental loss has occurred after that period. In either case, the resulting arrest of separation-individuation process perpetuates excessive dependency, keeping the individual psychologically in the position of a child. Splitting-off of aggression also depletes the central core of the ego of the assertive energy required to negotiate the adolescent passage. Of course, this is not an all-or-none matter. Ameliorative presences in the environment may help the orphaned child muster enough strength to separate from primary objects and form an autonomous identity. Yet, in most instances, some tendency toward splitting remains at the core and leads to the persistence of idealized and hated objects in the inner world.

If, however, the love–hate economy in the external surround is in favor of the former, a more integrated self can emerge. Even under such circumstances, one sees evidences that much of aggression has undergone repression and finds only limited expression in rational ways.

> Aggressive feelings are not confronted, labeled, mutually managed, and brought under modulated ego regulation by the child. Instead, they remain unchanged in the unconscious mind and are subjectively felt to be a potentially dangerous, internal liability. When stimulated by loss or threat of loss in a current important relationship, the repressed aggression threatens to breach the defense of repression and erupt in an uncontrolled aggressive act. Other defenses are then evoked to reinforce repression. (Settlage 2001, p. 62).

Prominent among such defenses are turning against the self (leading to self-neglect, self-sabotage, and self-destructiveness), projection (leading to fear of others), undoing (leading to superstitious and compulsive rituals), and reaction formation (leading to inordinate generosity and pathological altruism).[8] All in all, atrophy, splitting, and repression are mechanisms that form a hierarchy in the inner processing of early aggression in parentally deprived individuals. Keeping this spectrum in mind has implications for the treatment of orphaned adults (see details below).

12.2.5 Problems in the Realm of Love and Sexuality

Developing and sustaining attachments, especially in the realm of romance and marriage, are difficult for those who have lost parents in their childhood. The anxiety inherent in intimate bonds (e.g., abandonment, loss, mobilization of aggression) can tax their egos and lead to a reflexive avoidance of attachment or

---

[8]For a thoughtful discourse on the normal and pathological forms of altruism, see Seelig and Rosof (2001).

tenacious clinging to loved ones. Often there are oscillations between these poles. Or, the closeness–distance conflict (Akhtar 1992b) is displaced upon family pets, who are overindulged, or upon inanimate objects which are omnipotently controlled; deep discomfort at any change in their location or, conversely, constant rearrangement of furniture and art work on the wall, betray the underlying difficulties of attachment.

While there is no one-to-one correlation, the earlier the parental (especially maternal) death, the greater is the vulnerability of developing an 'oral fixation,' i.e., a hungry, yearning, and, mostly, passive orientation toward life with an entitled desire to be fed and taken care of. To escape from such dependent needs and fine alternate gratification, intense sexual strivings might develop prematurely. Kernberg (1975) emphasizes that such development powerfully reinforces oedipal fears by pregenital fears of the mother. Under these circumstances, a positive Oedipus complex is seriously interfered with. Adult sexuality is then characterized by either sexualized dependency or prominent negative oedipal trends. These manifest in greedy promiscuity and orally derived homosexuality among men, and among women, in an intensified penis envy, flight into promiscuity to deny penis envy, or a sexualized search for the gratification of oral needs from an idealized mother, leading to homosexuality.

12.2.6 Disturbances in the Subjective Experience of Time

Individuals who have lost a parent (especially the mother) during early childhood also display subtle—and sometimes, not so subtle—disturbances in the subjective experience of time. Now, we know that the origins of the sense of time are intricately bound with infantile experience of intervals between need and its gratification (Orgel 1965; Arlow 1984, 1986; Meissner 2007; Birksted-Breen 2009). And, we know that the mother's gratifying and frustrating responses are accompanied by intense emotions of pleasure and disappointment to that the "mother becomes the conveyor of time and timelessness (Erikson 1950, p. 246). In the Kleinian idiom,

> the baby endures and tolerates the separation because he/she can count on a good object that is firmly established inside himself; therefore, being able to identify with some aspects of this object. The ego builds up concomitantly to the initial notions of the present (which is based on the memory from the past) and it develops the ability to wait for the reappearance of the object in the future. The future emerges as a possibility of representing and waiting (instead of despairing), of repairing and affectively finding again the same emotional state of the contact between nipple and mouth (Bornholdt 2009, p. 101).

Among other factors that contribute to the consolidation of a sense of passing time are the "forward projection of narcissism" (Chasseguet-Smirgel 1984, p. 28) on the older generation and the associated injunction to wait (to marry, to be an adult) the oedipal children receive from their parents. All in all, it sees that parental availability and 'good-enough' parental functioning is essential for the evolution of a proper and realistic time sense in the child.

All this falls apart with the death of a parent. Not only the subtle structuring functions are lost, the child's ego is split between a developmentally pressured and inescapable forward movement in time and a stunned clinging to the object before it was lost. The former might go through post-trauma development with variable degrees of authentic participation and accruing of structure. The latter remains fixated upon a nostalgic longing for the now idealized past or a desperate conviction that the tragic loss can and will be totally undone. The former tendency is embodied in an 'if-only…' fantasy that claims that life would have been conflict-free were it not for the childhood parental loss. To be sure, there is some truth to this idea but the embellishment resides in feeling that life was devoid of all problems before the parental death and that everything would have turned out well had the tragedy not occurred.

A variant of the 'if-only..' fantasy is the 'someday..' fantasy whereby the orphan relentlessly expects to find and reunite with the parent whom, in a separate section of his mind, he recognizes to be dead. The manner in which such individuals seek a "fantasied reversal of a calamity that has occurred" (Renik1990, p. 234) and strive to materialize this 'someday' varies greatly (Akhtar 1996b). Some pursue it actively while others simply wait and turn toward spirituality. Abraham's (1924) observation, though made in a different context, is pertinent in this regard as well.

> Some people are dominated by the belief that there will always be some kind person – a representative of the mother, of course – to take care of them and to give them everything they need. This optimistic belief condemns them to inactivity (p. 399).

Frequently the 'if only..' and 'someday' fantasies (Akhtar 1996b) coexist and form a tandem theme. "If only this had not happened, life would have been all right, but someday this will be revealed and life will (again) become blissful." Such attitudes push the individual out of the present time; he shuttles between past and future, feeling nostalgic at one moment and hopeful at another but always out of tune with the calendar of actual life.

12.2.7 Attitudes Toward One's Own Mortality

The adult orphan often displays an attitude toward his own mortality that differs from his more fortunate counterparts in life. He is either inordinately afraid of dying or, equally likely, is idealizing of death and fascinated by the idea of his own mortality. Referring to the first constellation, Settlage (2001) declares that his

> clinical experience suggests that the inadequate structuring of object and self-constancy is an important factor in the fear of facing one's eventual mortality. Impairment of these structures deprives the individual of the inner sense of being loved and cared about that underlies emotional equanimity and being at peace with oneself. When present, this inner sense makes it easier to accept the reality of one's own death (p. 64).

I agree with this observation. However, I think that there is both a quantitative and qualitative difference in the fear of death experienced by normal persons and that felt by maternally deprived individuals. In the former, fear of death draws affective tributaries from the deepest remnants of annihilation anxiety, fear of separation from love objects, and castration fantasies. In those who have experienced childhood parental loss, all these factors are operative. In addition, there is a repudiated pressure to identify with the dead parent, give up the human aspects of identity, and return to an inanimate status (Lichtenstein 1963). Having, at times, been treated as inanimate by callously inattentive or enraged substitute caretakers has also blurred their inner boundaries between the animate and inanimate, and resulted in their fear that the latter will take over their entire existence. Finally, the despair at dying without having joyously lived is far more, as one would imagine, than at expecting death after having lived well.

The second outcome of having lost a parent in childhood is a tendency to be over-involved in thoughts about death and dying. Death can become idealized and, unconsciously, personified as a beckoning mother or lover (Wheelis 1966). One might pursue it actively (via gross or subtle self-destructive acts) or await its arrival with inordinate eagerness. The following poem by an East Coast-based psychotherapist eloquently captures the latter sentiment.

The train of death has started towards my city.
Only, it is at some distance right now.
Or, is it?
Thinking of death at thirty-seven,
Waiting on the train station,
I sense the aching of the tracks for the
Crushing embrace of oversized wheels. Can smell
The perspiration of the engine.
Am awed
At its dark surefootedness.
Yet, the cold certainty is familiar.
For thirty years,
I have waited on this station.
The pile of newspapers besides me growing each day
All the news of the world, cross word puzzles,
Cartoons, editorials, ads
My luggage for the journey to come.

The poem is titled *Thinking of Death at Thirty-Seven*, the age at which the individual (who prefers to remains anonymous, though has given permission to include this poem) wrote it. What became evident to him much later is that in writing "for thirty years/I have waited on this station," he had revealed that he was 7 years old at the time of his mother's death.

12.3 Some Caveats

The foregoing description of the psychopathological consequences of childhood parental loss needs 'softening' by a reminder that the outcome of such calamity is far from uniform. Many variables have to be taken into account with each having its own pathoplastic impact upon the inner goings on.

- The resemblance of what has been described above with certain features of severe character pathology (Kernberg 1975; Akhtar 1991a, 1992a) should not lead one to conclude that childhood parental loss always results in such disorders. The fact is that grown up orphans give evidence of a wide-range of personality functioning, ranging from severe to mild psychopathology and even mental health.[9] At the same time, it is true that a sector of their minds remain wounded forever, especially if the parental loss has occurred very early in life.
- Like all traumas, being orphaned may, at times, become the basis of personality strengths as well. Character traits of stoicism, ambition, and generativity especially can be intensified. Diminished fear of death, in some adults with childhood parental loss, can result in remarkable acts of courage and sacrifice.
- As a follow-up to the point above, the presence of 'God-given' talents (e.g., artistic inclination) and superior intelligence can greatly modify the impact of being orphaned. A healthy and ambitious nucleus of personality can get organized around such extraordinary abilities and lead to great fame and social success.[10]
- The impact of a parent's death varies with the child's age at the time of such loss (Bowlby 1961, 1963; Wolfenstein 1966; Furman 1974). The degree of psychic autonomy achieved, the particular developmental conflicts active at the time, and the level of ego maturity together determine how and to what extent would the trauma get adequately 'metabolized' and the nature of meanings that would be assigned to the tragedy.
- The death of a mother might have a greater or, at least, different affect upon a growing child than the death of a father. Provided all other variables remain the same, maternal death tends to deprive the child of 'a secure base' (Bowlby 1988)

[9]Few, if any, psychoanalytic texts describe 'mental health' explicitly, though implications about it are scattered throughout the corpus of our literature. Over three decades of absorption in this literature has led me to conclude that the following ten developmental achievements and ego capacities, if mostly intact most of the times, are sufficient to constitute mental health: (i) intact reality testing, (ii) capacity to experience and tolerate ambivalence, (iii) capacity for separateness, genuine attachment, and a mournful reaction upon separation, (iv) muted affects and reasonable degree of impulse control, (v) establishment of incest barrier, (vi) acceptance of generational boundaries, (vii) a well-internalized sense of morality, (viii) capacity to play, (ix) fusion of affection and erotic desire giving rise to a capacity for mature romantic love, and (x) a coherent sense of identity.

[10]An admittedly incomplete list of renowned orphans in the course of man's history includes *prophets* (e.g., Mohammad), *great philosophers* (e.g., Aristotle), *kings and conquistadors* (e.g., Julius Caesar), *musicians and singers* (e.g., Louis Armstrong, Johannes Sebastian Bach, and John Lennon), *writers and poets* (e.g., John Keats, Rudyard Kipling, and Leo Tolstoy,), *political leaders* (e.g., Bill Clinton, Nelson Mandela, and Malcolm X), and *film personalities* (e.g., Ingrid Bergman and Marilyn Monroe). The positive traits of courage, resilience, perseverance, imaginativeness, and creativity displayed by these individuals, though multiply-determined, might have been fueled by the trauma of childhood parental loss. A far less celebrated and yet profoundly impressive individual who could be added to this list was Korczak Ziolkowski (1908–1982), the Polish-American orphan from Boston who grew up to undertake the carving of the world's largest statue (in honor of the Native American chief, Crazy Horse) in South Dakota.

and a source of emotional refueling and the father's death robs the child of firm investment in external reality and the outer rind of the ego.

- The gender of the child might also play a role in the impact of parental loss. In general, girls tend to be more adversely affected by the loss of the mother than boys. The loss of mother deprives them not only of the primary love object and symbiotic partner but of a role model and scaffold for the elaboration of core gender identity. The same applies to the boy's losing a father during childhood.
- A major role in determining the outcome of parental loss is also played by the nature of relationship the child had with the parent before his or her death. Unresolved conflicts, especially those laden with aggression, tend to complicate the healing of the wounded psyche by adding a sense of guilt and responsibility for the parent's death (Volkan 1981).
- The socioeconomic status of the family can also impact upon what final shape the trauma of childhood parental loss would take. The availability of ample monetary resources can shield the child from the harshness of external reality while also providing access to better educational resources and institutions.
- The role of ameliorative influences is of paramount importance vis-à-vis childhood parental loss. The auxiliary ego support provided by the substitute parents (e.g., stepparents, grandparents) can go a long way in helping the orphaned child mourn, salvage self-esteem, and retain a sense of purpose in life. Extra-familial figures such as housekeepers, nannies, neighbors, school teachers, and clergy can also be of considerable help in mitigating the deleterious impact of such trauma. Much more important than all this is the behavior of the surviving parent. If he or she remains stable, continues the appropriate development-facilitating role, and attempts to compensate for the child's loss while also empathizing with it, the child can show remarkable resilience. A nonclinical anecdote captures this point very well. Recounted by a Pakistani colleague, Naeem Jaafri, the story goes like this:

> I was a little over seven when I lost my mother. It had a devastating impact upon me. But my father, an internist with a large private practice, was kind and loving and helped me a lot. A year or two later, he remarried. My step-mother was also good to me and yet I felt something was not quite right. I felt she never gave me sufficient food to eat. When I told this to my father, he did something remarkable. He told me that I could go and eat whatever and however much I liked at the corner restaurant down the street from his office, free of charge; he would pay the bill on a monthly basis without ever questioning me. I was at first flabbergasted, then thrilled, by this newfound power. I visited the restaurant at all sorts of times, ordering this and that item on the menu. The bills were always paid and no one raised an eyebrow. Within a few months, I got tired of the whole thing and stopped going to the restaurant. The complaint I had against my step-mother also withered away. Matters seemed more manageable and peaceful to me (personal communication, December 2009).

While it can be argued that my colleague's father should have sat him and his wife down and chatted about whatever was going on between them, such an expectation from a busy physician in 1950s Lahore is merely a psychoanalyst's dream. The fact is that the father intervened to restore the loss sense of omnipotence in his boy, most likely knowing (at least, on an unconscious level) that the matter had little to do with actual food. In doing so, he did help his child.

What this anecdote as well as the foregoing caveats demonstrate is that simply knowing that someone is an orphan is not enough. A larger number of biopsychosocial variables and their complex interplay with each other must be taken into account in order to grasp the deep psychological significance of childhood parental loss. In the words of Freud (1974)

> It is on the one hand the total character and personality of the child and on the other hand the totality of environmental circumstances which determine the outcome of the experience. Here, as in all other areas of the child's life, the interaction between internal and external forces decides between the possibility of normal developmental progress and the incidence of pathological developmental distortion or arrest (p. vii).

Armed with such nuanced empathy, one can approach the treatment of adult orphans in a meaningful manner.

12.4 Guidelines for Treating Orphaned Adults

Based upon my clinical experience with adults who have suffered the loss of one or both parents in childhood, I have delineated six technical guidelines for working with them. I must emphasize, though, that I am not recommending specific strategies, only a background for the "evenly suspended attention" (Freud 1912, p. 111) that is customary in our work.

12.4.1 Providing a Greater Amount of 'Illusion' and 'Holding'

Those who have lost a parent in early childhood have been introduced to 'reality' in a brutal manner. The illusion of absolute safety, afforded by parental 'holding' (Winnicott 1960), has been prematurely ruptured. Infantile omnipotence, instead of being renounced gradually and in a piecemeal fashion, has had to be given up abruptly. All this results in a longing—however dormant and disguised it may be—for a type of interpersonal relatedness in which one can truly relax and express oneself with little worry about the dyadic partner's needs. All one desires is to be fully accepted, cared for, and treated with exquisite empathy and devotion. Not that there is no aggression, hostility, and revenge fantasies contained in the patient's psyche but at the beginning stage of treatment, these are not fully accessible for the patient to experience and explore. That work will emerge but only after the patient has experienced an illusory 'dual unity' (Mahler et al. 1975) for a sufficiently long period of time.

The predominant therapeutic task with orphaned adults is therefore to create and sustain a proper 'holding environment' (Winnicott 1960). Besides the physical comfort and stability of the office where the two parties meet (for details see Akhtar 2009e), this includes a psychological ambience of trust, safety, nonjudgmental acceptance, and containment of affects while helping the patient's growth potential to be activated. To be sure, such provision is important in the treatment of all patients but it acquires greater valence in those with a background of childhood parental loss.

A concrete expression of such therapeutic attitude resides in seeing the patient in a face-to-face position. The availability of visual contact with the actual person of the analyst subliminally gratifies the 'real' object hunger of these patients to the extent that it becomes possible to discuss it. Even when a more traditional psychoanalytic treatment is undertaken, an initial period of sitting up for at least a few weeks is helpful; this leads to a certain amount of internalization of the analyst and diminishes the impact of the visual loss upon beginning to lie down on the couch (Akhtar 1992b). During the analytic treatment also, an atmosphere needs to be created whereby the patient feels comfortable to sit up from time to time; such departures from the recumbent position might be interpreted or benignly accepted depending upon the analyst's empathic sense of what is going on and how to handle it best. Celenza's (2005) recommendation that "every analysis should, at some point, include both modalities [sitting up and lying down] for some period of time" (p. 1656) is important to remember in this context. She notes that both lying down on the couch and sitting up on the chair have their own pros and cons and each can facilitate dialogue, even self-revelation, though in different ways.

Individuals who have suffered childhood parental loss also need a greater leeway with physically settling in the office and making it their own, so to speak. They often borrow magazines from the waiting room and, indeed, should be readily allowed to do so without making any interpretations. Abrams' (1978) concept of 'developmental intervention' is pertinent in this context. This refers to the analyst's supportively 'permitting' or underscoring the progressive trend when a hitherto thwarted capacity has emerged as a result of the analyst's 'holding' or interpretive activity. From this perspective, an orphaned adult's taking things from the office or the waiting room is seen as the resumption of the healthy sense of entitlement (over parents) that had been ruptured by the parental death. The analyst's upholding this newly acquired ability of the patient facilitates the emergence of experiential building-blocks necessary for further development.

12.4.2 *Validating the Importance and the 'Unfairness' of the Loss*

The therapist must offer empathic resonance to the adult orphan's loss and its profound effects upon him. If the patient asks whether it was 'fair' that his mother or father died when he was a little child, the therapist should not hesitate to say that it was certainly 'unfair.' Somewhat later in their work, the therapist might also point out that the question of something being 'fair' or 'unfair' is itself a concern of childhood; adult life is replete with randomness and unfairness both against and in favor of oneself. Subsequently, the therapist might add that, given the vantage point of a developing child it *is* unfair to have lost a parent and be left bereft of support and belonging. Such 'mirroring' (Kohut 1977) and 'affirmative' (Killingmo 1989) interventions can have healing effects of their own. Pine's (1997) remark that, at times, the seemingly nonspecific elements of technique acquire high individualized therapeutic effects is relevant in this context.

In working with such patients, one often comes across the fact that significant adults in their background did not help them mourn the death of the parent. In fact, they avoided the topic and acted as if everything had returned to normal very soon after the child's parent had died. The true subjective experience of the orphaned child was not validated. This, in turn, led to the child (and, subsequently, the adult) feeling even more lonely and isolated. The longing for genuine recognition became intensified and, at times, quite blatant.

Clinical Vignette: 3

Charles LeRoy (see Clinical Vignette: 1 above) had lost his mother at the age of seven and was soon abandoned by his father. Raised by aging grandparents and sundry relatives, Charles had no memory of any adult every talking to him about his mother's death. Everyone treated him kindly but this in itself was far removed from the shattered inner experience that he was going through. Charles once visited a remote uncle who worked as a superintendent of an old style orphanage. Upon seeing the place and the collective life of the institutionalized children, Charles felt a sharp pang of longing to be enrolled there. The environment mirrored his true self and held the promise of an authentic identity for him.

Listening to this kind of experience teaches us the importance of genuine mirroring and validation while dealing with orphaned adults. Any attempt to minimize the long-term, indeed lifelong, impact of childhood parental death negates the patients' subjectivity and erodes therapeutic alliance with them. At the same time, it should be underscored that validation is not restricted to verbal remarks. The well-timed raising of an eyebrow, the attuned leaning forward in the chair while talking to the patient and a confirming nod of the head often carries more weight than the therapist's words. Even a respectful acceptance of the patient's silence can make the patient feel deeply understood. The following observation of Klein (1963) eloquently captures this point.

> However gratifying it is in later life to express thoughts and feelings, to a congenial person, there remains an unsatisfied longing for an understanding without words – ultimately for the earliest relations with the mother. This longing contributes to the sense of loneliness and derives from the depressive feeling of an irretrievable loss (p. 301).

That this longing is much more intense in individuals who have lost parents (especially the mother) goes without saying.

12.4.3 Discerning the Defenses Against the Awareness of the Pervasive Impact of the Loss

Not infrequently, adults who have been orphaned as children enter psychotherapy and psychoanalysis for reasons that are overtly unrelated to their childhood trauma. They know the facts of their loss but do not realize how deep and pervasive its impact has been over them. The following cases illustrate how a background of pain pervades their lives and, in unconscious ways, contributes to their presenting symptoms.

Clinical Vignette: 4

Sol Ackerman, a thirty-five year old internist, became symptomatic a few months after the birth of his son. He was madly 'in love' with the baby and reacted with intense pain to the slightest in-attention of his wife towards the child. This led to friction between them which was fueled by Sol's repeatedly calling home from work to check on his infant son's welfare. The marital tension was not all, though. Sol was aware of some gnawing anguish that was threatening to break through his otherwise composed persona, a pain the true origins of which he could not fathom.

In the second session of his treatment, Sol reported the following dream: "I am flying a small plane, solo. Its engine is having some trouble. I land the plane on the North Pole and come out seeking help. There is snow everywhere. I walk. And then suddenly I come across this woman sitting on a bench. But there is something very peculiar about the woman. She is made entirely of small icicles. She is brittle and cannot move. Just as I am looking at her, my good friend Bob appears on the scene. He and I help the woman to rise up and begin walking. The scene changes. Now I am in Spain, a country I have never visited in reality. I am in a tavern. There is red wine being served. And, there are lively and beautiful women everywhere."

Sol's associations led to the memory of his mother's developing scleroderma when he was four years old and, over the next two years, developing contractures of skin and joints. She died, when Sol was six, in an immobile and 'frozen' state. Amidst sobs, Sol began to see how the dream revealed his wish to be helped by his analyst (represented by his friend, Bob) to thaw this frozen grief and move on with his life to more enjoyable activities. The analysis of this dream not only opened up the floodgates to the memories of his childhood loss (and how it had always remained with him) but also to associations that provided links between his maternal loss and his anxious insistence upon his wife remaining constantly available to his baby son.

Such stirring up of childhood loss at the time of becoming a parent is understandable. However, events that can trigger the trauma of orphanhood are diverse and, at times, far removed from the realm of parent–child interaction.

Clinical Vignette: 5

'Mary Thompson, a retired librarian in her mid- sixties, sought my help for panic attacks which interfered in her ability to function optimally. She had received ongoing but ultimately unhelpful treatment for the past twenty years. Mary had managed to function but her anxiety attacks had never gone away. She grew increasing disenchanted, angry, and depressed as she found herself unable to maintain the lifestyle that she had in the past.

Her symptoms appeared twenty years ago when she was bitten by a venomous snake while vacationing with her friends. She was treated by the local doctors with the appropriate anti-venom and flown home. However, upon her return she suffered a toxic reaction, which affected her body such that it swelled up and she was unable to move. Her medical doctor, unfamiliar with the particular anti-venom administered, put her through a series of tests that caused further incapacitation and left her feeling helpless and furious. Though the situation was eventually rectified, it precipitated the onset of her anxiety-related symptoms.

During the initial sessions of the treatment, Mary revealed the details of a tragic childhood. She lost both parents at three years of age. Her father bludgeoned Mary's mother to death. He then took a shotgun to his head and killed himself as his young daughter (Mary) and his infant son lay in a crib in the next room. The children were soon placed in an orphanage and, over time, adopted by different families. Mary, at age five, was sent from her native state to live with adoptive parents.

Mary grew very fond of her adoptive mother though she cared little for her adoptive father who was abusive both toward her and his wife. Mary moved out of the house during her late teens, when her adopted mother died. She then pursued a semiprofessional degree and found a job, which earned her a decent income. An avid sportswoman, she became active in the local women's soccer team. She also enjoyed writing poetry and had over the years written a fair amount of it. Though Mary had maintained some connection with her brother, spending her summer holidays with him, it was only after she became an adult did she have the freedom and flexibility to develop family ties of her own choosing. This consisted of a female lover with whom she had been living for over forty years.

Though Mary knew of her early parental loss, it was only during our work together that she began to connect that trauma with her current symptoms. Initially, she spoke of these losses through clenched teeth and tense posture, and responded with anger to my inquiries. I decided to stop asking questions and simply listen as her narrative unfolded. Mary was skeptical of any treatment and angry at the world of doctors. I listened patiently, affording her the space that she needed yet maintaining a neutral yet empathic stance towards her. I did not offer immediate relief, just the sense that that in time we would understand all this together.

In time, both Mary and I were able to link the onset of her symptoms to her early childhood trauma. The loss of her parents, which left her an orphan, introduced her to a profound sense of helplessness. She recalled hearing her father bludgeoning her mother and then the sound of the shotgun. While she attempted to run out of the house (at age three!) with her baby brother, the sense of being overwhelmed and without any support remained inside her. This feeling of helplessness emerged repeatedly during her stay in the orphanage. Such was the case when she had to abide by ideosyncratic 'house rules' and, more importantly, to witness her brother (and the little friends that had made there) being sent away for adoption. Mary could now begin to understand why the immobility following the snake bite episode had stirred a deep sense of anxiety in her. As she developed a deeper insight into the nature of her current symptoms and the childhood narrative that lay hidden in them, Mary began to feel less anxious and resumed some of her earlier activities.

While both foregoing cases portray anxiety-related symptoms as the presenting features that gradually led to the discerning of the long-term effects of childhood parental loss, the clinical picture in such situations varies greatly. At times, patients seek help because they have become depressed in the face of a current loss which triggers the earlier but dormant trauma. At other times, the clinical picture is one of self-destructive acting out that turns out to be a desperate cry for help.

Clinical Vignette: 6

Susan King, an college student in her mid-twenties was referred to me following a sudden onset of depression precipitated by the death of her maternal grandmother. Despite a trial of anti-depressants by her family physician, Susan's symptoms did not lessen. Instead, she found herself abruptly ending a relationship of five months. Her uncontrollable crying and inability to study finally brought her to my office.

I gathered that Susan had lost her mother in an automobile accident, when she was five years old. Following this, her father remarried and Susan was placed in the care of caretakers who came and went as the family struggled to deal with their departures. Susan later moved away from home to attend college. Following this, she procured a job in the adjoining state where I had my practice.

Later, Susan narrated a more complex history of her childhood and adult life. She had terminated a relationship of five months describing it as nothing but sexual and one that could not be sustained anyway. Prior to that, she had ended a meaningful relationship with a young man that had lasted five years. Though she described this relationship as being 'ideal' in many ways, she nevertheless engaged in destructive behaviors, including sexual promiscuity, that were bound to destroy the bond.

A picture of early childhood neglect also emerged. After her mother died, Susan was placed in a new school. Too ashamed to talk about her loss, she kept silent. She often went to school with a disheveled appearance receiving little supervision from her stepmother or the ever-changing cadre of housekeepers. The youngest of five siblings, she was often in the company of teenagers who overlooked her need to be supervised. She soon became a participant in their sexual play and this dominated most of her adolescent life.

As our work deepened, the pattern of self-destructive behaviors became more apparent. On one occasion, she, along with a girlfriend, went on a trip and 'played a game of roulette with the drug Ecstasy.' What this essentially entailed was taking the drug without knowing the vendor, off the street – an extremely dangerous thing to do. Susan had a history of some drinking and doing drugs but this was certainly out of character for her. At another time, she 'crashed 'party in her neighborhood wearing a short leather skirt, boots and a sexy top.' Again, this was out of character for her, as she frequented the church on weekends and was a devout Christian. Besides such dangerous enactments, there was a deepening attachment to me. Susan now began to have enormous difficulty leaving the office. She cried in almost every session as she recalled painful memories of her deceased mother. As a child, she was numb but clung to her housekeepers, becoming distraught when they would leave. This part was now present in my office.

Susan could now begin to connect her symptoms to her early childhood loss of her mother. It became clear that her counterphobic risk-taking was an unconscious cry for help; it betrayed a wish that I (as a parent) protect her from all dangers. The hitherto unrecognized and yet dominant role of the number five (e.g., her breakups at five months and five years, her going to the fifth floor of my building even though my office was located on the fifteenth floor) could be seen as a magical attempt to return to age five (when she lost her mother) in order to thaw the frozen grief within her.

Besides the sort of interpretative linkages described in the three vignettes above, the analyst must keep his ears attuned to listening for the subtle ways in which the death of a parent in childhood is denied and the full moving over it postponed. Here, the disarmament of the 'if-only' and 'someday' fantasies (Akhtar 1996b) acquires a central technical role. It is as if what the child could not mourn, the adult is refusing to mourn. That this needs holding, containing, unmasking, and interpreting goes without saying (for details of technique vis-à-vis such fantasies, see Akhtar 1996b).

Additionally, an eye must be kept on the vicissitudes of aggression in such patients. If one suspects a mal-development and atrophy of aggression in them, gentle questioning about it and encouragement to be more expressive might be indicated. Also useful might be unmasking the patient's lack of entitlement. With patients whose aggression has become split off from the main sector of the personality, it might help to make 'bridging interventions' (Kernberg 1975) that involve the analyst's display (by gentle verbal reminders or a subtle shift in the tone of voice) that he, at least, has not forgotten the transference configuration that is opposite to the one currently active. Finally, with patients in whom aggression has undergone massive repression, the customary work of defense analysis and transference interpretation is indicated.

12.4.4 Interpreting the Defensive Uses of One's Status as an Orphan

Another important task in the treatment of orphaned adults involves discerning the moments when the lament of loss is serving a 'screen' (Akhtar 2009b, p. 253) function and keeping even more troubling intrapsychic matters in abeyance. Often the 'pre-death' family environment has not been as tranquil as initially portrayed by the patient. In the case of one particular patient, for instance, there had been many shifts of family residence, the death of a beloved aunt, and a painful separation from the biological father *before* the patient lost his mother at age seven. The traumatic effects of the preceding incidents had, however, been glossed over by the patient who attributed all his difficulties to the death of his mother. Certainly there is little reason to regard this case to be exceptional in clinical practice.

Given the fact that orphanhood has diverse consequences and there is a dialectical relationship between the direct and indirect damage that has occurred as a result, it is hardly surprising that patients can use one as a defense against the other. Take, for instance, the patient's need for validation that he or she has suffered a major loss and this indeed has been a very unfortunate occurrence. This can acquire a sadomasochistic coloration. One who asks over and over again if it was 'good' or 'fair' that his parent(s) died during childhood is hardly looking for a mirroring confirmation. Such 'interrogation' is better responded to by clarifying its affective tone, unmasking the denial (of the therapist's having already stated that it was 'unfair') implicit in it, and interpreting the sadistic ('you do not believe me') and masochistic ('see how fate has dealt me a cruel blow') transferences inherit in it. The desperate object hunger, the near-addictive masochism, and the unconscious sadism can only then come to surface. Endlessly patient listening to repetitive material and going on and on with 'affirmative interventions' (Killingmo 1989) is not technically appropriate under such circumstances. Here I wish to reiterate an earlier comment of mine.

> Listening is good. Listening patiently for a long time is better. But listening forever to material that is all too familiar constitutes a collusion with the patient's sadomasochism and narcissism. Such listening is contrary to the purposes of psychoanalysis (Akhtar 2007, p. 13).

12.4.5 Paying Special Attention to Termination and Post-termination Phases of the Treatment

Though it is not possible to generalize, there is ample foundation to the thought that terminating treatment might be harder for those with a background of childhood parental loss. Letting go of the nurturing and development-enhancing relationship provided by psycho- analysis (or intensive psychotherapy) is likely to reawaken the wound of childhood loss. This can be mitigated by the judicious use—in varying and individually tailored combinations—of the following measures:

- Arriving at the decision to terminate more slowly than usual and with much greater attention to the patient's vulnerability in this regard.
- Having a longer interval between the day one agrees to terminate and the day one decides the actual date of termination.
- Setting the date of termination fairly in advance, i.e., at least 6 months or so still left to work together.
- Following Bergman's (2005) recommendations, conducting the last few hours of treatment with the patient sitting up and with the analyst and patient assessing what has been accomplished and what further work might still be there to do on one's own. "During this time, the two partners are speaking to each other more as equals than they did during the analysis itself" (p. 251).
- Following Schachter's (1990, 1992) recommendations, bringing up the possibility of post-termination contacts though leaving the choice to exercise this option and to initiate it to the patient.

These five guidelines seek to provide auxiliary ego support for the patient for whom separation and loss are especially painful. However, these are only pointers, not rules. Their use has to be tailored to individual situations, keeping the strengths and 'soft spots' of each particular patient in mind.

12.4.6 Managing the Countertransference Experience

Working with adults who have lost one or both parents in childhood can evoke powerful countertransference responses. Pertinent in this context is the following observation by Parens (2010), even though it is made in the context of children grieving over the death of a parent.

> Many empathic adults find it difficult to tolerate a young child's experiencing intense psychic pain. We know in our field that helping such a child deal with his/her feelings, thoughts, and fantasies is extremely painful not only for the remaining sensitive parent, but also for such teachers, and it is even taxing for therapists. Yet, we know that we cannot help a child cope with painful experiences without empathetically allowing the child's affects to resonate within our own psyche, with our own experiences of object loss, an experience unavoidably painful to a greater or lesser degree for each of us (p. 43).

Similar difficulties can arise in the treatment of adults who have suffered childhood parental loss. Their desperate hunger for the deceased parent, their wistful longing for the analyst to provide the guidance expected from the parent who is no more, their soul-wrenching pain at the inability to turn the clock back, and their recurring reminder about the unfairness of what happened, can together strain the analyst's work ego. The fact that the transferences of these patients have a markedly 'real' quality can also compromise his interpretive skills. The difficulty is compounded if the analyst has also suffered a similar childhood loss.

The resulting countertransferences can lead either to a defensive recoil from the patient's anguish or to an overidentification with the consciously avowed 'traumatized child' self. The former tendency can lead to viewing the patient's wailing mostly as a defense against other, more 'primitive' or more 'advanced' conflicts. The latter tendency can lead to over-gratification of the patient and nonactivation (hence, non-interpretation) of negative transference constellations. The former stance overlooks the patient's dependent strivings. The latter ignores the patient's resilience and creativity in face of the loss. The former type of countertransference leaning minimizes the patient's need for continuity and availability (e.g., for knowing where the analyst is going for vacation, for having some contact during long breaks in treatment). The latter type of countertransference leaning minimizes the patient's developmental need for autonomy and to bear a modicum of pain at separations. Clearly, both extremes are to be avoided. A sustained, though benevolent, vigilance toward one's own emotional participation in the therapeutic process goes a long way in assuring a balanced stance.

12.5 Concluding Remarks

In this chapter, I have surveyed the multilayered consequences of childhood parental loss. Employing the much avoided but direct and evocative designation 'orphan,' I have elucidated the lifelong struggles and vulnerabilities of individuals whose parents have died early on in their lives. The realms in which long-term consequences of this trauma can be found include those of aggression, narcissism, love and sexuality, subjective experience of time, and attitudes toward one's own mortality. However, a more central issue is the intrapsychic relationship the 'orphan' maintains with his or her lost parent. Never fully relinquished, this internal object-representation exerts a powerful influence on the individual, an influence that can be pathogenic (e.g., lifelong vulnerability to separation anxiety) or salutary (e.g., enhanced ambition and creativity). Clearly, the balance of outcome depends upon a large number of factors that include the age at which the loss occurred, the nature of relationship with the parent before he or she died, the constitutional talents of the child, the degree of love and reliability offered by the surviving parent and/or substitute parental figure(s), the availability of health-promoting role models, the monetary stability of the family and, the degree to which those around the child were willing and/or able to facilitate his mourning of the loss. This last mentioned factor cannot be overemphasized since many adults feel uncomfortable in seeing a child sad and distract him from the work of mourning instead of helping him with it.

All this has consequences for the treatment of adults who have lost one or both parents during childhood. A greater degree of 'illusion' and 'holding,' validation of the tragic nature of the loss, clarification and interpretation of defenses against mourning, unmasking of the defensive uses of the tragedy and of its consequences, and careful monitoring of the countertransference experience constitute the needed background for conducting psychotherapy and psychoanalysis with such patients.

While I have covered a fairly large territory of concerns, there still remain matters that need to be understood. Four unaddressed areas readily come to mind. *First*, and foremost, since childhood parental loss hardly ever occurs in isolation from other potentially pathogenic influences (e.g., destabilized family, compromised monetary situations, depressed caretakers), it is important that comparative long-term studies be made of 'real' versus 'psychic' orphans. The latter designation includes children abandoned by parents and raised in haphazard ways by this or that reluctant relative and children who were misinformed that their mother or father had died only to later find out the actual truth about the situation. Such comparative data might help distinguish the psychopathological impact of parental loss from other complicating factors that are often associated with it but are not specific to it. *Second*, while I have mentioned, in passing, the poignant depiction of orphans in literature, a thorough comparison of the personality characteristics attributed to them is still awaiting. Such pooling of the available 'data' might help in developing a finer and more sophisticated composite profile of the adult orphan's psychic functioning. *Third*, more knowledge is needed regarding whether the old style orphanages (or some contemporary reincarnation of them) are more ego-supportive of an orphan child or is it better that the child be shielded from orphanhood becoming a part of his identity? Investigations along this line might also yield strategies to help diminish what I call the 'shame of the motherless child' and to improve coping skills of the traumatized child. *Finally*, a critical revisiting of the psychoanalytic case reports dealing with orphaned children and adults—since it was last done over three decades ago (Furman, 1974)—is warranted in order to fine tune therapeutic strategies that best serve this clinical population. The technical guidelines I have offered in this chapter need to be examined, supported or refuted, and further elaborated upon by others.

As work along the lines suggested above evolves, the answer to the most frequently asked question in this realm ("does one every fully get over an early childhood parental loss?") might find further refinement and nuance. Meanwhile, Furman's (1974) observation remains valid: "Some may be better able to cope with this tragedy than others; for all, it becomes a life-long burden" (p. 172). At the same time, how one carries this 'burden' and to what extent the subterranean anguish fuels creative efforts also remain important. Georges Braque's (1882–1963) following statement is good to keep in mind in this context: "art is a wound turned to light".

References

Abraham, K. (1924). The influence of oral eroticism on character formation. In *Selected papers of Karl Abraham, M.D.* (pp. 393–406). New York, NY: Brunner/Mazel.

Abrams, S. (1978). The teaching and learning of psychoanalytic developmental psychology. *Journal of the American Psychoanalytic Association, 26*, 387–406.

Akhtar, S. (1987). Schizoid personality disorder: a synthesis of developmental, dynamic, and descriptive features. *American Journal of Pyschotherapy, 41*, 499–518.

Akhtar, S. (1991a). Three fantasies related to unresolved separation-individuation: a less recognized aspect of severe character pathology. In S. Akhtar & H. Parens (Eds.), *Beyond the symbiotic orbit: Advances in separation-individuation theory* (pp. 261–284). Hillsdale, NJ: The Analytic Press.

Akhtar, S. (1992a). *Broken structures: Severe personality disorders and their treatment.* Northvale, NJ: Jason Aronson.

Akhtar, S. (1992b). Tethers, orbits, and invisible fences: clinical, developmental, sociocultural, and technical aspects of optimal distance. In S. Kramer & S. Akhtar (Eds.), *When the body speaks: Psychological meanings in kinetic clues* (pp. 21–57). Northvale, NJ: Jason Aronson.

Akhtar, S. (1996b). "Someday… " and "if only. " fantasies: pathological optimism and inordinate nostalgia as related forms of idealization. *Journal of American Psychoanalytic Association, 44*, 723–753.

Akhtar, S. (2000). Mental pain and the cultural ointment of poetry. *International Journal of Psychoanalysis, 81*, 229–243.

Akhtar, S. (2007). The 'listening cure': An overview. In *Listening to others: Developmental and clinical aspects of empathy and attunement* (pp. 1–16). Lanham, MD: Jason Aronson.

Akhtar, S. (2009a). *Good feelings: Psychoanalytic perspectives on positive attitudes and emotions.* London, UK: Karnac Books.

Akhtar, S. (2009b). *Comprehensive dictionary of psychoanalysis.* London, UK: Karnac Books.

Akhtar, S. (2009c). *The damaged core: Origins, dynamics, manifestations, and treatment.* Lanham, MD: Jason Aronson.

Akhtar, S. (2009d). The schizoid wish to die and be reborn. In *The damaged core: Origins, dynamics, manifestations, and treatment* (pp. 67–86). Lanham, MD: Jason Aronson.

Akhtar, S. (2009e). The analyst's office. In *The damaged core: Origins, dynamics, manifestations, and treatment* (pp. 113–133). Lanham, MD: Jason Aronson.

Arlow, J. A. (1984). Disturbances of the sense of time with special reference to the sense of timelessness. *Psychoanalytic Quarterly, 53*, 13–37.

Arlow, J. A. (1986). Psychoanalysis and time. *Journal of the American Psychoanalytic Association, 34*, 507–528.

Bellow, S. (1953). *The adventures of Augie March.* New York, NY: Viking Press.

Ben Hur. (1959). Directed by William Wyler. A Metro-Goldwyn-Mayer (MGM) Production.

Bergman, M. (2005). Termination and re-analysis. In E. Person, A. Cooper, & G. Gabbard (Eds.), *The American Psychiatric Publishing Textbook of Psychoanalysis* (pp. 241–253). Washington, DC: American Psychiatric Press.

Birksted-Breen, D. (2009). 'Reverberation time', dreaming, and the capacity to dream. *International Journal of Psychoanalysis, 90*, 35–51.

Bornholdt, I. (2009). The impact of the time experience on the psychoanalysis of children and adolescents. In L. Glocer Fiorini & J. Canestri (Eds.), *The experience of time: Psychoanalytic perspectives* (pp. 97–116). London, UK: Karnac Books.

Bowlby, J. (1960). Grief and mourning in infancy and early childhood. *Psychoanalytic Study of the Child, 15*, 9–52.

Bowlby, J. (1961). Processes of mourning. *International Journal of Psychoanalysis, 42*, 317–340.

Bowlby, J. (1963). Pathological mourning and childhood mourning. *Journal of the American Psychoanalytic Association, 11*, 500–541.

Bowlby, J. (1969). *Attachment and loss: Vol I. Attachment.* New York, NY: Basic Books.

Bowlby, J. (1988). *A secure base*. New York, NY: Basic Books.
Carveth, D. L. (1992). Dead end kids: Projective identification and sacrifice in 'Orphans'. *International Review of Psychoanalysis, 19*, 217–227.
Celenza, A. (2005). Vis-à-vis the couch: where is psychoanalysis? *International Journal of Psychoanalysis, 86*, 1645–1660.
Chasseguet-Smirgel, J. (1984). *Creativity and perversion*. New York, NY: W. W. Norton.
Cournos, F. (2001). Mourning and adaptation following the death of a parent in childhood. *Journal of the American Academy of Psychoanalysis, 29*, 137–145.
Deutsch, H. (1942). Some forms of emotional disturbance and their relationship to schizophrenia. *Psychoanalytic Quarterly, 11*, 301–321.
Dickens, C. (1860). *Great expectations*. New York, NY: W.W. Norton, 1999.
Erikson, E. H. (1950). *Childhood and society*. New York, NY: W.W. Norton and Co.
Fichtner, G. (Ed.). (2003). *The Freud-Binswanger correspondence 1908–1938*. London, UK: Open Gate Press.
Fielding, H. (1749). *The history of Tom Jones, a foundling*. New York, NY, 2005.
Freud, S. (1895). Project for a scientific psychology. *Standard Edition, 1*, 295–343. London: Hogarth Press.
Freud, S. (1897). Letter to Wilhelm Fliess, October 3, 1897. In J. M. Masson (Eds.), *The complete letters of Sigmund Freud to Wilhelm Fliess* (p. 268). Cambridge, MA: Harvard University Press.
Freud, A. (1974). Foreword. In E. Furman (Ed.), *A child's parent dies* (p. vii). New Haven, CT: Yale University Press.
Freud, S. (1912). Recommendations to physicians practising psychoanalysis. *Standard Edition, 12*, 109–120.
Freud, S. (1916). Some character types met with during psychoanalytic work. *Standard Edition, 14*, 310–333.
Freud, S. (1917). Mourning and melancholia. *Standard Edition, 14*, 237–258.
Freud, S. (1926). Inhibitions, symptoms, and anxiety. *Standard Edition, 20*, 77–175.
Furman, E. (Ed.). (1974). *A child's parent dies*. New Haven, CT: Yale University Press.
Glauber, P. (1955). On the meaning of agoraphilia. *Journal of the American Psychoanalytic Association, 3*, 701–709.
Goldsmith, O. (1766). *The Vicar of Wakefield*. Oxford: Oxford University Press, 2008.
Gordon, K. H., & Sherr, P. C. (1974). Orphans in literature: a bibliography for the study of the adolescent. *Journal of the American Psychoanalytic Association, 22*, 537–541.
Hesse, H. (1919). *Demien: A dual language book* (S. Appelbaum, Trans.). Mineola, NY: Dover Publications, 2002.
Joffee, W. G., & Sandler, J. (1965). Pain, depression, and individuation. In J. Sandler (Ed.), *From safety to superego* (pp. 154–179). New York, NY: The Guilford Press.
Joseph, B. (1981). Towards the experiencing of psychic pain. In M. Feldman & E.B. Spillius (Eds.), *Psychic equilibrium and psychic change. Selected papers of Betty Joseph* (pp. 88–97). London, UK: Routledge, 1989.
Kernberg, O. F. (1975). *Borderline conditions and pathological narcissism*. New York, NY: Jason Aronson.
Khan, M. M. R. (1979). From masochism to psychic pain. In *Alienation in Perversions* (pp. 210–218). New York: International Universities Press.
Killingmo, B. (1989). Conflict and deficit: Implications for technique. *International Journal of Psycho-analysis, 70*, 65–79.
Klein, M. (1935). A contribution to the psychogenesis of manic depressive states. In *Love, guilt and reparation and other works—1921–1945* (pp. 262–289). New York, NY: The Free Press, 1975.
Klein, M. (1940). Mourning and its relation to manic-depressive states. *International Journal of Psychoanalysis, 21*, 125–153.
Klein, M. (1963). On the sense of loneliness. In *Envy and gratitude and other works—1946–1963* (pp. 300–313). New York, NY: The Free Press, 1975.

Kogan, I. (1990). A journey to pain. *International Journal of Psychoanalysis, 71*, 629–640.
Kohut, H. (1977). *Restoration of the self.* New York, NY: International Universities Press.
Lichtenstein, H. (1963). The dilemma of human identity: notes on self-transformation, self-objectivation, and metamorphosis. *Journal of American Psychoanalytic Association, 11*, 173–223.
Mahler, M. S., Pine, F., & Bergman, A. (1975). *The psychological birth of the human infant: Symbiosis and individuation*. New York, NY: Basic Books.
Masson, J. M. (Ed.). (1985). *The complete letters of Sigmund Freud to Wilhelm Fleiss*. Cambridge, MA: Harvard University Press.
Masur, C. (2001). Can women mourn their mothers? In S. Akhtar (Ed.), *Three faces of mourning: Melancholia, manic defense, and moving on* (pp. 33–46). Northvale, NJ: Jason Aronson.
Maugham, W. S. (1915). *Of human bondage* (p. 1999). New York, NY: Random House.
Meissner, W. (2007). *Time, Self, and Psychoanalysis*. Lanham, MD: Jason Aronson.
Meyers, H. (2001). Does mourning become Electra?: Oedipal and separation-individuation issues in a woman's loss of her mother. In S. Akhtar (Ed.), *Three faces of mourning: Melancholia, manic defense, and moving on* (pp. 13–31). Northvale, NJ: Jason Aronson.
Nagera, H. (1970). Children's reactions to the death of important objects. *Psychoanalytic Study of the Child, 25*, 369–392.
Orgel, S. (1965). On time and timelessness. *Journal of the American Psychoanalytic Association, 13*, 102–121.
Parens, H. (2010). Thoughts on children's understanding of death. In S. Akhtar (Ed.), *The wound of mortality: Fear, denial, and acceptance of death* (pp. 37–50). Lanham, MD: Jason Aronson.
Pine, F. (1979). The separation-individuation process. *International Journal of Psychoanalysis, 60*, 225–242.
Pine, F. (1997). *Diversity and direction in psychoanalytic technique*. New Haven, CT: Yale University Press.
Pollock, G. H. (1961). Mourning and adaptation. *International Journal of Psychoanalysis, 42*, 341–361.
Pontalis, J. B. (1981). *Frontiers in psychoanalysis: Between the dream and psychic reality*. New York, NY: International Universities Press.
Renik, O. (1990). Comments on the clinical analysis of anxiety and depressive affect. *Psychoanalytic Quarterly, 59*, 226–248.
Roland, A. (1988). Indians in American: Adaptation and the bicultural self. In P. H. Elovitz & C. Khan (Eds.), *Immigrant experiences: Personal narrative and psychological analysis* (pp. 148–157). Cranbury, NJ: Associated University Press.
Schachter, J. (1990). Post-termination patient-analysis contact: analyst's attitudes and experience. *International Journal of Psychoanalysis, 71*, 475–486.
Schachter, J. (1992). Concepts of termination and post-termination. Patient-analyst contact. *International Journal of Psychoanalysis, 73*, 137–154.
Seelig, B., & Rosof, L. (2001). Normal and pathological altruism. *Journal of the American Psychoanalytic Association, 49*, 933–959.
Settlage, C. (2001). Defenses evoked by early childhood loss: Their impact on life-span development. In S. Akhtar (Ed.), *Three faces of mourning: Melancholia, manic defense, and moving on* (pp. 47–94). Northvale, NJ: Jason Aronson.
Silverman, P., & Worden, J. (1993). Children's reactions to the death of a parent. In M. Stroebe, W. Stroebe, & R. Hansson (Eds.), *Bereavement, a sourcebook of research and intervention* (pp. 41–59). Cambridge, England: Cambridge University Press.
Spitz, R. (1946). Anaclitic depression: An inquiry into the genesis of psychiatric conditions in early childhood. *Psychoanalytic Study of the Child, 2*, 313–342.
Spitz, R. (1950). Anxiety in infancy: a study of its manifestations in the first year of life. *International Journal of Psycho-analysis, 31*, 138–143.
Spitz, R. (1965). *The first year of life*. New York, NY: International Universities Press.

Volkan, V. D. (1981). *Linking objects and linking phenomena: A study of the forms, symptoms, metapsychology, and therapy of complicated mourning*. New York, NY: International Universities Press.
Weiss, E. (1934). Bodily pain and mental pain. *International Journal of Psychoanalysis, 15*, 1–13.
Wheelis, A. (1966). *The illusionless man*. New York, NY: Harper Colophon.
Winnicott, D. (1935). The manic defense. In *Collected papers: Through paediatrics to psychoanalysis* (pp. 129–144). New York, NY: Basic Books, 1958.
Winnicott, D. (1960). Ego distortion in terms of true and false self. In *Maturational processes and the facilitating environment* (pp. 140–152). New York, NY: International Universities Press, 1965.
Wolfenstein, M. (1966). How is mourning possible? *Psychoanalytic Study of the Child, 21*, 93–123.

Part IV
Early Identification and Antecedents of Psychopathology

Chapter 13
Early Identification of Psychopathology

Miri Keren, Astrid Berg, Palvi Kaukonnen and Kai von Klitzing

Abstract This chapter deals with identification of psychopathology in the first 3 years of life. Early identification implies, by definition, the use of assessment tools. We will show how assessment must be tailored to the specific culture to which the infant and his/her parents belong: tools that fit Western cultures will probably not fit nonWestern cultures. As an instance of the Western culture, we describe the Infant Mental Health Assessment Form that was developed in Finland to help primary health care professionals identify infants and families in need of psychosocial support. The tool has two cutoffs: Exceeding the lower cut-off score indicates that the infant or the family needs further examination at the primary level of care, while the higher cut-off indicates that the infant and his/her parents needs a referral to a child psychiatric clinic. In contrast, the typical clinical situation in a nonWestern country such as South Africa is characterized by numerous

M. Keren (✉)
Geha Mental Health Hospital, Helsinki, Israel
e-mail: ofkeren@zahav.net.il

M. Keren
Tel Aviv University, Tel Aviv, Israel

A. Berg
Division of Child and Adolescent Psychiatry,
Red Cross War Memorial Children's Hospital and University of Cape Town,
Cape Town, South Africa
e-mail: a.berg5@icloud.com

P. Kaukonnen
Department for Social and Health Services,
Health Affairs, Ministry of Social Affairs and Health,
Meritullinkatu 8, Helsinki, Finland
e-mail: palvi.kaukonen@stm.fi

K. von Klitzing
Department of Women's and Children's Health,
University of Leipzig, Liebigstreet 20a, 04103 Leipzig, Germany
e-mail: kai.vonklitzing@uniklinik-leipzig.de

S. Malhotra and P. Santosh (eds.), *Child and Adolescent Psychiatry*,
DOI 10.1007/978-81-322-3619-1_13

challenges that do not allow for the usually known methods of assessment, such as a quiet, contained space, toys, and time. A simple, creative assessment tool, named the "biscuit game" has been developed in Capetown, as a cultural appropriate assessment tool that provided a useful adjunct to observing the infant with an eating disorder, as illustrated with a clinical vignette. Finally, early identification of psychopathology requires knowing about risk and protective factors in the infant, the parents, and their environment, as also illustrated by a clinical vignette. After reading this chapter, the reader will realize that early signs of psychopathology are already evident in infants and most of the major mental disorders like anxiety, depression, and behavioral disorders often have their origin already in this early age; the reader will also become more aware of the need to use culture appropriate assessment tools.

Keywords High-risk infants and parents · Early identification of psychopathology · Culture appropriate assessment tools

13.1 Introduction: Psychopathology Starts in Infancy

A seminal epidemiological study (Egger and Angold 2006) has shown that child psychiatry starts already in the first 3 years of life, as most of the disorders can be observed already then. Inline with the ecological perspective (Cichettiti and Aber 1988; Sameroff et al. 1987), the embedded nature of infant development, which include the child dispositions, the parenting style, the family structure, and the cultural milieu, is the determinant in healthy and pathological development. Emotional and behavioral disorders in infancy should be examined in relation to the infant's ecological context. Therefore, not only the level of infant biological and psychological adaptation needs to be assessed, but also, the characteristics of the caregiving environment need to be specifically and broadly evaluated. Specificity relates to the specific conditions under which a maladaptive pattern appears (e.g., only during feeding). Broad assessment refers to different manifestations of maladaptive patterns in different contexts (child non-compliance at home versus at nursery school), as well as assessment of the parents' strengths and weaknesses and the level of their co-parenting functioning. Assessment viewed from this broad perspective also removes infant mental health from its exclusive reliance on a medical model and on the diagnoses of disease, affording a broader view on the entire range of maladaptive symptoms—normal and pathological—typical of this age range.

Infants and toddlers are in the community, therefore our approach needs to be community-based. This, in turn, requires from the clinician to relate with other professionals who are part of the infant's ecological system, such as the pediatrician, the community nurse, the family's social worker. The community-based model calls for the integration of the medical and developmental approaches within a comprehensive framework. Most importantly, such an integration implies the ability to wear two different types of lenses concurrently while looking at observed information: the nosological one (i.e., the multiaxial Diagnostic Classification of Mental Health and Developmental Disorders of Infancy, and Early Childhood Revised (DC: 0-3R 2005), as well as the psychodynamic one (i.e., parental projections, defense mechanisms, and intergenerational transmission of conflictual issues).

There is no value in detection if it is not followed by assessment and diagnoses Categorical diagnostic evaluations are often necessary for practical purposes: They are typically required by healthcare agencies, serve as the basis for treatment, and sharpen the distinction between sets of maladaptive behaviors. Yet, giving psychiatric diagnoses to infants is a controversial topic in many countries. Kagan et al. (1989) suggested that the decision of whether to use a categorical or continuum approach to data collection is the scientist's choice, often reflecting the specific research framework of the observer. The complex task of evaluating the largely preverbal infant from a person-in-context perspective may benefit from the integration of these two traditions. Along the medical tradition, infant assessment can benefit from a differential, multiaxial diagnosis, from the epidemiological description of specific risk groups for various disorders, and from the attempt to devise treatment with measurable outcomes. Categorical assessment may be enhanced by multidimensional developmental information. Such information may include different levels of data collection (behaviors, representations), multiple informants, various contexts, and several settings that may provide convergent evidence on child adaptation and on the caregiving context.

In multicultural contexts, a mediating professional from the local culture is most often needed. Indeed, a behavior that constitutes a problem in the regulation of a basic function may be, to an extent, culturally defined. For instance, the regularity in which the child eats may be considered more or less normative in different cultures, as will more or less aggressive behavior. Cultural belief systems also dictate how parents perceive the referral, assessment, and proposed treatment in mental health clinics, and, should thus be considered prior to devising the treatment plan.

It is beyond the scope of this chapter to review all the categories of psychopathology in the first 3 years of life, as well as the core principles of developmental psychopathology (gene-environment interactions, trajectories of development, vulnerability, resilience, and more). We address those readers who are interested to deepen their knowledge in Infant Psychiatry to the Handbook of Infant Mental Health (Zeanah 2009). We bring here more of an approach to detection and early diagnosis in different contexts.

13.2 Early Identification of Psychopathology in a Western Context

Contrary to popular belief, mental health problems among infants and toddlers are as prevalent as mental health problems among older children. In Finland, assessed by general practitioners in primary health care, about 3 % of 4-, 8- and 18-month-old infants were found to be withdrawn, which is an early sign of psychosocial stress (Puura et al. 2010). Finnish parents have reported behavioral and emotional symptoms in 8–10 % of 3-year-old children (Sourander 2001). The prevalence of psychiatric problems in 18-to-60-month-old Romanian children was 9 % (Gleason et al. 2011) and in 4-year-old Norwegian children 7 % (Wichstrom et al. 2012). Among 0-to-3-year-old children in Bangalore, India, psychiatric morbidity, including epilepsy and mental retardation, was 13.8 % (Srinath et al. 2005).

These days we have access to a wide range of evidence-based early interventions, from supportive interventions to parenting programs and intensive parent–infant psychotherapies. Modern technology creates new possibilities to reach infant families and offer help regardless of time and place—in remote areas and outside working hours. Early interventions to prevent and reduce the psychosocial problems of infants, young children, and their families have a far-reaching beneficial impact on the development and well-being of the child and on the well-being of his or her family. The cost-effectiveness of early interventions has been proved to be high (Heckman et al. 2006). Thus, identifying infants and young children with psychosocial disorders as early as possible would be very important for infants and families and, from human and economic perspectives, also for societies. However, even in Western countries less than half of the children with psychiatric disorders are in contact with any psychosocial health care services (Sourander et al. 2008). In a Norwegian study, the rate of service use among young children with a behavioral or emotional disorder was 11 % at age 4 and somewhat higher, 25 %, at age 7 (Wichstrom et al. 2014).

Detection of early psychosocial problems in infants is a challenge for front-line professionals in primary healthcare services. The capacity for effective early detection depends on the organization and recourses of healthcare services, the education of healthcare professionals, cooperation between health care, social services, and early childhood education as well as on the cultural attitudes and awareness of parents and families. In many cultures, young families have a high threshold for seeking help for their infants and young children with psychosocial problems and for the whole family. For primary healthcare professionals, assessing the psychosocial well-being of infants is demanding due to the lack of easy-to-use assessment methods suitable for primary-level and front-line services. The infant's psychosocial symptoms and functioning must always be evaluated in the context of the parent–infant interaction and the strengths and stresses of his or her family. Identifying possible signs of psychopathology from the average course of early childhood psychosocial development is difficult. In addition, primary-level professionals rarely have sufficient access to suitable methods for early intervention, which may have an impact on their capacity to detect disorders.

Table 13.1 Items included in the Infant MHA

No.	Content
1.	Age-appropriate development
2.	Infant's/young child's somatic diseases
3.	Functioning at home
4.	Functioning in day care
5.	Functioning in social relationships
6.	Parent's ability to regulate emotions and behavior of the young child
7.	Internalized symptoms (joylessness, lack of play or interest, withdrawal, anxiety, fears)
8.	Externalized symptoms (aggressive, defiant or restless behavior that is excessive considering the infant's/young child's age-appropriate development)
9.	Danger to self or behavior that is harmful to self or others
10.	Significant disturbance in behavior, emotions or thinking or in the ability to engage in social relationships
11.	Assessment of parent–child interaction
12.	Family functioning or family factors affecting the infant/young child
13.	Family history of mental illness
14.	Parental substance use
15.	Domestic violence
16.	Parental concerns about the infant's/young child's emotional well-being, behavior, concentration, or ability to get along with others

A new method, Infant Mental Health Assessment Form (Infant MHA), was developed in Finland to help primary healthcare professionals identify infants and families in need of psychosocial support. The method contains 16 items on infant psychosocial development, functioning, symptoms, early interaction, parenthood, family factors, and parents' worries about the infant's psychosocial well-being (Table 13.1). The set of items includes all necessary information required for assessing the state of the psychosocial health of an infant aged between 0 and 3 years. The method also includes instructions for each item and their scoring. It can be used as a checklist for assessment in front-line services. The Infant MHA is intended for use by both public health doctors and nurses working alone and especially when they work together at well-baby clinics or child health clinics. The information needed in the assessment is gathered by interviewing the parent or parents and by observing the infant and his or her family or the infant–parent dyad during a health monitoring visit.

The method helps front-line professionals interpret and integrate all the available information into an understanding of the infant's psychosocial health and consider the need for further examination or primary-level intervention. Importantly, the method has two cut-offs. Exceeding the lower cut-off score indicates that the infant or the family needs further examination, support, or care within primary health care and social services, in day care, preschool or family services. It is important to build a co-operation network of primary-level professionals for planning and carrying out support and care for the infant and the family. The higher cut-off indicates that a child psychiatric consultation, interventions carried out in cooperation between primary care and child psychiatry, or a referral to a child psychiatric clinic should be considered. If the highest proportion of the total score originates from items related to family functioning and factors burdening the family (items 12–15), the primary alternative would be to guide the family to other specialized services, e.g., adult mental health services, services for substance abusers, or child protection.

Preliminary findings suggest that the Infant MHA well classifies the infants and young children in need for psychosocial support at the appropriate level of health care or social services, but a wider validation study is still needed. Primary healthcare professionals have evaluated the method to be easy to use, and the use of the method in health monitoring has also been well accepted by families. Parents and professionals alike expect it to promote a mutual understanding between the family and professionals on the infant's well-being and possible problems.

Asking parents by only one or a few questions about their perceptions of the child's behavioral and emotional difficulties has been found to be an essential source of information in recognizing children with psychosocial problems, especially if teachers are also asked the same questions (Ford et al. 2005). In a Finnish study on 4- to 9-year-old children (n = 2682; approximately 66 % aged between 4 and 6), the parent and the public health nurse were asked, during a regular health checkup of the child, by one question if the child had any difficulties in emotions, behavior, concentration, or being able to get on with other people (Borg et al. 2014). The nurses answered based on their overall clinical evaluation. These single questions to the parent and public health nurse proved to have an adequate capacity to discriminate between the low-risk and high-risk children in the sample. Combining the answers of parents and nurses produced even higher sensitivity compared to a single informant's report. Parents' awareness of psychological distress and their expressions of psychosocial problems in infants and young children seem to be culture dependent (Srinath et al. 2005) and somatic concerns are often easier to raise. The results of the above-mentioned studies suggest, however, that these kinds of one-question screening methods for parents and public health nurses or parents and teachers together could be considered as a firststep screening assessment in everyday clinical practice of professionals in front-line services.

In addition to measuring and examining physical health, monitoring the development and health of infants should always include the assessment of psychosocial development, well-being, and mental health. Professionals should have a low threshold for asking about parents' worries concerning infant mental health issues because parents usually are not the first ones to raise these questions. Detecting psychosocial problems as early as possible enables effective allocation of resources, help, support, and interventions. A multistage procedure for screening early problems in public front-line services would be cost-effective. A simple question to a parent and a public health nurse or teacher about concerns regarding an infant's psychosocial well-being has proved to be an easy to use and brief first-stage assessment tool. Specific assessment methods for primary-level and front-line services are the next step; they are more time-consuming but provide more information on the problem and options for interventions. A comprehensive diagnostic assessment requires a multi-informant and multi-method approach including standardized methods like questionnaires, interviews, observation and co-operation with other specialists in contact with the infant and his or her family. Overall, the aim of all assessment procedures is to ensure the beneficial development of infants and young children and to provide infants and their families with access to support and interventions according to their specific needs.

13.3 Early Identification of Psychopathology in a Nonwestern Context

It is important to realize that the professions of psychiatry and psychology are alien to a majority of the people living in a nonwestern context; there is indeed no universal language that speaks to problems of psychological and mental ill health. (Ramphele 2008) Mental illness, particularly of the more "neurotic" type is not easily talked about and does therefore not present itself. In Africa, generally speaking, emotional suffering is considered part of life and is borne in private. The challenge is thus to introduce the concept of infant mental health into an African setting and to find a way of intervention that is meaningful.

The infant mental health practitioner supports the notion that young children's needs are universal—for the baby this means that his/her parent regards him as a person who has individuality, preferences, and feelings from the beginning of life and that the relationship between mother or caregivers and child is of prime importance. Even if the culture does not regard the infant as a person at such an early stage of life, it is vital to impart the knowledge that has been gained through research which shows so clearly that babies are born into the world hardwired to relate and interact. Babies can hear, see, and feel and they do show what they like and what not from the beginning, irrespective of the culture into which they are born—the task is for the adults to recognize this.

One of the very early cases that were seen at a Parent–Infant Mental Health Service in Cape Town, South Africa, was of a toddler whose drop in weight coincided with the disruption of his primary attachment figure; once this was addressed through giving information and support, his weight improved. What however was important in terms of identifying the beginnings of this child's poor weight gain became apparent during the diagnostic session. The child was given a biscuit and it was noted that while he took a bit into his mouth, he kept it there and only swallowed it once; he was held and embraced. It was this small observation was a clue to why this child might not have been taking in sufficient food—he could have had doubts about being held in an ongoing, secure manner.

While this may be only a hypothesis which cannot be proven, it nevertheless allowed for the practitioner to look at the relationship between weight loss and a possible attachment disturbance in more detail. As a result of this and a few other, similar presenting cases, a drop in weight in an infant who was otherwise healthy became one the main reasons for referral to the infant mental health service. Faltering weight was a symptom the mother understood and was concerned about and there was an intuitive understanding that weight could be affected by emotional difficulties within the family. The time of the drop in weight provided a useful port of entry for the clinician to explore attachment relationships.

In the diagnostic classification, zero to three revised feeding behavior disorder is one of the categories used for an infant or toddler who has difficulty in establishing regular feeding patters.

The four stages described closely follow Chatoor's diagnostic classification (Chatoor 2002), namely

1. Feeding disorder of state regulation: difficulty with feeding evident during neonatal period—infant not able to reach state of calm alertness.
2. Feeding disorder of caregiver–infant reciprocity: 2–6 months "most exclusively social period of life" (Stern 1985) The infant may be emotionally "neglected" because of disturbance in mother.
3. Infantile Anorexia: 6 months–3 years: This often signifies difficulties with separation—Individuation and the cues of the infant may not have been understood.
4. Sensory food aversions: transitioning to table food where toddler is sensitive to the textures of the food.

In our community clinic setting, there is at most a bare room available; while patients may have been given dates for their appointments, these are often not kept and the clinical morning or afternoon does not follow a predictable pattern. There may be only one patient or there may be six—attendance at a clinic depends on many factors that mothers in harsh circumstances have to deal with. The barrier that exists in many communities where the health care professional is of a different language group adds to the challenges that face the community health practitioner. There can thus be difficulty in obtaining a detailed history or account of the presenting problems. If there are many patients waiting there may be no time for in-depth observation of mother and baby, or certainty of repeat visits. To bring a bag of diagnostic toys may also not be appropriate, unless the toy is available to be taken home by the child. In a setting where children do not have the privilege of toys, presenting an attractive object and then taking it away again would not help to establish a therapeutic alliance with the child.

What emerged out of the case example just cited was the use of a biscuit as a diagnostic tool or adjunct. It could be regarded as a similar procedure as described by Winnicott in The Set Situation.

The Set Situation (Winnicott 1941)

Winnicott described three stages which can be observed if infant is presented with new object. Anxiety influences how these stages manifest.

Stage 1: The "period of hesitation"

The baby "puts his hand to the spatula, but at this moment discovers unexpectedly that the situation must be given thought." (Winnicott 1941, p. 53) The gradual and spontaneous return of interest in the spatula is observed and noted.

Stage 2: Acceptance of reality of desire

"The child's acceptance of the reality of desire for the spatula is heralded by a change in the inside of the mouth…" (p. 54) The spatula is now available for purposes of "self-expression."

Stage 3: Stage of playfulness

This is the stage where the baby may first drops the spatula and is pleased when it is returned and real play may develop. "There is almost certainly a correlation between these and other variations from the norm and the infant's relation to food and to people." (p. 56).

13.4 The "Biscuit Game" as a Cultural Appropriate Assessment Tool

Winnicott asked how does the child approach and handle the spatula. In a similar vein the question can be asked: How does the infant approach and handle the biscuit? The following stages could be hypothesized when looking closely at how the infant approaches the new object which has been placed on the table within his/her reach.

1. No interest
2. Interest, but no approach
3. Interest, but hesitation
4. Interest and spontaneous reaching out
5. Eating
6. Mouthing and playing

Stages 1 and 2 could signify withdrawal, Stage 3 anxiety, while Stages 4, 5, and 6 could mean that the child is not withdrawn, is either hungry or is using the biscuit as a new object to explore and play with.

This simple method provided a useful adjunct to observe a young child in a clinic situation where the numerous challenges did not allow for the usually known methods of assessment, such as a quiet, contained space, toys, and time. Part of the diagnostic armamentarium that followed the clinical vignette here described was at all times box of biscuits—it was appropriate and humane to bring something physically nurturing for these children, an object which at the same time, could also serve the purpose of adding to the diagnostic assessment.

13.5 Early Identification of High-Risk Infants and Parents

The early identification of psychopathology in the early years of life requires knowledge about where to look for high-risk populations, i.e., groups of parents and infants where risk factors tend to cluster together and lead to poor developmental outcomes and/or to the emergence of psychopathology. Such risk factors are well-known nowadays, thanks to Sameroff's New York Longitudinal study and Transactional Model of development (Sameroff and Chandler 1975; Seifer and Sameroff 1983). Risk factors need to be identified in the infant, parents, and their environment, and the main categories are constitutional, biological, and experiential.

13.5.1 Risk Factors (Vulnerability) in the Infant

Constitutional risk factors, with which the infant was born, include difficult temperament and poor physiological regulation skills. Biological risk factors include any congenital or acquired medical condition, such as congenital heart disease, extreme prematurity, etc. Experiential risk factors relate to the infant's exposure to adverse stimuli, traumatic events (such as loss of a parent), and to poor parental functioning.

13.5.2 Risk Factors in the Parent

Poor maternal education, parental mental or physical illness, poor family functioning, severe personality psychopathology, are all risk factors for the infant's mental health because they directly impinge on the parent's availability and caregiving capacities. Parent's past of adverse, abusive interpersonal experiences with their own parents is a very significant risk factor for transgenerational transmission of insecure and disorganized attachment in the child.

13.5.3 Risk Factors in the Close Environment

Lack of social support is a major risk factor, unemployment, low socioeconomic status, and violent neighborhood.

Sameroff's longitudinal study has shown that the child's final outcome is the arithmetical sum of the risk factors in the infant, the parents, and their environment, minus the sum of the protective factors, also in the infant, the parents and their environment. The highest is the number of risk factors and the lowest is the number of protective factors; the more at risk is the young child.

The clinical implication of these findings is that, if we wish to detect early these infants at risk for early signs of emotional distress, we need to target our efforts on those families with a high number of risk factors. They are usually well-known to the social welfare services and the community pediatrician. An ongoing working relationship between the infant psychiatrist, the social worker and the pediatrician is therefore mandatory. At our IMH Unit in Israel, we have put in place a special "intensive care" model for infants at risk of neglect or abuse.

The first clinical challenge we meet with this specific group of parents is the low level of motivation for change the parents most commonly display when they are referred by the social services. Consequently, initial home visits are very often required as a first step of reaching out. Monitoring the level of change is often crucial, since these infants are at severe risk and may be about to be removed from home. In many of these cases, the court is involved and clinicians are requested to report. Hence, the pretreatment evaluation is based not only on clinical judgment, but also on standardized procedures, such as videotaped parent–infant dyadic play and feeding interactions, HOME observation (Caldwell and Bradley 1978), and parent insightfulness assessment (Oppenheim and Koren-Karie 2002). The infant's developmental level is assessed with Bailey test. Self-report questionnaires may also be filled by the parents, such as Self-report about individual psychopathology (SCL-90R), the social support questionnaire (Cutrona 1984), the Brief Infant and Toddler Social and Emotional Assessment (BITSEA; Version 2, Briggs-Gowan and Carter 2002), and the life events questionnaire.

Very recently, we have extended our scope of clinical work to the assessment of infants who have experienced a total parental failure and who have been placed out of home on an emergency basis. Until recently, these infants were routinely evaluated by a pediatrician for their physical and developmental status, but no professional attention was given to their psychological condition. Thanks to a pilot project we have initiated some 4 years ago, we have put in place an assessment battery for all the out-of-home placed infants, 1 month after their removal from the biological parents. Some of them continue to see their biological parents, while their final placement is discussed at court. The following case will illustrate the evaluation process we have put in place.

D., 2-years old and 10 months, was referred for evaluation at our Infant Mental Health Unit, 1 month after he had been removed from his biological parents' home to a shelter family.

Background: D.'s mother was a drug-addicted young woman, HIV positive, and his father was alcoholic and homeless. Both parents were known to the Social Welfare Services, and therefore, when D. was born, he was immediately put under the Child Protection surveillance. When D. was 3-months old, police was alerted by the neighbors because of unusually loud shouting. At entering the house, the policemen saw the baby lying in an unbelievable mess and dirt, and traces of blood were all around. Both parents were drunk and hitting one another. D. was immediately removed from the house, put in a shelter family, but returned home within a month because his parents agreed to enter an addiction program. At some point, father left the program and went back to street. When D. was 2 years and 8 months, passersby in the street reported to the police that D. was badly hit by his mother, who was under the influence of drugs. D. was removed again to a shelter family with three additional infants, and his mother definitely lost her parental rights upon him, except for supervised visitations once a week.

<u>History taking</u>: The evaluation started with a session with the shelter foster parents, aiming to get a description of D.'s general condition and behaviors since he arrived 2 months before. They described how D. looked dirty and neglected, cried most of the days and nights refused to sleep alone in his bed and would fall asleep only when the three other children of the shelter home joined hi, and continuously asked for food. Over 2 months, D. somehow calmed down, agreed to be touched and hold, and started to say a few words. Yet, he continued to eat strikingly large amounts of food, especially bread, poorly slept with frequent awakenings and crying. At the kindergarten (totally unfamiliar to him), he would play alone and bite his own fingers. The foster parents also mentioned D.'s recurrent pattern of regression that followed every visit to his biological mother.

<u>Clinical status</u>: The next session was dedicated to the child's mental status evaluation, done by the child psychiatrist at the Unit (MK). D. came once with his foster father, and once with his foster mother. D. appeared as a thin and sad toddler, with no dysmorphic features, and no abnormal movements. At both sessions, D. exhibited a disorganized pattern of attachment, even before the mini-separation procedure: he would stand "frozen" in the middle of the room, with no attachment behaviors nor exploratory behaviors. He never turned to the adults in the room for help. His affect was strikingly flat, only his eyes moved around ("gaze radar"). We were told that this behavior was typical of D. during the visitations with his biological mother. When the clinician said to the child "do not worry, you are not going to stay here, we will play a bit, and then you will go home with Y. and M. (foster parents' first names), D. relaxed a bit, and started to explore the room, more touching the toys than really playing. Yet, he never smiled.

<u>Developmental status</u>: The Bailey test (3rd edition) was conducted by the developmental psychologist of the Unit. It took three full sessions (an hour each) to complete it, because of D.'s extremely poor cooperation and lack of trust. His general level of functioning was 24 months (he was 2 years and 11 months at the time of the test), with a worse functioning at verbal tasks.

<u>Observation beyond the setting of the clinic</u>: The developmental psychologist, whom D. had encountered several times at the clinic, was the one who did the HOME and the kindergarten observations. In both contexts, D. looked less frightened than at the clinic, but his constricted affect and level of functioning was pervasive. So was his lack of play with peers (including with the other fostered children). We did not observe any attention-seeking behavior toward the shelter foster parents nor the kindergarten teacher, and he hardly spoke. The adults' efforts to approach him remained quite inefficient, except when they offered him sweets.

<u>Diagnostic formulation</u>: D.'s diagnoses of the DC 0-3R classification were the following:

Axis I: Deprivation and maltreatment disorder

Axis: No diagnosis was given on the axis of the parent relationship, since he had been only 2 months at the shelter foster home, and the caregiving figures were temporary, by definition of the shelter foster care system in Israel.

Axis III: Global developmental delay, especially language delay

Axis IV: S/p disruptions of attachment relationships, deprived, and abusive environment

Axis V: Did not reach level of socioemotional functioning expected at his chronological age

In psychodynamic terms, D.'s intrapsychic development was very severely impinged by the lack of maternal mirroring (impaired development of the child's primary narcissism and capacity of symbolization). Deprivation and maltreatment led to his striking lack of basic trust, and consequently, to impaired interpersonal relationships, in addition to global developmental delay. His insatiable hunger and craving for bread was understood as the metaphor for all what he needed and did not get from the adult world.

Treatment plan: Our recommendations to the Child Protection services, were contingent to the above diagnostic formulations, and included the following:

1. *Urgent placement in permanent home with less frequent visitations to biological mother, at least until some attachment is formed with the new caregivers.*
2. *Attachment-based child–parent psychotherapy with the new parents and the child.*
3. *Hearing test and speech therapist evaluation.*
4. *Therapeutic kindergarten*

To conclude, the link between growing up in a high-risk environment and the development of early psychopathology, especially depression, anxiety, and behavior problems, has been well established. As infant psychiatrists, our mission is to detect as early as possible these high-risk infants and parents, to diagnose their specific risk and protective factors, and to put in place an intensive intervention plan, including active reaching out.

13.6 Summary and Conclusions

Historically, there has been much debate in the scientific community as well as in the public opinion whether young children under 3 years may already suffer from mental problems and disorders. In this chapter, we have demonstrated that the scientific and clinical evidence is overwhelming: early signs of psychopathology are already evident and diagnosable in infants and most of the major mental disorders like anxiety, depression, and behavioral disorder often have their origin already in this early age.

This knowledge has major implications for psychiatry: first, there is an important need for a life cycle approach with respect to the assessment of mental disorders. Early regulatory problems of affect, motor development, and/or food intake have to be taken serious and diagnosed as possible early signs of affective, hyperactivity, behavior, and eating disorders. Second, our systems of describing and diagnosing psychopathology have to take development into account. For example, problems and disorders of affect regulation like depression certainly look different phenomenologically in a 1-year-old infant as compared to an individual in middle adulthood or in old age. Third, the younger the child, the more we need to include the relationship to the caregivers and the broader relational environment into our diagnostic considerations. Each mental health assessment has to comprise individual psychopathology as well as relational characteristics and symptoms. Fourth, early assessment should lead to early intervention because the earlier treatment starts the more effective.

There are lots of cultural and social resistances against these assumptions in industrialized, threshold as well as developing countries. In western industrialized countries, there exists a prevailing idealization of early childhood and mother happiness. We have the nice lovely baby in mind and his/her caring mother filled with joy and happiness. We think that we are borne innocent and free of any problems and we deny conflicts and aggression as common ingredients of early parent–infant relationships. In very poor countries and/or regions affected by war and violence, we consider basic needs like enough food, safety, and hygiene to be essential and mental health to be secondary.

But we know that humans are not free of conflict and aggression in any age and that negative biological and environmental influence can be detrimental for human life from conception on. Biological and mental aspects of development are closely interwoven especially during the first years. Taking care of basic needs like enough food, hygiene, and protection from violence is essential also for mental health development. But the case description above shows that for example the provision enough food does not lead the infant to a healthy development without a caring and holding relationship with a good enough care taker. Already R. Spitz (1945) has shown with his studies in North American baby homes that children suffer from severe disease or even die though they receive adequate food and live under excellent hygienic conditions if they do not experience adequate emotional resonance from vivid caring objects.

It does not make sense neither in economically well-developed nor in poverty-stricken regions of the world to split biological and mental health apart conceptually nor practically. We make a plea that it is important to take mental health conditions and concerns of young children serious all over the world. Such healthy conditions are even the basis of all social and economic development. Of course it is important to take the special social, cultural, and economic characteristics of each region as well as cultural meanings of mental suffering into account. But to take care of infant mental health needs is not a mere luxury of rich industrial countries, it is essential in every continent and every part of the world.

References

Borg, A-M., Salmelin, R., Joukamaa, M., & Tamminen, T. (2014). Cutting a long story short? The clinical relevance of asking parents, nurses, and young children themselves to identify children's mental health problems by one or two questions. *Scientific World Journal, 2014,* 2.

Briggs-Gowan, M. J., & Carter, A. S. (2002). *Brief infant-toddler social and emotional assessment (BITSEA): Manual. Version 2.0.* New Haven, CT: Yale University.

Caldwell, B., & Bradley, R. (1978). *Home observation for measurement of the environment*. Little Rock, AR: University of Arkansas.
Chatoor, I. (2002). Feeding disorders in infants and toddlers: Diagnosis and treatment. *Child and Adolescent Psychiatric Clinics, 11*, 163–183.
Cichettiti, D., & Aber, J. L. (1988). Editorial: Contexts and developmental psychopathology. *Development and Psychopathology, 10*, 137–141.
Cutrona, C. E. (1984). Social support and stress in the transition to parenthood. *Journal of Abnormal Psychology, 93*, 378–390.
Diagnostic Classification of Mental Health and Developmental Disorders of Infancy and Early Childhood (DC 0-3R), 2005, Zero to Three Press.
Egger, H., & Angold, A. (2006). Common emotional and behavioral disorders in preschool children: Presentation, nosology and epidemiology. *Journal of Child Psychology and Psychiatry, 47*, 313–337.
Ford, T., Sayal, K., Meltzer, H., & Goodman, R. (2005). Parental concerns about their child's emotions and behaviour and referral to specialist services: General population survey. *BMJ (Clinical Research Ed.), 331*(7530), 1435–1436. doi:331/7530/1435 [pii]
Gleason, M. M., Zamfirescu, A., Egger, H. L., Nelson, C. A., 3rd, Fox, N. A., & Zeanah, C. H. (2011). Epidemiology of psychiatric disorders in very young children in a Romanian pediatric setting. *European Child & Adolescent Psychiatry, 20*(10), 527–535. doi:10.1007/s00787-011-0214-0; 10.1007/s00787-011-0214-0
Heckman, J. J., et al. (2006). Skill formation and the economics of investing in disadvantaged children. *Science, 312*, 1900. doi:10.1126/science.1128898
Kagan, J., Reznick, J. S., & Gibbons, J. (1989). Inhibited an uninhibited types of children. *Child Development, 60*(4), 838–845.
Oppenheim, D., & Koren-Karie, N. (2002). Mothers' insightfulness regarding their children's internal worlds: The capacity underlying secure child-mother relationships. *Infant Mental Health Journal, 23*, 593–605.
Puura, K., Mäntymaa, M., Luoma, I., Kaukonen, P., Guedeney, A., Salmelin, R., & Tamminen, T. (2010). Infants' social withdrawal symptoms assessed with a direct infant observation method in primary health care. *Infant Behavior & Development, 33*(4), 579–588. doi:10.1016/j.infbeh.2010.07.009; 10.1016/j.infbeh.2010.07.009
Ramphele, M. (2008). How does one speak of social psychology in a nation in transition? *Journal of Analytical Psychology, 53*, 157–167.
Sameroff, A. J., & Chandler, M. J. (1975). Reproductive risk and the continuum of caretaking casualty. In F. D. Horowitz, M. Hetherington, S. Scarr-Salapatek, & G. Siegel (Eds.), *Review of child development research (vol 4)*. Chicago: University of Chicago Press.
Sameroff, A. J., Seifer, R., Barocas, R., Zax, M., & Greenspan, S. (1987). Intelligence quotient scores of 4 year-old children: Social-environmental risk factors. *Pediatrics, 79*, 343–350.
Seifer, R., & Sameroff, A. J. (1983). Multiple determinants of risk and invulnerability. In E. J. Anthony & B. J. Cohler (Eds.), *The invulnerable child*. New York: The Guilford Press.
Sourander, A. (2001). Emotional and behavioural problems in a sample of Finnish three-year-olds. *European Child and Adolescent Psychiatry, 10*(2), 98–104.
Sourander, A., Niemelä, S., Santalahti, P., Helenius, H., & Piha, J. (2008). Changes in psychiatric problems and service use among 8-year-old children: A 16-year population-based time-trend study. *Journal of the American Academy of Child and Adolescent Psychiatry, 47*(3), 317–327. doi:10.1097/CHI.0b013e318160b98f.
Spitz, R. (1945). Query hospitalism. An inquiry in the genesis of psychiatric conditions in early childhood. *Psychoanalytic Study of the Child, 1*, 53–74.
Srinath, S., Girimaji, S. C., Gururaj, G., Seshadri, S., Subbakrishna, D. K., Bhola, B., et al. (2005). Epidemiological study of child & adolescent psychiatric disorders in urban & rural areas of Bangalore, India. *Indian Journal of Medical Research, 122*, 67–79.
Stern, D. (1985). *The interpersonal world of the infant—a view from psychoanalysis and developmental psychology*. New York: Basic Books Inc.

Wichstrom, L., Belsky, J., Jozefiak, T., Sourander, A., & Berg-Nielsen, T. S. (2014). Predicting service use for mental health problems among young children. *Pediatrics, 133*(6), 1054–1060. doi:10.1542/peds.2013-3184.

Wichstrom, L., Berg-Nielsen, T. S., Angold, A., Egger, H. L., Solheim, E., & Sveen, T. H. (2012). Prevalence of psychiatric disorders in preschoolers. *Journal of Child Psychology and Psychiatry, and Allied Disciplines, 53*(6), 695–705. doi:10.1111/j.1469-7610.2011.02514.x; 10.1111/j.1469-7610.2011.02514.x

Winnicott, D. W. (1941). The observation of infants in a set situation. In *Through paediatrics to psychoanalysis—collected papers* (pp. 52–69). London: Karnac.

Zeanah, C. H., Jr. (2009). *Handbook of infant mental health* (3rd ed.). New York: The Guilford Press.

Chapter 14
Temperament: Clinical Relevance

Savita Malhotra and Soumya Jhanda

Abstract Temperament primarily signifies innate patterns of neurobehavioral reaction, inhibition, socialization, and emotionality evident very early in development. Neurobiological research findings denote temperament dimensions as endophenotypes with implications for risk and vulnerability in children. Several researchers have defined temperamental dimensions and described its relationship to development and psychopathology. There are associations between various temperamental traits with internalizing disorders as well as externalizing disorders, conversion and psychotic disorders. Study of temperamental individuality helps in understanding psycho-pathogenesis of disorders and also guiding intervention strategies. Management of various psychiatric disorders can address temperamental issues. It is evident that temperament is not merely a theoretical/explanatory concept, but also useful in practice for interventions and therapy.

Keywords Temperament · Development · Psychopathology · Prevention

Abbreviations

CNS	Central Nervous system
NYLS	New York Longitudinal Study
BAS	Behavioral Activation System
BIS	Behavioral Inhibition System
ACTH	Adrenal Corticotropic Hormone
CRH	Corticotrophin Releasing Hormone

S. Malhotra (✉) · S. Jhanda
Department of Psychiatry, Post Graduate Institute of Medical Education and Research, Chandigarh 160012, India
e-mail: savita.pgi@gmail.com

S. Jhanda
e-mail: soumyajhanda86@gmail.com

S. Malhotra and P. Santosh (eds.), *Child and Adolescent Psychiatry*,
DOI 10.1007/978-81-322-3619-1_14

14.1 Historical Overview

Temperament is an ancient concept including variations in physiological reactivity and behavioral patterns, rooted in centuries' old traditions in Eastern and Western thought to describe individual characteristics and personality types. The term "temperament" itself comes from the Latin *temperamentum* meaning a mixture of bodily humors; from *temperare:* to mingle in due proportion.

The initial attempts to link psychological characteristics to body structure was as early as fifth century BC by Hippocrates. He defined two physical types, *habitus apoplectus* (thick, muscular, and strong) and *habitus phthisicus* (delicate, thin, and weak). He said that the two body types differed temperamentally, and that muscular individuals were more prone to high blood pressure and thin individuals to tuberculosis. Several years later in the year 1941, continuing on the same note, Sheldon and Stevens gave the concept of endomorphic (soft, rounded), mesomorphic (hard, rectangular), and ectomorphic (linear, fragile) body types.

Following this period, wherein there was emphasis on the relationship between physique and behavior, the focus gradually shifted to link behavior with the properties of the central nervous system (Ruch 1992). Pavlov's research on the efficiency of conditioning in dogs drew his attention to the observation that there exist properties of excitation and inhibition of the CNS. He stated that combination of these properties constitute the physiological basis of temperament. He used the terms nervous system and temperament interchangeably. Pavlov (1951–1952) described three fundamental properties of the CNS: strength, balance (equilibrium) and mobility of the nervous system (excitation and inhibition). The strength of the CNS refers to the functional capacity (endurance), i.e., the ability to withstand prolonged excitation (or inhibition). The process of protective inhibition, expressed in decrease of performance under strong/prolonged stimulation, was regarded by Pavlov as the main indicator of the strength of excitation. Equilibrium was regarded as the property that results from the ratio between the strength of excitation and inhibition. Mobility means the speed and adequacy of reactions to the change in the surroundings. Pavlov said that the individuals who were able to continue to function under high intensity or prolonged exposure to stimulation before inhibition set in were characterized by "strong" nervous system; those with low thresholds for the same by "weak" nervous system.

Continuing on the work, Strelau (1983, 1996) proposed the Regulative Theory of Temperament. This theory states "temperament is defined as a set of relatively stable features of the organism that reveal themselves in formal traits of behavior. Being primarily determined by inborn physiological mechanisms, temperament is subjected to slow changes caused by maturation and by some environment factors."

Strelau (1983) proposed that temperament is less susceptible to change. However, like other psychological and physiological characteristics it does change with the process of maturation due to developmental and life span changes in the physiological mechanisms underlying temperament. Some changes in temperament characteristics may also occur under the influence of environmental factors, such as nutrition, stimulation, chronic deprivation, population density, etc. These changes under environmental influences do not occur from moment to moment or from day to day, instead take years.

The statement that temperament traits reveal themselves in the formal characteristics of behavior means that temperament traits manifest in every behavior, in all human actions, independent of their content and direction. Any behavior may be characterized by its intensity (magnitude) as well by its speed or duration. Hence these traits do not exist as isolated phenomena, but appear as a rule, as characteristics of reactions and behaviors. This means that the assessment of temperament is always involved in any given behavior.

Following this, Gray (1991) proposed the concept of **Behavior Activation and Inhibition** in relation to temperament. He described two operating systems: Behavioral Activation System (BAS) and Behavioral inhibition System (BIS). The BAS, as per Gray, responds to cues signaling reward, and the BIS to signals of punishment. Individuals differ in their strength of each, with the balance indicating differences in introversion (BIS greater than BAS) and extraversion (BAS greater than BIS). The BAS responds to incentive reward cues by activating approach and exploratory behaviors intended to locate the reward in question. Most of the traits grouped within extraversion are examples of approach or exploratory behavior, including activity, sociability, talkativeness, and assertiveness. Key brain regions involved in the BAS and linked to extraversion include orbitofrontal cortex and nucleus accumbens, regions strongly influenced by dopamine (DeYoung and Gray 2009; DeYoung et al. 2010). Hence, dopamine appears to be the primary neurotransmitter involved in the BAS. Another neurotransmitter system involved in reward and linked to Extraversion, but not central to the BAS, is the opioid system, which is associated with the pleasure experienced after acquiring rewards generally and with social bonding specifically (Depue and Morrone-Strupinsky 2005). This system is primarily involved in the experience of receiving reward, rather than in responding to incentive reward cues.

The BIS, in contrast, responds to stimuli that one desires to approach but that also contain threat, creating an approach-avoidance conflict. The output of the BIS is vigilance, rumination, and passive avoidance, which Gray described as symptoms of anxiety, and which may also be linked to depression.

Gradually, the research focused on neuro-hormonal responses on two adrenal systems—the sympathetic adrenal medullary axis and pituitary—adrenal cortical axis. The adrenal medulla being an extension of the sympathetic nervous system, synthesizes and secretes catecholamines (epinephrine and nor epinephrine). It is regulated by ACTH (adrenal corticotropic hormone) from the anterior pituitary, which in turn is regulated by CRH (corticotrophin releasing hormone) released from the hypothalamus. It was seen that increased serum cortisol in mother was found to be associated with negative emotionality in infant.

It was the first time in 1956, that Alexander Thomas and Stella Chess galvanized the interest of researchers and clinicians in the field of temperament. They began the classic New York Longitudinal Study and followed 136 infants from

84 educated families living in New York, USA, from 3 months of age to adulthood. They derived their list of temperamental traits based on a content analysis from interviews with the parents. The list of traits included nine dimensions (a) activity level (b) rhythmicity (c) approach/withdrawal (d) adaptability (e) sensory threshold (f) intensity of reaction (g) quality of mood (h) distractibility (i) attention span/persistence. This was the first time that clinical research on temperament highlighting aspects of children's behavior that could have implications in process of maladaptation and intervention as well as prevention was done.

Further, Buss and Plomin (1975) emphasized on the "phylogenetic" approach in defining temperament. They described that temperament traits show early in ontogenesis, "preferably in first two years of life," exhibit high "heritability" (i.e., the more heritable a given trait is, the more likely it is to be temperament) and "continuity," i.e., there is continuity into later personality.

Rothbart (1981) described temperamental traits to consist of constitutional differences in reactivity and self regulation. There were three major temperamental traits proposed by Rothbart: ***Surgency,*** i.e., tendencies toward high activity, a rapid approach style, expressions of positive emotions, and pleasure and excitement in social interaction. ***Negative Emotionality,*** i.e., children's tendencies toward sadness, fear, irritability and frustration, and difficulty with being quieted after high arousal. ***Effortful Control,*** i.e., the ability to sustain attention and inhibit behavior, the ability to persist in tasks, pleasure in low intensity situations, and sensitivity to perceptual experiences (Rothbart 1998, 2000a, b, 2001, 2006).

It was in 1994 that Cloninger gave a model of personality comprising of 4 temperamental and 3 character states:

The four temperamental traits as described by Cloninger are the following:

(1) **Novelty Seeking:** A personality trait associated with exploratory activity in response to novel stimulation, impulsive decision-making, extravagance in approach to reward cues, and quick loss of temper.

(2) **Harm Avoidance:** To respond by behavioral inhibition to signals of punishment or non reward.

(3) **Reward Dependence:** This trait is characterized as a tendency to respond markedly to signals of reward, particularly to verbal signals of social approval, social support, and learning to maintain and pursue behaviors which were previously associated with such rewards.

(4) **Persistence**: To be persistent and hardworking, despite frustration and fatigue.

The three character traits are as follows:

(1) **Self-directedness**: Self-determination and will power, the ability to control, regulate and adapt one's behavior in order to achieve personal goals
(2) **Cooperativeness**: The tendency of identification with and acceptance of other individuals
(3) **Self-transcendence**: Acceptance of ambiguity and uncertainty, spiritual acceptance and identification with the wider world

It was hypothesized that the temperament traits are evident early in ontogeny and are strongly genetically determined, whereas character traits develop later because they are determined by experience during development rather than primarily by genes.

14.2 Temperamental Characteristics

Taking into view the clinical research in temperament and the various temperamental models, following parameters describe childhood temperament (Zetner and Bates 2008):

1. Individual differences in normal behaviors pertaining to the domains of affect, activity, attention, and sensory sensitivity are understood as temperament.
2. These behavioral differences are typically expressed formally as response intensities, latencies, thresholds, and recovery times.
3. These appear in the first few years of life as early as infancy and full expression is evident by preschool age.
4. There is phylogenetic continuity with primates as well certain social mammals (Nettle 2006).
5. These are closely linked to biological mechanisms (e.g., neurochemical, neuroanatomical, genetic).
6. These are relatively enduring and predictive of certain outcomes during development.

14.2.1 Basic Temperament Traits

Temperament researchers have described various temperaments using different names for similar behavioral dimensions. Based on the commonalities of descriptions and underlying essence, it is possible to drive certain temperamental traits that fulfill the above mentioned criteria:

14.2.1.1 Activity Level

It refers to frequency and intensity of motor activity. Eaton and Enns (1986) have defined it as 'the individual's level of energy expenditure through movement.' Energy is expended faster when the pace of movements is rapid. A major component of activity is ***tempo***. Highly active children often gallop instead of walking, skip and hop frequently, run up and down stairs, talk faster and generally move at a quicker pace than those who are low in activity. An alternative means of expending energy is through ***vigor***, responses of high amplitude or greater intensity.

Highly active children tend to push open doors with force, bang hard on toys, talk louder and generally move with greater force than those who are low in intensity. These examples reveal that activity is mainly a stylistic trait. Style refers to the manner in which a response is delivered and not their content: the *how,* not the *what* of behavior. Thus, a handshake is a greeting response (content), but it can be delivered with a quick movement (tempo) or the hand can be grasped with force (vigor) (Fagot 1994).

14.2.1.2 Positive Emotionality/Extraversion

It is linked to frequencies and intensity of positive emotions, such as interest, eagerness, and associated behaviors such as approach. The subcomponents of positive emotionality are positive anticipation, sensation or novelty seeking, smiling, and laughter. Evidence suggests that the mechanisms underlying positive emotionality are linked to a number of neural circuits, such as midbrain dopamine systems projecting from the substantia nigra and the ventral tegmental area, as well as systems controlling locomotion such as the nucleus accumbens (Posner and Rothbart 2007; Gray 1991; Panksepp 1998; Burgdorf and Panksepp 2006). In infancy, individual differences in this trait are expressed, e.g. by the total amount of smiling, laughing, and motor acts, such as clapping hands and reaching when in a playful situation. Findings suggest that components of positive emotionality tend to be quite stable across the early childhood period, regardless of whether they are measured by laboratory observation or via parental reports (Lemery et al. 1999; Putnam 2005; Putnam et al. 2006). It is one of the most important behavior systems involved in the processing of information about potential rewards that are useful for our survival.

14.2.1.3 Negative Emotionality/Introversion

All schemas of temperament used to describe children include a negative emotionality concept. The major components of negative emotionality are fear and anger.

Fear: Fear has two components, affective and cognitive**. Affective** component describes strong autonomic arousal, specifically activation of the sympathetic division of the autonomic nervous system. Such arousal is accompanied by feelings of apprehension and worry, which comprise the ***cognitive*** component.

Socialization has only just begun when children are young, and so they express their emotions freely, especially in the face. The ***expressive*** component of fear, which can be distinguished from facial appearance of other emotions is believed to have evolved from the primate grimace. When afraid, children shrink back, inhibit motor activity or run away from the threatening stimulus. If the fear is sufficiently intense, children may subsequently avoid the fear stimulus. These various responses comprise the ***instrumental*** or ***motor*** component of fear. It is the most observable aspect of fear. Fearful children are regarded as being predisposed to become phobic as they mature.

Anger: Anger is primarily an ***affect***. Its physiological reactivity is regarded same as that of fear. The expressive component, especially the facial aspect, appears to be universal in our species and has evolved from the primate facial expression in anger, which it resembles. The cognitive component is transient dislike of others and the negative attributions to them, which comprise the reactions often labeled hostility.

14.2.1.4 Attention/Persistence

Attention span concerns the length of time a particular activity is pursued by the child. Persistence refers to the continuation of an activity in face of obstacles.

This ability is due to interplay between two major subcomponents: ***attentional control*** (the capacity to maintain attention on tasks as well as to shift attention when desired) and ***inhibitory control*** (the capacity to plan and to suppress inappropriate action). Infants and children differ greatly along these dimensions. Recent neuroimaging data suggest that these differences are associated with three biologically based attentional networks, or systems: the "**alerting attentional system**," the "**orienting attention system**," and the "**executive attention system**" (Posner and Rothbart 2007; Rothbart and Bates 2006; Rueda et al. 2004). Developmentally, the first attention system to appear is the alerting attention system, which is involved in achieving and maintaining a state of alertness. Evidence suggests that, anatomically, this system is supported by the locus coeruleus, the right frontal cortex, and the parietal cortex, with norepinephrine as the principal neuromodulator (Xu et al. 2015). The second system, the orienting system, is involved in the selection of information from sensory input. This system is associated with the superior parietal lobe, the temporal parietal junction, and the frontal eye field area, and is believed to be primarily regulated by the neurotransmitter acetylcholine. Finally, the third network, called the executive network, is involved in maintaining continuity of behavior in accordance with goals in the presence of possible distractions. Anatomically, the executive network is related to the anterior cingulate cortex, the basal ganglia, and the lateral prefrontal cortex, with dopamine as its prime neuromodulator (Posner and Rothbart 2007; Raz and Buhle 2006).

14.2.1.5 Sociability

Sociability is defined as a preference for being with others rather than remaining alone. The major component of sociability is *instrumental*—seeking out others and remaining in their company. There are the intrinsic social rewards that motivate this behavior. One reward is the *sharing of activities*. Children enjoy playing with other children. Sociable people prefer to eat, watch television, watch movies, etc., with others. There need be no interaction, just the company of others who are doing the same thing. A second intrinsic reward is *attention from others*. Sociable people strongly want to be listened to or at least have their presence noted by others looking at or talking to them. Finally, there is *responsivity from others*. The height of social interaction is exemplified by conversation: What I say partly determines what you say, which in turn is a stimulus for what I say. These three rewards, occur only when people are together.

14.2.1.6 Adaptability

This is also related to the concept of negative emotionality. Initial approach and eventual adaptability are separate variables in the Thomas and Chess system, but empirically they always tend to cluster together. The core idea is that there are individual differences in the extent to which children respond positively versus negatively to new people and other new stimuli. The child's adaptation to one kind of stimulus can covary to another kind of stimulus e.g., a child could be positive in response to new physical settings yet shy with new people. Inadaptability perceived in infancy tends to predict anxiety, internalizing behavior problems better than it predicts externalizing problems (Bates 1979, 1989, 1998, 2007).

14.2.2 Assessment of Temperament

There are four types of measures that are available to assess childhood temperament each with different strengths and weaknesses. Ideally more than one method should be used, to take advantage of the strengths of different methods and to counteract the weaknesses inherent in each (Kagan et al. 1988, 1999; Kagan and Fox 2006, Kagan and Snidman 2004; Kochanska et al. 1990, 1997, 2000). It is also important to include more than one informant when possible, as is true for assessing children's functioning in general (Thomas et al. 1963).

(1) **Questionnaires**: These are the most commonly used measures. Although questionnaires are most often administered to parents, they can also be used to obtain reports from peers, teachers, and other informants. Self-report questionnaires are available for older children. Questionnaires have a number of strengths—they aggregate information about children's behavior across a number of situations and over a period of time; they are inexpensive to administer and they efficiently gather a lot of information (Seifer et al. 1994; Keiley et al. 2003; Bishop et al. 2003).

(2) **Peer reports**: These can be obtained through peer nomination measures wherein peers nominate other students who are "best" or "least well" described by particular items.

(3) **Naturalistic observation**: These can be used to evaluate for children's behavioral tendencies. For example, home observation systems have been developed to assess temperament in preschoolers (Harman et al. 1997; Guerin et al. 2003; Henderson and Wachs 2007; Caspi et al. 1995, Caspi 2000).

(4) **Laboratory tasks**: These create specific situations in which children's behaviors can be observed, e.g., playroom observation (Fullard et al. 1984) .

The weaknesses of naturalistic observation and laboratory tasks are these methods are time limited, being vulnerable to situational effects on behavior and limiting the possibility of observing rare behaviors.

14.2.3 Goodness of Fit

Thomas and Chess gave the concept of "goodness of fit" which arises from an understanding that normal or pathologic psychological development does not depend on temperament alone. Rather, it is the nature of the interaction between temperament and the individual's other characteristics with specific features of the environment, which provides the basic dynamic influence for the process of development (McClowry et al. 2008).

There is goodness of fit when the child's temperament and other characteristics, such as motivations and levels of intellectual and other abilities, are adequate to master the successive demands, expectations and opportunities of the environment. If on the other hand the individual cannot cope successfully with the environmental demands, then there is poorness of fit (Huizink 2008). With a goodness of fit, psychological development and functioning progresses favorably. With a poorness of fit, the individual experiences excessive stress and failures of adaptation, and the development takes an unfavorable course.

It is important to note that goodness of fit does not imply an absence of stress or conflict. These are inevitable factors of the developmental process, in which new expectations and demands for change and progressively higher levels of functioning occur continuously as the child grows older. Demands, stresses, and conflicts, when in keeping with the person's developmental potentials and capacities for mastery, may be constructive in their consequences and should not be considered as an inevitable cause of behavioral disturbance. The issue involved in behavioral functioning is that of *excessive* stress resulting from poorness of fit between environmental expectations and demands and the capacities of the individual at a particular level of development.

This concept can be used practically in many ways in which the response of parents, teachers, mental health professionals, and pediatricians will foster either a goodness or poorness of fit for a child with a particular extreme level of one temperamental trait or another. In general, this special concern for a child's temperamental characteristics is required when it is either at a very high or very low level. In the average range of temperament, which will usually be consonant with environmental demands and expectations, usually no special management techniques are required. Occasionally, parents will expect that their child to function at an extreme level of temperament, e.g. with adaptability or persistence, when the child is only at an average level. This kind of excessive demand can also create poorness of fit, with unfavorable consequences.

14.3 Temperament and Child Psychopathology

14.3.1 Individual Disorders

14.3.1.1 Attention Deficit Hyperkinetic Disorder

Attention deficit hyperactivity disorder (ADHD) is an example of a disorder that appears in the upward range of temperamental traits related to activity level and attention span. Much of the public controversy surrounding this diagnosis is related to the view that what will be diagnosed as an illness are the temperamental traits at somewhat higher levels than are typically observed. It has been seen that *low levels of task persistence, attentional focusing* (Ruf et al. 2008) *and inhibitory control* (Goldsmith 1993; Goldsmith et al. 2000; Cole et al. 2004) *with higher levels of novelty seeking, extraversion is seen in ADHD* (Nigg et al. 2004; Castellanos 2008). The molecular genetic studies of novelty seeking and ADHD have converged on similar candidate genes, often related to dopaminergic transmission (Wood et al. 2007; Dick 2007).

It is found that children who have been classified as having *behavioral disinhibition* are more likely to develop later externalizing disorders. Many of these children with behavioral disinhibition, however, also go on to develop other types of psychopathology, such as mood disorders.

A recent study (Healey et al. 2016) evaluated the relationship between temperament, neuropsychological abilities, and global functioning in young hyperactive/inattentive 114 preschool children. This study indicated that higher verbal executive abilities were associated with better child functioning when parent-rated effortful control was high, but not when effortful control was low. Also, high levels of nonverbal executive skills were associated with higher child global functioning when both parent- and teacher-rated negative affect was low, but not when negative affect was high.

14.3.1.2 Conduct and Oppositional Defiant Disorder

In several studies on children with conduct disorder, difficult temperament in infancy was one of the major variables in the explanation of later aggressive behavior. According to these studies, children with a combination of *high novelty seeking, high negative emotionality, low harm avoidance, and low reward dependence* should be most at risk for the development of conduct and oppositional defiant disorder. Of these high novelty seeking and low harm avoidance have been consistently linked with externalizing symptoms like aggression and delinquency (Burke 2002; Schmeck 2001)

14.3.1.3 Anxiety and Mood Disorders

Anxiety and mood disorders are often collectively referred to as internalizing disorders. Although they are considered to be separate categories in the current classificatory systems, yet there is good evidence to support they are closely linked. Both have strongest association with dimensions of *negative emotionality, neuroticism, and harm avoidance*. Major depression has also been associated with the combination of *high negative emotionality, low extraversion, and low approach*. Behavioral inhibition also poses risk for development of anxiety disorders (Tackett 2006). High negative emotionality predicts emotional disorders only when individuals lack adequate levels of effortful control to be able to regulate their negative emotions and cognitive biases toward threatening information.

Bipolar Affective Disorder has been shown to be related to *high novelty seeking, high harm avoidance, and low persistence*. (Zaninotto et al. 2016). This pattern represents an "approach-avoidance" tendency, which is in contrast to the general population wherein novelty seeking is generally inversely related to harm avoidance.

Also, it was also found that bipolar disorder is associated with comorbid conditions like alcoholism and anxiety disorders, but differed from bipolar patients without these comorbid conditions on certain traits. Bipolar patients with comorbid alcoholism had high novelty seeking; and those with comorbid anxiety disorder had high scores of harm avoidance.

14.3.1.4 Substance Use Disorders

Certain traits may predispose an adolescent to participate in risk-taking behaviors. Impulsivity interferes with an adolescent's ability to make wise decisions, due to inability to enter into a cost/benefit analysis of the behavior or to foresee any negative consequences (Cooper 2003). Some adolescents have temperamental features that favor thrill and risk taking, i.e., high novelty seeking. Other characteristics of negative emotionality are also thought to put adolescents at risk for substance use disorders. Overall, adolescents with difficult temperaments, high levels of sensation seeking, anger/aggression, and impulsivity may be at particular risk of engaging in substance use disorders (Bonomo and Bowes 2001; Chassin 2004; Cooper 2003; Feldstein 2006).

14.3.1.5 Eating Disorders

Whereas most individuals with eating disorders share a preoccupation with weight and self-image, there appear to be substantial differences that generally fall along diagnostic lines, particularly between the restricting subtype of **anorexia nervosa (AN)** and **bulimia nervosa (BN),** and these may reflect underlying differences in temperament and personality. The results of a recently published meta-analysis of temperament in eating disorders (Atiye et al. 2015) report persistence to be significantly higher than controls in all eating disorders; highest levels being observed in AN. Correspondingly, the highest effect sizes for harm avoidance was seen in AN. Novelty seeking was significantly higher relative to controls only in BN. Harm avoidance was significantly lower, and reward dependence was significantly higher in individuals who had recovered from AN than in those who remained ill.

14.3.1.6 Somatoform and Dissociative Disorder

Temperamental traits of low activity, low emotionality, low rhythmicity, and low distractibility in children presenting with both somatoform disorder and dissociative disorder (Raghutaman and Cherian 2003).

14.3.1.7 Psychotic Disorders

Temperamental associations with psychotic disorders have been less studied. High harm avoidance though has been consistently found in both patients with schizophrenia and their relatives. Some authors suggest harm avoidance as schizophrenia-related endophenotype. An increased risk of schizophrenia may be associated with asociality (configured as high harm avoidance and low reward dependence) and schizotypy (configured as low self directedness, low cooperativeness and high self transcendence) (Smith and Cloninger 2008; Jetha and Zheng 2013)

14.3.2 Research in India

Considering the relevance of temperament in the theory of child development and its potential for practical application, efforts were made to systematically study temperament in India. Many questions arose when the temperament concept of NYLS workers derived from working middle class urban population of New York was applied to a section of population in India markedly different in sociocultural background. Thus, keeping in mind the relevant situations and based on the temperamental dimensions described by Thomas and Chess a Temperament Measurement Schedule was developed in Hindi and English (Malhotra et al. 1983a, b).

The Temperament Schedule thus devised and standardized on North Indian population has been used in many studies by the author and also been used by different centers across the country.

Relationship between temperament and psychopathology in childhood is analogous to the relationship between personality and psychiatric illness, where personality constitutes vulnerability to develop the disorder as well as exerts pathoplastic influence on it. Role of temperament in influencing the symptom pattern was examined in a systematic study (Malhotra 1989).

Malhotra (1989) studied the temperament characteristics of 30 children each with conduct disorder, conversion disorder, emotional disorder (diagnosed as per DSM III criteria), and normal controls. The children with conduct disorder showed a temperament profile of high-energy, i.e., high activity and intensity of reaction and persistently negative mood. Those diagnosed as conversion disorder had low distractibility, which overlaps with soothability. According to Rothbart (1986) soothability is a recovery parameter of distress. Low 'distractibility' in conversion disorder as was observed in this study indicates low soothability, i.e., such children temperamentally, take longer to come out of a distressed state. They remain in distress for relatively longer periods in times of distress. Positive and early attempts at soothing the child might help in preventing the distress into somatic symptoms.

Overall findings of this study revealed that temperament profile of conduct disorder children was most deviant, i.e., highest in energy and lowest in emotionality; for emotional disorders it was less deviant than conduct disorder, and in conversion disorders it closest to the normal group.

These findings supported the view that there is some link between particular temperament style and some of the clinical diagnostic entities seen in childhood, the nature of which needs to be explored. Does temperament represent specific neurophysiological vulnerability; or a continuum with psychopathology; or a stimulus for evolving particular pathological parenting responses or is there a common biological substrate for both; or is it simply pathoplastic influence, are some of the hypothesis offered.

In another study (Malhotra 1990) on temperament profile of 50 children with Mental Retardation it was found that children with mental retardation were found to be withdrawing, poorly adaptable, with predominantly negative mood, and low distractibility. These are characteristics of 'difficult' child temperament as described by Thomas and Chess. Moreover, these children exhibited significantly higher scores on all psychopathology factors as compared to normal children. Thus, it appears that mentally retarded children, having behavioral/emotional problems also show signs of 'difficult' temperament. Therefore, it can be hypothesized that intelligence and temperament being innate, determine the vulnerability to develop behavior/emotional problems during the course of development.

There were also studies conducted to evaluate the relationship between high risk to develop a psychiatric illness and temperament of children.

In a comparative study of Malhotra et al. (1993) temperamental characteristics of children of substance dependent fathers were compared with those of emotionally disturbed children as well as with general population norms (Malhotra et al. 1993), it was found that children with substance dependent fathers were found to be low in rhythmicity, less adaptable, having pronounced negative emotionality, tending to withdraw in social situations, less distractible and having lower threshold of responsiveness as compared to normal children. Differences were accentuated on rhythmicity and distractibility in those children whose fathers had greater severity of substance dependence. Variables implicating potential environmental factors, such as duration of exposure of child to father's illness, dysfunction in father, or depression in mother were not associated with child temperamental profile.

Given the 'high risk' background, it seems likely that study of temperament in this group might provide a way to understand how genetic predispositions may be translated into the risk behavior patterns. Also, a deviant temperament profile in childhood often indicates higher vulnerability to psychopathology in later life (Thomas and Chess 1977, 1984). Finally, a deviant profile of temperament makes parenting difficult. The difficulty is compounded by the fact that one of the parents may not be effective in the handling due to the problem of addiction. Thus, the issue of management and counseling of the parents with the aim of primary prevention in this high-risk category is highly important.

In another study Malhotra and Kaur (1997) studied the temperament characteristics of children born to parents suffering from a mental disorder. Two hundred children, one each of eighty parents with psychotic disorder, eighty parents with neurotic disorder (on ICD 10 criteria) and forty healthy parents were studied. The most significant finding of this study was that children of parents with psychotic as well as neurotic disorder showed low sociability, i.e., were withdrawing and less adaptable; had lower emotionality (persistently negative mood); lower energy, i.e., less activity and less intensity of emptions and less regular biological rhythms. In this study, the results showed that temperament of children had no relationship to the duration of illness of the parent, or to the child's age at first exposure to parental illness; to nature of illness whether psychosis or neurosis; or whether the father was ill or the mother was ill. The main effect on temperament was from being born to a psychotic or a neurotic patient.

Since children of parents with mental disorder are more likely to have psychiatric disorder, difficult temperamental traits may be the behavioral markers or the meditational variables between the predisposition and the manifest disorder. The clinical implications of these findings are significant. Genetic predisposition may manifest itself in temperamental variation in children which is no less significant than the environmental consequences of parental mental disorder determining the psychological adjustment of the children with mental disorder. Since temperament can be identified at an early age, children at risk for disorder later on could be identified early enough for possible primary prevention.

Most studies on emotional disorders in physically sick children have focused on the role of family factors and studies relating to temperament are very few. Malhotra (1989) studied temperament profile of 50 physically ill children (excluding brain diseases) and found that the psychological adjustment was determined to a significant extent by temperament particularly low distractibility rather than the disease parameters such as duration of illness or diagnosis. Low distractibility has been regarded to overlap with soothability (i.e., recovery from distress) parameter. It appears that children who temperamentally take longer to recover from state of distress (i.e., low distractibility) have greater likelihood of developing maladjustment.

14.4 Other Important Areas in Relation to Temperament

14.4.1 Temperament and School Functioning

With the onset of formal schooling, a new and more complex hierarchy of stimuli, demands, and expectations begin to influence the developmental process. The school makes a number of new demands on the child. These include the mastery of increasing complex cognitive tasks, and simultaneous requirements to adapt to new geographical setting, to strange adults in unfamiliar role and to a host of new rules and regulations.

Temperament plays an important role in shaping the course of a child's school functioning. Temperamental characteristics will help determine the individual child's response to a new and demanding cognitive school task, but so will his intellectual and perceptual capacities, level of motivation, teacher characteristics, and nature of peer social interactions.

The parents in the NYLS uniformly gave great importance to the children's school functioning and academic achievement. The general patterns of difficulty involving temperament that could be identified have been described below:

The Difficult Child with his slow adaptability and intense negative reaction to new situation presents the teacher with the same need for understanding and quite firm patience as was required of his parents at home. In those instances where parents had appreciated the temperamental issues and handled them adequately, they were often helpful in orienting the first teacher to the significance of the child's initial reaction to school. Hence, experienced and competent teachers and principals could often identify these children accurately and helped them eventually to adapt to school. When the parents, on the contrary, had become entangled in an unhealthy interaction with the child at home, the same sequence was more likely to occur at school.

The highly active or distractible child may also have similar problems adapting to the demands of the school as he did in home setting. Children with difficulties in sitting quietly or following directions without distraction can create annoyance and impatience in teachers as in parents. In several instances these children did poorly in very permissive unstructured school settings. When the highly active child was allowed to roam at will and the distractible youngster was permitted to turn his attention to whatever caught his eye or ear—the children did not settle down spontaneously, and learned little until structured, consistent, though flexible, demands were finally made on them.

The temperamental trait of low or high persistence and attention span usually presented minor problems in the preschool years at home, but sometimes made for greater difficulties at school. The needs and expectations of the family in the child's early years were generally not significantly affected whether his attention span was short or long or whether he stuck to a difficult task or gave up quickly. In school, however, prolonged concentration was usually expected in academic tasks, and this demand became excessively stressful for the child with low persistence and short attention span, especially combined with high distractibility. Sustained pressure by teacher and parent for the nonpersistent child to attain, inevitably led to anxiety, self-derogation and defensive techniques to avoid any difficult task performance. By contrast, when task assignments were structured so they did not exceed the child's concentration span, learning proceeded successfully.

The highly persistent child with a long attention span, on the other hand, often seemed to be made for learning. Parents and teachers only had to guide the child gently to maintain his steady and persistent effort to learn whatever was put before him. Problems did develop, however, if such a child insisted on continuing an activity and the teacher demanded that he shift to the next scheduled activity with the rest of the class. Such forcible interruption of his absorbed attention and effort, whether at home or school, is typically a source of intense frustration for a very persistent child. The expression of this frustration in tantrums or other explosive reactions sometimes led to the child being labeled by the school as anxious or a disciplinary problem.

Hence, knowledge of child's temperament will provide teachers with insights into children's behavior as well as understanding their own responses. The use of rewards and punishments also need to be tailored to child's temperaments. Thus, this will result in a "good fit" between the child and the school environment.

14.4.2 Temperament and Health Care Practices

The health care professional—pediatrician, general practitioner, or baby nurse is usually the most influential adviser to the parents, especially in the child's early years. It is this health care professional and not a psychiatrist, who is likely to be consulted consistently and frequently on the management of problems of feeding, sleeping, weaning, and toilet training.

The pediatrician's role with regard to the child's temperamental individuality can be considered under a number of headings: advice on child-care practices; reassurance to parents; routine examinations and procedures; management of minor problems; evaluation of the acutely ill/chronically ill child; and preventive counseling. In carrying out these activities it is necessary for the pediatrician to be able to assess the child's temperament characteristics.

An infant's responses to new people and procedures, especially if associated with discomfort or pain, are strongly influenced by his temperamental characteristics. Depending on his temperament, the child may fuss quietly and briefly, squirm a bit and then be immediately cheerful once the procedures are completed. Or he may howl loudly from the moment he enters the pediatrician's office, struggle violently during the physical examination, take up several hours to subside, and start up again even more intensely at the next visit. The child with low activity will sit quietly in the waiting room. The high activity child will fidget, jump around; try to poke in the drawers and closets long time before the doctor sees him.

The pediatrician who evaluates the temperament and understands its implications will be in a good position to minimize the distress of each child's office visit. With the Easy child, no special management approach is necessary. However, even such an adaptable child may be overwhelmed if the busy doctor rushes him too quickly through the procedures. The Slow-To-Warm-Up Child should be given time to get used to the waiting room, and further time in the examining room before proceeding with the physical examination. The highly active child should be seen quickly. If he has to wait, he should be given toys and space to move around in without disturbing others. The Difficult Child should also be given a warm-up period, but should still be expected to respond to the examination with loud and long protests.

In addition to dealing with aforementioned situations, many of the minor problems of a young child brought to the pediatrician's attention are also significantly related to temperamental issues. **Frequent night waking** is more likely to occur in an infant with a low sensory threshold. Carey suggests two possible explanations of this relationship: The low threshold child's greater responsiveness to daytime stimulation makes him more arousable at night; or the infant is more responsive to internal and external stimuli at night as well. Carey (1978) recommends dealing with the problem by reducing environmental stimulation before bedtime and during night.

The **prolonged loud crying spells** of the infant with **colic** presents a difficult and disturbing management problem to the parents. Carey's work (1994) suggests a relationship to a low sensory threshold in such a situation. The pediatrician can provide much needed reassurance and support parents in such cases.

The response of a child to the irritation of a **skin rash** can be significantly influenced by temperamental traits. The intense reactor may cry loudly and complain vigorously even if treatment is proceeding effectively, and this reaction should not lead doctor or parent into a misjudgment of the treatment progress. The child with a low sensory threshold may have great difficulty in obeying the instructions not to rub or scratch the irritated skin, and special measures may be necessary to reduce the sensory stimulation from the rash.

The above instances illustrate some of the ways in which the child's temperament influences the response to physical symptoms and management of minor ailments.

Finally, the pediatrician has to also **guide the family on a preventive level** for the benefit of the child's mental health. He is in a position to detect the first signs of unhealthy physical or emotional developmental trends and to advise the family as to the most desirable remedial measures.

With regard to psychological issues, especially in the young child, temperamental aspects play a significant role in prevention. Two goals are paramount: the achievement of a goodness of fit between parental attitudes and practices and child's temperamental traits; and the alleviation of inappropriate parental guilt and anxiety when the child behavioral patterns deviate from the normal.

14.4.3 Practical Implications

The child's temperament influences his responses to parental practices and attitudes and helps to shape parents' judgments and feelings toward him. Sibling and peer group relationships, school functioning and academic achievement, behavior responses to illness or other special stress—all can be significantly affected by specific temperamental traits (Rowe and Plomin 1977; Wachs 2000; Hart et al. 2005).

For adults also, temperamental characteristics frequently play an important role in determining personal and social functioning, work patterns, and adaptation to change (Diamond 1957; Eisenberg et al. 2000; Constantino et al. 2002; Roberts et al. 2007).

For the teacher, as well as for the mother, inappropriate burdens of responsibility can be lifted by the awareness that the child's school functioning can be influenced by his/her temperament. No matter how competent and committed the teacher may be, he/she will not be able to make a high activity child sit quietly or a distractible child concentrates for long periods of time.

The same situation applies to the pediatrician, nurse, and mental health professional. The health care professional has the responsibility of gathering and analyzing information on temperament before interpreting behavior and offering advice and treatment.

14.4.4 Parent Guidance

The concept of "goodness of fit" between the child's characteristics and environmental demands and expectations offers the basis for parent guidance procedures when a child presents evidence of a behavior disorder.

Parent guidance involves educating parents about child's temperamental traits followed by identification of those elements of parental behavior that appear to be exerting a harmful influence on the child's development. This is followed by the formulation of a program of altered parental functioning, which then modify/change the interactive pattern between the child and the parent in healthy direction.

The rationale of the guidance program is explained to the parents in terms of the necessity of a "goodness of fit" between the child's characteristics and the parent's functioning. The specific areas of undesirable parent–child interaction are identified, the specific temperamental traits of the child are described, and the parental behaviors, which are creating excessive stress, are pointed out. Throughout the discussion, the parents are assured that no judgment is being made that they are "bad parents," and that same behavior with a child with different characteristics might be positive instead of negative in its consequences.

References to concrete incidents in the child's life are made to illustrate each suggestion. For e.g., the initial intense negative responses to new situations and slow adaptability of a Difficult Child are documented by details of the child's history with new foods, new people, new activities, new school situations, etc. Harmful parental attitudes, such as guilt, anxiety and hostility, and undesirable management practices, such as impatience, inconsistency, and rigidity are identified, again with examples. As another example, the restlessness and shifts in attention of a highly active and distractible child are distinguished from willful inattention and lack of interest. Parental demands that the child can sit on a long trip or concentrate for long periods without distraction on homework are identified, and their undesirable consequences explained.

The parents are then offered specific suggestions and advice for changing the identified undesirable attitudes and practices. Several sessions may be required for them to grasp adequately the concept of temperamental individuality and its influence on the child's ability to cope with parental and other environmental demands and expectations.

A constructive approach by the parents to the child's temperament does not mean an acceptance or encouragement of all the child's behavior in all situations. The parent's goal should be to prevent any undesirable temperament- environment interaction. This involves two considerations: avoidance of demands or expectations that are substantially dissonant with the child's temperament, and the encouragement of those activities which will minimize any undesirable consequences of child's temperament. As an example of the latter goal, the high activity child should be guided to channel his motor activity into acceptable directions. The mildly expressive child should be taught to articulate his desires clearly and repetitively until they are noticed. The nonpersistent child should be encouraged to take breaks with a difficult task as often as necessary until mastery is achieved, rather than just giving up.

In some instances, psychopathology in the parents may be present so as to prevent their making the necessary changes in behavior. This will usually become evident quickly in the course of the guidance sessions and will differentiate from those in whom it reflects more easily remedial causes, such as ignorance, poor advice or transient situational difficulties. In the former cases, psychotherapy for the parent will be necessary whether it be individual psychotherapy, group or family therapy.

In addition to parent guidance, Muris and Ollendick (2005) have proposed that many cognitive behavioral treatment programs have as their goal the improvement of children's effortful control. CBT teaches techniques that help children to inhibit their maladaptive behaviors and to regulate their attention, thereby improving their effortful control. Preventive work may have a similar focus on strengthening children's basic skills in emotional regulation, self-control, and adjustment to the environment.

Thus, treatment and prevention may operate in different and complementary ways: by modifying basic tendencies or by helping youths cope better with those tendencies; and by parent guidance intervention programs.

14.5 Conclusions

Temperament denotes innate behavioral individuality or uniqueness of children evident very early in infancy that can be easily identified and also measured in clinical and nonclinical settings. Temperament has sound neurobiological underpinnings. Temperament has tremendous appeal as well as application in understanding the developmental trajectories and origins of psychiatric disorders in children and adolescents; and lends itself to intervention strategies. The entire approach involves goodness of fit between temperament and environment, skills training, emotional, and behavioral regulation. Integrating knowledge about individual differences into best clinical practices in treatment and prevention has the potential to make interventions more effective and holistic.

References

Atiye, M., Miettunen, J., & Raevuori-Helkamaa, A. (2015). A meta-analysis of temperament in eating disorders. *European Eating Disorders Review, 23*, 89–99.

Bates, J. E., Freeland, C. A. B., & Lounsbury, M. L. (1979). Measurement of infant difficultness. *Child Development, 50*, 794–803.

Bates, J. E., & Kohnstamm, R. (1989). Applications of temperament concepts. In E. Bates (Ed.), *Temperament in childhood*. New York: Wiley.

Bates, J. E., & Pettit, G. (2007). *Temperament, parenting and socialization*. Guilford, New York: Handbook of socialization.

Bates, J. E., Pettit, G. S., Dodge, K. A., & Ridge, B. (1998). Interaction of temperamental resistance to control and restrictive parenting in the development of externalizing behavior. *Developmental Psychology, 34*, 982–95.

Bishop, G., Spence, S. H., & McDonald, C. (2003). Can parents and teachers provide a reliable and valid report of behavioral inhibition? *Child Development, 74*, 1899–1917.

Bonomo, Y., & Bowes, G. (2001). Putting harm reduction into an adolescent context. *Journal of Paediatrics and Child Health, 37*, 5–8.

Burgdorf, J., & Panksepp, J. (2006). The neurobiology of positive emotions. *Neuroscience and Biobehavioral Reviews, 30*, 173–87.

Burke, J. D. (2002). Oppositional defiant disorder and conduct disorder: A review of the past 10 years, part II. *Journal of the American Academy of Child & Adolescent Psychiatry, 41*, 1275–93.

Buss, A., & Plomin, R. (1975). *Temperament theory of personality development*. New York: Wiley.

Campos, J., Frankel, C., & Camras, L. (2004). On the nature of emotion regulation. *Child Development, 75*, 377–94.

Carey, W. B., & McDevitt, S. C. (1978). Revision of the infant temperament questionnaire. *Pediatrics, 61*, 735–39.

Carey, W. B., & McDevitt, S. C. (1994). *Prevention and early intervention. Individual differences as risk factors for the mental health of children*. New York: A Festschrift for Stella Chess and Alexander Thomas.

Caspi, A. (2000). The child is father of the man: Personality continuities from childhood to adulthood. *Journal of Personality and Social Psychology, 78*, 158–72.

Caspi, A., Henry, B., McGee, R. O., Moffitt, T. E., & Silva, P. A. (1995). Temperamental origins of child and adolescent behavior problems: From age three to age fifteen. *Child Development, 66*, 55–68.

Castellanos, F. X. (2008). The relationship between attention deficit hyperactivity disorder and child temperament. *Journal of Applied Developmental Psychology, 29*, 157–169.

Chassin, L. (2004). Trajectories of alcohol and drug use and dependence from adolescence to adulthood: The effects of familial alcoholism and personality. *Journal of Abnormal Psychology, 113*, 483–498.

Chess, S., & Thomas, A. (1984). *Origins and evolution of behavior disorders*. New York: Bruner/Mazel.

Cloninger, C. R. (1987). A systematic method for clinical description and classification of personality variants. *Archives of General Psychiatry, 44*, 573–88.

Cole, P. M., Martin, S. E., & Dennis, T. A. (2004). Emotion regulation as a scientific construct: Methodological challenges and directions for child development research. *Child Development, 75*, 317–33.

Constantino, J. N., Cloninger, C. R., Clarke, A. R., Hashemi, B., & Przybeck, T. (2002). Application of the seven-factor model of personality to early childhood. *Psychiatry Research, 109*, 229–43.

Cooper, C. L. (2003). Inappropriate prescription of methylphenidate. *The New Zealand Medical Journal, 116*, 1183.

Depue, R. A., & Morrone-Strupinsky, J. V. (2005). A neurobehavioral model of affiliative bonding: Implications for conceptualizing a human trait of affiliation. *Behavioral and Brain Sciences, 28*, 313–50.

DeYoung, C. G., & Gray, J. R. (2009). Personality neuroscience: Explaining individual differences in affect, behavior, and cognition. In P. J. Corr & G. Matthews (Eds.), *The Cambridge handbook of personality psychology*. New York: Cambridge University Press.

DeYoung, C. G., Hirsh, J. B., Shane, M. S., Papademetris, X., Rajeevan, N., & Gray, J. R. (2010). Testing predictions from personality neuroscience. *Brain structure and the big five, 21*, 820–8.

Diamond, S. (1957). *Personality and temperament*. New York: Harper.

Dick, D. (2007). Identification of genes influencing a spectrum of externalizing psychopathology. *Current Directions in Psychological Science, 16*, 331–35.

Eaton, W., & Enns, L. (1986). Scheme for observing activity level: Reliability and convergent validity. *Journal of Psychoeducational Assessment, 3*, 273–80.

Eisenberg, N., Fabes, R. A., Guthrie, I. K., & Reiser, M. (2000). Dispositional emotionality and regulation: Their role in predicting quality of social functioning. *Journal of Personality and Social Psychology, 78*, 136–57.

Fagot, B. I., & Brian, M. (1994). Activity level in young children. *Merrill-Palmer Quarterly, 40*, 378–90.

Feldstein, S. (2006). Substance use and risk taking among adolescents. *Journal of Mental Health, 15*, 633–43.

Fullard, W., McDevitt, S. C., & Carey, W. B. (1984). Assessing temperament in one-to-three-year-old children. *Journal of Pediatric Psychology, 9*, 205–16.

Goldsmith, H. H. (1993). *Temperament: Variability in developing emotion systems*. Handbook of emotion New York: Guildford Press.

Goldsmith, H. H., Lemery, K. S., Aksan, N., & Buss, K. A. (2000). Temperament substrates of personality development. In V. J. Molfese & D. L. Molfese (Eds.), *Temperament and personality development across the life-span* (pp. 1–32). New Jersey: Erlbaum.

Gray, J. A. (1991). *The neuropsychology of temperament. International perspectives on theory and measurement*. New York: Plenum Press.

Guerin, D. W., Gottfried, A. W., Oliver, P. H., & Thomas, C. W. (2003). *Temperament. Infancy through adolescence*. New York: Kluwer Academic.

Harman, C., Rothbart, M. K., & Posner, M. I. (1997). Distress and attention in early infancy. *Motivation and Emotion, 21*, 27–43.

Hart, D., Burock, D., London, B., Atkins, R., & Santiago, G. (2005). The relation of personality types to physiological, behavioral and cognitive processes. *European Journal of Personality, 19*, 391–407.

Healey, D. M., Rajendran, K., O'Neill, S., Gopin, C. B., & Halperin, J. M. (2016). The interplay among temperament, neuropsychological abilities, and global functioning in young hyperactive/inattentive children. Br J Dev Psychol, Feb 11 (Epub ahead of print).

Henderson, H. H., & Wachs, T. D. (2007). Temperament theory and the study of cognition-emotion interactions across development. *Developmental Review,* 396–427.

Huizink, A. (2008). Prenatal stress exposure and temperament: A review. *European Journal of Developmental Science, 2,* 77–99.

Jetha, M. K., & Zheng, X. (2013). Shyness and emotional face processing in schizophrenia: An ERP study. *Biological Psychology, 94,* 562–74.

Kagan, J. (2008). The biological contributions to temperaments and emotions. *European Journal of Developmental Science, 2,* 38–51.

Kagan, J., & Fox, N. (2006). Biology, culture, and temperamental biases. In W. Damon & R. Lerner (Series Eds.), & N. Eisenberg (Vol. Ed.), *Handbook of child psychology, Vol. 3. Social, emotional, and personality development* (6th ed., pp. 99–166). New York: Wiley.

Kagan, J., Reznick, J. S., & Snidman, N. (1988). Biological bases of childhood shyness. *Science, 24,* 167–71.

Kagan, J., & Snidman, N. (2004). *The long shadow of temperament.* Cambridge, MA: Harvard University Press.

Kagan, J., Snidman, N., Zentner, M. R., & Peterson, E. (1999). Infant temperament and anxious symptoms in school age children. *Development and Psychopathology, 11,* 209–24.

Keiley, M. K., Lofthouse, N., Bates, J. E., Dodge, K. A., & Pettit, G. S. (2003). Differential risks of covarying and pure components in mother and teacher reports of externalizing and internalizing behavior across ages 5 to 14. *Journal of Abnormal Child Psychology, 31,* 267–83.

Kochanska, G. (1997). Multiple pathways to conscience for children with different temperaments: From toddlerhood to age 5. *Developmental Psychology, 33,* 228–40.

Kochanska, G., Coy, K. C., Tjebkes, C. T., & Husarek, S. (1990). Individual differences in emotionality in infancy. *Child Development, 69,* 375–90.

Kochanska, G., Murray, K., & Harlan, E. T. (2000). Effortful control in early childhood: Continuity and change, antecedents, and implications for social development. *Developmental Psychology, 36,* 220–32.

Lee, C. L., & Bates, J. E. (1985). Mother–child interaction at age two-years and perceived difficult temperament. *Child Development, 56,* 1314–25.

Lemery, K. S., Goldsmith, H. H., Klinnert, M. D., & Mrazek, D. A. (1999). Developmental models of infant and childhood temperament. *Developmental Psychology, 35,* 189–204.

Malhotra, S. (1989). Temperamental characteristics of children with conduct and conversion disorders. *Indian Journal of Psychiatry, 31,* 168–72.

Malhotra, S. (1990). Temperamental characteristics of mentally retarded children. *Indian Journal of Pediatrics, 57,* 213–18.

Malhotra, S., Aga, V. M., Bedi, B., & Gupta, N. (1999). Comparison of conduct disorder and hyperkinetic conduct disorder, a retrospective clinical study from North India. *Indian Journal of Psychiatry, 41,* 22–32.

Malhotra, S., Basu, D., Bhagat, A., & Malhotra, A. (1993). Temperament in children of addicts: A preliminary report. *Journal of Hongkong College of Psychiatrists, 3,* 5–8.

Malhotra, S., & Kaur, R. (1997). Temperament study of children of mentally ill parents. *Journal of Hongkong College of Psychiatrists, 7,* 39–45.

Malhotra, S., & Malhotra, A. (1990). Psychological adjustment of physically sick children; relationship with temperament. *Indian Pediatrics, 27,* 577–84.

Malhotra, S., Malhotra, A., & Randhawa, A. (1983a). Children's temperament: Factorial validity. *Indian Journal of Clinical Psychology, 24,* 399–406.

Malhotra, S., Malhotra, A., & Randhawa, A. (1983b). Temperament as discriminating variable between emotionally disturbed and normal children. *Indian Journal of Clinical Psychology, 10,* 79–83.

Malhotra, S., & Randhawa, A. (1982). A schedule for measuring temperament in children: Preliminary data on development and standardization. *Indian Journal of Clinical Psychology, 9,* 203–16.

Malhotra, S., Varma, V. K., & Verma, S. K. (1986). Temperament as determinant of phenomenology of childhood psychiatric disorders. *Indian Journal of Psychiatry, 28*, 263–76.

McClowry, S. G., Rodriguez, E., & Koslowitz, R. (2008). Temperament-based intervention: Re-examining goodness-of-fit. *European Journal of Developmental Science, 2*, 120–35.

Muris, P., & Ollendick, T. H. (2005). The role of temperament in the etiology of child psychopathology. *Clinical Child and Family Psychology Review, 8*, 271–89.

Nettle, D. (2006). The evolution of personality variation in humans and other animals. *American Psychologist, 61*, 622–31.

Nigg, J. T., Goldsmith. H., & Sachek, J. (2004). Temperament and attention deficit hyperactivity disorder: The development of a multiple pathway model. *Journal of Clinical Child and Adolescent Psychology, 33*, 42–53.

Panksepp, J. (1998). *Affective neuroscience: The foundations of human and animal emotions*. New York: Oxford University Press.

Pavlov, I. P. (1951–1952). *Complete works* (2nd ed.). Moscow: USSR Academy of Sciences (in Russian).

Posner, M. I., & Rothbart, M. K. (2007). Research on attention networks as a model for the integration of psychological science. *Annual Review of Psychology, 58*, 1–23.

Putnam, S. P., Gartstein, M. A., & Rothbart, M. K. (2006). Measurement of fine-grained aspects of toddler temperament: the early childhood behavior questionnaire. *Infant Behavior and Development*, 29, 386–401.

Putnam, S. P., & Stifter, C. A. (2005). Behavioral approach-inhibition in toddlers: Prediction from infancy, positive and negative affect components, and relations with behavior problems. *Child Development, 76*, 212–26.

Raghutaman, G., & Cherian, A. (2003). Temperament of children and adolescents presenting with unexplained physical symptoms. *Indian Journal of Psychiatry, 45*, 43–7.

Raz, A., & Buhle, J. (2006). Typologies of attentional networks. *Nature Reviews Neuroscience, 7*, 367–69.

Roberts, B. W., Kuncel, N. R., Shiner, R., Caspi, A., & Goldberg, L. (2007). The power of personality: The comparative validity of personality traits, socioeconomic status, and cognitive ability for predicting important life outcomes. *Perspectives on Psychological Science, 4*, 313–45.

Rothbart, M. K. (1981). Measurement of temperament in infancy. *Child Development, 52*, 569–78.

Rothbart, M. K. (1986). Longitudinal observation of infant temperament. *Developmental Psychology, 22*, 356–365.

Rothbart, M. K., Ahadi, S. A., & Evans, D. E. (2000a). Temperament and personality: Origins and outcomes. *Journal of Personality and Social Psychology, 78*, 122–35.

Rothbart, M. K., & Bates, J. E. (1998). Temperament. In W. Damon (Series Ed.) & N. Eisenberg (Vol. Ed.), *Handbook of child psychology. Vol. 3. Social, emotional and personality development* (5th ed., pp. 105–176). New York: Wiley.

Rothbart, M. K., & Bates, J. E. (2006). Temperament. In W. Damon & R. Lerner (Series Eds.), & N. Eisenberg (Vol. Ed.), *Handbook of child psychology, Vol. 3. Social, emotional, and personality development* (6th ed., pp. 99–166). New York: Wiley.

Rothbart, M. K., Chew, K. H., & Gartstein, M. A. (2001). Assessment of temperament in early development. In L. T. Singer & P. S. Zeskind (Eds.), *Biobehavioral assessment of the infant* (pp. 190–208). New York: Guilford Press.

Rothbart, M. K., & Derryberry, P. (1981). Development of individual differences in temperament. In M. E. Lamb & A. Brown (Eds.), *Advances in developmental psychology* (Vol. 1, pp. 37–86). Hillsdale, NJ: Erlbaum.

Rothbart, M. K., Derryberry, D., & Hershey, K. (2000b). Stability of temperament in childhood: Laboratory assessment to parent reports at seven years. In V. J. Molfese & D. L. Molfese (Eds.), *Temperament and personality development across the life-span* (pp. 85–120). Hillsdale, NJ: Erlbaum.

Rowe, D. C., & Plomin, R. (1977). Temperament in early childhood. *Journal of Personality Assessment, 41*, 150–56.

Ruch, W. (1992). Pavlov's types of nervous system, Eysenck's typology and the Hippocrates-Galen experiments: An empirical examination of asserted correspondence of three temperamental typologies. *Personality and Individual Differences, 13*, 1259–71.

Rueda, M. R., Fan, J., McCandliss, B. D., Halparin, J. D., Gruber, D. B., Lercari, L. P., et al. (2004). Development of attentional networks in childhood. *Neuropsychologia, 42*, 1029–40.

Ruf, H. T., Schmidt, N. L., Lemery-Chalfant, K., & Goldsmith, H. H. (2008). Components of childhood impulsivity and inattention: Child, family, and genetic correlates. *European Journal of Developmental Science, 2*, 52–76.

Schmeck, K. (2001). Temperament and disruptive behavior disorders. *Psychopathology, 34*,159–63.

Schwartz, C. E., Wright, C. I., Shin, L. M., Kagan, J., & Rauch, S. L. (2003). Inhibited and uninhibited infants "grown up": Adult amygdalar response to novelty. *Science, 300*, 1952–53.

Seifer, R., Sameroff, A., Barrett, L. C., & Krafchuk, E. (1994). Infant temperament measured by multiple observations and mother report. *Child Development, 65*, 1478–90.

Sharma, N. K., Malhotra, S., & Malhotra, A. (1983). Temperament correlates of I.Q. *Indian Journal of Clinical Psychology, 10*, 407–15.

Smith, M., & Cloninger, R. (2008). Temperament and character as schizophrenia-related endophenotypes in non-psychotic siblings. *Schizophrenia Research, 104*, 198–205.

Strelau, J. (1983). *Temperament-personality-activity*. London: Academic Press.

Strelau, J. (1996). The regulative theory of temperament: Current status. *Personality and Individual Differences, 20*, 131–42.

Tackett, J. L. (2006). Evaluating models of the personality-psychopathology relationship in children and adolescents. *Clinical Psychology Review, 26*, 584–99.

Thomas, A., & Chess, S. (1977). *Temperament and development*. New York: Brunner/Mazel.

Thomas, A., Chess, S., Birch, H., Hertzig, M., & Korn, S. (1963). *Behavioral individuality in early childhood*. New York: New York University Press.

Wachs, T. D. (2000). *Necessary but not sufficient: The respective roles of single and multiple influences on individual development*. Washington, D.C.: American Psychological Association.

Wood, A. C., Saudino, K. J., Rogers, H., Asherson, P., & Kuntsi, J. (2007). Genetic influence on mechanically assessed activity level in children. *Journal of Child Psychology and Psychiatry, 48*, 695–702.

Xu, J., Yin, X., Ge, H., Han, Y., Pang, Z., Tang, Y., et al. (2015). Attentional performance is correlated with the local regional efficiency of intrinsic brain networks. *Frontiers in Behavioral Neuroscience, 9*, 200.

Zaninotto, L., Solmi, M., Toffanin, T., Veronese, N., Cloninger, C. R., & Correll, C. U. (2016). A meta-analysis of temperament and character dimensions in patients with mood disorders: Comparison to healthy controls and unaffected siblings. *Journal of Affective Disorders, 194*, 84–97.

Zetner, M., & Bates, J. (2008). Child temperament: An integrative review of concepts, research programs and measures. *European Journal of Development Science, 2*, 7–37.

Chapter 15
Childhood Antecedents of Personality Disorders

Pratap Sharan and Sathya Prakash

Abstract Early life influences have for long been suspected to play a crucial role in shaping adult life. A significant body of literature now supports the effect of early life influences on adult medical conditions such as obesity and heart disease. In psychiatry too, evidence now suggests a similar phenomenon. This is especially true for personality disorders which are now seen as a continuity of the patterns of tendency to feel and behave observed in childhood. A number of factors ranging from psychological to socio-economic and biological have been postulated as causal factors, mediating factors or simply associated factors. The present chapter attempts to discuss some of the basic theoretical foundations, the commonly cited factors involved, and the utility and implications for clinical practice.

Keywords Childhood antecedents · Personality disorders · Conduct disorder · Attention deficit hyperactivity disorder · Life span approach

Abbreviations

ADHD	Attention deficit hyperactivity disorder
APA	American Psychiatric Association
COMT	Catechol-O-methyl transferase
DOHaD	Developmental origins of health and disease
MAO A	Monoamine oxidase
WHO	World Health Organization

P. Sharan (✉) · S. Prakash
Department of Psychiatry, All India Institute of Medical Sciences, New Delhi 110029, India
e-mail: pratapsharan@gmail.com

S. Prakash
e-mail: dr.sathyaprakashtbts@gmail.com

S. Malhotra and P. Santosh (eds.), *Child and Adolescent Psychiatry*,
DOI 10.1007/978-81-322-3619-1_15

15.1 Introduction

Early life influences and its effects have always been an area of great interest in psychiatry. The classical psychoanalysts referred to the formative years of life as having great significance in the development of personality and causation of a range of psychiatric disorders. From a more biological standpoint too, it appeals to reason that minor 'defects' produced in early life or prenatally, can produce potentially devastating consequences in later life. Over the years though, the emphasis seems to have shifted away from this line of thinking for a variety of reasons. One potential reason could be the way the diagnostic criteria for personality disorders are structured in the current classificatory systems (World Health Organization 1992). The current classificatory systems seem to give an impression of personality being relevant or assessable only after middle to late adolescence (Salekin 2016). This could have potentially hindered research in this area. However, in the recent years there is an acknowledgement of a lifespan approach to personality pathology, best exemplified by many of the structural changes proposed in the appendix of DSM-5 for further study (American Psychiatric Association 2013).

Traditionally, personality disorders were discussed as categorical entities; and were broadly categorized into three 'clusters': Cluster A or the 'eccentric' cluster, cluster 'B' or the 'dramatic' cluster and cluster 'C' or the 'fearful' cluster. Categorical arrangements do seem to have some validity. While cluster analytic studies failed to replicate this three cluster model; many environmental factors influencing personality clusters fit into a three factor solution roughly coinciding with the clusters A, B, and C described above (Mervielde et al. 2005).

However, issues related to comorbidity; overlap between personality disorders and normal personality as well as between personality disorders that led to a plethora of not otherwise specified diagnosis; and the similarities between structure of personality and personality disorders led to the consideration of dimensional conceptualization of personality disorders. In the debate on whether psychiatric disorders are categorical or dimensional, the broader consensus is that both apply to differing extent and also depending upon the disorder in question. However, personality disorders as a group is more often considered as dimensional rather than categorical (Zimmerman and Spitzer 2009). In view of the limitations in the diagnostic criteria in current classificatory systems, several researchers have attempted to study childhood presentations using various modifications of the existing criteria. However, the validity of such modified criteria has often been questioned. Among the other ways of assessment, the one that has the highest empirical support is the five-factor model (Mervielde et al. 2005). The five factors are extraversion, conscientiousness, agreeableness, neuroticism, and openness. Minor variations of this model have been widely used. The terms personality, temperament, and character have been used somewhat interchangeably by many but are conceptually somewhat different (Cloninger and Svrakic 2009). Allport (1963) defined personality as the 'dynamic organization of one's psychophysical symptoms determining his/her adjustment to the environment.' Temperament refers to 'body's innate biases in conditioned behavioral response to stimuli' whereas character refers to 'what one voluntarily makes of oneself.' Cloninger has proposed four types of temperament—novelty seeking, reward dependence, persistence and harm avoidance and three dimensions of character—self directed, cooperative and self-transcendent (Cloninger and Svrakic 2009).

15.2 Conceptual Framework for the Role of Antecedents

15.2.1 The Developmental Origins of Health and Disease (DOHaD) Hypothesis

Developmental Origins of Health and Disease (DOHaD) hypothesis is an interesting hypothesis and has gained much ground in recent years (Kubota et al. 2015). In simple terms, it refers to the observation that less than optimal environmental condition during early life may permanently change the structure and function of various body parts, such that, the individual gets predisposed to various chronic conditions in later life. Such an alteration is believed to occur via various mechanisms, for instance, alteration of feedback mechanisms and altered maladaptive stress responses. From a homeostatic standpoint, such a reaction serves to salvage the organism in its early life, which may have evolutionary significance. However, such short term gains occur at the cost of long term losses. The multi-factorial causation of various medical conditions such as cardiovascular disorders and diabetes are believed to be in keeping with such a hypothesis (Moore 2016). Among psychiatric disorders, schizophrenia has been the best studied disorder within the DOHaD framework. Meta-analytic studies (Cannon et al. 2002) have verified that indicators of suboptimal early life environment such as low birth weight and smaller head circumference predict risk of schizophrenia. A number of factors have been proposed as possible explanations, including altered complement activity and excessive oxidative and nitrosative stress (Mhillaj et al. 2015). Personality disorders being chronic conditions of adult life automatically attract research attention in this regard. Indeed, there is now a considerable body of evidence supporting such a view, though, as has been previously mentioned, some inconsistencies exist. Some of these inconsistencies could be attributed to the potentially nonlinear relationships between markers of early life adversity and adult conditions. The classic example of such a phenomenon is birth weight. While low birth weight predisposes to various adult disorders, weight beyond 4 kg also increases risk for such disorders.

15.3 Childhood Antecedents of Personality Disorders

A number of antecedents have been described in relation to personality disorders; some of them specific to certain clusters or disorders, while others posing a general risk to personality disorders as a group while still others increasing risk for several psychiatric disorders. Some of the better researched antecedents are described below.

15.3.1 Parity and Maternal Age

Children born to mothers in their teenage or third or more in the birth order have been reported to demonstrate an increased evidence of personality disorders (Fazel et al. 2012). Other studies have demonstrated that this increased risk may be especially for the cluster B (dramatic cluster) of personality disorders (Kuja-Halkola et al. 2012; Mitrou et al. 2010). But as in case of previously discussed antecedents, this finding too is not without inconsistency. Some longitudinal studies have found no effect of teenage births on future risk of personality disorders (Kantojärvi et al. 2008). Similarly, parity beyond the sixth pregnancy did not increase risk of personality disorders but did so for other psychiatric disorders (Kemppainen et al. 2000). This again highlights the nonlinear nature of risk factor-outcome relationship.

15.3.2 Growth in Early Life

Pre- and post-natal growth (growth in early life) is another important antecedent that is often linked to personality disorders (Samuel and Widiger 2008). Studies have looked into several different temperamental traits in relation to this characteristic. Negative affectivity and harm avoidance have been found in several studies to be linked to the measures of poor early growth such as 'thinness' (Pesonen et al. 2006) and lower birth weight, length, and head circumference (Pesonen et al. 2009). However, other studies have demonstrated that very low birth weight babies went on to develop higher levels of conscientiousness, agreeableness (Pesonen et al. 2008) and behavioral inhibition (Pyhälä et al. 2009) and lower levels of openness to experience. There is some evidence to suggest that sex may have a modifying role to play but evidence on the exact nature of this is conflicting and inconclusive (Moilanen et al. 2010; Lahti et al. 2008).

15.3.3 Temperament

Temperament refers to the organism's innate bias in responding to the external stimuli. They include its spontaneous and characteristic ways of reacting to stimuli such as danger, novelty, challenges and reward (Basaglu et al. 2011). Temperamental traits are generally believed to have a strong genetic component and heritability and also to be precursors of adult personality. A number of studies including several longitudinal studies have shown a 'continuity of pattern' in behavior from early childhood to adulthood. For instance, measures such as irritability, attention span, lability and negativism measured from as early as 6 months of age to five years predicted borderline personality symptoms at age twelve and beyond (Belsky et al. 2012). Similarly, poor behavioral control at 3 years of age predicted antisocial personality at 21 years of age (Caspi et al. 1996). Along similar lines, low inhibition and fearfulness at 3 years of age also predicted psychopathic behavior in adulthood in another study. Persistent overestimation of self confidence after age 10 is a predictor of narcissistic personality. In the same vein, persistence of illogical thinking and loose associations beyond age 7, poor attention and executive functioning, and, disorganized verbal responses predict schizotypal disorder-related communication impairments in adulthood. Reduced involvement in extracurricular activities and less popularity in school reflects temperamental inclination towards adult avoidant personality. On the contrary, several studies have shown that many temperamental features are not stable and may change over an individual's life span. It has been suggested that certain 'core' features do not change whereas 'secondary' features may change over a period of time. However, as can be seen, most of the work till date is focused on the dramatic cluster, that too mainly borderline and antisocial personality disorders and there is a dearth of research related to other personality disorders.

15.3.4 Parenting Style and Neighborhood

Maladaptive parenting style is another important antecedent of personality disorders. Again, most studies have focused on borderline and antisocial personality disorders. Measures of poor parenting style such as hitting, shouting, hostility, resentment, physical, and emotional abuse have all been associated with increased subsequent development of personality disorder symptoms, especially borderline (Waylen et al. 2008; Johnson et al. 2006). Other features such as low closeness to parents, maternal over-control and disorganized attachment patterns have also been noted to have similar associations. A wide oscillation from hostile over-control to passive aloofness is often seen in mothers with borderline personality pathology and this raises the risk of personality disorders for their children (Stepp et al. 2011).

Neighborhood also seems to play an important role in shaping personality and this is best exemplified by studies related to antisocial personality disorder. Presence of delinquent peers in the neighborhood along with an environment of socio-economic adversity, crime and violence has been reported to promote the continuation of conduct and antisocial personality symptoms (Piehler and Dishion 2008). Similar observations have been made in case of borderline personality, especially with regard to self-injurious behaviors (Prinstein et al. 2000).

15.3.5 Parental Psychopathology

History of substance use in parents and presence of parental psychopathology are also known antecedents for personality disorders, usually of the borderline type. As shall be described in a subsequent section, presence of personality disorders in parents, especially of the dramatic cluster, tend to increase risk of developing the same in their children (Stepp et al. 2011). Presence of schizophrenia in parents increases risk for development of the eccentric cluster of personality disorders in their children. As is the case for many of the other previously discussed antecedents, the possibility of confounding exists here too. Presence of substance use and psychopathology in parent is often linked to separation, divorce, lower socioeconomic status, and poor parenting style; all known antecedents of personality disorders.

15.3.6 Psychiatric Disorder in Childhood

Early development of many psychiatric disorders increases the risk for further development of personality disorders. In some cases, this represents a continuity of the same symptoms with age appropriate changes into adulthood. In others, the development of personality problems may be viewed as reactive. A third possibility is that of shared risk between the said psychiatric disorders and personality disorders. Finally, the possibility of a flawed diagnostic system artificially dividing a single disorder into multiple parts, giving an impression of one disorder being the antecedent of the other is also possible. Some of the better described associations are discussed below.

15.3.6.1 Conduct Disorder

Conduct disorder or symptoms represent one of the most well studied antecedents of personality disorders, specifically for the antisocial type (Hill 2003). A number of parameters are available to identify those who are likely to have greater problems within this group. Some of these factors include earlier development of antisocial behavior, greater number of conduct symptoms, greater severity of conduct symptoms and longer persistence of such symptoms. It was conventionally believed that children with conduct symptoms who remitted actually 'recovered,' i.e., did not retain the risk of developing antisocial personality; however, this may not be entirely true. Some evidence suggests that although the risk of developing a syndromal antisocial personality disorder is definitely reduced, such children do develop a number of problems in adulthood. Such problems typically included poor educational and occupational performance, social isolation, depression and anxiety-related problems (Hill 2003). As is the case with other antecedents, it is only logical to assume numerous confounders in relation to presence of conduct disorder, e.g., lower socio-economic status, substance use, parental separation, separation and so on. However, there is some evidence to suggest that the risk attributable to conduct disorder is over and above, and independent of such factors (Hill 2003).

15.3.6.2 Attention Deficit Hyperactivity Disorder (ADHD)

The association between ADHD and future personality disorders is somewhat controversial. ADHD is often closely associated with conduct or oppositional defiant disorder leading to the confusion. However, careful longitudinal studies have shown that ADHD in itself does not elevate risk for criminality—in other words, the rates of criminality are similar in those with conduct disorder alone versus those with both conduct disorder and ADHD (Mordre et al. 2011).

15.3.6.3 Other Disorders

Depressive disorders in childhood have been found to increase the risk of personality disorders across all three clusters (Cohen et al. 2005). Similarly, childhood anxiety disorders impart an increased risk of adult paranoid and anankastic personality disorders (Kasen et al. 2001). Childhood anxiety disorders also increased risk of suicidal attempts across various personality disorders across clusters (Rudd et al. 2004).

15.3.7 Socio-economic Adversity

A number of studies have looked into the effects of socio-economic status in early childhood on development of personality disorders in adulthood. The findings are somewhat inconclusive. A longitudinal study found increased risk for borderline and antisocial personality disorders in children exposed to economic adversities (Crawford et al. 2009; Lahey et al. 2005). Widom et al. (2009) on the other hand, did not find any such association. Such discrepancies may be attributed to several factors such as small effect of the adversity on future personality making differences of power between studies important. Socio-economic status may act as a confounding factor influencing many other variables; for instance weight and other anthropometric disadvantages. Similarly, family conflict, abuse, separation may all be influenced by socio-economic status. Further, socio-economic status is known to modify effects of separation from parents (Tieman et al. 2005). Other methodological differences include varying definitions of socio-economic strata and varying impact of a particular status in different countries, regions or cultures.

15.3.8 Parental Separation

A major limitation of studies on parental separation is that they are of a retrospective nature. Available evidence suggests that a number of personality disorders of varying severity occur in relation to parental separation, especially of the dramatic cluster (Lahti et al. 2008). Parental separation could be of various types depending upon the extent and severity of separation. Being separated from both parents versus living with a single parent can have different impacts on the child. Similarly, some studies suggest that the duration of separation and the age at separation can potentially impact development of personality pathology.

Presence of a single parent or separation by the age of 14 years was found to considerably increase the risk of Cluster B (dramatic) personality disorders (Mäkikyrö et al. 1998; Kantojärvi et al. 2008). The risk was particularly increased for borderline and antisocial personality disorders. Moreover, there is some evidence to suggest that separation before the age of 5 years predisposes to borderline personality disorder (Crawford et al. 2009) whereas even earlier separation (before 3 years of age) may lead to 'psychopathic' personality (Gao et al. 2010b) in later life. Long periods of separation in the first 2 years of life have been found in some studies to heighten risk of schizotypal disorder (Anglin et al. 2008).

15.3.9 Biological Variables

A number of biological factors have been postulated as indicative of specific personality disorders. Again, they are best studied for borderline and antisocial personality disorders. Many of the variables described below are either actually or potentially involved in mediating the role of various antecedents discussed so far. As shall be seen, these biological variables play crucial roles in various aspects of the functioning of the developing brain, including how various environmental stimuli are perceived and handled, and, what impact such stimuli have on modeling future cognitions and behaviors, and eventually the personality itself.

15.3.9.1 Monoamine Oxidase A (MAO-A)

The plausibility of the role for enzymes degrading the major brain neurotransmitters such as serotonin, dopamine, nor-adrenaline and acetylcholine in various psychiatric conditions was always evident to researchers. One such enzyme, the MAO-A, has been studied in relation to antisocial personality disorders (Reti et al. 2011). Evidence suggests that among Caucasians, the high activity allele of MAO-A was protective against antisocial personality disorder amongst those without a history of physical abuse (Reti et al. 2011).

15.3.9.2 Serotonin Transporter

The serotonin transporter gene is among the most widely studied genes in all of psychiatry. Its regulation of synaptic serotonin levels implies obvious relevance to numerous psychiatric disorders. There is preliminary evidence to suggest that the serotonin transporter gene mediates the effect of various previously mentioned antecedents on the risk of development of antisocial personality disorder (Douglas et al. 2011). African-American women, with homozygous low activity alleles of the serotonin transporter gene were found to have higher risk of developing antisocial personality disorder (Douglas et al. 2011).

15.3.9.3 Catechol-O-Methyl Transferase (COMT)

As is well known, the COMT enzyme is a key enzyme in the metabolism of various monoamine neurotransmitters. Thus, alteration in its genetic structure has been studied in various psychiatric disorders. The replacement of valine for methionine results in a version of the enzyme that is more active. This plausibly could cause lowered dopamine levels in the brain. A study found that antisocial personality traits were much higher in those carrying the valine substituted COMT gene than in controls (Thapar et al. 2005). Also, preliminary evidence for a gene-environment interaction of the COMT gene and low birth weight was found in males (Thapar et al. 2005). It is being speculated that the counterpart of the same in females is borderline personality disorder (Beauchaine et al. 2009).

15.3.9.4 Amygdalar Structure and Fear Conditioning

The amygdale is a crucial structure in the brain related to various aspects of fear recognition and response. Since, consequence of a given action is an important variable that determines future repetition (or absence of) of the act, fear has been considered to be an important factor in shaping behavior and personality. In well adjusted individuals, it is believed that antisocial acts during childhood result in consequences that induce fear, which in turn, results in learning that such behaviors are not desirable and are not to be performed. In individuals with various constitutional and environmental factors favoring eventual development of antisocial personality, fear conditioning is poor and leads to a failure in modifying the antisocial behaviors. In a landmark study (Gao et al. 2010a), investigators measured fear conditioning at 3 years of age. Twenty years later, the relationship of fear conditioning with adult criminal behavior was assessed. Poor to no fear conditioning was found in them, in keeping with the aforementioned hypothesis. Low levels of amygdalar activation and an inability to recognize cues signaling threat as well as fearful facial expressions were also seen, giving clues to potential mechanisms of antisocial behavior. However, it must be remembered that these findings are at the group level and cannot be extrapolated to individuals. Criminal behavior of an individual is a combined effect of a multitude of factors. Indeed, in certain studies, excessive activation of the amygdale have been linked to antisocial personality questioning the previously mentioned hypothesis, or alternatively, suggesting that different mechanisms may be at work in different groups of individuals (Meyer-Lindenberg et al. 2006). One such explanation is that the increased activation represents heightened anxiety related to pathological aggression.

15.3.9.5 Epigenetics

It is known that many psychiatric disorders including personality disorders have a strong 'genetic' basis. Such a basis is typically polygenic, meaning that a number of genes, each with a small effect act together to account for the variation. Indeed, such an assumption has been made for many other psychiatric disorders as well. This has often been interpreted as fixed genes present at birth that pose a certain vulnerability, which when combined with other influences such as environmental, result in the disorder in question. However, more recent research suggests that this is partly true and partly false. Although born with a certain chromosomal quota, the non DNA elements can be altered to influence the downstream effects of genes—a phenomenon that epigenetics deals with. The best known of such mechanisms are the acetylation or methylation of histones. It was earlier believed that such epigenetic changes are possible only in early infancy. However, now it is known to occur at much older ages too (Champagne 2008). This potentially represents one of the mechanisms by which the environment influences development of a psychiatric disorder, including personality disorders. It has also become increasingly clear over the years that such epigenetic influences may be much more than initially imagined. In fact the current consensus is that most behavior traits are shaped epigenetically by way of gene-environment interactions. Thus, an individual begins with certain broad dispositions which progressively branch out to generate more specific and subtle variations defining individual personality traits (Templeton 2006). Thus, effects of a 'bad environment' may be undone by the effects of a 'good environment.' Such epigenetic changes may be partially transmitted to further generations, or altered by counteracting environmental influences; all without any change in the DNA sequence. Such changes are not detectable by traditional quantitative genetics, explaining its elusive nature (Templeton 2006). This is an area of active research interest with the potential to identify newer ways of understanding human behavior.

15.3.9.6 Others

Several other genes have been postulated in the etiology of personality disorders for which clear and direct evidence are lacking. These genes have been typically speculated to increase risk for some of the key traits common to several personality disorders. For instance, dopamine receptor D4 (DRD4), dopamine transporter (DAT1) and dopamine receptor D2 (DRD2) have been considered as influencing impulsivity and in turn increasing risk of borderline and antisocial personality disorders, besides other psychiatric disorders such as ADHD (Beauchaine et al. 2009).

15.4 Future Directions

Further studies need to assess interactions between genetic and environmental factors contributing to development of personality disorders. The exact neurobiological mechanisms through which these factors work also need to be explored. Prospective studies collecting data on genome and epigenome, HPA axis, and different early life stressors will help in identifying the possible etiological roles played by each of these factors and the interactions among them. Moderating and mediating roles of different etiological factors should also be simultaneously assessed. Functional brain imaging methods could help in identifying the abnormalities in brain functioning associated with these disorders characterized by potentially reduced brain growth in prenatal life. Above all, use of this knowledge to design early intervention programs is also the need of the hour. Some work has already been done in this area, particularly for borderline personality disorder. Its close association with mood disorders has encouraged an integrated early intervention program based on clinical staging (Chanen et al. 2016).

15.5 Conclusions

Traditionally, there has been some reluctance in acknowledging that personality disorders have antecedents in childhood and need to be described and understood since the early years of life. However, over the past few years, this view has garnered wider acceptance and some of the traditional views have become untenable. The DSM-5 too, has now considered personality from a life cycle perspective. In keeping with the DOHaD hypothesis, a range of adult conditions are now being viewed from a developmental perspective and search is on to find out their antecedents, or even better, their etiological factors. Such a search has also instilled some hope that such disorders may not necessarily have a chronic and relentless course. Future studies must actively look into the various antecedents with the eventual goal of building capabilities to intervene early enough to delay, retard, or completely prevent these disorders.

References

Allport, G. (1963). *Pattern and growth in personality*. Pennsylvania: Harcourt College Publishers.

American Psychiatric Association. (2013). *The diagnostic and statistical manual* (5th ed.). Washington DC: American Psychiatric Association.

Anglin, D. M., Cohen, P. R., & Chen, H. (2008). Duration of early maternal separation and prediction of schizotypal symptoms from early adolescence to midlife. *Schizophrenia Research, 103*, 143–150.

Basaglu, C., Oner, O., Ates, A., Algul, A., Bez, Y., Cetin, M., et al. (2011). Synaptosomal associated protein 25 gene polymorphisms and antisocial personality disorder: association with temperament and psychopathy. *Canadian Journal of Psychiatry, 56*, 341–347.

Beauchaine, T. P., Klein, D. N., Crowell, S. E., Derbidge, C., & Gatzke-Kopp, L. (2009). Multifinality in the development of personality disorders: a Biology x Sex x Environment interaction model of antisocial and borderline traits. *Development and Psychopathology, 21*, 735–770.

Belsky, D. W., Caspi, A., Arseneault, L., Bleidorn, W., Fonagy, P., Goodman, M., et al. (2012). Etiological features of borderline personality related characteristics in a birth cohort of 12-year-old children. *Development and Psychopathology, 24*, 251–265.

Cannon, M., Jones, P. B., & Murray, R. M. (2002). Obstetric complications and schizophrenia: historical and meta-analytic review. *American Journal of Psychiatry, 159*, 1080–1092.

Caspi, A., Moffitt, T. E., Newman, D. L., & Silva, P. A. (1996). Behavioral observations at age 3 years predict adult psychiatric disorders. Longitudinal evidence from a birth cohort. *Archives of General Psychiatry, 53*, 1033–1039.

Champagne, F. A. (2008). Epigenetic mechanisms and the transgenerational effects of maternal care. *Frontiers in Neuroendocrinology, 29*, 386–397.

Chanen, A. M., Berk, M., & Thompson, K. (2016). Integrating early intervention for borderline personality disorder and mood disorders. *Harvard Review of Psychiatry,* Epub ahead of print.

Cloninger, C. R., & Svrakic, D. M. (2009). Personality disorders. In B. J. Sadock, V. A. Sadock, & P. Ruiz (Eds.), *Kaplan and Sadock's comprehensive textbook of psychiatry* (9th ed., pp. 2197–2240). Philadelphia: Lippincott Williams and Wikins.

Cohen, P., Chen, H., Kasen, S., Johnson, J. G., Crawford, T., & Gordon, K. (2005). Adolescent cluster A personality disorder symptoms, role assumption in the transition to adulthood, and resolution or persistence of symptoms. *Development and Psychopathology, 17*, 549–568.

Crawford, T. N., Cohen, P. R., Chen, H., Anglin, D. M., & Ehrensaft, M. (2009). Early maternal separation and the trajectory of borderline personality disorder symptoms. *Developmental Psychopathology, 21*, 1013–1030.

Douglas, K., Chan, G., Gelernter, J., Arias, A. J., Anton, R. F., Poling, J., et al. (2011). 5-HTTLPR as a potential moderator of the effects of adverse childhood experiences on risk of antisocial personality disorder. *Psychiatric Genetics, 21*, 240–248.

Fazel, S., Bakiyeva, L., Cnattingius, S., Grann, M., Hultman, C. M., Lichtenstein, P., et al. (2012). Perinatal risk factors in offenders with severe personality disorder: A population-based investigation. *Journal of Personality Disorders, 26*, 737–750.

Gao, Y., Raine, A., Chan, F., Venables, P. H., & Mednick, S. A. (2010a). Early maternal and paternal bonding, childhood physical abuse and adult psychopathic personality. *Psychological Medicine, 40*, 1007–1016.

Gao, Y., Raine, A., Venables, P. H., Dawson, M. E., & Mednick, S. A. (2010b). Association of poor childhood fear conditioning and adult crime. *The American Journal of Psychiatry, 167*, 56–60.

Hill, J. (2003). Early identification of individuals at risk for antisocial personality disorder. *The British Journal of Psychiatry, Supplement, 44*, S11–S14.

Johnson, J. G., Cohen, P., Chen, H., Kasen, S., & Brook, J. S. (2006). Parenting behaviors associated with risk for offspring personality disorder during adulthood. *Archives of General Psychiatry, 63*, 579–587.

Kantojärvi, L., Joukamaa, M., Miettunen, J., Läksy, K., Herva, A., Karvonen, J. T., et al. (2008). Childhood family structure and personality disorders in adulthood. *European Psychiatry, 23*, 205–211.

Kasen, S., Cohen, P., Skodol, A. E., Johnson, J. G., Smailes, E., & Brook, J. S. (2001). Childhood depression and adult personality disorder: alternative pathways of continuity. *Archives of General Psychiatry, 58*(3), 231–236.

Kemppainen, L., Mäkikyrö, T., Jokelainen, J., Nieminen, P., Järvelin, M. R., & Isohanni, M. (2000). Is grand multiparity associated with offsprings' hospital-treated mental disorders? A 28-year follow-up of the North Finland 1966 birth cohort. *Social Psychiatry and Psychiatric Epidemiology, 35*, 104–108.

Kubota, T., Miyake, K., Hariya, N., & Mochizuki, K. (2015). Understanding the epigenetics of neurodevelopmental disorders and DOHaD. *Journal of Developmental Origins of Health and Disease, 6*, 96–104.

Kuja-Halkola, R., Pawitan, Y., D'Onofrio, B. M., Långström, N., & Lichtenstein, P. (2012). Advancing paternal age and offspring violent offending: A sibling-comparison study. *Developmental Psychopathology, 24*, 739–753.

Lahey, B. B., Loeber, R., Burke, J. D., & Applegate, B. (2005). Predicting future antisocial personality disorder in males from a clinical assessment in childhood. *Journal of Consulting and Clinical Psychology, 73*, 389–399.

Lahti, J., Räikkönen, K., Heinonen, K., Pesonen, A. K., Kajantie, E., Forsén, T., et al. (2008). Body size at birth and socio-economic status in childhood: implications for Cloninger's psychobiological model of temperament at age 60. *Psychiatry Research, 160*, 167–174.

Mäkikyrö, T., Isohanni, M., Moring, J., Hakko, H., Hovatta, I., & Lönnqvist, J. (1998). Accuracy of register-based schizophrenia diagnoses in a genetic study. *European Psychiatry, 13*, 57–62.

Mervielde, I., De Clercq, B., De Fruyt, F., & Van Leeuwe, K. (2005). Temperament, personality, and developmental psychopathology as childhood antecedents of personality disorders. *Journal of Personality Disorders, 19*, 171–201.

Meyer-Lindenberg, A., Buckholtz, J. W., Kolachana, B., Hariri, A. R., Pezawas, L., Blasi, G., et al. (2006). Neural mechanisms of genetic risk for impulsivity and violence in humans. *Proceedings of the National Academy of Sciences of the United States of America, 103*, 6269–6274.

Mhillaj, E., Morgese, M. G., & Trabace, L. (2015). Early life and oxidative stress in psychiatric disorders: What can we learn from animal models? *Current Pharmaceutical Design, 21*, 1396–1403.

Mitrou, F., Gaudie, J., Lawrence, D., Silburn, S. R., Stanley, F. J., & Zubrick, S. R. (2010). Antecedents of hospital admission for deliberate self-harm from a 14-year follow-up study using data-linkage. *BMC Psychiatry, 10*, 82.

Moilanen, K., Jokelainen, J., Jones, P. B., Hartikainen, A. L., Järvelin, M. R., & Isohanni, M. (2010). Deviant intrauterine growth and risk of schizophrenia: A 34-year follow-up of the Northern Finland 1966 Birth Cohort. *Schizophrenia Research, 124*, 223–230.

Moore, S. E. (2016). Early life nutritional programming of health and disease in Gambia. *Journal of Developmental Origins of Health and Disease, 7*, 123–131.

Mordre, M., Groholt, B., Kjelsberg, E., Sandstad, B., & Myhre, A. M. (2011). The impact of ADHD and conduct disorder in childhood on adult delinquency: A 30 years follow-up study using official crime records. *BMC Psychiatry, 11*, 57.

Pesonen, A. K., Räikkönen, K., Heinonen, K., Kajantie, E., Forsén, T., & Eriksson, J. G. (2008). Reproductive traits following a parent-child separation trauma during childhood: a natural experiment during World War II. *American Journal of Human Biology, 20*, 345–351.

Pesonen, A. K., Räikkönen, K., Kajantie, E., Heinonen, K., Strandberg, T. E., & Järvenpää, A. L. (2006). Fetal programming of temperamental negative affectivity among children born healthy at term. *Developmental Psychobiology, 48*, 633–643.

Pesonen, A. K., Räikkönen, K., Lano, A., Peltoniemi, O., Hallman, M., & Kari, M. A. (2009). Antenatal betamethasone and fetal growth in prematurely born children: Implications for temperament traits at the age of 2 years. *Pediatrics, 123*, e31–e37.

Piehler, T. F., & Dishion, T. J. (2008). Interpersonal dynamics within adolescent friendships: Dyadic mutuality, deviant talk, and patterns of antisocial behavior. *Child Development, 78*, 1611–1624.

Prinstein, M. J., Boergers, J., Spirito, A., Little, T. D., & Grapentine, W. L. (2000). Peer functioning, family dysfunction, and psychological symptoms in a risk factor model for adolescent inpatients' suicidal ideation severity. *Journal of Clinical Child Psychology, 29*, 392–405.

Pyhälä, R., Räikkönen, K., Pesonen, A. K., Heinonen, K., Hovi, P., Eriksson, J. G., et al. (2009). Behavioral inhibition and behavioral approach in young adults with very low birth weight? The Helsinki study of very low birth weight adults. *Personality and Individual Differences, 46*, 106–110.

Reti, I. M., Xu, J. Z., Yanofski, J., McKibben, J., Uhart, M., Cheng, Y. J., et al. (2011). Monoamine oxidase A regulates antisocial personality in whites with no history of physical abuse. *Comprehensive Psychiatry, 52*, 188–194.

Rudd, M. D., Joiner, T. E., & Rumzek, H. (2004). Childhood diagnoses and later risk for multiple suicide attempts. *Suicide and Life-Threatening Behavior, 34*, 113–125.

Salekin, R. T. (2016). Psychopathology in childhood: Toward better informing the DSM-5 and ICD-11 conduct disorder specifiers. *Personality Disorders, 7*, 180–191.

Samuel, D. B., & Widiger, T. A. (2008). A meta-analytic review of the relationships between the five factor model and DSM-IV-TR personality disorders: a facet level analysis. *Clinical Psychology Review, 28*, 1326–1342.

Stepp, S. D., Hallquist, M. N., Morse, J. Q., & Pilkonis, P. A. (2011). Multimethod investigation of interpersonal functioning in borderline personality disorder. *Personality Disorders, 2*, 175–192.

Templeton, A. (2006). *Population genetics and microevolutionary theory*. New Jersey: Wiley.

Thapar, A., Langley, K., Fowler, T., Rice, F., Turic, D., Whittinger, N., et al. (2005). Catechol O-methyltransferase gene variant and birth weight predict early-onset antisocial behavior in children with attention-deficit/hyperactivity disorder. *Archives of General Psychiatry, 62*, 1275–1278.

Tieman, W., van der Ende, J., & Verhulst, F. C. (2005). Psychiatric disorders in young adult intercountry adoptees: an epidemiological study. *American Journal of Psychiatry, 162*, 592–598.

Waylen, A., Stallard, N., & Stewart-Brown, S. (2008). Parenting and health in mid-childhood: A longitudinal study. *European Journal of Public Health, 18*, 300–305.

Widom, C. S., Czaja, S. J., & Paris, J. (2009). A prospective investigation of borderline personality disorder in abused and neglected children followed up into adulthood. *Journal of Personality Disorders, 23*, 433–446.

World Health Organization. (1992). *International classification of diseases* (10th ed.). Geneva: World Health Organization.

Zimmerman, M., & Spitzer, R. L. (2009). Psychiatric classification. In B. J. Sadock, V. A. Sadock, & P. Ruiz (Eds.), *Kaplan and Sadock's comprehensive textbook of psychiatry* (9th ed., pp. 1108–1139). Philadelphia: Lippincott Williams and Wikins.

Part V
Pharmacological and Biological Treatments

Chapter 16
Psychopharmacology for Children and Adolescents: A Paradigm Shift

Gordon Harper, Peter Parry, Jared Ng and Shekhar Seshadri

Abstract Background: The introduction of psychoactive medications for children and adolescents has changed practice worldwide. Debate continues about the indications for such practice, in particular about the possibility of unnecessary or contraindicated prescription. Such a debate usually assumes that changes in practice follow advances in the *knowledge base*—new scientific knowledge, coupled with new medications; but practice responds to changes in other areas as well. These other areas include public attitudes, the conditions of practice, and the regulatory environment. All of these are affected by the relationship between clinicians and the psychopharmaceutical industry (aka Pharma). Methodology: This paper reviews changes in factors, along with changes in the evolving knowledge base, which are transforming medication practice with children and adolescents. These

Based on a presentation at the 7th Congress of the Asian Society of Child and Adolescent Psychiatry and Allied Professions (ASCAPAP), 28 September 2013, New Delhi

G. Harper (✉)
Harvard Medical School, 128 Crafts Road, Chestnut Hill, MA 02467, USA
e-mail: Gordon_harper@hms.harvard.edu

P. Parry
Department of Psychiatry, University of Queensland, Brisbane, Australia
e-mail: p.parry1@uq.edu.au

P. Parry
Department of Psychiatry, Flinders University, Adelaide, Australia

P. Parry
Lady Cilento Children's Hospital, South Brisbane, QLD 4101, Australia

J. Ng
Institute of Mental Health, 10 Buangkok View, Singapore 539747, Singapore
e-mail: jared_ng@imh.com.sg

S. Seshadri
National Institute of Mental Health & Neurosciences (NIMHANS), Bangalore 560029, India
e-mail: shekhar@nimhans.ac.in

S. Malhotra and P. Santosh (eds.), *Child and Adolescent Psychiatry*,
DOI 10.1007/978-81-322-3619-1_16

changes, beginning in the United States, are affecting practice worldwide. Results: Changes in the knowledge base, public attitudes, the conditions of practice, and the regulatory environment amount to a *paradigm shift*. Conclusion: The implications of the emerging paradigm for practice and policy are reviewed.

Keywords Children and adolescents · Medication · Medical ethics · Paradigm shift · Psychopharmacology

16.1 Introduction

Child psychiatrists are committed to improve the lives of troubled children and their families. In the last quarter century, pharmacotherapy has become a part of their practice, a major addition to the array of services previously offered. Such evolving patterns, as in other areas of medicine, are usually thought to derive from an evolving knowledge base—we know more, we do more—while affected as well by pharmaceutical promotion (Drake et al. 2008; Spielmans and Parry 2010).

The evolving knowledge base can be called the evidence environment. Also relevant are the public attitude environment, the practice environment, and the regulatory environment, each influenced to some extent by Pharma. Within the US, these are changing at such a rate and with such deep effects, as to constitute a *Paradigm Shift*. These changes have not occurred to the same degree in European and Australian and New Zealand psychiatry—an instructive difference for child psychiatry in Asia. This chapter applies the concept of the paradigm to the use of psychoactive medications in children and adolescents, asking two questions: Are patterns shifting? Is a shift needed?

16.2 First, a Case

R R, a 4-year-old girl, had been diagnosed at age 2.5 with ADHD and by age 3 with comorbid "pediatric bipolar disorder." She had been treated with clonidine, quetiapine, and valproate. She died of clonidine toxicity. (This case summary is based on public data, not clinical records; media reports are cited in the references under Rebecca Riley.) Her parents were tried and convicted—the father of 1st degree homicide, the mother of second-degree homicide. The public learned, from the media and from the trial, that the prescribing child psychiatrist, at a teaching hospital, was well respected and proud of keeping up with the literature.

Postmortem investigation also disclosed previously unrecognized domestic violence, parental deceit about the child's behavior, and inadequate communication between child protection, medical providers, schools and dispending pharmacies. Many concluded that the care of such children requires more use of collateral data (beyond parent report), improved liaison among child-serving agencies like clinics, schools and child protection, and increased readiness among physicians to *dis*-believe what parents report.

The case also prompted questions, among professionals and the public, about the *context* of prescribing. Child psychiatry, like other fields, may not *see* the context in which it operates. Kuhn (1962) described the (often unrecognized) *context* in which we work as a *paradigm* defined by the terms in the text box. While scientific inquiry looks unfettered, argued Kuhn, in fact, it is tightly restricted.

Defining the Paradigm

- Unspoken values, beliefs, techniques
- Shared by a professional community
- Define problems to study
- Define acceptable interventions
- Define criteria for accepting new data

After Kuhn, The Structure of Scientific Revolutions

In child psychiatry, particularly in pharmacotherapy, what is the *context* of prescribing? Is a *paradigm* shifting?

In the 1980s, a prominent American child & adolescent psychiatrist, Leon Eisenberg, described a paradigm shift from a post-World War-II era dominated by psychoanalysis, the era of "brainless psychiatry," to an era dominated by biomedicine, which he chided as "mindless psychiatry" (Eisenberg 1986). Resistance to psychotropic medication for children and adolescents persisted somewhat longer, but an era of easy acceptance can be said to have begun around 1990. An era of increasing scrutiny can be said to have begun around 2005. [Increased scrutiny was evident in a 2006 report from the American Psychological Association (2006)]. The change from one Era to another is a paradigm shift.

Here we will look at these two Eras in terms of four relevant environments: The evidence environment, the public attitude environment, the practice environment, and the regulatory environment. The relationship between prescribers and Pharma is part of each Environment.

First, the Evidence Environment.

The Evidence Environment		
Era of Easy Acceptance (c 1990 – 2005)		Era of Increasing Scrutiny (2005 -)
Mostly, drug-placebo trials, selectively published and edited	What's the Knowledge Base?	All-trial registries; practical clinical trials; reports neutrally edited
Pharmaceuticals, contractors	Who pays, does trials?	Increasingly, public entities like the NIMH
Mostly, missing Little on brain effects; adult-derived taxonomy	Developmental focus?	More on developing CNS, growth and symptoms over time focus on attachment and trauma
Family and context irrelevant	Context relevant?	Family engagement and view of child
Often, injudicious generalization	How are data used?	With caution; looking for data matched to populations served

During the Era of Easy Acceptance, most new "evidence" came from clinical trials supported by the manufacturers purporting to demonstrate clinical efficacy of single medications compared to placebos. Reports starting as early as 2000 (Gilbody and Song 2000) pointed to publication bias: studies showing positive outcomes were selectively published, those showing no beneficial effect frequently not published at all (Turner et al. 2008; Parry 2009; Jureidini et al. 2008). The evidence base was also overly dependent on short-term trials in which the raw data, "commercial property" owned by the sponsors, were not publicly available. For example, increased suicidality in a study of paroxetine in adolescent depression was not reported as such in the published article (Keller et al. 2001). The original study data have been reanalyzed and published in the BMJ with opposite conclusions to the article published in the Journal of the American Academy of Child and Adolescent Psychiatry (LeNoury et al. 2015). This raises serious questions about the evidence base and ultimately the need for open data access (Doshi 2015; Godlee 2015).

The problem was not confined to psychiatry. Later reviews (Chan 2008; McGauran et al. 2010) indicated widespread publication bias and lack of transparency in the academic medical literature. A former chief-editor of the British Medical Journal called medical journals "an extension of the marketing arm of pharmaceutical companies" (Smith 2005) and recommended independent analysis of drug trial methodology and results, similar to a proposal by the editors of the Journal of the American Medical Association (JAMA) (DeAngelis and Fontanarosa 2008). A current international campaign—"AllTrials"—moves toward this goal by lobbying for enforceable regulated trial registries. The World Health Organization, in line with the "AllTrials" goals, recommends that all results including those from past research be made available (Moorthy et al. 2015).

In addition to this change in the publication of research, sponsorship of research has also been changing, from reliance on Pharma to greater use of public funds. To this end, the US National Institutes of Mental Health (NIMH 2015) has sponsored the TADS Study (Kennard et al. 2009), the TORDIA study (Emslie et al. 2010), and follow-up of the MTA study from the 1990s (e.g. Molina et al. 2009; Fernandez de la Cruz et al. 2015).

The way children are studied is also changing. For example, despite a warning by Coyle (2000) that children were not just miniature adults, most clinical trials in the era of easy acceptance used categorical diagnoses (like bipolar disorder) derived from adult practice, with little modification to reflect the developing brain or the developmentally shifting clinical presentations of children. Examples of such differences appear, for example, in neuroimaging (Pavuluri et al. 2009; DelBello 2009). Right orbitofrontal hypoactivation and amygdala hyper-reactivity in children, taken as indications of bipolar disorder, are also seen in children with developmental trauma (Schore 2002). Such trauma and disorders of attachment were rarely considered in industry-funded research (Parry 2012).

The last decade has also seen studies comparing pharmacological and other interventions, like the TORDIA study. Future work must address more fully the effect of context, especially family, including parents' understanding of and attitudes toward the child, as mediating or modulating variables.

The evidence environment has also changed with the introduction of "practical clinical trials" (March et al. 2005). These studies, in contrast to trials done on selected populations in clinical research centers, use clinical settings and populations similar to those among whom the study results are likely to be applied.

These reforms in research hopefully herald a different kind of evidence-based practice. In the meantime, long-term outcome data in pediatric psychopharmacology are sparse and post-marketing pharmacovigilance has been erratic and poorly reported. These factors should be considered when prescribing. Well-conducted longitudinal research is needed when considering the effects of psychotropic medication on growing brains.

Next. the Public Attitude Environment.

The Public Attitude Environment		
Era of Easy Acceptance (c 1990 – 2005)		Era of Increasing Scrutiny (2005 -)
Promotions, some guidelines, direct-to-consumer ads (DTCA)	What shapes public attitudes?	Increasingly, unbiased sources; news about Pharma
Assumed benign, not disclosed	Pharma money to MDs	Transparency required; some gifts illegal; conflict of interest bars panel membership
Mostly, trust	View of Child Psychiatrists?	Increasing distrust
Enthusiasm, confidence	View of Pharma	Skepticism, apprehension

Public attitudes toward child psychopharmacology have changed dramatically in the last decade, a change that is a part of the paradigm shift.

A triggering event in this change was the rise and fall of Vioxx. Rofecoxib (marketed as Vioxx) had been promoted as a dramatic breakthrough in the treatment of pain and gastrointestinal distress. Its introduction was even cited in medical schools as an example of the application of physiology to drug discovery ("more specific targeting…"). Sales rose to US$billions. But rofecoxib also increased the rate of heart attacks. By the time the evidence of that risk was revealed, dozens had died. Vioxx was withdrawn from the market, with huge fiscal consequences for its manufacturer (nearly $5 billion to settle lawsuits). The dramatic rise and fall of this heavily promoted agent received considerable attention in the media (Grant 2009), some frankly accusatory. The history of Vioxx and its effect on the public was recently reviewed (Rosenbaum 2015).

But the effects of the Vioxx story went beyond that one medication. In retrospect, "Easy Acceptance" was seen to have characterized not just the general public and the media, but medical journals as well. Easy acceptance was fostered at times by deceit. For instance, the international medical publishing company, Elsevier, published six journals that were secretly sponsored but falsely presented to readers as peer-reviewed (Grant 2009). At least one clinician listed on the editorial board of such a journal was unaware of the journal's existence (Rout 2009).

In addition to articles in the medical literature, several books reflected a new skepticism and criticism of the reliance of the profession and the public on the pharmaceutical industry (Abramson 2004; Angell 2004; Avorn 2005; Whitaker 2010). Their titles reflect both concern and the new skepticism: "Overdosed America: the broken promise," "The Truth about the Drug Companies," "Powerful Medicines," "Anatomy of an Epidemic."

Several consequences: as noted above, medical journals took the lead in disclosing drug company sponsorship of research; in establishing sponsor-neutral ("all payors") databases, and in policing conflicts of interest. To address possible conflicts of interest, guidelines and policies established a firewall between manufacturers and academic journals, a strict separation recently coming under review (Drazen 2015).

Child psychiatrists as a profession also suffered a degradation in public trust, largely as a consequence of perceived pharmaceutical influence (Anders 2008). In response, some have emphasized the burden of untreated illness and the effectiveness of interventions (Warner 2010; for a critical reply, see Gopnik 2010).

Next, the Practice Environment.

The Practice Environment		
Era of Easy Acceptance (c 1990 – 2005)		Era of Increasing Scrutiny (2005 -)
Mostly, medications	What's needed?	Multimodal care: psychoeducation, family treatment, CBT, ACT
Medication alone often indicated; Stimulants safe; SSRI's safe and widely indicated; SGA's a "standard of care" and "revolutionary" advance over FGAs	How medications are seen	A complement to non-drug therapies; Wider recognition of side-effects (stimulant abuse potential; suicidality, discontinuation syndrome and sexual SEs with SSRIs; metabolic syndrome with SGAs); SGAs effectiveness ~ FGAs
Disorders in the individual child reification of diagnostic labels; Multiple co-morbid diagnoses; Adult perspective	How are children's troubles seen?	Biopsychosocial formulation; dimensional developmental perspective; symptoms in
Individual, pharmacotherapy	Focus of child mental health	Population focus, supports for family; support for PCPs
Payment tied to diagnoses, fee-for-service, "medical necessity"	Funding/reimbursement	Bundled payments based on outcomes, as in Triple Aim
Often, little link between prescriber and other clinicians	Is care integrated?	Increasing liaison between treating team/clinicians
Approve what's proposed; parents influenced by DTCA demand medication	Consumers' and parents' role	Shared decision-making; parents receptive to biopsychosocial formulation and treatments
Often continues to be prescribed, unquestioned	Once a medication is prescribed...	First ask, what's the evidence of benefit and risk?

The practice environment in the US has changed in many ways. In the era of easy acceptance, care was often limited to the prescription of medications, particularly for children from disadvantaged backgrounds and children in protective custody (Burcu et al. 2014; Safer et al. 2015; Government Accountability Office 2011). Such pharmaco-limited practice has been criticized in the media (Wilson 2010) and by federal officials (Government Accountability Office 2014). States, which administer public services and services for foster children, are now required to demonstrate how they are managing medication use, not relying on medication treatment alone [Department of Health and Human Services (HHS)]. Multimodal care may include psychoeducation, family treatment, and non-medication treatments such as trauma-informed care and cognitive-behavioral treatment.

Attitudes toward the second-generation antipsychotics (SGAs, also called "atypical antipsychotics") have also changed. Where previously the SGAs were seen as a "standard of care," a "revolutionary" advance over first-generation antipsychotics (FGAs), with minimal side-effects, and with minimal within-class differences, studies like the CATIE study (Lieberman et al. 2005; Rosenheck et al. 2006) have shown within-class differences, demonstrated serious metabolic effects and weight gain, and demonstrated equal or better adherence with older agents. While SGA's have brought some advantages, the market dominance of the SGA's has been described as due to marketing rather than evidence (Tyrer and Kendall 2009). Older off-patent medications like clonidine, that do not have metabolic or extrapyramidal side-effects, are worth considering for managing disruptive behavior, though toxicity (as in the case of R.R.) needs to be carefully considered in terms of parents' capacity to supervise. Regarding stimulants for ADHD, the immediate benefits may lessen over time (Molina et al. 2009), warranting an accompanying non-drug approach to ADHD. Concerns of over-diagnosis of ADHD and over-prescription of stimulants have been debated in the media (Schwarz and Cohen 2013).

Concerns over the SSRI's and the agitation reaction, uncommon but life-threatening, led to the FDA "black box" warning label in 2004. Debate continues over the merits of this warning but data indicate that SSRI's produce increased suicidal ideation at double the rate of placebo (National Institutes of Mental Health). Suicidality and agitation aside, SSRI's may foster dependency more than was originally believed. There is also evidence for a discontinuation syndrome (Fava et al. 2015). Sexual side-effects of SSRI's are common and can be distressing to adolescents who are developing their sexual identities. A recent case review suggests potentiation of SSRI's with alcohol (Menkes and Herxheimer 2014) and warrants discussion with adolescents, who may tend to minimize alcohol risks.

Interest in the whole child, not just brain receptors, has increased—encompassing appreciation of strengths, of developmental status, and of context—school, family, and parental attitudes. Publicly insured children benefit from a federal requirement that the states must provide early periodic screening diagnosis and treatment (EPSDT). Such initiatives, often the result of class-action litigation, has strengthened a focus on whole populations, not just the individual child, and led to increased supports for comprehensive services including family (Department of Health and Human Services 2011).

The characterization of children's troubles has also changed, from the use of multiple categorical "comorbid" disorders, sometimes as many as five or six, often seen as younger versions of adult disorders, to embrace a developmental, dimensional, and contextual approach. Some see a renaissance of the biopsychosocial model (Frances 2014) and a return to the art of biopsychosocial diagnostic case formulations (Nurcombe 2014). Such formulations complement DSM or ICD diagnoses and provide a better description of the child's reality, pointing to a range of contributing factors and providing a better guide to treatment planning. On the other hand, the reclassification in DSM5 of ADHD as a neurodevelopmental disorder, emphasizing its biological side, may lead to increased use of medications as a sole intervention.

Efforts are underway, though still at an early stage, to shift payments from fee-for-service reimbursement based on categorical diagnoses, with preference for concrete services like pharmacotherapy, to outcomes-based reimbursement, in which payment is based on how children, even groups of children, are functioning. Fee-for-service reimbursement has not provided an incentive for coordination of care between prescriber and other clinicians. As a result, the prescribing child psychiatrist might visit a program for a brief visit once per week, with little interaction with other members of the team.

More integrated care will address another problem of the Era of Easy Acceptance—disconnection between acute hospitals, where medications were started, often in addition to those prescribed pre-admission, in response to the acute symptoms that led to admission. Those caring for the child post-admission would often continue the new as well as the previous medications, without questioning what had been prescribed inpatient. "After all," was the prevalent attitude, "in the hospital they've got the most time and the most expertize." As a result, medicines were added, and much less often taken away. In addition, the perception of symptoms as the first signs of a lifetime disorder led to the assumption that medications, once prescribed, would need to be continued indefinitely. In the era of increased skepticism, the possibility of a reactive, phase-specific condition, as opposed to a lifetime disorder, is taken more seriously.

Changes in the regulatory environment are another part of the Paradigm Change. The role of the State (aka public authority), as represented above (Fig. 16.1), is moving from a position of laissez-faire to one of increasing vigilance and regulation.

The Regulatory Environment		
Era of Easy Acceptance (c 1990 – 2005)		Era of Increasing Scrutiny (2005 -)
Completely, autonomy not questioned	How autonomous are prescribers?	Shared responsibility and oversight
Drug ads, studies sponsored by Pharma	Where do prescribers get information?	Guidelines from public, professional sources
Largely, laissez-faire	FDA role on claims in ads	Increasingly, vigilant and demanding
Prescribers don't know, payers deem inevitable, State doesn't question	Medication costs: Who knows? Who needs to know?	Increasing awareness of private and public costs; readiness to challenge
Assume medication is indicated and benign; pay the bills	What do public agencies and insurers do?	Actively monitor quality, aggregate and individually: Is treatment safe? Is it effective?

The position of the prescriber changes from total autonomy toward one of *shared* responsibility and oversight, the details of which vary from State to State and country to country. Practitioners who want the latest information, and who

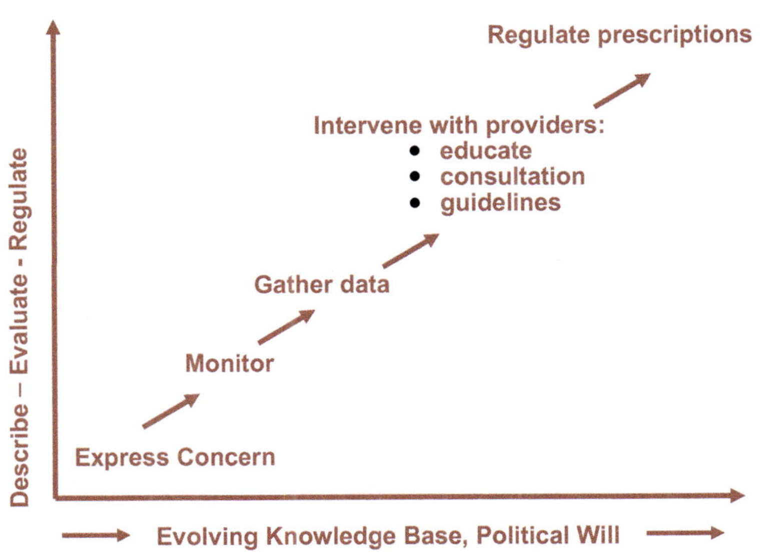

Fig. 16.1 The evolving state role regarding psychoactive medications. Adapted from Harper (2014)

want to integrate what is new with existing knowledge, no longer depend entirely or largely on pharmaceutical promotion, but use guidelines from public, professional sources.

In some jurisdictions, this change also entails greater awareness among prescribers of the costs of care. Many physicians grew up professionally at a time when knowing what care costs was considered outside the doctor's role. The state, whether as payor or regulator, is moving from not knowing costs and simply paying the bills, to one of actively seeking (and requiring) cost information and data regarding safety and effectiveness.

16.3 Comparison of United States with Other Countries

Child psychiatry in the US has undergone a dramatic paradigm shift. The change has not been so great in Australia and New Zealand, the UK and Europe, and in economically developed regions of East and South Asia.

One measure of this difference is that the pediatric bipolar diagnosis was not widely adopted outside the US (Parry et al. 2014). Several reasons are given for this difference. One is the absence in the other countries of direct-to-consumer advertising (DTCA)—so that parents are less likely to expect a pharmacological fix for a child's problems. New Zealand is the only other nation to allow DTCA, but its small market has meant little DTCA in practice. Another difference is that reimbursement outside the US is not tied to categorical diagnoses and to narrowly defined "medical necessity" criteria that are most easily met by prescribing and adjusting medications. In addition, in other countries research and academia are not dominated by "key opinion leaders" with industry ties, as still occurs in the US. And a strong psychodynamic and contextual emphasis continues to prevail in much of the world. That psychodynamic perspective, once the strength of US psychiatry, languished in parts of the USA during the era of easy acceptance (Tasman 1999), nonetheless practice varies. For example, Australian pediatricians and general practitioners in busy clinics often experience greater pressure to prescribe, whereas child psychiatrists are reimbursed for longer consultations.

In East and South Asia, vast differences in those served—genetic, environmental, socioeconomic, and cultural—challenge the facile generalization, based on evidence and attitudes in the West, of medication practices from the era of easy acceptance. Immense differences also exist in professional development and service availability. Generalizations are difficult, but attitudes to Psychiatry are changing (Thirunavukarasu et al. 2012), some studies of the developing child are beginning (Chiang et al. 2015), and services developed (Lim and Vitiello 2015; Lim et al. 2015; Zheng and Zheng 2015).

Recommendations have been made for psychiatric practice among "Asians," partly based on clinical experience in the West. For instance, some Asian populations metabolize drugs in the CYP450 2D6 system more slowly than other ethnic groups and, with lower body weight, may respond to lower doses of antipsychotics and experience side-effects at lower doses than are seen in other ethnic groups (Chen et al. 2002). Such differences seen in adults are likely relevant to Asian children as well.

In the meantime, even in less-resourced areas, child and adolescent mental health services are increasingly in demand from a rapidly industrializing population beset by the same factors that contribute worldwide to increasing symptoms and to their recognition. In some settings, medications may be the most available (or the only) service on offer.

Polarization regarding medication use may also be seen. For instance, in India, children seen in settings with little capacity to offer psychosocial interventions (clinical "set-ups") may be given multiple medications, even for minor anxieties, while in Child Guidance clinics with strong developmental orientation, children, even those who would benefit from medications, will be offered only psychosocial interventions. Integrated care may be available only in select institutions. A priority is for providers who are trained to recognize, diagnose, and help.

In short, a narrowly medicalized response to these rising demands for help, while sometimes better than no help at all, has its problems. We hope that this discussion of two Eras in the West—of Easy Acceptance and Increased Scrutiny—will be useful in these rapidly changing and expanding fields of practice.

16.4 Conclusion

This review shows how the efforts of child and adolescent psychiatrists on behalf of troubled children are shaped not only by an evolving knowledge base, but by public opinion, evolving conditions of practice, and regulation. The resulting paradigm shift revives the biopsychosocial model, enhanced through advances in developmental psychology and neuroscience, with increased understanding of the biology of attachment and developmental trauma. In this new paradigm, focus on the child's psychosocial environment is paramount and pharmacotherapy becomes adjunctive to psychosocial interventions.

A globalizing profession of child and adolescent psychiatry can avoid the pitfalls of both "mindless" and "brainless" psychiatry by explicitly emphasizing the psychosocial environment's interaction with temperament and other innate vulnerabilities. Psychiatry training, practice and research need to always pay heed to the biopsychosocial model and integrative paradigm. In addition, a healthy skepticism toward commercial influences on the academic research literature and clinical practice is vital if child psychiatry worldwide is to avoid the "Era of Easy Acceptance." Professional child psychiatry colleges and associations have a duty to uphold high standards of medical and scientific ethics. Advocating for global data-access initiatives (such as AllTrials) will assist in an evidence-based future. New data need to be appraised and integrated into the knowledge base within a biopsychosocial paradigm that draws upon traditional wisdom from developmental psychology and psychopathology. Child and adolescent psychiatrists in their daily practice need to be highly sophisticated across a broad field of knowledge and therapeutic modalities.

References

Abramson, J. (2004). *Overdosed America: The broken promise of American medicine*. New York: Harpercollins. AllTrials, Accessed May 3, 2015 at http://www.alltrials.net/find-out-more/all-trials/

American Psychological Association. (2006). *Report of the working group on psychotropic medication*. Washington: American Psychological Association.

Anders, T. F. (2008). Child and adolescent psychiatry: The next 10 years. *Psychiatric Times*. Accessed on May 1, 2008 at http://www.psychiatrictimes.com/articles/child-and-adolescent-psychiatry-next-10-years/

Angell, M. (2004). *The truth about the drug companies: How they deceive us and what to do about it*. New York: Random House.

Avorn, J. (2005). *Powerful medicines: The benefits, risks, and costs of prescription drugs*. New York: Random House Vintage Books.

Burcu, M., Zito, J. M., Ibe, A., & Safer, D. J. (2014). Atypical antipsychotic use among Medicaid-insured children and adolescents: Duration, safety, and monitoring implications. *Journal of Child and Adolescent Psychopharmacology, 24*, 112–119.

Chan, A.-W. (2008). Bias, spin, and misreporting: Time for full access to trial protocols and results. *PLoS Medicine, 5*(11), e230. doi:10.1371/journal.pmed.0050230, http://journals.plos.org/plosmedicine/article?id=10.1371/journal.pmed.0050230

Chen, J.-P., Lin, K.-M., & Chung, H. (2002). Prescribing medication for Asians with mental disorders. *Western Journal of Medicine, 176*, 271–275.

Chiang, Y.C., Lin, D.C., Lee, C.Y., & Lee, M.C. (2015). Effects of parenting role and parent-child interaction on infant motor development in Taiwan Birth Cohort Study. *Early Human Development, 91*(4), 259–264.

Coyle, J. T. (2000). Psychotropic drug use in very young children. *Journal of the American Medical Association, 283*, 1059–1060.

DeAngelis, C. D., & Fontanarosa, P. B. (2008). Impugning the integrity of medical science: The adverse effects of industry influence. *Journal of the American Medical Association, 299*(15), 1833–1835.

DelBello, M. (2009). The neurobiology of pediatric bipolar disorder. In *Proceedings of American Academy of Child & Adolescent Psychiatry, 56th Annual Meeting*, October 27–November 1 2009, Honolulu, Hawaii.

Department of Health and Human Services. (2011). *Letter to state departments of child welfare*. Accessed at http://childwelfare.gov/pubPDFs/jointlettermeds.pdf.

Doshi, P. (2015). No correction, no retraction, no apology, no comment: Paroxetine trial reanalysis raises questions about institutional responsibility. *British Medical Journal, 351*, h4629.

Drake, R., Skinner, J., & Goldman, H. H. (2008). What explains the diffusion of treatments for mental illness? *American Journal of Psychiatry, 165*, 1392–1395.

Drazen, J. M. (2015). Revisiting the commercial-academic interface. *New England Journal of Medicine, 372*, 1853–1854.

Eisenberg, L. (1986). Mindlessness and brainlessness in psychiatry. *British Journal of Psychiatry, 148*, 497–508.

Emslie, G. J., Mayes, T., Porta, G., Vitiello, B., Clarke, G., Wagner, K. D., et al. (2010). Treatment of resistant depression in adolescents (TORDIA): Week 24 outcomes. *American Journal of Psychiatry, 167*, 291–782.

EPSDT. Information available at http://mchb.hrsa.gov/epsdt/

Fava, G. A., Gatti, A., Belaise, C., Guidi, J., & Offidani, E. (2015). Withdrawal symptoms after selective serotonin reuptake inhibitor discontinuation: A systematic review. *Psychotherapy and Psychosomatics, 84*, 72–81.

Fernandez de la Cruz, L., Simonoff, E., McGough, J. J., Halperin, J. M., Arnold, L. E., & Stringaris, A. (2015). Treatment of children with attention-deficit/hyperactivity disorder (ADHD) and irritability: Results from the multimodal treatment study of children with ADHD (MTA). *Journal of the American Academy of Child and Adolescent Psychiatry, 54*, 62–70.

Frances, A. (2014). Resuscitating the biopsychosocial model. *The Lancet Psychiatry, 1*, 496–497.

Gilbody, S. M., & Song, F. (2000). Publication bias and the integrity of psychiatric research. *Psychological Medicine, 30*, 253–258.

Godlee, F. (2015). Editor's choice: Study 329. *British Medical Journal, 351*, h4973.

Gopnik, A. (2010). To drug or not to drug: Judith Warner misses the real questions about medicating children. *Slate Magazine*, 22.

Government Accountability Office (GAO). (2011). *Foster children: HHS guidance could help states improve oversight of psychotropic prescriptions.* Accessed at http://www.gao.gov/products/GAO-12-270T

Government Accountability Office (GAO). (2014). *Foster children: Additional federal guidance could help states better plan for oversight of psychotropic prescriptions administered by managed-care organizations.* Accessed at http://www.gao.gov/products/GAO-14-362

Grant, B. (2009). Merck published fake journal. *The Scientist*, April 30, 2009. Accessed at http://www.the-scientist.com/?articles.view/articleNo/27376/title/Merck-published-fake-journal/

Harper, G. (2014). Child and adolescent mental health policy. In J. M. Rey (Ed.), *IACAPAP e-textbook of child and adolescent mental health.* Geneva: International Association for Child and Adolescent Psychiatry and Allied Professions. Accessed at http://iacapap.org/wp-content/uploads/J.6-POLICY-2014.pdf

Jureidini, J. N., McHenry, L. B., & Mansfield, P. R. (2008). Clinical trials and drug promotion: Selective reporting of study 329. *International Journal of Risk and Safety in Medicine, 20*, 73–81.

Keller, M. B., Ryan, N. D., Strober, M., Klein, R. G., Kutcher, S. P., Birmaher, B., et al. (2001). Efficacy of paroxetine in the treatment of adolescent major depression: A randomized, controlled trial. *Journal of the American Academy of Child and Adolescent Psychiatry, 40*, 762–772.

Kennard, B. D., Silva, S. G., Tonev, S., Eohsw, P., Hughes, J. L., Vitiello, B., et al. (2009). Remission and recovery in the treatment for adolescents with depression study (TADS): Acute and long-term outcomes. *Journal of the American Academy of Child and Adolescent Psychiatry, 48*, 186–195.

Kuhn, T. S. (1962). *The structure of scientific revolutions.* Chicago: University of Chicago Press.

LeNoury, J., Nardo, J. M., Healy, D., Jureidini, J., Raven, M., Tufanaru, C., et al. (2015). Restoring study 329: Efficacy and harms of paroxetine and imipramine in treatment of major depression in adolescence. *British Medical Journal, 351*, h4320.

Lieberman, J. A., Stroup, T. S., McEvoy, J. P., Swartz, M. S., Rosenheck, R. A., Perkins, D. O., et al. (2005). Effectiveness of antipsychotic drugs in patients with chronic schizophrenia. *New England Journal of Medicine, 353*, 1209–1223

Lim, C. G., Ong, S. H., Chin, C. H., & Fung, D. S. S. (2015). Child and adolescent psychiatry services in Singapore. *Child and Adolescent Psychiatry and Mental Health, 9*, 7–14.

Lim, C. G., & Vitiello, B. (2015). Child psychiatry services in Asia: evolving state of affairs? *Child and Adolescent Psychiatry and Mental Health, 9*, 12–14. doi:10.1186/s13034-015-0044-9

March, J. S., Silva, S. G., Compton, S., Shapiro, M., Califf, R., & Krishnan, R. (2005). The case for practical clinical trials in Psychiatry. *American Journal of Psychiatry, 162*, 836–846.

McGauran, N., Weisler, B., Kreis, J., Schüler, Y. B., Kölsch, H., Kaiser, T. (2010). Reporting bias in medical research—A narrative review. *Trials, 11*, 37. http://www.trialsjournal.com/content/11/1/37

Menkes, D., & Herxheimer, A. (2014). Interaction between antidepressants and alcohol: Signal amplification by multiple case reports. *International Journal of Risk & Safety in Medicine, 26*, 163–170.

Molina, B. S. G., Hinshaw, S. P., Swanson, J. M., Arnold, L. E., Vitiello, B., Jensen, P. S., et al. (2009). The MTA at 8 years: Prospective follow-up of children treated for combined type ADHD in a multisite study. *Journal of the American Academy of Child & Adolescent Psychiatry, 48*, 484–500.

Moorthy, V. S., Karam, G., Vannice, K. S., & Kieny, M.-P. (2015). Rationale for WHO's new position calling for prompt reporting and public disclosure of interventional clinical trial results. *PLoS Medicine, 12*(4), e1001819. doi:10.1371/journal.pmed.1001819.

National Institute for Mental Health (NIMH). (2015). *Antidepressant medication for children and adolescents: Information for parents and care-givers*. http://www.nimh.nih.gov/health/topics/child-and-adolescent-mental-health/antidepressant-medications-for-children-and-adolescents-information-for-parents-and-caregivers.shtml. Accessed May 23, 2015.

Nurcombe, B. (2014). Diagnosis and treatment planning in child and adolescent mental health problems. In J. M. Rey (Ed.), *IACAPAP e-textbook of child and adolescent mental health*. Geneva: International Association for Child and Adolescent Psychiatry and Allied Professions. Accessed at http://iacapap.org/wp-content/uploads/A.11-TREATMENT-PLAN-2014.pdf

Parry, P. (2009). Internal company documents regarding 3 atypical antipsychotic drugs. *Healthy Skepticism International News*, December 2009, published earlier at: http://www.healthyskepticism.org/documents/Antipsychotics.php

Parry, P. I. (2012). Paediatric bipolar disorder: Are attachment and trauma factors considered? In: J. Barnhill (Ed.), Bipolar disorder—A portrait of a complex mood disorder. InTech, Rijeka, Croatia 2012. http://www.intechopen.com/books/bipolar-disorder-a-portrait-of-a-complex-mood-disorder/paediatric-bipolar-disorder-are-attachment-and-trauma-factors-considered

Parry, P. I., Allison, S., Bastianpillai, T. (2014). Reification of the paediatric bipolar hypothesis in the USA. *The Lancet Psychiatry*. (Published **Online** December 1, 2014). http://dx.doi.org/10.1016/S2215–0366(14)00075-3

Pavuluri, M. N., Passarotti, A. M., Harral, E. M., & Sweeney, J. A. (2009). An fMRI study of the neural correlates of incidental versus directed emotion processing in pediatric bipolar disorder. *Journal of the American Academy of Child and Adolescent Psychiatry, 48*, 308–319.

Rebecca Riley Story on CBS News. http://www.cbsnews.com/news/what-killed-rebecca-riley/

Rebecca Riley Story on Wikipedia. http://en.wikipedia.org/wiki/Rebecca_Riley

Rosenbaum, L. (2015). Reconnecting the dots—Reinterpreting industry-physician relations. *New England Journal of Medicine, 372*, 1860–1864.

Rosenheck, R. A., Leslie, D. L., Sindelar, J., et al. (2006). Cost-effectiveness of second-generation antipsychotics and perphenazine in a randomized trial of treatment for chronic schizophrenia. The *American Journal of Psychiatry, 163*, 2080–2089

Rout, M. (2009). Doctor not told about Vioxx "role". *The Australian*, May 09. http://www.theaustralian.com.au/news/doctor-not-told-about-vioxx-role/story-e6frg6n6-1225734663308

Safer, D. J., Rajakannan, R., Burcu, M., & Zito, J. M. (2015). Trends in subthreshold psychiatric diagnosis for youth in community treatment. *Journal of the American Medical Association Psychiatry, 72*, 75–83.

Schore, A. (2002). Dysregulation of the right brain: A fundamental mechanism of traumatic attachment and the psychopathogenesis of posttraumatic stress disorder. *Australian and New Zealand Journal of Psychiatry, 36*(1), 9–30. ISSN 0004-8674.

Schwarz, A., Cohen, S. (2013). ADHD seen in 11 % of US children as diagnosis rises. *New York Times,* March 31, 2013. Available at: http://www.nytimes.com/2013/04/01/health/more-diagnoses-of-hyperactivity-causing-concern.html?_r=0. Accessed May 23, 2015.

Smith, R. (2005). Medical journals are an extension of the marketing arm of pharmaceutical companies. *PLoS Medicine, 2*(5), e138. doi:10.1371/journal.pmed.0020138, http://journals.plos.org/plosmedicine/article?id=10.1371/journal.pmed.0020138

Spielmans, G. I., & Parry, P. I. (2010). From evidence-based medicine to marketing-based medicine: Evidence from internal industry documents. *Journal of Bioethical Inquiry, 7*(1), 13–29.

Tasman, A. (1999). Teaching psychodynamic psychiatry during medical school and residency. *Journal of Psychotherapeutic Practice and Research, 8*, 187–189.

Thirunavukarasu, M., Cherukuri, S. D., Pragatheeshwar, K. D., Thirunavukarasu, P. (2012). Public perception of psychiatry in India: A changing landscape. *Indian Journal of Psychiatry, 54*, 6–7.

Turner, E. H., Matthews, A. M., Linardatos, E., Tell, R. A., & Rosenthal, R. (2008). Selective publication of antidepressant trials and its influence on apparent efficacy. *New England Journal of Medicine, 358*, 252–260.

Tyrer, P., & Kendall, T. (2009). The spurious advance of antipsychotic drug therapy. *The Lancet, 373*(9657), 4–5.

Warner, J. (2010). *We've Got Issues: Children and parents in the age of medication*. New York: Riverhead.

Whitaker, R. (2010). *Anatomy of an Epidemic: Magic bullets, psychiatric drugs, and the astonishing rise of mental illness in America*. New York: Random House Crown Publishing.

Wilson, D. (2010). Child's ordeal reveals risks of psychiatric drugs in young. *The New York Times*, September 2, 2010.

Zheng, X., & Zheng, Y. (2015). Current state and recent developments of child psychiatry in China. *Child and Adolescent Psychiatry and Mental Health, 9*, 10–20. doi:10.1186/s13034-015-0040-0.

Chapter 17
Pediatric Psychopharmacology: Perspectives from Low Resource Countries

Devashish Konar and Srinivas Balachander

Abstract Systematic research and evidence to guide prescribing practices for children and adolescents with psychiatric disorders, have seen tremendous growth in the last two decades. Despite the lack of trained personnel and capabilities for multidisciplinary care in low resource countries, use of psychopharmacological treatments in children has seen wide dissemination. Mostly guided by data from the West, there are a few contributions in the field of pediatric psychopharmacology from India. For a rational prescriber, the most sought-after knowledge would be regarding proper diagnosis, selection of the right medicine, pharmacokinetics, pharmacodynamics, proper dosage, dose titration schedule, side effects, and drug interactions of the relevant drugs. Better characterization of childhood psychiatric disorders; advances in developmental neurobiology; cellular and molecular mechanisms of neuronal functions; and advent of newer and more specifically targeted psychotropic drugs have contributed to the advancements in pediatric psychopharmacology.

Keywords Pediatric psychopharmacology · Challenges low resource countries · Pharmacokinetics pharmacodynamics · Drug interactions · Psychiatric disorders · Pharmacotherapies

D. Konar
Mental Health Care Centre, Burdwan, Kolkata, West Bengal, India
e-mail: devkon59@yahoo.com

S. Balachander (✉)
Department of Psychiatry, National Institute of Mental Health and Neuro Sciences, Bengaluru, Karnataka, India
e-mail: srinivasbalachander@gmail.com

S. Malhotra and P. Santosh (eds.), *Child and Adolescent Psychiatry*,
DOI 10.1007/978-81-322-3619-1_17

17.1 Introduction

Historically, pediatric pharmacology in general, and pediatric psychopharmacology in particular, have received much less research interest and funding than their adult counterparts. As a consequence, relatively few drugs are licensed for use in child and adolescent populations (Coghill and Sinita 2014). There is growing evidence that the use of psychopharmacological agents in children and adolescents has increased manifold and gained widespread acceptance (Zito et al. 2008; Huline-Dickens 2014). Alongside this, the debate whether this trend may be truly beneficial or harmful in the long run, still rages on (Rapoport 2013).

Childhood and adolescence, being a period of key biological, psychological and social growth, renders individuals more vulnerable to disruptions in healthy development. It has been reported that nearly 50 % of all adult psychiatric disorders manifest as early as age 14, and 75 % manifest by age 24 (Kessler et al. 2005). Nearly two-thirds of mental disorders that have their onset in childhood or adolescence are likely to be moderate to severe, and most of them continue into adulthood (Kessler et al. 2012). Thus, it is crucial that these disorders are identified and treated early, so as to minimize disruptions in the individual's developmental trajectory and hence reduce suffering (Correll et al. 2013).

17.2 The Chronology of Progress

A number of developments in the treatment of psychiatric disorders in children and adolescents have occurred, especially in the last two decades, which have been groundbreaking. Psychological and behavioral interventions were once the mainstay of treatment in child psychiatric disorders. But psychopharmacological approaches have provided important biological management tools. In recent years, child psychopharmacology is thus becoming more important day by day.

To promote research in the field of child psychopharmacology, the US Congress in 1997 authorized the United States Food and Drug Administration (US FDA) to grant an additional 6 months of drug exclusivity in return for conducting specific studies in children. Also, the US FDA, by its "Best Pharmaceuticals for Children Act" mandates that clinical trials are to be conducted in pediatric population by the pharmaceutical industry, especially when there is a possibility that the drugs may be of use in the children and adolescents. Research Units on Pediatric Psychopharmacology (RUPPs) under the leadership of the National Institute of Mental Health (NIMH) have formed. These measures have contributed to the remarkable increase in research relevant to child psychopharmacology since the last two decades (Vitiello 2006).

17.3 Low Resource Countries—The Challenges Faced

(1) **Paucity of Psychiatrists with Specialized Training in Child and Adolescent Psychiatry**

Mental health issues are being recognized more and more at an earlier age. The shortage of psychiatrists with specialized training is always the main constraint in case of developing countries. Current models that rely on psychiatrists to deliver direct care are unsuitable for low and middle income countries, where number of mental health professional is limited. A shift to a collaborative care model has been proposed, wherein the role of a psychiatrist is to provide training, supervision, and tertiary-level care. The majority of the service delivery, which comprises of treating common mental disorders, is to be provided by primary care professionals and community health workers, who would receive training and supervision from the tertiary care centers (Becker and Kleinman 2014; Malhotra and Padhy 2015).

(2) **Lack of Professionals to Aid in Psychosocial Interventions**

There is a huge dearth of personnel trained to provide evidence-based psychological, social, and educational therapies, which are essential to holistic treatment and rehabilitation of psychiatric illnesses especially in children. Very few centers have an infrastructure to provide multidisciplinary care, which is a basic standard in most high-income countries. The burden of providing, or coordinating these also rests upon the psychiatrist.

The increasing prevalence of childhood psychiatric disorders, along with constraint of resources makes work difficult in real-life situation, and may necessitate some practical changes. In order to cope with large numbers of patients in need of psychiatric treatment with acutely deficient manpower, clinical work-up has to be brief; therapeutic sessions may have to be cut down to simpler modules involving counseling; and parents and families have to become therapeutic allies as well as co therapists Medication thus assumes a more critical role in treatment, with possibly involving the nonspecialist psychiatrists/pediatricians; and a tendency to overrely and over-prescribe medications. This partly also stems from clinicians' wish to be helpful with whatever resources available at hand. Judicious evidence-based prescribing, slow titration and never, ever, overprescribing, needs be emphasized to improve treatment outcomes in children.

(3) **Availability and Regulation of Psychotropics**

Most antipsychotics, antidepressants, mood stabilizers, and benzodiazepines are easily available in most low resource countries. This is partly due to measures by the World Health Organization to include these as "essential medications," and mostly due to the pharmaceutical industry. Even stimulant medications, though not as readily available as other psychotropics, are generally within reach of most populations and at affordable costs. The main challenge in developing countries, however, has been poor regulation of prescription and sale of psychotropics. Polypharmacy, off-label use of medications, is rampant. Along with the lack of training and resources for monitoring adverse effects, the onus on clinicians to use more discretion in treating children is thus much larger.

(4) **Cultural Factors, Knowledge, and Attitudes of Parents and Teachers**

On the one hand, there are problems of lack of knowledge and failure of timely referral for psychiatric consultation. Furthermore, spiritual and magico-religious beliefs lead parents to take their children to faith healers for psychological problems causing treatment delays. All too often, a psychiatric consultation is sought only when there is an acute deterioration of clinical status, such as catatonic symptoms or suicide, or when the patient or family starting to lose hope in other treatments and turns to medications "as a last resort" (Shrivastava et al. 2013). Educating patients and families that prolong the duration of untreated symptoms and waiting for the illness to become more severe may decrease the likelihood of response or remission of symptoms, which is part of the clinician's overall responsibility (Stroeh and Trivedi 2012).

On the other hand, stigmatization and criticism of certain diagnoses and treatments (especially attention-deficit hyperactivity disorder [ADHD]) and stimulant medications in particular) in media and in the internet infusing negative attitudes amongst people, and reluctance of families to expose children to "mind altering drugs" in middle and upper socioeconomic groups is equally strong.

In summary, caregivers need to be educated to bring children early for assessment, adopt a more rational and informed approach to acceptance of psychopharmacology in children.

17.4 Treatment Gap and Need for an Indigenous Service Model

Children and adolescents with psychiatric illness in developing economies is a grossly under-cared section of population. By rough estimates, 6–20 % of children and adolescents have a diagnosable mental health disorder (Malhotra and Patra 2014). Very few have access to specialist services. The treatment gap is huge.

An indigenous service delivery model needs to be developed. More than in developed economies, training general psychiatrists, pediatricians, and family physicians may be required to bridge the gap. The bare minimum skills that they need to be sensitized about are proper identification of childhood psychiatric disorders, evidence-based medication choice and dosing, monitoring for adverse effects, along with basic counseling and psychoeducation abilities.

Transmitting information in this collaborative model has to be specifically very restricted and simple. General physicians and pediatricians have to be acquainted with a restricted number of medicines. In the case of antipsychotics, possible drugs are risperidone, aripiprazole, and quetiapine; in case of antidepressants, fluoxetine, sertraline, and escitalopram; among mood stabilizers, lithium, and divalproex and among drugs for ADHD, methylphenidate, and atomoxetine.

An innovative model that has been studied in the Post-Graduate Institute of Medical Education and Research (PGIMER), Chandigarh is the use of automated clinical decision support system through telepsychiatry services to facilitate diagnosis, treatment at the primary care level along with collaboration, and referral for more complicated cases (Malhotra et al. 2015) can be a viable option.

17.5 The Research Gap

Owing to the above-mentioned factors, research in child psychopharmacology from low resource countries has been minimal (Malhotra and Padhy 2015; Malhotra and Kate 2015a, b), though studies have started to emerge over the last few years (Malhotra and Kate 2015a, b; Malhotra and Banerjee 2009a, b). Much of the available research is in the form of case reports or open-label trials. Clinicians have to rely almost exclusively on evidence from studies in western populations to guide their selection of drugs, dosages, interactions, etc. There are likely to be differences in pharmacokinetic and dynamics owing to various genetic, biological factors, which may affect treatment. Other factors, such as treatment seeking and adherence also need to be addressed, as they also have a significant impact on management.

Below is a brief review of the available evidence in pediatric psychopharmacology, including research from lower-resource countries (mostly India), wherever available.

17.6 General Principles of Prescribing for Children

It is not easy or straightforward to formulate principles of prescribing psychotropic medications in children. Many a times, illnesses do not fully evolve, such that "syndromic" diagnosis may be difficult to make. Thus, more often than not, it is "symptoms" that are targeted, rather than underlying disease processes. Also, as presence of comorbidity is a "rule rather than an exception," diagnoses become more complicated.

The dictum for prescribing psychotropics in children has always been "begin with less, go slow and be prepared to end with more." The ideal way to decide the dose is mg/kg per day, but this should be child-specific data and not one extrapolated from adults. Also, even though monotherapy is preferred, polypharmacy may often be required. Off-label use of medications may quite often be necessary. Whether it is monotherapy, polypharmacy, or off-label use of medication, the rationale for including a drug in treatment plan, has to be based on a sound scientific basis.

In addition, regular monitoring of treatment in childhood and adolescence is very important. Ample time for an adequate trial of treatment should be considered, and wherever possible, only one drug at a time has to be changed or modified. Outcomes are better monitored in more than one setting, like home, school, and the playground.

As the aphorism goes, "children are not half, quarter or one-tenth adults," they need to be studied separately for their own data. One cannot just extrapolate data from adults to children. Simple body weight basis of drug dose fixation is not adequate. Pharmacodynamics and pharmacokinetic considerations are important. Most importantly, the possibility that long-term use of certain medications may cause deleterious effects on the developing brain have to be kept in mind, and need to be studied further (Karanges and McGregor 2011; Marrus et al. 2014).

17.7 Pharmacodynamics

Serotonin, dopamine, norepinephrine, and GABAergic networks are the main targets of most currently used psychotropic medications. These neurotransmitter systems undergo numerous developmental changes (Rho and Storey 2001; Chugan et al. 2001), the impact of which may have major implications on the efficacy and tolerability of psychotropics in children. This is evident from various studies, which have shown in children that tricyclic antidepressants have no antidepressant effect (Hazell et al. 1995); stimulants are less likely to produce euphoria; susceptibility to the metabolic side effects of antipsychotics is much higher (Correll et al. 2009); serotonergic antidepressants may induce suicidal ideations and attempts (Hammad et al. 2006; Stone et al. 2009). The relative lack of efficacy and tolerability of methylphenidate in pre-school age children (between 3 and 5 years of age), as compared to older children (Greenhill et al. 2006) also highlights this fact. It is also well known that first-generation antipsychotics produce acute dystonic reactions much more commonly in children and adolescents, especially males, than in adults. This clearly elucidates the need for separate drug trials in younger age groups. Only such evidence can inform rational, safer, and better prescribing and hence better treatment outcomes for children with psychiatric illnesses (Vitiello 2014).

17.8 Pharmacokinetics

Beginning from absorption of the drug till the process of excretion, there are numerous differences between adults and children, which need to be kept in mind while prescribing for children.

Absorption:

Although the extent of drug absorption for most medications is similar in children and adults, the rate of absorption may be faster in children and peak levels are reached earlier. Absorption is also dependent on the form in which it is administered, i.e., liquid versus tablet, and levels peak faster for liquid preparations (Santosh 2009). Ionized drugs (many of which are weak acids) may be less well absorbed from a child's less acid stomach (Taylor 2015).

Metabolism:

The normal rate of hepatic metabolism is high in children until the time of puberty. The result is that most medications are aggressively metabolized in the liver and rapidly excreted. Because what ultimately matters is how much of the drug enters the bloodstream, treatment of pre-pubertal children may require dose that approach or equal those for adults. The use of seemingly high doses for young children may seem counterintuitive to many parents, and thus it will be helpful for clinicians to explain the role of increased rate of drug metabolism.

During the entry into puberty, the rate of hepatic metabolism significantly slows down. For this reason, young children who have been on long-term maintenance doses of psychiatric medications and were tolerating it well may start to have worsening adverse effects around the time of puberty when this lowering of the hepatic metabolic rate occurs. Dosage adjustments may then be required, to minimize side effects (Preston et al. 2015a).

Distribution:

Children differ from adults in the proportions of extracellular water volume and body fat. The proportion of extracellular water decreases substantially from birth through early adolescence, resulting in a relatively larger distribution volume for water-soluble drugs in younger children, who therefore require a relatively higher dose to achieve a comparable plasma concentration (Johnson et al. 2015).

Blood—brain barrier:

The blood–brain barrier is possibly more permeable in children than in adults (Benedetti and Baltes 2003). The greater permeability of the blood–brain barrier in children may mean a greater proportion of the drug reaches the brain in a shorter duration of time, thus leading to greater than predicted efficacy or adverse reactions with smaller dosages (Taylor 2015).

Excretion:

Most psychotropics are eliminated mainly through the kidneys, biliary excretion; and excretion through skin and lungs account for a smaller proportion. It should be noted that although the absolute clearance is usually lower in children than in adults, the weight-adjusted clearance is greater. This is possibly because children have greater renal and liver parenchymal volumes relative to the body size as compared to adults. As the drugs are eliminated faster, plasma half-lives are often of shorter durations in children than in adults. A shorter elimination half-life means that plasma steady state is reached sooner during repeated administration, and that withdrawal symptoms upon discontinuation are more likely. Thus, in children, a more frequent dosing may be needed in order to maintain stable therapeutic levels and avoid withdrawal symptoms between dosing (Vitiello 2014).

17.9 Clinical Guidelines

Unlike in adults, there are very few evidence-based practice guidelines for children. The practice parameters provided by the American Academy of Child and Adolescent Psychiatry (AACAP) are perhaps the most widely used and quoted. The National Institute of Clinical Excellence (NICE) also provides clinical guidelines for most child psychiatric disorders.

The numerous above-mentioned complexities of pharmacokinetic and pharmacodynamic factors always have to be taken into account. In every case, it is necessary that the dose be very gradually titrated against the desired clinical response. Wherever possible, blood levels should be monitored, especially of those medications that have an unpredictable or a narrow therapeutic window. Some of these drug levels, e.g., lithium and anticonvulsants, are very useful in monitoring the optimum dose of the drugs. Maintenance level for lithium is 0.6–1.2 mEq/L. Therapeutic level for carbamazepine is 8–12 ng/ml and for valproic acid is 50–125 μg/ml (Cobert 2013a).

17.10 Preventive Measures to Avoid Drug Interactions

It is important to obtain a detailed medication history including over-the-counter (OTC) drugs and compounds from alternative approaches than modern medicine. As young patients constitute high-risk group, usage drugs with minimum interaction potential is preferred.

Avoid polypharmacy, whenever possible. Educate patient and their families, include written instruction, when appropriate, and keep detailed, updated references on important potential drug interactions (Konar 2005).

17.11 Common Conditions Requiring Pharmacotherapies

Common pharmacotherapies for some of the common pediatric psychiatric disorders are covered here. Readers are also referred to the next chapter in this book written by Dr. Jatinder Singh and Dr. Paramala J. Santosh, which is an excellent review of treatment of neurodevelopmental disorders in children.

Anxiety Disorders

Both cognitive behavioral therapy (CBT) and selective serotonin reuptake inhibitors (SSRIs) are effective treatments for anxiety disorders in children and adolescents. Studies of tricyclic antidepressants (TCAs) have not shown efficacy (Chrzanowski et al. 2014). There is little evidence to support the use of non-antidepressant medication (Vallance and Fernandez 2014). Benzodiazepines should be prescribed only when other pharmacological approaches have failed, or to cover for the latency of onset of action of SSRIs when anxiety is severe. They should be prescribed only for weeks, and not months. Buspirone, a nonbenzodiazepine anxiolytic (5-HT_{1A} partial agonist), has been found to be of comparable efficacy to the benzodiazepines, with fewer adverse events, in several open-label trials in children with anxiety disorders. However, no controlled data are available for either safety or efficacy (Sinita and Coghill 2014).

Obsessive Compulsive Disorder (OCD)

Several randomized controlled studies have established the efficacy of serotonin reuptake inhibitors (clomipramine, fluoxetine, sertraline, fluvoxamine) in the treatment of OCD in children, with no demonstrable superiority of any particular agent apart from clomipramine (Geller et al. 2003; Preston et al. 2015b). The Pediatric OCD Treatment Study (POTS) showed that combined treatment (CBT + sertraline) was superior to either CBT or sertraline alone, there was no treatment emergent suicidality in the study (Franklin et al. 2011).

There are a few studies from India on the clinical profile, course, and outcome of juvenile-onset OCD (Reddy et al. 2010). However, as of yet, there are no studies evaluating its pharmacotherapy.

Autism Spectrum Disorders

A wide range of medications have been tried in autism to improve various target symptoms such as aggression, comorbid disorders such depression and OCD, and also core features such as deficient social communication and stereotypies. These medications include psychotropics (antipsychotics, antidepressants, stimulants) and naltrexone, oxytocin and nutritional supplements just to name a few.

Children who were taking risperidone showed significant improvement in behaviors including aggression, self-injury, and tantrums, and 87 % of risperidone-treated subjects showed global improvement in their conditions, compared to 40 % of subjects treated with placebo. Mean dosage: 1.17 mg/day. Maximum allowable dose: 0.06 mg/kg/day (King and Bostic 2006). As such, risperidone and aripiprazole are the only drugs currently approved by the US FDA for this target symptom domain in children and adolescents with autism (Stigler 2014).

In a double-blind randomized placebo-controlled trial using risperidone in children with autism (Nagaraj et al. 2006), it was found that children in risperidone group showed improvement in the symptoms of social responsiveness, nonverbal communication, hyperactivity, and aggression with few side effects. Another study from India compared 40 children diagnosed with autism randomized to a 16-week trial of either risperidone or fluoxetine. The risperidone group showed significant improvement in irritability and hyperactivity, while the fluoxetine group showed significant improvement in speech deviance, social withdrawal, and stereotypy (Desousa 2010).

Attention-Deficit Hyperactivity Disorder (ADHD)

Neurochemical dysfunction in ADHD is in the dopaminergic and adrenergic systems. Mainstay of treatment is psychostimulants and atomoxetine. Bupropion, modafinil, and TCAs have secondary role in treatment. Clonidine is useful in ADHD with comorbid conduct or oppositional defiant disorder, tic disorders, and sleep disturbances (Prince 2006).

Usual range for methylphenidate is 0.3–0.7 mgs per kg per dose rounded to nearest 2.5 or 5 mgs. In some cases, the dose may need rise to as high as 15 mg of methylphenidate three times a day, before response is seen. Dexamphetamine often has a longer duration of action than methylphenidate, permitting less frequent doses but its disadvantages include greater risk of growth retardation, appetite suppression, compulsive behavior, and higher potential for abuse by the patient's peer and family.

Clonidine is initiated at a dose of 25–50 mcgs at bedtime and the dose is titrated gradually over several weeks up to 150–300 mcg per day in 3–4 divided doses. Pulse and blood pressure should be monitored for bradycardia and hypotension (Santosh 2005).

Atomoxetine is a potent NAergic-specific reuptake inhibitor; is not a stimulant and not a controlled substance (no-abuse). 0.5–1.8 mg/kg/day once daily or bid is the usual dose. The best response in child and adolescents is seen with 1.2–1.8 mg/kg/day. It is well tolerated in long-term follow up of 1 yr. Severe liver injury and failure, has been reported though rare; so the drug must be discontinued if there is jaundice or an increase in liver function parameters. Increased risk of suicidal thinking and behavior in child and adolescents has been reported; weigh risks/benefits before starting; monitor closely for worsening depression or emergence of suicidal thoughts/behaviors especially early in treatment or after increased dose. Monitor for anxiety, agitation, panic attacks, insomnia, irritability, hostility, impulsivity, akathisia, mania, and hypomania. Expect mild increase in pulse and diastolic BP and mild decrease in appetite (Cobert 2013b).

Indian research on pharmacological management in ADHD is surprisingly very sparse. Malhotra and Santosh (1998) showed that buspirone had a favorable side effect profile and significantly reduced the symptoms of ADHD. Another study comparing effects of methylphenidate and atomoxetine showed that treatment response was observed in 90.7 % patients from methylphenidate group and 86.2 % patients of atomoxetine group at an average dose of 0.45 and 0.61 mg/kg/d, respectively (Garg et al. 2014).

Conduct Disorder or Oppositional Defiant Disorder

A crucial part of assessment in children with conduct or oppositional defiant disorder is to determine whether there is an underlying comorbid disorder, especially one of the following: significant situational stress, bipolar disorder, major depression, ADHD, emotional dyscontrol secondary to neurological injury, or substance abuse. The pharmacological treatments used for pure CD only target symptoms such as aggression, irritability, and impulsivity. These medications include atypical antipsychotics such as risperidone, SSRIs, stimulants, clonidine, etc. (Preston et al. 2015c).

Childhood-Onset Schizophrenia (COS)
There is strong evidence for continuity between childhood-onset and adult-onset forms: it is assumed that many treatments used in adults will also apply to children. Typical antipsychotics, like, haloperidol and chlorpromazine can be used. Dystonia, extrapyramidal symptoms (EPS) and akathisia and tardive dyskinesia are the main side effects, which children are likely to be more susceptible to as compared to adults. Atypical antipsychotics, like, risperidone, olanzapine, quetiapine, aripripazole, and clozapine can also be used. With these drugs, tardive dyskinesia (TD) and neuroleptic malignant syndrome (NMS) are rare. Metabolic syndrome and increased prolactin could be some of the important concerns. Investigations are to be routinely pursued (Cobert 2013c). With clozapine, total white blood cell and differential count has to be done at prescribed interval. Evidence has been emerging that clozapine's superiority to other antipsychotics especially in COS may outweigh the risks, and that early initiation of clozapine may lead to better outcomes in COS.

Though research from low resource countries on pharmacological management of COS is sparse, a few studies from India are worthy of a mention. An early study by Bassa (1961) demonstrates the efficacy of trifluoperazine to treat psychosis in children with cerebral palsy. In a 6-week trial of olanzapine in children diagnosed with acute and transient psychotic disorders, 61 and 35 % of children showed marked and good improvement, respectively. (Agarwal and Sitholey 2006). An open trial of clozapine was carried out in five patients with childhood-onset schizophrenia in which it was found that there was improvement in positive symptoms, but not negative symptoms and ritualistic behavior. No side effects such as seizures or leukopenia were encountered in any of the patients (Malhotra et al. 2000). An open-label trial comparing aripiprazole to haloperidol and found both to be equally efficacious, with aripiprazole having significantly lower rates of extrapyramidal symptoms and weight gain (Banerjee et al. 2007).

The Schizophrenia Prodrome
Schizophrenia prodrome can be identified with certain clinical presentations such as:

1. Attenuated positive symptoms
2. Fully psychotic but very brief and intermittent positive symptoms
3. A substantial recent fall in functioning along with genetic risk

Drug treatment of prodromal schizophrenia is controversial. Omega-3 fatty acid or psychotherapies could potentially benefit these children. Atypical antipsychotics in doses lower than those employed for chronic schizophrenia are used sometime. Additional research is needed before the balance of long-term risks and benefits can be decided in support of drug treatment of schizophrenia (Thomas and Woods 2006).

Major Depressive Disorder and Dysthymia

Dysthymia, major depressive disorder in children is usually treated with SSRIs. Though most SSRIs have been studied, fluoxetine and escitalopram are the only ones that are approved by the US FDA for use in children. For psychotic depression, an atypical antipsychotic may be added. SSRIs and suicidality have been one of the most talked about issues in child psychiatry during recent times. In February 2004, the US FDA held meeting with parents. On October 15, 2004, the FDA issued the "Black Box:" warning regarding use of SSRI. Finally on February 9 2005, this warning was made milder (Rey and Martin 2006).

Three important trials of depression in children, TADS (Treatment of Adolescents with Depression Study), TORDIA (Treatment of SSRI-Resistant Depression in Adolescents), and ADAPT (Adolescent Depression and Psychotherapy Trial) found that a combination of medication with CBT was always more efficacious than either treatment alone. The TORDIA study, did not find any difference in efficacy between Venlafaxine and a switch to another SSRI (Brent et al. 2008).

TCAs, on the other hand, have been largely found to be inefficacious for managing depression in pre-adolescent children. Even in adolescents, there might be only marginal efficacy, despite robust evidence in adults (Hazell and Mirzaie 2013).

There again is a lack of data with respect to efficacy and effectiveness of antidepressants in patients with depression from India. One double-blind randomized controlled trial evaluated the usefulness of loading dose of imipramine in treatment of depression in adults, where high bolus doses of imipramine led to reduction in depressive features within 72 h (Malhotra and Santosh 1996). However there is no such data on children and adolescents.

Mania and Bipolar Disorder

Currently available antimanic medications intended to reduce symptoms of, and to prevent the occurrence of, hypo/mania include: (i) lithium, (ii) second-generation antipsychotic medications (SGAs) and (iii) antiepileptic medications (AEDs, for example, valproate and carbamazepine). Recent RCTs support the following conclusions: (i) SGAs are effective, and potentially superior to other antimanic agents, in the treatment of bipolar disorder (BD). However, such medications are associated with significant side effects, most notably impairing weight gain and metabolic abnormalities: (ii) lithium's role in BD children is less clear than in BD adults, though further study is warranted, given studies showing its efficacy in pediatric patients with extreme aggression; and (iii) AEDs may be less efficacious than other antimanic agents for children with BD. For an individual, a stepwise approach is often needed, involving trying different antimanic agents if initial attempts are unsuccessful. The treatment of acute mania may require augmentation with anxiolytic medications for short-term (Leibenluft and Dickstein 2015).

Usual mood stabilizers are lithium carbonate, divalproex sodium, carbamazepine when mania is predominant and lamotrigine when depression is predominant. Atypical antipsychotics are also used as mood stabilizer. Combining is possible (Kowatch and DelBello 2006).

Tic Disorders and Tourette's Syndrome
Some less severe and transient ones will not need medication. Atypical and typical antipsychotics, α-adrenergic agents and brief treatment with clonazepam have been found useful. Haloperidol, olanzapine, risperidone, all in small dose, may be useful. Alpha 2 receptor agonists are less effective, possible adverse effects are drowsiness, headache, irritability, and hypotension. Clonidine and guanfacine both are in use (Cobert 2013d).

Sleep Disorders (Insomnia, Hypersomnolence, Parasomnia)

Insomnia:

Although behavioral interventions should be the primary intervention and have a robust evidence base, exogenous melatonin is now the 'first-line' medication prescribed for childhood insomnia. The effect size for sleep latency is much greater than that for total sleep time, confirming that melatonin is of most use for sleep initiation, rather than sleep maintenance. Though melatonin is a hormone that is produced by the pineal gland in a circadian manner, its therapeutic use is not without side effects. Common side effects include headache, depression, restlessness, confusion, nausea, tachycardia and pruritus. The common dose is between 500 μg and 5 mg. Increasing doses above 5 mg is likely to involve the sedative effects for melatonin, rather than its sleep-phase shifting properties (Jan et al. 1999).

Parasomnias:

Sleep terror disorder and sleepwalking disorder occur in the transition from deep delta-wave sleep to light sleep. Benzodiazepines may be effective in these disorders. They work by reducing both delta-wave sleep and arousals between sleep stages. The medications should be used temporarily and only in severe cases, because tolerance to the medications develops. Cessation of these medications can lead to severe rebound worsening of the disorders, and reducing delta sleep in children may have deleterious effects (Sadock et al. 2015a, b).

Parasomnias like sleep walking, sleep talking, and night terrors are usually treated with benzodiazepines and tricyclic antidepressant (Santosh 2005).

Hypersomnolence:

Modafinil and stimulants can be used for hypersomnolence (Stahl 2014).

Enuresis
Patients can be treated with medicine when behavioral treatments fail. Imipramine and DDAVP (1-desamine-8-D-arginine-vasopressin) are commonly used in enuresis. Imipramine and amitriptyline have been used in the treatment of encopresis (Cobert 2013e). Two open-label trials from India evaluated the usefulness of imipramine in enuresis (Chatterjee and Khandpur 1965) and behaviorally disturbed children (Mahendru et al. 1970) and reported positive results with few side effects.

Substance Use Disorders in Adolescents
Psychopharmacological interventions for adolescent alcohol and drug users are still in their early stages (Sadock et al. 2015a, b). The mainstay of treatment of substance use disorders in adolescence, as in adults, continues to be non-pharmacological treatment. However, medication can play an important role. It should be noted that medications for substance abuse have been studied almost exclusively in adults, so that suggested uses are based on extrapolation from adult data and must be viewed with caution (Preston et al. 2015c).

17.12 Common and Useful Pharmacotherapies

In order to be a good practitioner of child and adolescence psychiatry, some of the more useful drugs for children need to be understood in greater detail.

Stimulants and Other ADHD Medications
Stimulants are sympathomimetic drugs that act by enhancing dopaminergic and noradrenergic transmission in the prefrontal cortex. Methylphenidate is the most commonly used stimulant in India, while Dexmethamphetamine and Lisdexmethamphetamine are not available in the market. As pharmacokinetics plays a key role in the effectiveness of stimulants, there is a range of formulation options (plain, sustained release and extended release) with half-lives ranging from four to about 12 h. Commonly reported side effects are anorexia, insomnia, headaches, dysphoria, and gastrointestinal upset. There is also controversy that long-term use of stimulants may cause a delay or stunting of growth. Other rare side effects include arrhythmias, seizures, worsening of tics, hallucinations, etc. Although rare, in some specific individuals sudden cardiac death has been reported when using stimulants. However, currently, no routine pretreatment cardiology evaluation is indicated unless the patient has a cardiac disorder and/or symptoms.

Atomoxetine, selective inhibitor of presynaptic norepinephrine transporters, also increases dopamine and norepinephrine in prefrontal cortex. Despite a plasma half-life of just four hours, it is effective in treating ADHD for 24 h. Though not as efficacious as stimulants (effect size 0.9), atomoxetine has an effect size of 0.6–0.7, with a latency of around 6–8 weeks to its onset of action (Banaschewski et al. 2006). Sedation, fatigue, somnolence, and dizziness, along with anorexia, weight loss, nausea and gastrointestinal symptoms are the common side effects. Nonclinical elevations in heart rate and blood pressure have also been seen. Treatment emergent suicidal thinking has also been reported, for which the FDA has issued a black box warning.

The α–adrenergic agents (clonidine and guanfacine) are presynaptic adrenergic agonists that appear to stimulate inhibitory presynaptic autoreceptors in the central nervous system. Although most commonly used in Tourette's disorder and ADHD, these agents may be useful in controlling aggression, particularly in patients with developmental disorders. Sedation, hypotension, dry mouth, depression, and confusion are potential side effects. Abrupt withdrawal can result in rebound hypertension. Guanfacine appears to be less sedating and to have a longer duration of action than clonidine (DeMaso and Walter 2011).

Antidepressants

Antidepressant drugs act on pre- and post-synaptic receptors affecting the release and reuptake of brain neurotransmitters, including norepinephrine, serotonin, and dopamine. Major depressive disorder, anxiety disorders, and obsessive compulsive disorders are the three main indications.

SSRIs are generally the first-line of antidepressants used for most patients, as on the whole they have a favorable safety profile and minimal cardiovascular effects. Common side effects include gastrointestinal symptoms, headaches, irritability, restlessness insomnia, appetite changes and diaphoresis. Withdrawal or "discontinuation" symptoms are more common in short-acting SSRIs such as paroxetine and fluvoxamine. Reports of behavioral activation along suicidal thoughts warrant close monitoring for these adverse effects, especially in the first few weeks of treatment.

The TCAs have a broader mechanism of action, blocking both serotonin, and norepinephrine reuptake (e.g., clomipramine is primarily serotonergic; imipramine is both noradrenergic and serotonergic), along with anticholinergic and antihistaminic effects. The use of TCAs in children has declined significantly after the advent of SSRIs, and meta-analyses showing lack of efficacy studies (particularly in depression). They have a narrow therapeutic index, with overdoses being potentially fatal. Anticholinergic symptoms (e.g., dry mouth, blurred vision, and constipation) are the most common side effects. TCAs can have cardiac conduction effects in doses higher than 3.5 mg/kg. Blood pressure and electrocardiographic monitoring are indicated at doses above this level. The few common indications in children for which TCAs are used nowadays are obsessive compulsive disorder (clomipramine), enuresis (imipramine), and certain pain disorders (amitriptyline and nortriptyline).

The atypical antidepressants include bupropion, venlafaxine, and trazodone; they are second-line medications for anxiety and depressive disorders. Bupropion has also been used for smoking cessation and ADHD. Bupropion appears to have an indirect mixed agonist effect on dopamine and norepinephrine transmission. Common side effects include irritability, nausea, anorexia, headache, and insomnia. Venlafaxine has both serotonergic and noradrenergic properties. Side effects are similar to SSRIs, including irritability, insomnia, headaches, anorexia, nervousness, dizziness, and blood pressure changes (DeMaso and Walter 2011).

Anxiolytic Agents

Anxiolytic agents (including lorazepam, clonazepam, buspirone, and hydroxyzine) have all been effectively used for acute situational anxiety. Their efficacy as chronic medication is poorer, particularly when used as a monotherapy agent (DeMaso and Walter 2011).

Antipsychotics

Based on their mechanism of action, antipsychotic medication can be divided into typical (blocking dopamine D2 receptor) and atypical (mixed dopaminergic and serotoninergic activity) agents.

Atypical antipsychotics have lesser binding at the D2 receptors but relatively strong antagonistic effects with 5-HT2 receptors. Variable activity at central adrenergic, cholinergic, and histaminic sites account for the varying side effects noted among these agents. These medications have an evidence base for the treatment for psychotic disorders, moderate to severe agitation, and increasingly for monotherapy in bipolar disorder. The most commonly used medications of this class are risperidone, olanzapine, quetiapine, amisulpiride, aripiprazole, and clozapine. Common side effects of these medications include sedation, weight gain, and metabolic syndrome, extrapyramidal symptoms (e.g., restlessness and dyskinesias), hyperprolactinemia. Rare side effects include hematologic adverse effects (e.g., leukopenia or neutropenia), seizures, hepatotoxicity, neuroleptic malignant syndrome, and cardiovascular effects (QTc) prolongation. Monitoring metabolic profile, which includes weight, body mass index and waist circumference, blood pressure, fasting blood glucose, fasting lipid profiles, is essential while using atypical antipsychotics.

Typical (first-generation) antipsychotics that are still in use are haloperidol, chlorpromazine, trifluoperazine, and pimozide. The most commonly used amongst these is haloperidol, which is a high-potency butyrophenone. Its main indications are psychosis, Tourette's syndrome, and severe agitation. Side effects are drowsiness and extrapyramidal symptoms (dystonia, rigidity, tremor, and akathisia) and NMS. There is a risk of tardive dyskinesia with chronic administration (DeMaso and Walter 2011). As earlier mentioned, children are much more susceptible to both EPS and tardive dyskinesia, so these agents are preferably avoided or used with extreme caution.

Mood Stabilizers

Several medications have been shown to be potentially helpful in children experiencing significant mood instability and/or mania, although the evidence base is again sparse.

Lithium's mechanism of action is not well understood, though proposed theories relate to neurotransmission, endocrine effects, circadian rhythm, and cellular processes. Common side effects include polyuria and polydipsia and central nervous system symptoms (tremor, somnolence, and memory impairment). Periodic monitoring of lithium levels along with thyroid and renal function is needed. Lithium serum levels of 0.8–1.2 mEq/L are targeted for acute episodes and 0.6–0.9 mEq/L are targeted for maintenance therapy.

Valproic acid is an anticonvulsant with some evidence supporting its use in the treatment of mania. The therapeutic plasma concentration range is 50–100 μg/ml. Common side effects include sedation, gastrointestinal symptoms, and hair thinning. Idiosyncratic bone marrow suppression and liver toxicity have been reported, necessitating monitoring of blood counts as well as liver and kidney function.

Lamotrigine is another anticonvulsant that may be useful in the treatment of adolescent bipolar depression. It has been associated with potentially life-threatening Stevens-Johnson syndrome (DeMaso and Walter 2011).

17.13 Specific Issues Related to Pediatric Pharmacology

A few pertinent issues in the treatment of children and adolescents need discussion. First is the diagnosis versus target symptom approach. Though a categorical approach to diagnosis is easier to use; a dimensional approach by rating target symptoms that are functionally impairing may be a better approach to deal with the clinical situation. In child psychiatry, two common encountered circumstances favor a target symptom approach, when the disorder is poorly defined or when there are several comorbid conditions. Effective pharmacotherapists should be mindful of this, and should as much as possible, use medication to treat underlying disease states while regularly monitoring target symptoms as an index of progress (Bostic and Rho 2006). One cannot over emphasize the need for a good diagnosis, to the best of our understanding and ability, keeping differential diagnoses in mind and giving careful attention to comorbidities. These are a must in tailoring a rational prescription for the child.

Therapeutic alliance is a bit more complicated in the context of child psychiatry. Clinicians should strive to include both the child and his or her parents/guardian into the working alliance, and involve all of them in treatment plan (Joshi 2006). One should also keep in mind the need for autonomy in older children and adolescents, and be respectful of the same.

Children's concept about medications is also to be acknowledged and addressed. They may be concerned about "physical properties" of the medication itself like name, form, size, color, taste, etc. This may lead to certain wrong kind of notions about medicine. They may also harbor beliefs that only children who are "sick" or "bad" have to be on medications. Dosing schedules (like, morning, evening or during school dosage) also have to be kept in mind (Joshi 2006), to ensure availability of parents or guardians.

As earlier mentioned, comorbidity is more a rule than exception in children. For example, intellectual disability, autism, ADHD, ODD, epilepsy, anxiety disorders, depression, all come in different combinations of one another. Greater awareness of this has led to a dramatic increase in the use of polypharmacy in children. One has to be more cautious, look at drug interactions because children have a much higher propensity for seizure and EPS.

Adverse events are more likely when multiple drugs are used, and interactions can be unpredictable. Combining drugs from the same pharmacological class is rarely indicated, except when cross-tapering when switching drugs. Combining drugs can be rational when their pharmacological actions are complementary, although the side effect burden is usually higher. Examples include quetiapine augmentation of SSRIs to treat depression where there is good RCT evidence or a second antipsychotic with clozapine for poor response in treatment resistant schizophrenia. If a second drug is added to counteract an adverse effect, strong justification is needed for not swapping drug if drugs are from the same broad class (e.g., aripiprazole to reduce raised prolactin caused by another antipsychotic). A careful weighing of risks and benefits is required if they are from different classes (e.g., antimuscarinic drugs for EPSE on antipsychotics). Polypharmacy requires pharmacological expertise and should usually be supervised by a specialist (Haddad and Wieck 2016).

17.14 Conclusion

Our basic commitment is to the patient, whom we should be treating "as a whole" and not just the disease or symptoms. We must remember, pharmacotherapy, no matter how effective, should only be a part of a larger, multimodal treatment plan.

Equal consideration must be given to all aspect of child's life-like psychosocial, educational, and family interventions. Almost every major clinical trial and practice guideline has shown that combination treatments are more effective. Though this may not be feasible in most settings in low resource countries, clinicians should work toward equipping themselves or developing an infrastructure for the same.

There is great concern today that children are being over treated with medication, especially in the US (Rapoport 2013). By contrast, many countries make so little use of medications, that it very likely that many children who could profit have no access to it or do not receive it. Undertreatment is perhaps a bigger problem globally than overmedication.

Great international differences in the use of psychopharmacological agents stem from differences in professional and cultural attitudes. In the light of these differences, clinicians need to always try and formulate treatment plans that are empirically informed and evidence based. As research in the field of pediatric psychopharmacology has been expanding rapidly over the last decade, it has become more important for clinicians to stay apace with the latest developments. In addition, pediatric pharmacovigilance for psychotropic agents are essential and more studies on efficacy in this population is necessary (Santosh 2009).

Research from low resource countries in this area has been very meager, though is likely to emerge in the next few years. With limited availability of professionals, the developing economies need to keep their focus on training professionals, developing infrastructure to enhance service delivery to reach to the widest population.

References

Agarwal, V., & Sitholey, P. (2006). A preliminary open trial of olanzapine in pediatric acute and transient psychotic disorders. *Indian Journal of Psychiatry, 48*, 43–46.

Banaschewski, T., et al. (2006). Long-acting medications for the hyperkinetic disorders: A systematic review and European treatment guideline. *European Child and Adolescent Psychiatry, 15*, 476–495.

Banerjee, M., Ram, D., & Das, A. (2007). An open label comparison of aripiprazole versus haloperidol for the treatment of childhood and adolescent psychotic disorders. *Indian Journal of Psychiatry, 49*(Suppl), 3.

Bassa, O. M. (1961). Some early observations on the use of Trufluoperazine (Eskazine) in children. *Indian Journal of Psychiatry, 3*, 243–250.

Becker, A. E., & Kleinman, A. (2014). In J. P. Raynaud, S. H. F. Gau, & M. Hodes (Eds.). *Mental health and global agenda, from research to practice in child and adolescent mental health* (pp. 3–14). New York: Rowman & Littlefield.

Benedetti, S. M., & Baltes, E. L. (2003). Drug metabolism and disposition in children. *Fundamental and Clinical Pharmacology, 17*, 281–299.

Bostic, J. Q., & Rho, Y. (2006). Target symptom psychopharmacology: Between the forest and trees. *Child and Adolescent Psychiatric Clinic of North America, 15*, 289–302.

Brent, D., Emslie, G., Clarke, G., Wagner, K. D., Asarnow, J. R., Keller, M., et al. (2008). Switching to another SSRI or to venlafaxine with or without cognitive behavioral therapy for adolescents with SSRI-resistant depression. *JAMA, the Journal of the American Medical Association, 299*(8), 901–913.

Chatterjee, A. K., & Khandpur, S. S. (1965). Tofranil in enuresis of children. *Indian Journal of Psychiatry, 7*, 243–245.

Chrzanowski, D. T., Guthrie, E. B., Perkins, M. B., & Rynn, M. A. (2014). In J. L. Cutler (Ed.), *Child and adolescent psychiatry* (3rd ed., p. 489). Oxford: Oxford University Press.

Chugan, D. C., Muzik, O., Juhasz, C., et al. (2001). Postnatal maturation of human GABAA receptors measured with positron emission tomography. *Annals of Neurology, 49*, 618–626.

Cobert, J. (2013a). *Laboratory and diagnostic testing, assessment and diagnosis, tarascon pediatric psychiatrica*. Burlington MA: Jones & Bartlett Learning. 47.

Cobert, J. (2013b). *Attention deficit hyperactivity disorder, psychiatric disorder, tarascon pediatric psychiatrica* (pp. 83–98). Burlington MA: Jones & Bartlett Learning.

Cobert, J. (2013c). *Childhood schizophrenia, psychiatric disorders, tarascon pediatric psychiatrica* (pp. 130–152). Burlington MA: Jones & Bartlett Learning.

Cobert, J. (2013d). *Tic disorders, disorder affecting somatic functions, tarascon pediatric psychiatrica* (pp. 225–226). Burlington MA: Jones & Bartlett Learning.

Cobert, J. (2013e). *Disorder of elimination: Enuresis and encopresis, disorder affecting somatic functions, tarascon pediatric psychiatrica* (pp. 226–229). Burlington MA: Jones & Bartlett Learning.

Coghill, D., & Sinita, E. (2014). In S. Huline-Dickens (Ed.), *Pharmacology for attention deficit hyperactivity disorder, tourette syndrome and autism spectrum disorder, clinical topics in child and adolescent psychiatry* (p. 74). Glasgow, UK: Bell & Brain Limited.

Correll, C. U., Gerhard, T., & Olfson, M. (2013). Prescribing of psychotropic medications to children and adolescents: Quo vadis? *World psychiatry, 12*(2), 127–128.

Correll, C. U., Manu, P., Olshanskiy, V., et al. (2009). Cardiometabolic risk of second-generation antipsychotic medications during first-time use in children and adolescents. *Journal of the American Medical Association, 302*, 1765–1773.

DeMaso, D. R., & Walter, H. J. (2011). In Kliegman et al. (Eds.), *Psychopharmacology, Nelson textbook of pediatrics* (19th ed, pp. 60–65). Philadelphia: Saunders, Elsevier.

Desousa, A. (2010). An open-label trial of risperidone and fluoxetine in children with autistic disorder. *Indian Journal of Psychological Medicine, 32*(1), 17–21.

Franklin, M. E., Sapyta, J., Freeman, J. B., Khanna, M., Compton, S., Almirall, D., et al. (2011). Cognitive behavior therapy augmentation of pharmacotherapy in pediatric obsessive-compulsive disorder: The pediatric OCD treatment study II (POTS II) randomized controlled trial. *JAMA, 306*(11), 1224–1232.

Garg, J., Arun, P., & Chavan, B. S. (2014). Comparative short term efficacy and tolerability of methylphenidate and atomoxetine in attention deficit hyperactivity disorder. *Indian Pediatrics, 51*(7), 550–554.

Geller, D. A., Biederman, J., Stewart, S. E., Mullin, B., Martin, A., Spencer, T., & Faraone, S. V. (2003). Which SSRI? A meta-analysis of pharmacotherapy trials in pediatric obsessive-compulsive disorder. *The American Journal of Psychiatry, 160*(11), 1919–1928.

Greenhill, L. L., Abikoff, H., Chuang, S., et al. (2006). Efficacy and safety of immediate-release methylphenidate treatment for preschoolers with ADHD. *Journal of the American Academy of Child and Adolescent Psychiatry, 45*, 1284–1293.

Haddad, P. M., & Wieck, A. (2016). Prescribing in clinical practice. In I. M. Anderson & R. H. M. Williams (Eds.), *Fundamentals of clinical psychopharmacology* (pp. 215–217). CRC Press.

Hammad, T. A., Laughren, T., & Racoosin, J. (2006). Suicidality in pediatric patients treated with antidepressant drugs. *Archives of General Psychiatry, 63*, 332–339.

Hazell, P., O'Connell, D., Heathcote, D. et al. (1995). Efficacy of tricyclic drugs in treating child and adolescent depression: a meta-analysis. *British Medical Journal, 310*, 897–901.

Hazell, P., & Mirzaie, M. (2013). Tricyclic drugs for depression in children and adolescents. *The cochrane database of systematic reviews, 18*, CD002317.

Huline-Dickens, S. (Ed.). (2014). *Clinical topics in child and adolescent psychiatry* (p. XXI). Glasgow, UK: Bell & Brain Limited.

Jan, J. E., Freeman, R. D., & Fast, D. K. (1999). Melatonin treatment of sleep–wake cycle disorders in children and adolescents. *Developmental Medicine and Child Neurology, 41*(7), 491–500.

Johnson, M. R., Hatzis, N. M., Dulcan, M. K., Crawford, G. C., & Cozza, S. J. (2015). In R. E. Hales, S. C. Yudofsky, L. W. Roberts (Eds.), *Treatment of children and adolescent, text book of psychiatry* (6th ed., p. 1192). Washington, D.C., London: American Psychiatric Publishing.

Joshi, S. V. (2006). Team work: The therapeutic alliance in pediatric pharmacotherapy. *Child and Adolescent Psychiatric Clinic of North America, 15*, 239–262.

Karanges, E., & McGregor, I. (2011). Antidepressants and adolescent brain development. *Future Neurology, 6*, 783–808.

Kessler, R. C., Avenevoli, S., Costello, J., Green, J. G., Gruber, M. J., McLaughlin, K. A., et al. (2012). Severity of 12-month DSM-IV disorders in the national comorbidity survey replication adolescent supplement. *Archives of General Psychiatry, 69*(4), 381–389.

Kessler, R. C., Berglund, P., Demler, O., Jin, R., Merikangas, K. R., & Walters, E. E. (2005). Lifetime prevalence and age-of-onset distributions of DSM-IV disorders in the national comorbidity survey replication. *Archives of General Psychiatry, 62*(6), 593–602.

King, B. H., & Bostic, J. Q. (2006). An update on pharmacologic treatments for autism spectrum disorders. *Child and Adolescent Psychiatric Clinic of North America*, 161–175.

Konar, D. (2005). In S. Malhotra (Ed.), *Mental disorders in children and adolescents needs and strategies for intervention* (pp. 132–137). Delhi: CSB Publishers & Distributors.

Kowatch, R. A., & DelBello, M. P. (2006). Pediatric bipolar disorder: Emerging diagnostic and treatment approaches. *Child and Adolescent Psychiatric Clinic of North America, 15*, 73–108.

Leibenluft, E., & Dickstein, D. P. (2015). Bipolar disorder in childhood (Chapter 62). In A. Thapar et al. (Ed.). *Rutter's child and adolescent psychiatry* (6th ed., pp. 866–867). Wiley Blackwell.

Mahendru, B. K., Gupta, S. C., Agarwal, A. K., & Sethi, B. B. (1970). Imipramine as an effective tool in the management of behavioural disorders in children. *Indian Journal of Psychiatry, 12*, 238–243.

Malhotra, S., & Banerjee, A. (2009a). Research in child and adolescent psychiatry in India Part I: Psychaitric disorders. In V. K. Varma, A. K. Kala, N. Gupta (Eds.), *Culture, personality and mental illness: A perspective of traditional societies* (pp. 298–322). Jaypee Brothers.

Malhotra, S., & Banerjee, A. (2009b). Research in child and adolescent psychiatry in India Part II: Assessment, intervention and services. In V. K. Varma, A. K. Kala, N. Gupta (Eds.), *Culture, personality and mental illness: A perspective of traditional societies* (pp. 323–341). Jaypee Brothers.

Malhotra, S., Chakrabarti, S., Shah, R., Mehta, A., Gupta, A., & Sharma, M. (2015). A novel screening and diagnostic tool for child and adolescent psychiatric disorders for telepsychiatry. *Indian Journal of Psychological Medicine, 37*(3), 288–298.

Malhotra, S., Gupta, N., & Singh, G. (2000). Clozapine in childhood-onset schizophrenia: A report of five cases. *Clinical Child Psychology and Psychiatry, 5*, 403–410.

Malhotra, S., & Kate, N. (2015a). Research endeavours in child psychiatry in India-I. In Malhotra & Chakrabarti (Eds.), *Developments in psychiatry in India: Clinical, research and policy perspectives* (pp 215–232). India: Springer.

Malhotra, S., & Kate, N. (2015b). Research endeavours in child psychiatry in India-II. In Malhotra & Chakrabarti (Eds.), *Developments in psychiatry in India: Clinical, research and policy perspectives* (pp. 233–254). India: Springer.

Malhotra, S., & Padhy, S. K. (2015). Challenges in providing child and adolescent psychiatric services in low resource countries. *Child and adolescent psychiatric clinics of North America, 24*(4), 777–797.

Malhotra, S., & Patra, B. N. (2014). Prevalence of child and adolescent psychiatric disorders in India: a systematic review and meta-analysis. *Child and Adolescent Psychiatry and Mental Health, 8*, 22.

Malhotra, S., & Santosh, P. J. (1996). Loading dose imipramine—New approach to pharmacotherapy of melancholic depression. *Journal of Psychiatric Research, 30*, 51–58.

Malhotra, S., & Santosh, P. J. (1998). An open clinical trial of buspirone in children with attention-deficit/hyperactivity disorder. *Journal of the American Academy of Child and Adolescent Psychiatry, 37*(4), 364–371.

Marrus, N., Bell, M., & Luby, J. L. (2014). Psychotropic medications and their effect on brain volumes in childhood psychopathology. *Child and Adolescent Psychopharmacology News, 19*(2), 1–8.

Nagaraj, R., Singhi, P., & Malhi, P. (2006). Risperidone in children with autism: Randomized, placebo-controlled, double-blind study. *Journal of Child Neurology, 21*, 450–455.

Preston, J. D., O'Neal, J. H., & Talaga, M. C. (2015a). Issue in psychopharmacological treatment of children and adolescents. *Child and adolescent clinical psychopharmacology made simple* (3rd ed., p. 9). New Harbinger Publications, Inc.

Preston, J. D., O'Neal, J. H., & Talaga, M. C. (2015b). Anxiety disorder. *Child and adolescent clinical psychopharmacology made simple* (3rd ed., pp. 59–60). New Harbinger Publications, Inc.

Preston, J. D., O'Neal, J. H., & Talaga, M. C. (2015c). Miscellaneous disorders. *Child and adolescent clinical psychopharmacology made simple* (3rd ed., pp. 101–114). New Harbinger Publications, Inc.

Prince, J. B. (2006). Pharmacotherapy of attention deficit hyperactivity disorder in children and adolescents: Update on new stimulant preparations, atomoxetine and novel treatments. *Child and Adolescent Psychiatric Clinic of North America, 15*, 13–50.

Rapoport, J. L. (2013). Pediatric psychopharmacology: Too much or too little? *World Psychiatry, 12*(2), 118–123.

Reddy, Y. C. J., Rao, N. P., & Khanna, S. (2010). An overview of Indian research in obsessive compulsive disorder. *Indian Journal of Psychiatry, 52*(Suppl 1), S200–S209.

Rey, J. M., & Martin, A. (2006). SSRIs and suicidality in juveniles: Review of the evidence and implications for clinical practice. *Child and Adolescent Psychiatric Clinic of North America, 15*, 221–237.

Rho, J. M., & Storey, T. W. (2001). Molecular ontogeny of major neurotransmitter receptor systems in the mammalian central nervous system: Norepinephrine, dopamine, serotonin, acetylcholine, and glycine. *Journal of Child Neurology, 16*, 271–279.

Sadock, J. B., Sadock, V. A., & Ruiz, P. (2015a). *Pharmacotherapy, child psychiatry, synopsis of psychiatry (Behavioral science and clinical psychiatry)* (11th ed., p. 1300). USA: Wolters Kluwer.

Sadock, J. B., Sadock, V. A., & Ruiz, P. (2015b). *Adolescent substance abuse, child psychiatry, synopsis of psychiatry (Behavioral science and clinical psychiatry)* (11th ed., p. 1278). USA: Wolters Kluwer.

Santosh, P. J. (2005). Pharmacotherapy of psychiatric disorder in childhood and adolescence. In S. Malhotra (Ed.), *Mental disorders in children and adolescents need and strategies for intervention* (pp. 138–167). Delhi: CSB Publishers & Distributors.

Santosh, P. J. (2009). Medication for children and adolescents: Current issues. In M. G. Gelder, N. C. Andreasen, J. J. Lopez-Ibor Jr, & J. R. Geddes (Eds.), *New oxford textbook of psychiatry* (2nd ed., Vol. 2, pp. 1793–1799). Oxford: Oxford University Press.

Shrivastava, S. R., Shrivastava, P. S., & Ramasamy, J. (2013). Childhood and adolescence: Challenges in mental health. *Journal of the Canadian Academy of Child and Adolescent Psychiatry, 22*(2), 84–85.

Sinita, E., & Coghill, D. (2014). Pharmacology for anxiety and obsessive—compulsive disorders, affective disorders and schizophrenia. In S. Huline-Dickens (Ed.), *Clinical topics in child and adolescent psychiatry* (pp. 94–95). Glasgow, UK: Bell & Brain Limited.

Stahl, S. M. (2014). *Essential psychopharmacology, prescriber's guide* (5th ed., pp. 466–469). Cambridge: Cambridge University Press.

Stigler, K. A. (2014). Psychopharmacologic management of serious behavioral disturbance in ASD. *Child and Adolescent Clinic of North America*, 73–82.

Stone, M., Laughren, T., & Jones, M. L. (2009). Risk of suicidality in clinical trials of antidepressants in adults: Analysis of proprietary data submitted to US food and drug administration. *British Medical Journal, 339*, b2880.

Stroeh, O., & Trivedi, H. K. (2012). Appropriate and judicious use of psychotropic medications in youth. *Child and Adolescent Psychiatric Clinics of North America, 21*(4), 703–711.

Taylor, E. (2015). Pharmacological, medically–led and related treatments (Chapter 43). In A. Thapar et al. (Ed.), *Rutter's child and adolescent psychiatry* (6th ed., p. 564). Wiley Blackwell.

Thomas, L. E., & Woods, S. W. (2006). The schizophrenia prodrome: A developmentally informed review and update for psychopharmacologic treatment. *Child and Adolescent Psychiatric Clinic of North America, 15*, 109–133.

Vallance, A. K., & Fernandez, V. (2014). Anxiety disorder. In S. Huline-Dickens (Ed.), *Clinical topics in child and adolescent psychiatry* (p. 178). Glasgow, UK: Bell & Brain Limited.

Vitiello, B. (2006). An update on publicly funded multisite trials in pediatric psychopharmacology. *Child and Adolescent Psychiatric Clinic of North America, 15*, 1–12.

Vitiello, B. (2014). Principles in using psychotropic medication in children and adolescents (Chapter A.7). In M. Rey Joseph (Ed.), *IACAPAP text book of child and adolescents mental health* (pp. 7–8). Geneva: International Association for Child and Adolescent Psychiatry and Allied Professions, IACAPAP.

Zito, J. M., Safer, D. J, de Jong-van den Berg, L. T., et al. (2008). A three-country comparison of psychotropic medication prevalence in youth. *Child and Adolescent Psychiatry and Mental Health, 2*, 26.

Chapter 18
Psychopharmacology of Neurodevelopmental Disorders in Children

Jatinder Singh and Paramala Santosh

Abstract Recent advances in genetics and psychopharmacology have begun to illuminate the key players that contribute to neurodevelopmental disorders in children such as attention deficit hyperactivity disorder (ADHD), autism spectrum disorder (ASD), Tourette's syndrome (TS) and rare diseases such as Rett syndrome (RTT). Clinical guidelines and data from clinical trials mainly focus on management of single disorders whilst most patients present with multiple, chronic, co-occurring developmental disorders. Neurodevelopmental disorders often present with a myriad of neuropsychiatric, emotional and behavioural problems and have neurochemical and neuro-circuitry problems underpinning this. Evidence from meta-analyses have indicated the efficacy of different treatments and some studies show benefit in improving co-occurring symptoms in children with ADHD, ASD or TS. It is increasingly being recognized that emotional, behavioural and autonomic dysregulation (EBAD) is central to difficult presentations in children and adolescents with rare diseases, and those with multiple co-occurring disorders. An incremental treatment approach should be adopted starting with non-pharmaceutical intervention followed by implementation of drug treatments. When drug treatments are used, a multimodal treatment strategy to neurodevelopmental disorders in children should be used in order to provide flexible medication regimens where one is able to select and adjust medication that achieves maximum benefit with the least possible side effects so that treatment can be personalized. Cross-lifespan approaches and web-based clinical and research medication-monitoring systems, such as the HealthTracker™, an e-health web-based platform, can assist in the triaging and management of cases across specialist and community clinics.

J. Singh · P. Santosh
Department of Child and Adolescent Psychiatry, Institute of Psychiatry, Psychology and Neuroscience (IoPPN), King's College London, London, UK

P. Santosh (✉)
Centre for Interventional Paediatric Psychopharmacology and Rare Diseases (CIPPRD), National and Specialist Child and Adolescent Mental Health Services,Michael Rutter Centre, Maudsley Hospital, London, UK
e-mail: paramala.1.santosh@kcl.ac.uk

S. Malhotra and P. Santosh (eds.), *Child and Adolescent Psychiatry*,
DOI 10.1007/978-81-322-3619-1_18

Pharmacological management of neurodevelopmental disorders can present with challenges in Asia, where many of the commonly used medications such as stimulants are more difficult to access. Recent advances in the treatment of ADHD, ASD and TS in children are presented and when applicable discussed in line with experiences from Asia. Innovative strategies working with children and families such as the effective dosing with minimum side effects (EDMS) strategy, and the use of wearable sensor technology to assist in the management of a patient with RTT are described.

Keywords Attention deficit hyperactivity disorder (ADHD) · Autism spectrum disorder (ASD) · Effective dosing with minimum side effects (EDMS) strategy · Emotional behavioural and autonomic dysregulation (EBAD) · HealthTracker™ · Psychopharmacology · Rett syndrome (RTT) · Tourette's syndrome (TS) · Web-based health monitoring · Wearable sensor technology

18.1 Introduction

Neurodevelopmental disorders such as attention deficit hyperactivity disorder (ADHD), autism spectrum disorder (ASD) and Tourette's syndrome (TS) are multifactorial disorders and some of their symptoms can be attributed to abnormalities in neurotransmitter pathways within the central nervous system. These abnormalities can manifest in impediments in social, personal and academic function. Research into ADHD, ASD and TS has proceeded at a geometric rate and whilst the precise molecular targets remain to be elucidated, recent genetic advances have paved the way for genetic variants that predispose certain individuals with an increased risk of neurodevelopmental disorders. Despite this, there is a general notion that phenotypically the clinical picture remains blurred and common molecular and genetic targets across disorders have not yet been identified. To broach this conundrum, some recent evidence has shed light on characterizing the genetic loci for complex neuropsychiatric disorders as was shown for schizophrenia and components of the complement cascade (Sekar et al. 2016).

In this chapter, the pertinent observations of neurodevelopmental disorders in children will be focused upon with an emphasis on the psychopharmacology of ADHD, ASD and TS in children. Increasingly, managing emotional, behavioural and autonomic dysregulation (EBAD) is becoming central to improving the quality of life in individuals with neuropsychiatric disorders such as Rett syndrome (RTT) (see Sect. 18.6.1). We describe novel strategies such as the effective dosing with minimum side effects (EDMS), and the use of wearable sensor technology to assist in managing a patient with RTT. The need for low-dose initiation with gradual increase of dosage, and frequent monitoring of impact of medication in children and adolescents will be emphasized. Specific issues that affect pharmacological and non-pharmacological interventions in Asia are highlighted as necessary.

18.2 The Art of Prescribing Medication

To begin with, apart from the chemical effect, the response to medication also depends on an inherent 'placebo response', as well as the 'therapeutic alliance' achieved by obtaining agreement and acceptance of why the medication is prescribed and what is the expected response. The role of the prescriber is to make the patient/parents/carers feel understood and jointly agree the treatment plan, that is, there is concordance between the world view of the clinician, patient, parents/carers, regarding the illness and its treatment. Treatment regimen(s) should be closely monitored with medication given in small doses, gradually increased and monitored for adverse effects regularly.

18.3 Attention Deficit Hyperactivity Disorder (ADHD)

Attention deficit hyperactivity disorder (ADHD) according to the Diagnostic and Statistical Manual of Mental Disorders (DSM-5) (DSM-5 2013) or Hyperkinetic Disorder (HKD) according to the International Classification of diseases (ICD-10) [10th edition; ICD-10, World Health Organization (WHO 1992)] is a common condition characterized by inattention and hyperactivity/impulsivity, with a strong genetic component, that is present in the child population on a continuum of severity. Hyperkinetic Disorder is a narrower diagnosis, which requires the presence of inattention, impulsivity <u>and</u> hyperactivity, with symptoms starting before the age of 6 years and being present in more than one setting. The presence of another disorder, such as anxiety or depression, is in itself an exclusion criterion—the expectation is that most cases will have a single diagnosis. This restricted categorization makes HKD a subgroup of the broader ADHD group and could be considered as 'severe ADHD'. ADHD typically occurs with a prevalence of about 3–5 % and HKD around 1.5 %. Specific guidelines for the treatment of ADHD are presented elsewhere (National Institute for Health and Care Excellence [NICE] guidelines GC 72 2013) and in the following sections the key principles in managing ADHD will be described.

The complexity of ADHD is compounded as it frequently presents with one or more co-occurring conditions such as conduct disorder, oppositional defiant disorder, anxiety and/or depressive disorder and there is considerable symptom overlap between ADHD and comorbid disorders. Perturbations in synaptic plasticity within certain regions of the brain are thought to play a key role. Evidence has shown that patients with ADHD have a delay in regional cortical maturation within the prefrontal cortex (Shaw et al. 2007) and large-scale neural network analyses have revealed other important areas of the brain implicated in the pathogenesis of the disorder (Castellanos and Proal 2012). Others have indicated deficits in neural circuits in children with ADHD (Nagel et al. 2011; Cha et al. 2015). These brain regions and the associated neural connections are highly sensitive to modulations in neurochemical pathways, and it is highly likely that even relatively benign fluctuations in catecholamine and serotoninergic signalling pathways can produce marked changes in attention, behaviour and emotion. The genetic heritability of ADHD symptoms is approximately 70 % in children and adolescents, and about 30 % in adults (Boomsma et al. 2010); however, other non-genetic factors, for example, pre-natal smoking and alcohol abuse, prematurity/low birth weight and other drug/environmental factors, are thought to increase the risk of ADHD (Purper-Ouakil et al. 2011). Epigenetic modulation is likely to be key factor in the causation of ADHD. Whether this is genetic and/or drug/environmental, it is probably likely that multiple epigenetic mechanisms coalesce and contribute to the complexity of ADHD resulting in differing degrees of severity and comorbidities that are often observed in individuals with ADHD.

18.3.1 Pharmacotherapeutic Strategy in Managing ADHD

In this section, we provide an overview of the pharmacotherapeutic strategy when managing ADHD in children.

- First-line Medication: methylphenidate (MPH) (immediate release MPH, Concerta XL, Medikinet XL, etc.), dexamphetamine (immediate release dexamphetamine; mixture of amphetamine salts—Adderall [immediate release and XR]); prodrug of dexamphetamine—Lisdexamfetamine [Elvance]); atomoxetine.
- Second-line Medication: guanfacine, bupropion, clonidine, imipramine, nortriptyline.
- Third-line Medication: carbamazepine, risperidone, aripiprazole, buspirone, venlafaxine.

18.3.1.1 Stimulants

In ADHD, the diagnosis and management NICE guidelines (NICE guidelines GC 72 2013), advocates group-based parent-training/education programmes as the first-line treatment for parents/carers of children and adolescents of school-going age with ADHD and moderate impairment. It is further recommended for older age cohorts that individual psychological treatment may be deemed acceptable if group behavioural or psychological approaches are found to be un-effective, or have been refused. Finally, drug treatment ought to be held in reserve for those with moderate impairment who have rejected non-drug interventions, or whose symptoms have not adequately responded to the first-line interventions (NICE guidelines GC 72 2013).

Medication is usually necessary when treating HKD or severe ADHD or if psychological treatments have been insufficient alone in managing symptoms. Greater hyperactivity, inattention and clumsiness in the absence of emotional disorder predict greater positive response to MPH (Taylor et al. 1987). Similarly, those with HKD show greater response to MPH (Santosh et al. 2005). However, it has also been shown that symptoms in those with less severe ADHD improve more completely. NICE recommends drug treatment as the first-line treatment for school-aged children and young people with severe ADHD (hyperkinetic disorder) and severe impairment. Where drug treatment is considered appropriate, MPH, atomoxetine and dexamphetamine can be used. Of note, the choice of drug should be guided by comorbidities and adverse events. Specific issues that may affect compliance and whether there is a potential for drug diversion and/or substance misuse should also be considered. Finally, the wishes of the child/adolescent and their parent or guardian should also be taken into account (NICE guidelines GC 72 2013).

The literature on stimulant medications MPH, dexamphetamine, and lisdexamfetamine and their use in the treatment of ADHD is voluminous. In most cases a stimulant is the first choice medication. Its onset of action is rapid, the dosage easy to titrate and positive response(s) can often be predicted from a single dose. Delayed delivery systems, such as Diffucaps MPH system, spheroidal oral drug absorption system (SODAS) and osmotically controlled-release oral delivery system (OROS) for MPH and mixed amphetamine salts extended-release systems have allowed treatment without medication having to be dispensed in school, and have the potential to decrease the abuse potential of stimulant agents. Lisdexamfetamine dimesylate is an amphetamine prodrug that is inactive until ingested and metabolized (Gamo et al. 2010), and is an effective treatment for ADHD.

The multimodal treatment of ADHD (MTA) study was a 14-month longitudinal trial that compared the effectiveness of pharmacotherapy and behavioural therapy in children aged 7.0–9.9 years with combined ADHD (inattention and hyperactivity/impulsivity) (MTA Cooperative Group 1999). The findings from the MTA indicated that the combination of pharmacological and behavioural therapy did not confer additional benefit when compared to pharmacological treatment alone for core ADHD symptoms, but the combination or multimodal treatment offered some benefit with regards to associated symptoms such as academic achievement, conduct problems and parental satisfaction (Swanson et al. 2001; Conners et al. 2001). A re-analysis of the MTA data using the ICD-10 classification of HKD showed that the effect size of stimulants was significantly greater in those with a diagnosis of HKD, compared to those who had non-HKD ADHD (Santosh et al. 2005).

Stimulant medications are the most commonly prescribed medication for children and at present the most extensively studied treatment for ADHD. The use of MPH is based on a substantial evidence base, summarized by a recent Cochrane review that analysed 38 parallel group trials ($n = 5111$, median treatment duration 49 days) and 147 crossover trials ($n = 7134$, 14 days), with an average age across all studies of 9.7 years (Storebø et al. 2015). The analysis suggested a beneficial effect of MPH on teacher rated symptoms in 19 parallel group trials (standardized mean difference [SMD] −0.77, $n = 1698$), and teacher rated general behaviour (SMD −0.87, five trials, $n = 668$), and may improve parent-reported quality of life (SMD 0.61, three trials, n = 514) (Storebø et al. 2015). There was no evidence that MPH was associated with an increase in serious adverse events (risk ratio 0.98, nine trials, n = 1532). MPH was associated with a small but increased risk of non-serious adverse events namely decreased appetite and poor sleep (risk ratio 1.29, 21 trials, n = 3132) (Storebø et al. 2015). They however rate the likelihood of bias as being high in most of the studies included in the analyses (Storebø et al. 2015).

A Cochrane review of the use of amphetamines in children and adolescents with ADHD (Punja et al. 2016) showed that amphetamines were effective. When comparing the effectiveness of stimulants such as MPH to amphetamines, a meta-analysis has shown that the effect size for amphetamines was greater than MPH (Charach et al. 2013). Furthermore, a more recent meta-analysis showed that the effectiveness of reducing ADHD symptoms in children and adolescents was the greatest for lisdexamfetamine followed by MPH, atomoxetine and bupropion (Stuhec et al. 2015).

Precautions with Stimulants

When managing the symptoms of ADHD in children, any treatment should be given with precaution and regular safety and tolerability monitoring should be routinely done. The main precautions are emphasized below.

- When children are started on stimulants, one needs to monitor pulse, blood pressure and heart rate (HR) at each dose increase and at every 6 months. Weight and height should also be monitored carefully using standardized charts at the minimum of 6-month intervals. Tics, depression, irritability, lack of spontaneity, withdrawal and excessive perseveration should be monitored at each visit. Routine haematological tests are unnecessary.
- Stimulants are contraindicated in schizophrenia, hyperthyroidism, cardiac arrhythmias, angina pectoris, glaucoma or a history of hypersensitivity to drug.
- There is no evidence that stimulants decrease seizure threshold. They can be used in well-controlled epilepsy. If seizures appear or worsen, change to dexamphetamine and avoid atomoxetine.
- Stimulants can reduce height and weight centiles over time. It is advisable not to start stimulants in children who are short or are biologically predisposed to short stature.
- Many anti-ADHD medications can increase HR and blood pressure and therefore electrocardiograms should be done and evaluated regularly. This is of particular importance in high-risk groups such as those with structural cardiac defects. Adderall should be avoided in cardiac high-risk groups.
- Stimulants can be abused by anyone with access to it. Self-initiated increase in dose by emotionally unstable patients with substance use disorders is possible, and should be monitored. Where substance abuse is suspected, atomoxetine, bupropion or Concerta XL (drug-delivery system makes it difficult to abuse) can be used, as they are safer in this scenario.

- Stimulants can induce or worsen psychotic experience. Therefore, stimulant use should be avoided in those who have first-degree relatives with a psychotic disorder or in children who have psychotic or quasi-psychotic experiences. Atomoxetine, tricyclic antidepressants, clonidine, bupropion, aripiprazole or risperidone can be used instead.

18.3.1.2 Atomoxetine

Atomoxetine was the first non-stimulant drug approved for the treatment of ADHD. Whilst the precise therapeutic effects of atomoxetine in the treatment of ADHD remain unclear, atomoxetine is thought to bring about its effect by acting as a selective norepinephrine inhibitor. The plasma half-life is usually about 4 h; an active metabolite, 4-hydroxyatomoxetine, is excreted in urine after glucuronidation. In 5–10 % of people, a polymorphism of the cytochrome enzyme P450 2D6 leads to a longer plasma half-life of up to 19 h. Randomized double-blind placebo-controlled trials in children and adolescents demonstrate atomoxetine's effectiveness in treating ADHD (Michelson et al. 2001, 2002; Bushe and Savill 2014). Atomoxetine was noted to be significantly more effective compared to placebo on both the parent and teacher scales. The primary adverse effects noted with atomoxetine were gastrointestinal upset, decreased appetite, fatigue, dizziness and mild increases in pulse and systolic blood pressure. Despite its relatively short half-life, atomoxetine can be used as either a once daily or twice daily dose and is generally quite safe. It produces minimal increase in blood pressure, HR and gastrointestinal symptoms (nausea and vomiting are possible especially during the early part of treatment). It may be useful in those with comorbid tics, anxiety/depression, or in those who have not responded to stimulants (although at present there have been no clear studies indicate this as yet). Symptoms take about 6 weeks to improve with atomoxetine (unlike stimulants), and hence parents have to be informed about this at start of treatment. Dosage can be initiated at half the required total dose in order to decrease the chances of side effects (especially upper gastrointestinal effects). Anecdotally, there have been some reports that suggest extremely rare, but serious liver dysfunction in patients treated with atomoxetine.

18.3.1.3 Clonidine and Guanfacine

Clonidine and Guanfacine are central acting alpha-2-adrenergic agonists commonly used as adjuncts in the treatment of pediatric ADHD. A meta-analysis summarizes the evidence base of clonidine in the treatment of ADHD (Connor et al. 1999). Several of these studies involved patients with ADHD and a comorbid psychiatric illness (conduct disorder, developmental disorder or tic disorder). Positive effects were reported on ADHD symptoms from all of these studies across parent, teacher and clinician raters. The effect size on ADHD symptoms was 0.58 ± 0.16, which corresponds to a moderately positive clinical effect (Connor et al. 1999). In support of this finding, a recent meta-analysis of ADHD in youth has shown that clonidine XR (extended release) was more superior in comparison to placebo for total ADHD symptoms (Hirota et al. 2014). Seven prospective randomized controlled trials (RCTs) using guanfacine XR (extended release) for the treatment of ADHD in children and adolescents showed superiority over placebo on the primary outcome measure (Rizzo and Martino 2015). Based on this evidence, guanfacine, especially XR, appears to be an effective and safe treatment option in children and adolescents with ADHD (Rizzo and Martino 2015). There is no evidence to suggest a difference in efficacy between clonidine and guanfacine for total ADHD symptoms (Hirota et al. 2014).

Side effects frequently noted with these medications include sedation, hypotension, tachycardia and dizziness. Pulse and blood pressure should be monitored for bradycardia and hypotension in those treated with guanfacine (Ruggiero et al. 2014). Of note, when discontinuing clonidine, the dose needs to be carefully tapered rather than stopped all of a sudden to avoid rebound hypertension. Unpredictable compliance with clonidine elevates the risk of adverse cardiovascular events and this factor needs to be discussed with families. In general, the clinician needs to consider whether clonidine should be prescribed if it cannot be taken reliably. Depression and impairment of glucose tolerance can also occur.

18.3.1.4 Combination of a Stimulant and Non-stimulant

The problems presented by severe hyperactivity can be very severe and families may become desperate. Clinicians often feel pressed to prescribe unduly high dosages (for which there is no evidence base of value) and combinations of drugs, sometimes to target different aspects of the symptom complex. This can be justifiable in extreme cases, but the concurrent use of inadequately evaluated drugs can create hazards and warrants specialist advice and careful monitoring.

18.3.2 Developmental Trajectory and Medication Response

ADHD in Pre-schoolers: Behavioural interventions such as parent-training approaches are useful. Stimulants are less effective in school-going children and are associated with greater side effects. The evidence base is stronger for parent-based behaviour training interventions in comparison to MPH treatment in pre-schoolers at increased risk for ADHD (Charach et al. 2013).

ADHD in School-going Children: Medication is superior to behavioural interventions in this age group. Behavioural interventions are essential when treating comorbidity in ADHD.

ADHD in Adolescence: Non-compliance with medication is a greater problem in treatment of adolescents due to their desire to avoid taking medication during

school hours and the increased prevalence of stimulant-related dysphoria. The risk of misuse of stimulants is also elevated in adolescents. Giving or selling medication to peers is more common than abuse by the patients themselves. The drug interactions that could result from undisclosed substance misuse should always be borne in mind. Concerta XL or atomoxetines are good options in this group.
ADHD in Adults: It becomes difficult from a clinical perspective on how to manage adult ADHD without the necessary experience regarding the presentation of the disorder in childhood. Adult ADHD has a prevalence of about 5 % (Bonvicini et al. 2016) and evidence suggests that adult ADHD might be a distinct entity, i.e. without childhood ADHD (Moffitt et al. 2015). Nowadays, it is becoming more frequent for adult patients to seek treatment and management of their ADHD symptoms, and in this view clinicians are in the need for robust practice guidelines. An important factor to consider is that adult ADHD frequently presents differently from ADHD seen in childhood and can be comorbid with other disorders. When compared to children, adults with ADHD present with more inattentive symptoms and show less hyperactivity or impulsivity (Volkow and Swanson 2013). Hence, from this viewpoint it is important to recognize the different diagnoses. Physicians and other professionals should work with patients in a concerted manner in order to provide the most appropriate feedback about their symptoms, to empower them about ADHD, and to set realistic treatment goals. Both stimulants and atomoxetine are effective and well tolerated in adults with ADHD (Santosh et al. 2011) and RCTs using these treatments show favourable clinical effect sizes ranging from 0.4 to 0.7 (Asherson et al. 2016).

If hyperactivity is present only in one situation, i.e. at school or at home, then stresses in that situation should be sought and alleviated as the first line of management. With *school specific problems*, specific learning disabilities should be sought carefully through the assessment of a clinical or educational psychologist. If present, then adjustment of educational techniques and expectations should be given a try before anti-hyperactivity treatments. If hyperactive behaviour is *confined to the home situation*, then the possibility of adverse parenting influences should be considered, leading to a parent-training approach. In pervasive and severe cases, without autistic or affective comorbidity, a multimodal treatment approach will be needed. Medication should be initiated with proper monitoring of target symptoms. *Patients without hyperactivity (ADD)* may benefit from and tolerate lower doses of stimulants.

18.3.3 Experiences from the Indian Context

High-quality pharmacological research in neurodevelopmental disorders is currently sparse from Asia. Some studies exploring this topic from India have been highlighted here.

The significant lack of knowledge about the causes of academic impairments associated with ADHD and specific learning disorders (SLDs) among school-aged children in India often goes unrecognized (Mukherjee et al. 2016). This is despite the prevalence of ADHD as assessed through questionnaire data in 6–11 year olds in India that shows rates of 16.33 % among the lower socio-economic group and 6.84 % among middle socio-economic group, highlighting the increased risk for ADHD from those at a socio-economic disadvantage (Venkata and Panicker 2013). This might have some significance because a case control study of newly diagnosed cases with ADHD has indicated that serum ferritin to be substantially lower in children with ADHD as compared to controls. Moreover, a statistically significant negative correlation between serum ferritin levels and oppositional sub-score on the Conners Rating Scale was observed (Juneja et al. 2010). This is important in countries with high rates of hookworm infestations and iron deficiency anaemia, often associated with poor socio-economic status. Despite this evidence, further work would be warranted in a much larger sample size before making any confirmatory claim(s) linking lower serum ferritin levels to ADHD causation and severity. The prevalence of ADHD and associated psychological problems among college students in Chandigarh, India showed that 5.48 % of the students fulfilled the criteria for adult ADHD. These students experienced significantly higher emotional instability and low self-esteem than those without ADHD but did not differ in the occurrence of depression, social problems and substance abuse (Jhambh et al. 2014).

Despite availability of effective treatments for ADHD in India, a substantial proportion of the patient population has unsatisfactory access to care or face protracted delays when seeking help (Arya et al. 2015). Patients with ADHD attending tertiary outpatient psychiatric services in India showed a mean delay of 3.96 years in seeking help for ADHD symptoms, due to a lack of recognition of ADHD by qualified practitioners (other than teachers), leading to delayed referral to Child and Adolescent Mental Health Services (CAMHS). Sociocultural beliefs of parents also influenced help seeking (Arya et al. 2015). There remains significant non-adherence to treatment in children with ADHD in India with 62.5 % being non-adherent and social factors contributing to non-adherence in 75.7 % (Antony 2016).

From a pharmacotherapy perspective, an open-label clinical trial of buspirone, a full 5HT1A agonist at the somatodendritic auto-receptor and a partial agonist at the post-synaptic 5HT1A receptors, conducted in a tertiary hospital setting in north India suggested that it can help to improve hyperactivity, impulsivity and oppositionality (Malhotra and Santosh 1998). The short-term efficacy and tolerability of MPH and atomoxetine in children with ADHD was explored using an open-label randomized parallel group clinical trial in a tertiary care hospital in north India using MPH (0.2–1 mg/kg/d) or atomoxetine (0.5–1.2 mg/kg/d) for 8 weeks. Methylphenidate and atomoxetine were both efficacious in Indian children with ADHD at lower doses than conventionally reported in the West. The dose needed was 0.45 mg/kg/d for MPH and 0.61 mg/kg/d for atomoxetine, and their efficacy and tolerability were comparable (Garg et al. 2014). In the subgroup with ADHD and oppositional defiant disorder (ODD) ($n = 37$), 80 % of the patients from MPH group and 64.3 % patients from atomoxetine group ceased to fulfil the criteria for the presence of ODD at 8 weeks (Garg et al. 2015). In an interesting Indian study of 18 subjects recruited with early onset of substance dependence to at least two substances (alcohol, tobacco and other drug dependence), atomoxetine supplementation to treatment as usual led to significant reduction in externalizing symptoms, longer abstinence, shorter turnaround time and better quality of life (Benegal et al. 2013). Further work would be required in a much larger sample size to warrant generalization of these findings.

In summary, although some findings require confirmation in larger studies, in general, the following points should be considered in developing countries such as India:

- Psychoeducation regarding diagnosis and treatment of ADHD of professionals coming in contact with children and adolescents, parents and children should become a priority.
- Correction of iron deficiency should become an important component of the treatment package of ADHD in India.
- The difficulties associated in obtaining stimulants for treating ADHD have led to non-stimulants such as atomoxetine, tricyclic antidepressants, clonidine and non-allopathic medicines being used. Easing access to first-line treatments such as long-acting stimulants and making it affordable to patients should be aimed for in countries such as India.
- Non-adherence to treatment remains high and needs targeting.
- Lower doses of MPH and atomoxetine have been reported to produce comparable improvements in ADHD and ODD symptoms, suggesting that dose titration start at lower doses than suggested from studies conducted in the West.
- Screening high-risk groups such as adolescents and young adults with alcohol or substance misuse for ADHD (and treating it if present) should become part of holistic alcohol or substance misuse treatment programmes.

18.4 Autism Spectrum Disorder (ASD)

At its core, ASD is a disorder that impacts on the several aspects of socialization. The disorder is characterized by impairments in communication, social reciprocity, and by restrictive and repetitive patterns (DSM-5 2013). The mean prevalence of ASD is currently estimated as being 1 in 68 children (Wingate et al. 2014). Due to its inherent pleiotropic heterogeneity, teasing out the precise neurotransmitter receptor systems implicated in the pathophysiology of ASD makes it less tractable to pharmacological manipulation. Epigenetic dysregulation has been linked to a wide range of neurodevelopmental disorders (Petronis 2010) and it is likely that in ASD, modulation of epigenetic factors responding to internal and external environmental cues manifest in the disease and contribute to the divergent symptomology. Current evidence indicates that mid-foetal human cortical neurons (Willsey et al. 2013; Miller et al. 2014) are an important area for the co-expression of candidate genes, and as described below, these candidate genes have a crucial role in the integrity of divergent synaptic pathways. Studies on candidate genes have provided valuable molecular insights into ASD. Defects in the gene encoding the adhesive junction-associated d-catenin protein (CTNND2) were shown to be associated with severe autism (Turner et al. 2015). Moreover, restoration of the gene *Shank3* that encodes SH3 and multiple ankyrin repeat domains 3 (SHANK3), a post-synaptic scaffold protein important for synaptic function and plasticity, and responsible of about 1 % of all ASD cases, rescued ASD like phenotypes in adult mice including certain behaviour abnormalities such as social interaction and repetitive grooming behaviour deficits (Mei et al. 2016). Despite these single-gene mutations providing important insight into molecular mechanisms, as mentioned above, the heterogeneity of ASD underscores the fact that the aetiology of about 70 % of ASD cases is still unknown (O'Roak and State 2008; Devlin et al. 2012). A recent study has shed light on possible epigenetic biomarkers associated with ASD and has implicated mutations of the gene *ERMN* that codes Ermin, an oligodendroglia-specific protein integral for myelinogenesis (Brockschnieder et al. 2006), in ASD susceptibility (Homs et al. 2016). Other studies in mice have shown that impairments in patched domain containing 1 (PTCHD1) within the thalamic reticular nucleus could have an important role in propagating the adverse symptomology across neurodevelopmental disorders such as ASD (Wells et al. 2016). Whilst promising, further work needs to be done in terms of how the findings conducted in animal models may extrapolate to humans. The road to clinical translation is beset with obstacles and data in animal models do not necessary yield the same outcomes as in clinical trials involving human subjects.

Whilst there is no established literature for prevention or cure, it is well agreed upon that defects in the core features of autism can be mitigated by focused behavioural interventions coupled with pharmacological treatments to reduce the co-occurring symptoms (Santosh and Singh 2016). In fact, ASD frequently presents with one or more comorbid problem (Simonoff et al. 2008). A number of different pharmacological treatments are used to treat the co-occurring disorders associated with ASD such as antidepressants, antipsychotics, anticonvulsants and stimulants. Despite their widespread use, there is paucity in the literature whether such treatment regimens can treat the underlying core symptoms in children with ASD.

18.4.1 Treatment Strategies in ASD

When planning treatment strategies in individuals with ASD, in particular children, an important factor to consider is compliance to medication. This is because individuals with ASD are likely to have cognitive rigidity and atypical sensory symptoms that can influence treatment compliance. Hence, medication may not be taken due to its smell or taste in those with ASD. In this scenario, prescribing needs to be individualized (Santosh and Singh 2016) to the patients' needs and the EDMS would be useful in this regard (Santosh 2014). In this context, the dose can be titrated to provide maximum effectiveness with the minimum of side effects. In the UK, evidence-based guidelines inform clinicians and other healthcare practitioners' different ways of treating and managing children and adolescents with ASD (NICE guidelines GC 170 2013). An all-encompassing multimodal approach is essential for the treatment and management of ASD. This is particularly important in children. In children with ASD, medication should form only a part of a comprehensive treatment programme that also includes behavioural and psychological therapies. In the following sections, we discuss the treatments strategies when managing the frequent comorbidities seen in children with ASD.

In comparison to the UK and other developed countries, children in South Asia have little or if any access to treatment. The number of children with ASD is the highest in South Asia, and in particular, current estimates in India indicate that >5million children aged between 2–9 years of age have ASD (Rahman et al. 2016). Evidence has further emphasized the lack of an evidence base for treatment interventions that have been adapted from high-income countries and their practicability in countries such as India. Furthermore, the need for specialists to deliver these interventions, particularly for those in rural populations, where the treatment gap is nearly 100 % (Patel et al. 2013) also presents another barrier to treatment. Recent evidence has indicated that non-specialist interventions adapted from those used in high-income countries for children with ASD could be the way forward for countries such as India. Parent-mediated intervention was shown to be feasible and effective for the treatment of ASD in children in India and Pakistan (Rahman et al. 2016) and warrants the case for testing other non-specialist interventions in these and other regions of South Asia.

18.4.1.1 Treating Aggression, Irritability and Agitation

One of the most damaging comorbidities associated with ASD is aggression. Prevalence rates of aggression in children with ASD are variable. In one study involving 1380 children aged 4–17 years with ASD, it was reported that 56 % engaged in some form of aggression ranging from mild to severe towards caregivers and 32 % towards non-caregivers (Kanne and Mazurek 2011). Another study in 169 children aged 1.5–5.8 years with ASD, 22.5 % of children displayed aggression that was deemed to be clinically significant (Hartley et al. 2008). Despite these variations, it is clear that aggression and irritability can manifest as extreme non-compliance and socially inappropriate behaviours. This often leads to high risk and jeopardizes the core elements of ordinary personal experience for people with ASD such as living with their families, and attending local schools (Hodgetts et al. 2013).

The atypical antipsychotics risperidone and aripiprazole can be useful in treating aggression and irritability in ASD. In a study by McCracken et al. (2002), risperidone was safe, well tolerated and effective for treating aggression in 101 youth aged 5–17 years with ASD. Following on from this, in 2004, the effectiveness of risperidone for treating aggression and irritability was confirmed in 79 children aged 5–12 years old with ASD in an 8-week placebo-controlled double-blind RCT (Shea et al. 2004). Another study has shown that risperidone was efficacious in reducing hyperactivity and aggression in children (Nagaraj et al. 2006). Similarly, studies have shown that aripiprazole was effective for the treatment of irritability in children with autistic and aggressive behaviour (Owen et al. 2009; Ching and Pringsheim 2012) and had positive effects on secondary outcome measures in individuals aged 6–17 years old with ASD (Findling et al. 2014). Taken together, these findings show that treatments with risperidone and aripiprazole are effective in reducing aggression and irritability in children and adolescents with ASD. Both risperidone and aripiprazole have been approved by the United States Food and Drug Administration for the treatment of irritability in youth with ASD. From a safety perspective, a systematic review has shown that aripiprazole has a more favourable metabolic safety profile than risperidone (De Hert et al. 2011); however, there is no evidence that risperidone or aripiprazole is more effective than the other (Ghanizadeh et al. 2014).

Some case reports have also suggested a positive safety and efficacy profile of clozapine when treating aggression in youth with ASD (Chen et al. 2001; Lambrey et al. 2010). In a recent meta-analysis, the effectiveness of pharmacological treatment for irritability and aggression in children and adolescents aged 2–17 years of age with ASD was evaluated (Fung et al. 2016). The primary outcome measure was the reduction in the Aberrant Behavior Checklist-Irritability (ABC-I) in the treatment group when compared to placebo. Forty-six (46) placebo-controlled RCTs were identified and in comparison to placebo, risperidone, aripiprazole followed by *N*-acetylcysteine showed the greatest improvement in ABC-I scores with effect sizes of 0.9, 0.8 and 0.7, respectively (Fung et al. 2016).

18.4.1.2 Treating Hyperactivity and Inattention

ASD presents with a plethora of symptoms and whilst not all will be described in this chapter, as with aggression, however, inattention and hyperactivity reflect symptoms that are frequently encountered in children with ASD. Indeed, evidence has suggested that in some cases, these symptoms are so severe that a diagnosis of ADHD is justified (Lee et al. 2014).

Although they might present as different disorders, recent evidence suggests that there is considerable aetiological overlap between the genes that cause ASD and those that cause ADHD (Smoller et al. 2013). That said, there are commonalities in the medication used for the treatment of hyperactivity and inattention in those with ASD comorbid for ADHD and those with ADHD. Good symptom reduction using MPH was observed in children and adolescents with ADHD comorbid for ASD in an open-label trial (Santosh et al. 2006). Moreover, MPH was shown to improve social communication and self-regulation in children aged 5–13 years old with pervasive development disorder and hyperactivity (Jahromi et al. 2009).

There is a dearth in the literature when assessing the effectiveness of amphetamines in children and adolescents with ASD. The evidence base suggests that amphetamines are useful for treating ADHD in children with ASD. Lisdexamfetamine dimesylate is useful in improving outcomes in children with ADHD (Coghill et al. 2013) and therefore its use in treating ADHD in ASD might be warranted; however, further work in studies of sufficient power and sample size would be needed to corroborate this.

In children with ASD, the overall strength of evidence for atomoxetine in improving hyperactivity and inattention is low. In children aged 6–17 years with ASD and ADHD, atomoxetine appears to have no effect on social functioning but might improve stereotyped behaviours and communication (Harfterkamp et al. 2014). Further work from this group showed no evidence of predictors of response to atomoxetine (Harfterkamp et al. 2015). Despite these findings, before making definitive claims on the effectiveness of atomoxetine in children with ASD, clearly there is a case that more RCTs of atomoxetine in children with ASD are needed.

Some studies have evaluated the efficacy of the alpha-2 adrenergic agonists clonidine and guanfacine in improving comorbid symptoms in children with ASD. In one double-blind placebo-controlled crossover study using transdermal clonidine, Fankhauser et al. (1992) showed that transdermal clonidine improved hyperactivity in autistic subjects aged 5–33 years old. Caution should be stressed when extrapolating this finding as the sample size was very small (nine males) and duration of the trial was short (4 weeks). Others have questioned the validity of clonidine for treating hyperactivity in individuals with ASD (Hazell 2007). Further work would be needed before confirming the effectiveness of clonidine in treating ADHD in those with ASD. Conversely, the evidence base for guanfacine is stronger. Recently, extended release guanfacine was shown to improve hyperactivity in children (mean age: 8.5 years) with ASD. Sixty-two (62) subjects were enrolled in a multi-site RCT and in the guanfacine treatment group; there was a 43.6 % decline in the ABC-hyperactivity score compared to a 13.2 % decrease in the placebo treatment group (Scahill et al. 2015). It is hoped that the advancement of treatments that aim to ameliorate core symptoms in ASD and ADHD will provide therapeutic inroads in not only combating the core deficits but also in addressing the associated psychiatric comorbidities.

18.4.1.3 Treating Anxiety and Depression

Elevated anxiety and depression are frequent occurrences in children with ASD. Anxiety ranges from 40 to 84 % for any anxiety disorder to 5–23 % for generalized anxiety and 13–29 % for social anxiety (Sukhodolsky et al. 2013). Parent-reported data has shown beneficial treatment effects of cognitive behavioural therapy (CBT) on anxiety in young adolescents aged 11–15 years of age with ASD (Wood et al. 2015). Treatment for anxiety would usually involve the use of serotonin reuptake inhibitors (SSRIs), and in this vein although, not specifically investigated in children with ASD, SSRIs together with CBT have been shown to decrease the severity of anxiety in children (Walkup et al. 2008). Based on these data, it is likely that treatment for anxiety in children with ASD would follow a combined approach involving both medication and parent-led behavioural therapies.

18.4.2 Targeting the Core Symptoms of ASD

Currently, nearly all treatment strategies are directed towards managing the comorbid symptoms of ASD. No drug in routine clinical practice has as yet been found that is efficacious in improving the core impairments in ASD. Evidence from some preliminary studies indicates, however, that some might be useful in ameliorating the core symptoms of ASD. The molecules that aim to target core symptoms of ASD are quite broad and range from antibiotics that have been used previously for the treatment of tuberculosis, hormonal neuropeptides, to plant-based compounds.

The antibiotic D-cycloserine has been around for nearly 60 years for its use as a treatment in tuberculosis. More recently, it has emerged as a potential player in targeting core deficits in ASD and was shown to have positive effects on stereotypies and social deficits in patients aged 14–25 years old with ASD (Urbano et al. 2014, 2015). In another study, however, no differences between the placebo and D-cycloserine treatment groups were seen for the primary and secondary outcome measures in 34 children aged 5–11 years with ASD (Minshawi et al. 2016). Despite this finding, an improvement was seen for total raw scores in the social responsiveness scale from baseline to treatment end (Minshawi et al. 2016). These data warrant additional investigation before the role of D-cycloserine in ASD can be confirmed.

Oxytocin is a hormone secreted from the posterior pituitary gland and polymorphisms in the oxytocin receptor gene are thought to be associated with individual differences in social functioning observed in humans, including the social impairments seen in children with ASD (Parker et al. 2014). The potential of oxytocin for improving core deficits in ASD has garnered significant traction in recent years. In part, this momentum has been driven largely by single-dose studies of oxytocin that have yielded positive effects on core ASD symptoms in particular those related to social communication and interaction. In terms of single-dose studies, Hollander et al. (2003) was the first to show a significant beneficial effect following a single intravenous dose of oxytocin in 15 adults with ASD. Studies in children have shown that intranasal administration of single-dose oxytocin improved brain function for social stimuli in 17 children aged 8–16.5 years with high functioning ASD (Gordon et al. 2013). Further, in a crossover RCT, single-dose oxytocin administered for 5 weeks in 31 children aged 3–8 years with ASD led to significant improvement in caregiver-rated social responses when compared to placebo (Yatawara et al. 2015). Conversely, other studies using multiple doses of oxytocin have shown less effectiveness in individuals with ASD. Intranasal oxytocin did not improve outcomes in adolescents aged 7–16 years of age when given over 4 days (Dadds et al. 2014) nor administered bid for 8 weeks in youth aged 12–18 years (Guastella et al. 2015) with ASD.

N-acetylcysteine is an antioxidant that has a key role in regulating extracellular glutamate levels (Deepmala et al. 2015). There is a strong evidence base suggesting that abnormalities in the glutamatergic neurotransmission system could play an important role in ASD (James et al. 2006; Canitano and Scandurra 2014). Modulators of extracellular glutamate levels such as *N*-acetylcysteine have shown some benefit in treating irritability in children with ASD (Hardan et al. 2012; Fung et al. 2016). Furthermore, together with risperidone, *N*-acetylcysteine showed a positive improvement in treating irritability in youth with ASD (Ghanizadeh and Moghimi-Sarani 2013; Nikoo et al. 2015). Despite these findings, recently it was shown in youth with ASD that *N*-acetylcysteine had no significant impact on social impairment (Dean et al. 2016; Wink et al. 2016). The small sample sizes, the doses used in the studies together with different instruments used to capture changes preclude definitive inferences on the effectiveness of *N*-acetylcysteine from being made. Further larger scale studies that are sufficiently powered and are able to predict treatment response are warranted to confirm the efficacy of *N*-acetylcysteine in the childhood ASD population.

Sulforaphane is an extract derived from broccoli and one recent study in 44 young men aged 13–27 years randomized roughly 2:1 and diagnosed with moderate to severe ASD, showed that sulforaphane derived from the consumption of broccoli sprouts at levels usually found in the diet for 18 weeks, significantly (and reversibly) improved core behaviour in comparison to patients on placebo (Singh et al. 2015). This improvement regressed upon cessation of treatment. The interest in sulforaphane has amplified following the extensive epidemiological evidence from many countries demonstrating that consumption of Brassica vegetables (such as broccoli and rocket) was associated with a lower incidence of several human cancers, in particular of the prostate and breast. It is thought that sulforaphane can do this in part by up-regulating antioxidant genes involved in control mechanisms through the Keap1-Nrf2 cyto-protective signalling pathway. Moreover, it is well documented that sulforaphane can counteract many of the molecular processes inherent to neurodevelopmental disorders including oxidative stress, mitochondrial dysfunction and neuro-inflammation (Liu et al. 2016a) which are critical for the integrity of synaptic transmission and plasticity (Hagerman et al. 2010, 2011).

These disorder modifying compounds in ASD show promise in improving the core symptoms in ASD, however, before they can realize their full potential as novel clinical treatments, certain challenges need to be addressed. First, optimizing the dose would be imperative as well as the length of drug administration. Second, there are no 'gold standard', outcome measures that can capture changes in the core symptoms of ASD. Third, larger studies of a sufficient sample size are needed.

18.5 Tourette's Syndrome

As with ADHD and ASD, Giles de la Tourette syndrome (TS) has a multifactorial aetiology. About 0.85–1 % of the pediatric population worldwide is affected by TS (Robertson 2009, 2015) and is more frequent in males (male to female ratio 3:1 or 4:1) (Robertson et al. 1988). Whilst the precise causes remain to be established, it is likely that multiple immunological, genetic and environmental factors combine and interact with one another to establish susceptibility. Some studies have identified candidate genes that although might only account for a small proportion of cases, can still provide important information on understanding the disease at the molecular level. One candidate gene is Slit- and Trk-like family member 1 (*SLITRK1*) and members of the *SLITRK* gene family have a key role in promoting neurite outgrowth and development (Whitford et al. 2002). SLITRK1 is a transmembrane protein that is highly expressed in neuroanatomical regions of the brain commonly associated with TS such as the cortical, thalamic and basal nuclei regions (Proenca et al. 2011). A loss of function in the *SLITRK1* gene is thought to be associated with TS (Abelson et al. 2005) and some have suggested that the role of *SLITRK1* in TS causation might have been under estimated (Karagiannidis et al. 2012). Others have suggested that mutations in the *HDC* gene that codes for an enzyme involved in histamine biosynthesis (L-histidine decarboxylase) links disordered histaminergic neurotransmission to TS (Ercan-Sencicek et al. 2010; Karagiannidis et al. 2011). At the neuroimaging level, the evidence base suggests that the decreased size of the caudate nucleus maybe responsible for TS symptomatology (Robertson 2015). In youth with TS, others have shown immaturity and anomalous patterns of functional connectivity in control networks mostly in the fronto-parietal network of the brain (Church et al. 2009).

Tourette's syndrome is referred to as a syndrome (Robertson and Eapen 2014) and for a diagnosis to be fulfilled multiple motor tics together with one or more vocal/phonic tics for a duration of more than 1 year are required to be present (DSM-5 2013). The mean age of onset is about 7 years and typically motor tics tend to appear sooner (~7 years) than vocal/phonic tics (~11 years) (Robertson 2015). The overall opinion is that TS lessens in severity with age but does not completely disappear. Despite this, the comorbidities and psychopathologies that are associated with TS remain, which can have an impact on the treatment trajectory of the patient.

Tourette's syndrome can be demarcated into those with (i) pure TS, i.e. patients who present with solely motor and vocal tics but without any other co-occurring conditions or (ii) those who present with co-occurring conditions. About 12–13.5 % of diagnosed patients have pure TS (Robertson 2015); however, patients with TS frequently present with comorbidities such as ADHD, obsessive–compulsive disorder (OCD) and depressive disorder. Findings from 3500 patients with TS demonstrated that 88 % of patients had comorbidities or other psychopathologies (Freeman et al. 2000). In this study, the most common comorbid disorder was ADHD, followed by OCD and males were more at risk of developing comorbid disorders than females (Freeman et al. 2000). ADHD is present in about 60 % of individuals with TS (Rothenberger and Roessner 2013). TS and its associated comorbidities can have a disabling impact on the quality of life of the individual from both an academic and social functioning perspective (Eapen et al. 2016).

18.5.1 Treatment Strategies in TS

As with other neurodevelopmental disorders, medication should not be the only factor that is considered when offering care. In the UK, unlike ADHD and ASD, there are at present no NICE guidelines for the treatment and management of TS in children. The general opinion is that behavioural therapies should be used as first choice in children with TS. These include habit reversal training (HRT) and exposure and response prevention (ERP) therapies (Verdellen et al. 2011). In terms of management, comprehensive behavioural intervention in comparison to education and supportive therapy was shown to give greater improvement in tic severity in children with TS (Piacentini et al. 2010). Aripiprazole can be used to provide symptomatic relief in TS with few side effects (Davies et al. 2006) especially in refractory cases. A recent meta-analysis has indicated that aripiprazole was safe and effective in reducing tics in children and adolescents with TS (Liu et al. 2016b). Low-dose aripiprazole is increasingly considered as the first medication choice in TS. Others have shown clonidine and guanfacine should be considered as first-line treatments for tics in children and adolescents with TS (Whittington et al. 2016). In a systematic review, pooled analysis from four placebo-controlled RCTs favoured the use of clonidine and guanfacine for the treatment of tics in children with moderate effect sizes (SMD = −0.71; 95 % CI −1.03, −0.40; n = 164) (Whittington et al. 2016). Sulpiride is useful when managing the symptoms in patients with TS (Robertson et al. 1990), whilst fluoxetine has been shown to be beneficial in managing the obsessive symptoms (Eapen et al. 1996). In treatment refractory and severe cases, deep brain stimulation appears to be another treatment option available for TS (Deeb et al. 2016).

18.5.2 Cross-Cultural Perspectives

From an Asian perspective, TS and its associated features have been less well studied in comparison to Western populations. Nevertheless, TS exhibits remarkable similarity across cultures in terms of comorbidity, associated conditions and treatment outcomes (Staley et al. 1997). There are, however, some variations amongst cultures particularly with regards to associated features and comorbidities (Robertson et al. 2009). Less obsessive–compulsive behaviour was seen in 30 South Korean patients (Min and Lee 1986) and a higher incidence of TS in Japanese males has been documented (Nomura et al. 1992) when compared to

Western counterparts. The incidence of inappropriate and involuntary swearing (coprolalia) in TS might also vary across cultures, with broad occurrence rates ranging from 4 to 11 % in Japan (Nomura and Segawa 1979; Nomura et al. 1992) to 60 % in Hong Kong (Lieh-Mak et al. 1982). Moreover, in 39 case reports across cultures, the occurrence of coprolalia was 74 % (Staley et al. 1997). Despite these findings, it is unclear whether these variations across cultures are a true reflection of TS. Differences in diagnostic instruments, sample selection methods coupled with the small sample sizes used across studies hinder accurate comparisons across cultures from being made. At present, only one study has explored cultural differences in TS patients using the same diagnostic instruments (Eapen and Robertson 2008). In this study, 35 patients with TS of Arab heritage from the United Arab Emirates (UAE) where compared to age and gender matched 35 white Caucasian patients with TS from the United Kingdom (UK). Apart from rates of coprolalia being higher in the white Caucasian cohort, the clinical characteristics such as male preponderance, site of initial tic location and mean age of onset were similar amongst the UK and UAE cohorts (Eapen and Robertson 2008). Taken together, these findings suggest that when adopting treatment strategies for patients with TS, cultural factors and potential variations in TS symptomatology across populations must also be taken into consideration whenever applicable.

18.6 Neuropsychiatric Symptoms in Rare Diseases (for Example, Rett Syndrome [RTT])

Rett syndrome (RTT), a pervasive neurological disorder (Rett 1966; Hagberg et al. 1983), is characterized by compromised brain functions leading to language and learning disabilities, repetitive stereotyped hand movements and developmental regression. This condition is being discussed as an example of how one can manage neuropsychiatric symptoms accompanying many rare genetic diseases that present within developing countries.

Rett syndrome is predominantly found in young females with an incidence of 1: 20,000 live births (Kozinetz et al. 1993) although cases have been documented in males (Moog et al. 2003; Reichow et al. 2015). RTT presents with a complex clinical picture. Cianfaglione et al. (2015) provided evidence for a definable behavioural phenotype in individuals with RTT including hand stereotypies, breathing abnormalities, night-time unrest, anxiety and inappropriate fear. Hand stereotypies (hand wringing) appeared to be the most characteristic amongst individuals with RTT when compared to the contrast group that consisted of individuals with intellectual disability associated with a variety of genetic syndromes other than RTT.

The vast majority of patients with RTT have a loss of function in the methyl-CpG binding protein 2 (*MeCP2*) gene (Bienvenu et al. 2000), with some cases of RTT arising from mutations in CDKL5 and FOXG1 genes (Evans et al. 2005; Philippe et al. 2010). More recently, others have identified novel candidate genes not previously associated with RTT such as those encoding ankyrin repeat containing proteins or neuronal acetylcholine receptor subunit alpha 5 subunits (Lucariello et al. 2016). MeCP2 is a highly conserved nuclear protein that is expressed widely in the mammalian brain (Lewis et al. 1992). Loss of MeCP2 does not result in neuronal cell death as the phenotype is reversible in mice models of RTT (Guy et al. 2007) and in *MECP2* duplication syndrome (Sztainberg et al. 2015).

Literature evidence suggests that MeCP2 is a critical epigenetic modulator in the brain, controlling mechanisms such as DNA methylation and post-translational mechanisms (see Katz et al. 2016). These processes regulate gene expression without altering DNA sequences, and in mature neurons others have suggested that the role of MeCP2 is to dampen transcriptional noise (Skene et al. 2010). Most likely, dysfunction in MeCP2 causes defective transcriptional repression mechanisms, possibly in part governed by differential post-translational modification of MeCP2 at serine 164 (Stefanelli et al. 2016). MeCP2 also appears to be critical loci for other proteins. Recently, mutation in the gene *switch-insensitive 3 family member A* (*SIN3A*), a MeCP2 interactor and transcriptional repressor that has an important role in cortex development, causes intellectual disability and ASD (Witteveen et al. 2016). Moreover, the $MeCP2^{R306C}$ mutation prevents it from interacting with the NCoR/histone deacetylase 3 (HDAC3) complex which causes impairments in social and cognitive functioning in animal models (Nott et al. 2016).

The general consensus is that MeCP2 dysfunction causes deleterious gene expression which in turn has a marked impact on post-natal neuronal development and contributes to the disease pathophysiology in individuals who present with the classical RTT phenotype. Recently, it was shown that mutations in MeCP2 cause neurological dysfunction by specifically disrupting long gene expression within the brain (Gabel et al. 2015). Phenotypically, RTT is quite heterogeneous in nature and it is likely that post-translational modifications of long genes implicated in neuronal development regulate the functional and developmental versatility of MeCP2 (Bellini et al. 2014; Gabel et al. 2015). In RTT, the clinical picture ranges from individuals who are high functioning, to those who are severely disabled. Individuals with RTT appear to develop normally up to 6–18 months of age. However, this is followed by a period of developmental stagnation and regression with significant loss of speech and social interaction.

At the neuronal level, the architecture of brains in patients with RTT is altered, with dysfunction and general paucity in dendritic branching and spines, which contribute to the abnormal synaptic morphology (Armstrong et al. 1995; Chapleau et al. 2009). In support of these findings, there is also likely to be altered expression of both excitatory and inhibitory synaptic receptors in the brain of RTT patients, supporting the premise that disordered homeostasis of excitatory (Meng et al. 2016) and inhibitory (Ure et al. 2016) signaling coupled with perturbations in neuronal architecture contribute to disordered modulation and maintenance of critical synaptic pathways in RTT brains (Dani et al. 2005; Chao et al. 2010).

Pre-clinical animal models provide a window of opportunity to explore the complex facets of RTT. Recently, SUMOylation, a type of post-translational modification, of MeCP2 was shown to restore behavioural abnormalities in an animal model of RTT (Tai et al. 2016) and deep brain simulation can rescue cognitive dysfunction (Hao et al. 2015) and hippocampal circuit impairment (Lu et al. 2016) in RTT mice. Furthermore, using different pharmacological agents, defects in synaptic architecture and breathing have been restored in MeCP2 null mice (Bittolo et al. 2016; Gogliotti et al. 2016; Patrizi et al. 2016). Others have shown in mouse models of RTT that some of the core features of RTT related to social interaction and anxiety-like behaviour might be caused by abnormal neuronal wiring of the peripheral nervous system (Orefice et al. 2016). Taken at face value, these studies provide very important therapeutic gateways into clinical trials. However, as was shown for Fragile X (Berry-Kravis et al. 2016), which shares some commonalities with RTT such as intellectual disability and ASD, how effectively these animal models translate into studies involving RTT patients remains unclear.

18.6.1 Emotional, Behavioural and Autonomic Dysregulation (EBAD)

Autonomic dysregulation also known as dysautonomia refers to an imbalance between the sympathetic and parasympathetic elements of the autonomic nervous system (ANS) or more broadly speaking refers to any abnormality of the autonomic nervous system. Some examples are vasovagal syncope, neuroleptic malignant syndrome and autonomic dysreflexia but also effects due to medication such as serotonin syndrome (Schwantes and O'Brien 2014). There are several medical conditions that present with ANS imbalances (Baguley 2008); however, what are not readily obvious are the emotional and behavioural components of autonomic dysfunction. Emotional and behavioural dysregulation is common across diagnostic groups and occurs in children with early maltreatment, multiple co-occurring neurodevelopment disorders (such as borderline personality disorder, bipolar disorder, ASD, ADHD and disorders of mixed emotional conduct), acquired brain injury and many rare disorders (Dvir et al. 2014; McLaughlin et al. 2015; Mandavia et al. 2016; Shaw et al. 2014; Li and Liu 2013). Despite this evidence base, there is a scarcity in the literature in terms of evaluating the impact of the autonomic component on these disorders. Autonomic dysregulation has implications for treating and managing the sympathetic and parasympathetic disequilibrium in patients alongside behaviour and emotional dysregulation. Clinically, this situation is often found in treatment non-responders and those with significant functional disability. When emotional and behavioural dysregulation co-occurs in the context of autonomic dysregulation, the term EBAD (**E**motional, **B**ehavioural and **A**utonomic **D**ysregulation) has been coined.

It has become increasingly clear at the Centre for Interventional Paediatric Psychopharmacology and Rare Diseases (CIPPRD), a National Specialist Child and Adolescent Mental Health Service based at the Maudsley Hospital, London, UK, that managing EBAD is central to reducing impairment in complex neuropsychiatric disorders (Santosh et al. 2016), such as those encountered in many rare diseases. When dealing with rare diseases with a limited patient population, it is important that patients can be stratified using phenotype and biomarkers (such as those obtained through wearable sensor monitoring). Ideally, responsive adaptive clinical trial designs using Bayesian approaches that boost the statistical power and reduce the number of patients required for a rare-disease trial should be used (Hampson et al. 2015). Using rare-disease-specific outcome measures as primary end-points and surrogate biomarkers as secondary outcomes will improve the identification of compounds that produce an improvement in this emerging field of research.

When managing rare diseases, EBAD is important to consider as impairments occur in multiple overlapping body systems which can give rise to abnormal physiological responses. RTT can be considered as a congenital dysautonomia (Julu et al. 2001). Genes that are important in regulation of the ANS are likely to be effected in RTT and in these children, understanding the individual physiological reactions (biomarkers of EBAD) would be a critical part when planning treatment strategies, using web-based health monitoring and wearable sensor technology. In Sect. 18.6.1.3, a case will be presented to demonstrate how wearable sensor technology in conjunction with treatment with the 5HT1A partial agonist buspirone can be used to manage EBAD in a 15-year-old girl with RTT who presented with significant emotional and behavioural dysregulation, and autonomic dysfunction. We show that treatment with buspirone improved the autonomic dysfunction and EBAD in this patient.

18.6.1.1 Autonomic Function in RTT

Dysautonomia, i.e. a dysregulation of the parasympathetic and sympathetic components of the ANS, occurs in as much as 75 % of patients with RTT (Sansom et al. 1993) and the subsequent sympathovagal imbalance is thought to be a unique to individuals with RTT (Halbach et al. 2016). Dysautonomia is a leading cause of sudden death (Guideri and Acampa 2005) in RTT. Typically, the autonomic dysregulation can manifest as palpitations, panic attacks and diaphoresis. Evidence has indicated that brainstem immaturity (Julu and Witt Engerström 2005; Julu et al. 1997, 2001) in particular underdevelopment of nascent serotoninergic neurotransmission pathways (Guideri et al. 2004; Paterson et al. 2005) is a major underlying component causing the autonomic dysregulation in those with RTT. Autonomic dysfunction has been explored previously in patients with RTT (Naidu 1987; Paterson et al. 2005) and HR variability has been used as a tool for assessing sympathovagal imbalance in RTT (Dotti et al. 2004; Guideri and Acampa 2005). HR variability provides an indirect measure of autonomic regulation and is usually signified by the low frequency (LF) and high frequency (HF) ratio (LF/HF). However, the relationship between the sympathetic and parasympathetic components of the ANS and their effect on LF/HF (i.e. HR variability) is nonlinear and therefore not entirely obvious (Billman 2013). Nevertheless, although, having some opponents (Hopf et al. 1995; Eckberg 1997; Houle and Billman 1999; Billman 2013), the LF/HF ratio has been used widely as an index for the assessment of autonomic regulation of the cardiovascular system, whereby increases in LF/HF are thought to reflect a shift towards sympathetic activity and conversely decreases signify a shift towards parasympathetic activity (Billman 2013). In RTT, breathing dysrhythmia is one of the characteristic clinical features (Halbach et al. 2016), with forceful, feeble or apneustic breathing (Julu et al. 2008; Smeets et al. 2006; Julu and Witt Engerström 2005), with some having defective control of carbon dioxide metabolism (Halbach et al. 2011). These factors are important when assessing EBAD in RTT given the premise that it has been widely documented that respiratory parameters can modify HR variability (i.e. LF/HF) independent of changes exerted by the ANS (Billman 2013) and that carbon dioxide levels through interaction with chemoreceptors can also modulate in parallel sympathetic and parasympathetic components of the ANS (Eckberg 1997).

18.6.1.2 Using Web-Based Health Monitoring and Wearable Sensor Technology

The rates of development of digital health platforms and risk stratification strategies have rapidly increased in recent years and are widely adopted in medicine to assist in clinical decision-making. The CIPPRD uses a suite of instruments to monitor outcomes using the web-based HealthTracker™ health-monitoring platform—the HealthTracker™ (Santosh et al. 2016). The HealthTracker™ is a web-based health monitoring platform that allows for routine capture of symptoms, side effects, quality of life (QoL), patient experience and life-time response to individualized treatment episodes, using a multi-informant, multimodal methodology. It allows tracking of ongoing medical treatments and assists in optimal shared treatment decision-making and longitudinal patient centred outcome monitoring. The HealthTracker™ provides clinicians with baseline and longitudinal overview of symptom, side effects, QoL, patient experience and treatment response for each patient (Santosh and Singh 2016). Advances in wearable sensor technology have allowed it to be used by children with complex neurodevelopmental disorders such as in RTT. The technology is non-invasive, child-friendly, and allows real-time monitoring of biometric physiological data (heart rate [HR], skin conductance, blood volume pressure, perspiration and temperature) and how they might relate to medication use as well as external factors. In subjects with intellectual disability, poor communication and EBAD, mapping the physiological responses using sensor technology allows for a biometric proxy measure to assist in improving the dysregulation in EBAD.

The CIPPRD is pioneering the use of wearable sensor technology and uses real-time biometric physiological data obtained from different devices in patients with RTT and uses the captured biometric measures as biomarkers to assist in patient management. Once the physiological dysregulation has been identified, the clinician teaches parent/carer(s) to use the wearable sensor technology to track changes that require intervention and, for example, to understand what activities produce physiological stress and what activities/interventions help to normalize the physiological state. The sensor technology allows for colour-based alerts which show whether the HR is too high for the child in question, leading to parents/carers understanding that the child might be experiencing distress and so can use calming strategies for the patient. We have been able to help parents, carers and teachers who become aware of the situation sooner (often before behavioural meltdowns) via the biometric signals from the wearable sensor technology so that timely therapeutic action, i.e. stress-reducing strategies, can be taken (Santosh and Singh 2016).

18.6.1.3 Case

The subject was a 15-year-old girl with a clinical and genetic diagnosis of RTT who presented with significant emotional and behavioural dysregulation with concomitant autonomic dysfunction. Wearable sensor technology was used to monitor biometric physiological biomarker (HR variability and electro-dermal activity [EDA]) and the data for pre-treatment and post-treatment (30 mg/day buspirone) is presented in Fig. 18.1A1–A4 [pre-treatment] and B1–B4 [post-treatment]).

EDA at 1-h time intervals of pre- and post-treatment was analysed using Excel and SPSS software, and as described by Benedek and Kaernbach (2010). Whilst at pre-treatment there was significant variability in EDA (Fig. 18.1A1), this variability reduced significantly with buspirone treatment (Fig. 18.1B1). Heart rate (HR) variability at given time sessions was analysed with Kubios software (version 2.2) (http://kubios.uef.fi.) using time-domain, frequency-domain and nonlinear methods as described in Tarvainen et al. (2014). As noted in the time-domain histogram (Fig. 18.1A2), at pre-treatment, the average HR was 99.67 ± 18.79 beats/min. Following 30 mg/day buspirone, the average HR decreased to 82.20 ± 12.35 beats/min (Fig. 18.1B2).

Evaluable literature supports the premise that the HF component is associated solely with cardiac parasympathetic activity, whilst the LF component, although more complex, is thought reflect a more dominant sympathetic profile (Berntson et al. 1997; Billman 2011). Increases in LF/HF are thought to reflect a shift towards sympathetic activity and conversely decreases signify a shift towards parasympathetic activity (Billman 2013).

The data presented in Fig. 18.1 show a tendency to a shift towards parasympathetic dominance following treatment with buspirone. At 30 mg mg/day buspirone, the HR variability is far less (Fig. 18.1B2). This finding is further corroborated by the width of the Poincaré plot (Fig. 18.1B4) as this is greater than when compared

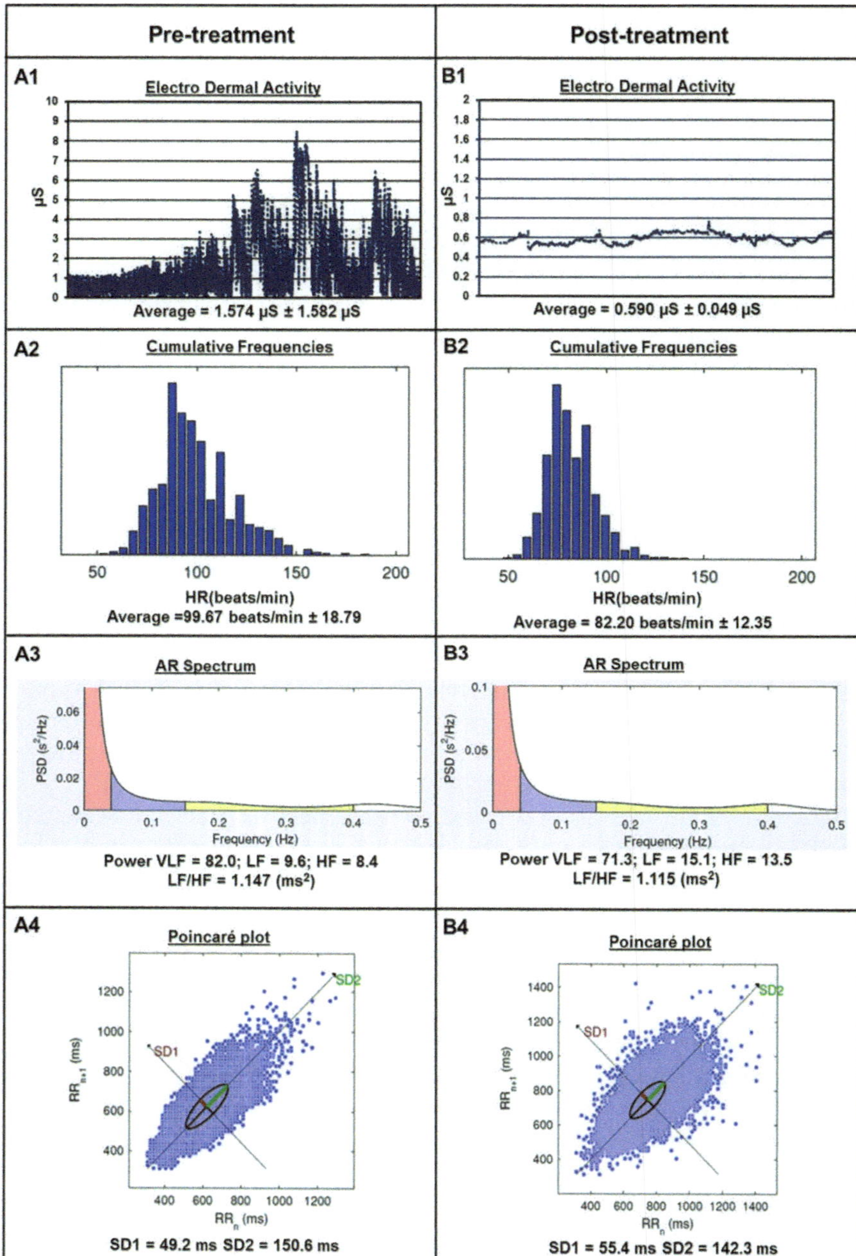

Fig. 18.1 Wearable sensor based biometric physiological data in a 15-year-old girl with Rett syndrome. *Notes* For frequency-domain results, spectral factorization was not used for the AR spectrum (AR model order = 16). Results were calculated from the non-detrended selected RR series. In panel A1, A2, B1 and B2, the data is presented as averages ± standard deviation (SD). *Abbreviations* Autoregressive (AR); High Frequency (HF); Low Frequency (LF); Standard Deviation (SD); Very Low Frequency (VLF)

to the Poincaré plot at baseline (Fig. 18.1A4). The width of the Poincaré plot can be used as a useful quantitative visual index of parasympathetic activity (Kamen et al. 1996). Taken together, these findings show that there was a recalibration of the autonomic equilibrium from pre-treatment to post-treatment. Buspirone 30 mg/day reduced the HR variability and EDA variability (measures of autonomic dysregulation), alongside emotional and behavioural symptoms—that is, an improvement in EBAD. This case represents an example, whereby monitoring and understanding the physiological responses is important when managing EBAD. This strategy is currently being tested in the CIPPRD and needs to be validated in other routine clinical settings.

18.7 Concluding Remarks

Neurodevelopmental disorders persist through development across the age range. It is necessary to combine pharmacological and non-pharmacological interventions together in order to optimize treatment outcomes. At present most treatments focus on symptomatic management, for example, hyperactivity and inattention; irritability, aggression and agitation; anxiety and low mood; tics; mood lability; psychotic symptoms; etc., rather than treatments being disorder-specific. The core symptoms of ASD have not shown response to pharmacological treatments till recently. These studies have shown some improvement of core symptoms (see Santosh and Singh 2016) and it would be of value to build upon the pertinent findings.

It is suggested that emerging technologies can provide biomarkers that can be useful in determining which subjects are most likely to respond and provide early detection of treatment effectiveness. Neuroimaging-based biomarkers would also be a useful adjunct to consider. Neuroimaging-based biomarkers developed using machine learning algorithms can help to unravel and identify pertinent neural phenotypes. Recently, this approach was used to show that a small number of abnormal brain connections were predictive for adult ASD (Yahata et al. 2016). Advancement of optogenetic tools may also shed light on pin-pointing circuit-level understanding of neuronal activity in neurodevelopmental disorders and may help to unravel complex neural mechanisms especially during social interaction (Gunaydin et al. 2014). It is also important to consider a balanced safety and efficacy profile in treatments that are used. In this regard, the EDMS strategy should be adopted to achieve the most acceptable improvement of symptoms with the least minimal side effects (Santosh and Singh 2016). Managing EBAD using wearable sensor technology would also be useful in the management of complex neuropsychiatric disorders especially in the case of individuals with rare diseases.

When treating neurodevelopmental disorders, it is likely that cross-cultural differences between Asian and Western cultures exist. From an Asian perspective, medication might not be readily available and cost of medication per patient would also need to be taken into account. Other factors that need to be considered are the lack of evidence base, in particular the paucity in the number of randomized placebo-controlled double-blind trials conducted in Asia. This coupled with the insufficient numbers of child psychiatrists and behavioural pediatricians for the populations served makes managing patients less straightforward in comparison to Western counterparts.

To summarize, in children and adolescents, a holistic approach should be adopted for managing care. Pharmacology should be used as an adjunct together with psychosocial, language and behavioural intervention therapies. Careful monitoring of pharmacological treatment is paramount and EDMS strategy together with wearable sensor technologies are important avenues for consideration. Research in the neurodevelopment field is expanding quickly and the heterogeneity of these disorders is an important obstacle that requires careful consideration. There is hope, however, that having opened up new inlets, researchers might soon provide ways to overcome such obstacles. Epigenetic strategies would be a useful foil to adopt. Targeting epigenetic dysregulation of neurodevelopmental disorders would be an important step when navigating forward and can help to bridge the gap in our understanding of genetic and environmental basis of disease mechanisms.

Acknowledgments We would like to thank our colleagues at the Centre for Interventional Pediatric Psychopharmacology and Rare Diseases (CIPPRD). In particular, we are indebted to Dr. Federico Fiori for his statistical analysis and Dr. Kate Lievesley for all of her helpful project management work.

Informed consent was obtained from the parent of the child with Rett syndrome.

Declaration of Interest: Dr. Paramala Santosh is the Head of the Centre for Interventional Pediatric Psychopharmacology and Rare Diseases (CIPPRD), Maudsley Hospital, London and is also the co-inventor of the HealthTracker™ and is a Director and shareholder in HealthTracker Ltd.

Dr. Jatinder Singh has no conflicts of interest to declare.

References

Abelson, J. F., Kwan, K. Y., O'Roak, B. J., et al. (2005). Sequence variants in SLITRK1 are associated with Tourette's syndrome. *Science, 310*, 317–320.

Antony, A. (2016). Study of factors influencing treatment adherence in childhood attention deficit hyperactivity disorder in a tertiary healthcare facility. *Indian Journal of Psychological Medicine, 38*, 20–24.

Armstrong, D., Dunn, J. K., Antalffy, B., & Trivedi, R. (1995). Selective dendritic alterations in the cortex of Rett syndrome. *Journal of Neuropathology and Experimental Neurology, 54*, 195–201.

Arya, A., Agarwal, V., Yadav, S., et al. (2015). A study of pathway of care in children and adolescents with attention deficit hyperactivity disorder. *Asian Journal of Psychiatry, 17*, 10–15.

Asherson, P., Buitelaar, J., Faraone, S. V., & Rohde, L. A. (2016). Adult attention-deficit hyperactivity disorder: Key conceptual issues. *The Lancet Psychiatry, 3*, 568–578.

Baguley, I. J. (2008). The excitatory:inhibitory ratio model (EIR model): An integrative explanation of acute autonomic overactivity syndromes. *Medical Hypotheses, 70*, 26–35.

Bellini, E., Pavesi, G., Barbiero, I., et al. (2014). MeCP2 post-translational modifications: A mechanism to control its involvement in synaptic plasticity and homeostasis? *Frontiers in Cellular Neuroscience, 13*(8), 236.

Benedek, M., & Kaernbach, C. (2010). A continuous measure of phasic electrodermal activity. *Journal of Neuroscience Methods, 190*, 80–91.

Benegal, V., Viswanath, B., Narayanaswamy, J. C., et al. (2013). The efficacy of atomoxetine as adjunctive treatment for co-morbid substance use disorders and externalizing symptoms. *Asian Journal of Psychiatry, 6*, 544–547.

Berntson, G. G., Bigger, J. T., Eckberg, D. L., et al. (1997). Heart rate variability: Origins, methods, and interpretive caveats. *Pyschophysiology, 34*, 623–648.

Berry-Kravis, E., Des Portes, V., Hagerman, R., et al. (2016). Mavoglurant in fragile X syndrome: Results of two randomized, double-blind, placebo-controlled trials. *Science Translational Medicine13, 8*(321): 321ra5.

Bienvenu, T., Carrie, A., de Roux, N., et al. (2000). MECP2 mutations account for most cases of typical forms of Rett syndrome. *Human Molecular Genetics, 9*, 1377–1384.

Billman, G. E. (2011). Heart rate variability—a historical perspective. *Frontiers in Physiology, 2*, 86.

Billman, G. E. (2013). The LF/HF ratio does not accurately measure cardiac sympatho-vagal balance. *Frontiers in Physiology, 20*(4), 26.

Bittolo, T., Raminelli, C. A., Deiana, C., et al. (2016). Pharmacological treatment with mirtazapine rescues cortical atrophy and respiratory deficits in MeCP2 null mice. *Scientific Reports, 6*, 19796.

Bonvicini, C., Faraone, S. V., & Scassellati, C. (2016). Attention-deficit hyperactivity disorder in adults: A systematic review and meta-analysis of genetic, pharmacogenetic and biochemical studies. *Molecular Psychiatry, 21*, 872–884.

Boomsma, D. I., Saviouk, V., Hottenga, J. J., et al. (2010). Genetic epidemiology of attention deficit hyperactivity disorder (ADHD index) in adults. *PLoS ONE, 5*, e10621.

Brockschnieder, D., Sabanay, H., Riethmacher, D., et al. (2006). Ermin, a myelinating oligodendrocyte-specific protein that regulates cell morphology. *Journal of Neuroscience, 26*, 757–762.

Bushe, C. J., & Savill, N. C. (2014). Systematic review of atomoxetine data in childhood and adolescent attention-deficit hyperactivity disorder 2009–2011: Focus on clinical efficacy and safety. *Journal of Psychopharmacology, 28*, 204–211.

Canitano, R., & Scandurra, V. (2014). Glutamatergic agents in autism spectrum disorders: Current trends. *Research in Autism Spectrum Disorders, 8*, 255–265.

Castellanos, F. X., & Proal, E. (2012). Large-scale brain systems in ADHD: Beyond the prefrontal-striatal model. *Trends in Cognitive Sciences, 16*, 17–26.

Cha, J., Fekete, T., Siciliano, F., et al. (2015). Neural correlates of aggression in medication-naive children with ADHD: Multivariate analysis of morphometry and tractography. *Neuropsychopharmacology, 40*, 1717–1725.

Chao, H. T., Chen, H., Samaco, R. C., et al. (2010). Dysfunction in GABA signalling mediates autism-like stereotypies and Rett syndrome phenotypes. *Nature, 468*, 263–269.

Chapleau, C. A., Calfa, G. D., Lane, M. C., et al. (2009). Dendritic spine pathologies in hippocampal pyramidal neurons from Rett syndrome brain and after expression of Rett-associated MECP2 mutations. *Neurobiology of Diseases, 35*, 219–233.

Charach, A., Carson, P., Fox, S., et al. (2013). Interventions for preschool children at high risk for ADHD: A comparative effectiveness review. *Pediatrics, 131*, e1584–e1604.

Chen, N. C., Bedair, H. S., McKay, B., et al. (2001). Clozapine in the treatment of aggression in an adolescent with autistic disorder. *Journal of Clinical Psychiatry, 62*, 479–480.

Ching, H., & Pringsheim, T. (2012). Aripiprazole for autism spectrum disorders (ASD). *Cochrane Database of Systematic Reviews, 5*: CD009043.

Church, J. A., Fair, D. A., Dosenbach, N. U., et al. (2009). Control networks in paediatric Tourette syndrome show immature and anomalous patterns of functional connectivity. *Brain, 132*, 225–238.

Cianfaglione, R., Clarke, A., Kerr, M., et al. (2015). A national survey of Rett syndrome: Behavioural characteristics. *The Journal of Neurodevelopmental Disorders, 7*, 11.

Coghill, D., Banaschewski, T., Lecendreux, M., et al. (2013). European, randomized, phase 3 study of lisdexamfetamine dimesylate in children and adolescents with attention-deficit/hyperactivity disorder. *European Neuropsychopharmacology, 23*, 1208–1218.

Conners, C. K., Epstein, J. N., March, J. S., et al. (2001). Multimodal treatment of ADHD in the MTA: An alternative outcome analysis. *Journal of the American Academy of Child and Adolescent Psychiatry, 40*, 159–167.

Connor, D. F., Fletcher, K. E., & Swanson, J. M. (1999). A meta-analysis of Clonidine for symptoms of attention-deficit hyperactivity disorder. *Journal of the American Academy of Child and Adolescent Psychiatry, 38*, 151–159.

Dadds, M. R., MacDonald, E., Cauchi, A., et al. (2014). Nasal oxytocin for social deficits in childhood autism: A randomized controlled trial. *Journal of Autism and Developmental Disorders, 44*, 521–531.

Dani, V. S., Chang, Q., Maffei, A., et al. (2005). Reduced cortical activity due to a shift in the balance between excitation and inhibition in a mouse model of Rett syndrome. *Proceedings of the National Academy of Sciences of the United States of America, 102*, 12560–12565.

Davies, L., Stern, J. S., Agrawal, N., & Robertson, M. M. (2006). The successful use of aripiprazole in a cohort of patients with Tourette's syndrome, refractory to treatment with other neuroleptics and habit reversal training. *Human Psychopharmacology, 21*, 447–453.

De Hert, M., Dobbelaere, M., Sheridan, E., et al. (2011). Metabolic and endocrine adverse effects of second-generation antipsychotics in children and adolescents: A systematic review of randomized, placebo controlled trials and guidelines for clinical practice. *European Psychiatry, 26*, 144–158.

Dean, O. M., Gray, K. M., Villagonzalo, K. A., et al. (2016). A randomised, double blind, placebo-controlled trial of a fixed dose of *N*-acetyl cysteine in children with autistic disorder. *Australian and New Zealand Journal of Psychiatry*. Jun 17.

Deeb, W., Rossi, P. J., Porta, M., et al. (2016). The international deep brain stimulation registry and database for Gilles de la Tourette syndrome: How does it work? *Frontiers in Neuroscience, 10*, 170.

Devlin, B., Scherer, S. W., Emanuel, B., et al. (2012). Genetic architecture in autism spectrum disorder. *Current Opinion in Genetics & Development, 22*, 229–237.

Dotti, M. T., Guideri, F., Acampa, M., et al. (2004). Autonomic dysfunction in mental retardation and spastic paraparesis with MECP2 mutation. *Journal of Child Neurology, 19*, 964–966.

DSM-5. (2013). American Psychiatric Association. *Diagnostic and statistical manual of mental disorders: DSM-5*. Washington, D.C.: American Psychiatric Association.

Dvir, Y., Ford, J. D., Hill, M., & Frazier, J. A. (2014). Childhood maltreatment, emotional dysregulation, and psychiatric comorbidities. *Harvard Review of Psychiatry, 22*, 149–161.

Eapen, V., Cavanna, A. E., Robertson, M. M. (2016). Comorbidities, social impact, and quality of life in Tourette syndrome. *Frontiers in Psychiatry, 7*: 97.

Eapen, V., & Robertson, M. M. (2008). Clinical correlates of Tourette's disorder across cultures: A comparative study between the United Arab Emirates and the United Kingdom. *Primary Care Companion Journal of Clinical Psychiatry, 10*, 103–107.

Eapen, V., Trimble, M. R., & Robertson, M. M. (1996). The use of fluoxetine in Gilles de la Tourette syndrome and obsessive compulsive behaviours: Preliminary clinical experience. *Progress in Neuropsychopharmacology and Biological Psychiatry, 20*, 737–743.

Eckberg, D. L. (1997). Sympathovagal balance: A critical appraisal. *Circulation, 96*, 3224–3232.

Ercan-Sencicek, A. G., Stillman, A. A., Ghosh, A. K., et al. (2010). L-histidine decarboxylase and Tourette's syndrome. *New England Journal of Medicine, 362*, 1901–1908.

Evans, J. C., Archer, H. L., Colley, J. P., et al. (2005). Early onset seizures and Rett-like features associated with mutations in CDKL5. *European Journal of Human Genetics, 13*, 1113–1120.

Fankhauser, M. P., Karumanchi, V. C., German, M. L., et al. (1992). A double blind, placebo controlled study of the efficacy of transdermal clonidine in autism. *Journal of Clinical Psychiatry, 53*, 77–82.

Findling, R. L., Mankoski, R., Timko, K., et al. (2014). A randomized controlled trial investigating the safety and efficacy of aripiprazole in the long-term maintenance treatment of pediatric patients with irritability associated with autistic disorder. *Journal of Clinical Psychiatry, 75*, 22–30.

Freeman, R. D., Fast, D. K., Burd, L., et al. (2000). An international perspective on Tourette syndrome: Selected findings from 3500 individuals in 22 countries. *Developmental Medicine and Child Neurology, 42*, 436–447.

Fung, L. K., Mahajan, R., Nozzolillo, A., et al. (2016). Pharmacologic treatment of severe irritability and problem behaviors in autism: A systematic review and meta-analysis. *Pediatrics, 137*(Suppl 2), S124–S135.

Gabel, H. W., Kinde, B., Stroud, H., et al. (2015). Disruption of DNA-methylation-dependent long gene repression in Rett syndrome. *Nature, 522*, 89–93.

Gamo, N. J., Wang, M., & Arnsten, A. F. (2010). Methylphenidate and atomoxetine enhance prefrontal function through α2-adrenergic and dopamine D1 receptors. *Journal of the American Academy of Child and Adolescent Psychiatry, 49*, 1011–1023.

Garg, J., Arun, P., & Chavan, B. S. (2014). Comparative short-term efficacy and tolerability of methylphenidate and atomoxetine in attention deficit hyperactivity disorder. *Indian Pediatrics, 51*, 550–554.

Garg, J., Arun, P., & Chavan, B. S. (2015). Comparative efficacy of methylphenidate and atomoxetine in oppositional defiant disorder comorbid with attention deficit hyperactivity disorder. *International Journal of Applied and Basic Medical Research, 5*, 114–118.

Ghanizadeh, A., & Moghimi-Sarani, E. (2013). A randomized double blind placebo controlled clinical trial of *N*-Acetylcysteine added to risperidone for treating autistic disorders. *BMC Psychiatry, 13*, 196.

Ghanizadeh, A., Sahraeizadeh, A., & Berk, M. (2014). A head-to-head comparison of aripiprazole and risperidone for safety and treating autistic disorders, a randomized double blind clinical trial. *Child Psychiatry and Human Development, 45*, 185–192.

Gogliotti, R. G., Senter, R. K., Rook, J. M., et al. (2016). mGlu5 positive allosteric modulation normalizes synaptic plasticity defects and motor phenotypes in a mouse model of Rett syndrome. *Human Molecular Genetics*, 1–15.

Gordon, I., Vander Wyk, B. C., Bennett, R. H., et al. (2013). Oxytocin enhances brain function in children with autism. *Proceedings of the National Academy of Sciences of the United States of America, 110*, 20953–20958.

Guastella, A. J., Gray, K. M., Rinehart, N. J., et al. (2015). The effects of a course of intranasal oxytocin on social behaviors in youth diagnosed with autism spectrum disorders: A randomized controlled trial. *Journal of Child Psychology and Psychiatry, 56*, 444–452.

Guideri, F., & Acampa, M. (2005). Sudden death and cardiac arrhythmias in Rett syndrome. *Pediatric Cardiology, 26*, 111.

Guideri, F., Acampa, M., Blardi, P., et al. (2004). Cardiac dysautonomia and serotonin plasma levels in Rett syndrome. *Neuropediatrics, 35*, 36–38.

Gunaydin, L. A., Grosenick, L., Finkelstein, J. C., et al. (2014). Natural neural projection dynamics underlying social behavior. *Cell, 157*, 1535–1551.

Guy, J., Gan, J., Selfridge, J., et al. (2007). Reversal of neurological defects in a mouse model of Rett syndrome. *Science, 315*, 1143–1147.

Hagberg, B., Aicardi, J., Dias, K., et al. (1983). A progressive syndrome of autism, dementia, ataxia, and loss of purposeful hand use in girls: Rett's syndrome: Report of 35 cases. *Annals of Neurology, 14*, 471–479.

Hagerman, R., Au, J., & Hagerman, P. (2011). FMR1 premutation and full mutation molecular mechanisms related to autism. *Journal of Neurodevelopmental Disorders, 3*, 211–224.

Hagerman, R., Hoem, G., & Hagerman, P. (2010). Fragile X and autism: Intertwined at the molecular level leading to targeted treatments. *Molecular Autism, 1*, 12.

Halbach, N. S. J., Smeets, E. E. J., Bierau, J., et al. (2011). Altered carbon dioxide metabolism and creatine abnormalities in Rett syndrome. *Journal on Inherited Metabolic Disease Reports, 3*, 117–124.

Halbach, N., Smeets, E. E., Julu, P., et al. (2016). Neurophysiology versus clinical genetics in Rett syndrome: A multicenter study. *American Journal of Medical Genetics Part A, 170*, 2301–2309.

Hampson, L. V., Whitehead, J., Eleftheriou, D., et al. (2015). Elicitation of expert prior opinion: Application to the MYPAN trial in childhood polyarteritis nodosa. *PLoS ONE, 30*(10), e0120981.

Hao, S., Tang, B., Wu, Z., et al. (2015). Forniceal deep brain stimulation rescues hippocampal memory in Rett syndrome mice. *Nature, 526*, 430–434.

Hardan, A. Y., Fung, L. K., Libove, R. A., et al. (2012). A randomized controlled pilot trial of oral *N*-acetylcysteine in children with autism. *Biological Psychiatry, 71*, 956–961.

Harfterkamp, M., Buitelaar, J. K., Minderaa, R. B., et al. (2014). Atomoxetine in autism spectrum disorder: No effects on social functioning; some beneficial effects on stereotyped behaviors, inappropriate speech, and fear of change. *Journal of Child and Adolescent Psychopharmacology, 24*, 481–485.

Harfterkamp, M., van der Meer, D., van der Loo-Neus, G., et al. (2015). No evidence for predictors of response to atomoxetine treatment of attention deficit/ hyperactivity disorder symptoms in children and adolescents with autism spectrum disorder. *Journal of Child and Adolescent Psychopharmacology, 25*, 372–375.

Hartley, S., Sikora, D., & McCoy, R. (2008). Prevalence and risk factors of maladaptive behaviour in young children with autistic disorder. *Journal of Intellectual Disability Research, 52*, 819–829.

Hazell, P. (2007). Drug therapy for attention-deficit/hyperactivity disorder like symptoms in autistic disorder. *Journal of Paediatrics and Child Health, 43*, 19–24.

Hirota, T., Schwartz, S., & Correll, C. U. (2014). Alpha-2 agonists for attention-deficit/hyperactivity disorder in youth: A systematic review and meta-analysis of monotherapy and add-on trials to stimulant therapy. *Journal of the American Academy of Child and Adolescent Psychiatry, 53*, 153–173.

Hodgetts, S., Nicholas, D., & Zwaigenbaum, L. (2013). Home sweet home? Families' experiences with aggression in children with autism spectrum disorders. *Focus on Autism Developmental Disabilities, 28*, 166–174.

Hollander, E., Novotny, S., Hanratty, M., et al. (2003). Oxytocin infusion reduces repetitive behaviors in adults with autistic and Asperger's disorders. *Neuropsychopharmacology, 28*, 193–198.

Homs, A., Codina-Solà, M., Rodríguez-Santiago, B., et al. (2016). Genetic and epigenetic methylation defects and implication of the ERMN gene in autism spectrum disorders. *Translational Psychiatry, 6*, e855.

Hopf, H. B., Skyschally, A., Heusch, G., & Peters, J. (1995). Low-frequency spectral power of heart rate variability is not a specific marker of cardiac sympathetic modulation. *Anesthesiology, 82*, 609–619.

Houle, M. S., & Billman, G. E. (1999). Low-frequency component of the heart rate variability spectrum: A poor marker of sympathetic activity. *American Journal of Physiology Heart and Circulatory Physiology, 267*, H215–H223.

Jahromi, L. B., Kasari, C. L., McCracken, J. T., et al. (2009). Positive effects of methylphenidate on social communication and self-regulation in children with pervasive developmental disorders and hyperactivity. *Journal of Autism and Developmental Disorders, 39*, 395–404.

James, S. J., Melnyk, S., Jernigan, S., et al. (2006). Metabolic endophenotype and related genotypes are associated with oxidative stress in children with autism. *American Journal of Medical Genetics Part B: Neuropsychiatric Genetics, 141B*, 947–956.

Jhambh, I., Arun, P., & Garg, J. (2014). Cross-sectional study of self-reported ADHD symptoms and psychological comorbidity among college students in Chandigarh, India. *Indian Journal of Psychiatry, 23*, 111–116.

Julu, P. O., Kerr, A. M., Apartopoulos, F., et al. (2001). Characterization of breathing and associated central autonomic dysfunction in the Rett disorder. *Archives of Disease in Childhood, 85*, 29–37.

Julu, P. O., Kerr, A. M., Hansen, S., et al. (1997). Functional evidence of brain stem immaturity in Rett syndrome. *European Child and Adolescent Psychiatry, 6*(Suppl 1), 47–54.

Julu, P. O., & Witt, Engerström I. (2005). Assessment of the maturity-related brainstem functions reveals the heterogeneous phenotypes and facilitates clinical management of Rett syndrome. *Brain and Development, 27*(Suppl. 1), S43–S53.

Julu, P. O., Witt Engerström, I., Hansen, S., et al. (2008). Clinical update addressing the cardiorespiratory challenges in medicine posed by Rett syndrome: The Frösö declaration. *Lancet 371*, 1981–1983.

Juneja, M., Jain, R., Singh, V., & Mallika, V. (2010). Iron deficiency in Indian children with attention deficit hyperactivity disorder. *Indian Pediatrics, 47*, 955–958.

Kamen, P. W., Krum, H., & Tonkin, A. M. (1996). Poincaré plot of heart rate variability allows quantitative display of parasympathetic nervous activity in humans. *Clinical Science (London), 91*, 201–208.

Kanne, S. M., & Mazurek, M. O. (2011). Aggression in children and adolescents with ASD: Prevalence and risk factors. *Journal of Autism and Developmental Disorders, 41*, 926–937.

Karagiannidis, I., Dehning, S., Sandor, P., et al. (2011). Support of the histaminergic hypothesis in Tourette syndrome: Association of the histamine decarboxylase gene in a large sample of families. *Journal of Medical Genetics, 50*, 760–764.

Karagiannidis, I., Rizzo, R., Tarnok, Z., et al. (2012). Replication of association between a SLITRK1 haplotype and Tourette Syndrome in a large sample of families. *Molecular Psychiatry, 17*, 665–668.

Katz, D. M., Bird, A., Coenraads, M., et al. (2016). Rett syndrome: Crossing the threshold to clinical translation. *Trends in Neurosciences, 39*, 100–113.

Kozinetz, C. A., Skender, M. L., MacNaughton, N., et al. (1993). Epidemiology of Rett syndrome: A population-based registry. *Pediatrics, 91*, 445–450.

Lambrey, S., Falissard, B., Martin-Barrero, M., et al. (2010). Effectiveness of clozapine for the treatment of aggression in an adolescent with autistic disorder. *Journal of Child and Adolescent Psychopharmacology, 20*, 79–80.

Lee, Y. J., Oh, S. H., Park, C., et al. (2014). Advanced pharmacotherapy evidenced by pathogenesis of autism spectrum disorder. *Clinical Psychopharmacology and Neuroscience, 12*, 19–30.

Lewis, J. D., Meehan, R. R., Henzel, W. J., et al. (1992). Purification, sequence, and cellular localization of a novel chromosomal protein that binds to methylated DNA. *Cell, 69*, 905–914.

Li, L., & Liu, J. (2013). The effect of pediatric traumatic brain injury on behavioral outcomes: A systematic review. *Developmental Medicine and Child Neurology, 55*, 37–45.

Lieh-Mak, F., Chung, S. Y., Lee, P., & Chen, S. (1982). Tourette syndrome in the Chinese: A follow-up of 15 cases. In A. Friedhoff & T. Chase (Eds.), *Gilles de la Tourette syndrome* (pp. 281–283). New York (NY): Raven.

Liu, Y., Ni, H., Wang, C., et al. (2016a). Effectiveness and tolerability of aripiprazole in children and adolescents with Tourette's disorder: A meta-analysis. *Journal of Child Adolescent Psychopharmacology, 5*, 436–441.

Liu, H., Talalay, P., & Fahey, J. W. (2016b). Biomarker-guided strategy for treatment of autism spectrum disorder (ASD). *CNS and Neurological Disorders: Drug Targets, 15*, 602–613.

Lu, H., Ash, R. T., He, L., et al. (2016). Loss and gain of MeCP2 cause similar hippocampal circuit dysfunction that is rescued by deep brain stimulation in a Rett syndrome mouse model. *Neuron, 91*, 739–747.

Lucariello, M., Vidal, E., Vidal, S., et al. (2016). Whole exome sequencing of Rett syndrome-like patients reveals the mutational diversity of the clinical phenotype. *Human Genetics, 135*, 1343–1354.

Malhotra, S., & Santosh, P. J. (1998). An open clinical trial of buspirone in children with attention-deficit/hyperactivity disorder. *Journal of American Academy of Child and Adolescent Psychiatry, 37*, 364–371.

Mandavia, A., Robinson, G. G., & Bradley, B. (2016). Exposure to childhood abuse and later substance use: Indirect effects of emotion dysregulation and exposure to trauma. *Journal of Traumatic Stress, 29*, 422–429.

McCracken, J. T., McGough, J., Shah, B., et al. (2002). Risperidone in children with autism and serious behavioural problems research units on pediatric psychopharmacology autism network. *New England Journal of Medicine, 347*, 314–321.

McLaughlin, K. A., Peverill, M., Gold, A. L., et al. (2015). Child maltreatment and neural systems underlying emotion regulation. *Journal of the American Academy of Child and Adolescent Psychiatry, 54*, 753–762.

Mei, Y., Monteiro, P., Zhou, Y., et al. (2016). Adult restoration of Shank3 expression rescues selective autistic-like phenotypes. *Nature, 530*, 481–484.

Meng, X., Wang, W., Lu, H., et al. (2016). Manipulations of MeCP2 in glutamatergic neurons highlight their contributions to Rett and other neurological disorders. *Elife, 5*, pii: e14199.

Michelson, D., Allen, A. J., Busner, J., et al. (2002). Once-daily atomoxetine treatment for children and adolescents with attention deficit hyperacivity disorder: A randomized, placebo-controlled study. *American Journal of Psychiatry, 159*, 1896–1901.

Michelson, D., Faries, D., Wernicke, J., et al. (2001). Atomoxetine in the treatment of children and adolescents with attention-deficit/hyperactivity disorder: A randomized, placebo-controlled, dose-response study. *Pediatrics, 108*(5), e83.

Miller, J. A., Ding, S. L., Sunkin, S. M., et al. (2014). Transcriptional landscape of the prenatal human brain. *Nature, 508*, 199–206.

Min, S. K., & Lee, H. (1986). A clinical study of Gilles de la Tourette's syndrome in Korea. *British Journal of Psychiatry, 149*, 644–647.

Minshawi, N. F., Wink, L. K., Shaffer, R., et al. (2016). A randomized, placebo-controlled trial of *D*-cycloserine for the enhancement of social skills training in autism spectrum disorders. *Molecular Autism, 14*(7), 2.

Moffitt, T. E., Houts, R., Asherson, P., et al. (2015). Is adult ADHD a childhood-onset neurodevelopmental disorder? Evidence from a four-decade longitudinal cohort study. *American Journal of Psychiatry, 172*, 967–977.

Moog, U., Smeets, E. E., van Roozendaal, K. E., et al. (2003). Neurodevelopmental disorders in males related to the gene causing Rett syndrome in females (MECP2). *European Journal of Paediatric Neurology, 7*, 5–12.

MTA Cooperative Group. (1999). Fourteen-month randomized clinical trial of treatment strategies for attention-deficit hyperactivity disorder. *Archives of General Psychiatry, 56*, 1073–1086.

Mukherjee, S., Shah, H. R., Ramanathan, S., & Dewan, M. (2016). Knowledge and attitudes about attention-deficit/hyperactivity disorder and specific learning disorder in an urban Indian population. *The Journal of Nervous and Mental Disease, 204*, 458–463.

Nagaraj, R., Singhi, P., & Malhi, P. (2006). Risperidone in children with autism: Randomized, placebo-controlled, double-blind study. *Journal of Child Neurology, 21*, 450–455.

Nagel, B. J., Bathula, D., Herting, M., et al. (2011). Altered white matter microstructure in children with attention-deficit/hyperactivity disorder. *Journal of the American Academy of Child and Adolescent Psychiatry, 50*, 283–292.

Naidu, S. (1987). Rett syndrome: New observations. *Brain Development, 9*, 525–528.

National Institute for Health and Care Excellence (2013). *Attention deficit hyperactivity disorder: Diagnosis and management of ADHD in children, young people and adults*. Guideline 72, Issued: September 2008, last modified: March 2013. https://www.nice.org.uk/guidance/cg72

National Institute for Health and Care Excellence (2013). *Autism: The management and support of children and young people on the autism spectrum* (Clinical Guideline GG170). https://www.nice.org.uk/Guidance/CG170

Nikoo, M., Radnia, H., Farokhnia, M., et al. (2015). N-acetylcysteine as an adjunctive therapy to risperidone for treatment of irritability in autism: A randomized, double-blind, placebo-controlled clinical trial of efficacy and safety. *Clinical Neuropharmacology, 38*, 11–17.

Nomura, Y., Kita, M., & Segawa, M. (1992). Social adaptation of Tourette syndrome families in Japan. *Advances in Neurology, 58*, 323–332.

Nomura, Y., & Segawa, M. (1979). Gilles de la Tourette syndrome in oriental children. *Brain Development, 1*, 103–111.

Nott, A., Cheng, J., Gao, F., et al. (2016). Histone deacetylase 3 associates with MeCP2 to regulate FOXO and social behavior. *Nature Neuroscience, 19*, 1497–1505.

O'Roak, B. J., & State, M. W. (2008). Autism genetics: strategies, challenges, and opportunities *Autism Research, 1*, 4–17.

Orefice, L. L., Zimmerman, A. L., Chirila, A. M., et al. (2016). Peripheral mechanosensory neuron dysfunction underlies tactile and behavioral deficits in mouse models of ASDs. *Cell, 166*, 299–313.

Owen, R., Sikich, L., Marcus, R. N., et al. (2009). Aripiprazole in the treatment of irritability in children and adolescents with autistic disorder. *Pediatrics, 124*, 1533–1540.

Parker, K. J., Garner, J. P., Libove, R. A., et al. (2014). Plasma oxytocin concentrations and OXTR polymorphisms predict social impairments in children with and without autism spectrum disorder. *Proceedings of the National Academy of Sciences of the United States of America, 111*, 12258–12263.

Patel, C., Kieling, C., Maulik, P. K., & Divan, G. (2013). Improving access to care for children with mental disorders: A global perspective. *Archives of Disease in Childhood, 98*, 323–327.

Paterson, D. S., Thompson, E. G., Belliveau, R. A., et al. (2005). Serotonin transporter abnormality in the dorsal motor nucleus of the vagus in Rett syndrome: Potential implications for clinical autonomic dysfunction. *Journal of Neuropathology and Experimental Neurology, 11*, 1018–1027.

Patrizi, A., Picard, N., Simon, A. J., et al. (2016). Chronic administration of the *N*-methyl-*D*-spartate receptor antagonist ketamine improves Rett syndrome phenotype. *Biological Psychiatry, 79*, 755–764.

Petronis, A. (2010). Epigenetics as a unifying principle in the aetiology of complex traits and diseases. *Nature, 465*, 721–727.

Philippe, C., Amsallem, D., Francannet, C., et al. (2010). Phenotypic variability in Rett syndrome associated with FOXG1 mutations in females. *Journal of Medical Genetics, 47*, 59–65.

Piacentini, J., Woods, D. W., Scahill, L., et al. (2010). Behavior therapy for children with Tourette disorder: A randomized controlled trial. *JAMA, 303*, 1929–1937.

Proenca, C. C., Gao, K. P., Shmelkov, S. V., et al. (2011). Slitrks as emerging candidate genes involved in neuropsychiatric disorders. *Trends in Neurosciences, 34*, 143–153.

Punja, S., Shamseer, L., Hartling, L., et al. (2016). Amphetamines for attention deficit hyperactivity disorder (ADHD) in children and adolescents. *Cochrane Database of Systematic Reviews Issue 7*: CD009996.

Purper-Ouakil, D., Ramoz, N., Lepagnol-Bestel, A. M., et al. (2011). Neurobiology of attention deficit/hyperactivity disorder. *Pediatric Research, 69*, 69R–76R.

Rahman, A., Divan, G., Hamdani, S. U., et al. (2016). Effectiveness of the parent-mediated intervention for children with autism spectrum disorder in south Asia in India and Pakistan (PASS): A randomised controlled trial. *The Lancet Psychiatry, 3*, 128–136.

Reichow, B., George-Puskar, A., Lutz, T., et al. (2015) Brief report: systematic review of Rett syndrome in males. *Journal of Autism and Developmental Disorders, 45*, 3377–3383.

Rett, A. (1966). On a unusual brain atrophy syndrome in hyperammonemia in childhood. *Wiener Medizinische Wochenschrift, 116*, 723–726.

Rizzo, R., & Martino, D. (2015). Guanfacine for the treatment of attention deficit hyperactivity disorder in children and adolescents. *Expert Review of Neurotherapeutics, 15*, 347–354.

Robertson, M. M. (2009). The prevalence and epidemiology of Gilles de la Tourette syndrome. Part 1: The epidemiological and prevalence studies. *Journal of Psychosomatic Research, 65*, 461–472.

Robertson, M. M. (2015). A personal 35 year perspective on Gilles de la Tourette syndrome: Prevalence, phenomenology, comorbidities, and coexistent psychopathologies. *The Lancet Psychiatry, 2*, 68–87.

Robertson, M. M., & Eapen, V. (2014). Tourette's: Syndrome, disorder or spectrum? Classificatory challenges and an appraisal of the DSM criteria. *Asian Journal of Psychiatry, 11*, 106–113.

Robertson, M. M., Eapen, V., & Cavanna, A. E. (2009). The international prevalence, epidemiology, and clinical phenomenology of Tourette syndrome: A cross-cultural perspective. *Journal of Psychosomatic Research, 67*, 475–483.

Robertson, M. M., Schnieden, V., & Lees, A. J. (1990). Management of Gilles de la Tourette syndrome using sulpiride. *Clinical Neuropharmacology, 13*, 229–235.

Robertson, M. M., Trimble, M. R., & Lees, A. J. (1988). The psychopathology of the Gilles de la Tourette syndrome: A phenomenological analysis. *British Journal of Psychiatry, 152*, 383–390.

Rothenberger, D., & Roessner, V. (2013). The phenomenology of attention deficit hyperactivity disorder in Tourette Syndrome. In D. Martino, J. F. Leckman (Eds.), *Tourette Syndrome* (pp. 26–49). Oxford: Oxford University Press.

Ruggiero, S., Clavenna, A., Reale, L., et al. (2014). Guanfacine for attention deficit and hyperactivity disorder in pediatrics: A systematic review and meta-analysis. *European Neuropsychopharmacology, 24*, 1578–1590.

Sansom, D., Krishnan, V. H., Corbett, J., & Kerr, A. (1993). Emotional and behavioural aspects of Rett syndrome. *Developmental Medicine and Child Neurology, 35*, 340–345.

Santosh, P. J. (2014). Medication in autism spectrum disorder. *Cutting Edge Psychiatry in Practice, 4*, 143–155.

Santosh, P. J., Baird, G., Pityaratstian, N., et al. (2006). Impact of comorbid autism spectrum disorders on stimulant response in children with attention deficit hyperactivity disorder: A retrospective and prospective effectiveness study. *Child: Care, Health and Development, 32*, 575–583.

Santosh, P. J., Bell, L., Fiori, F., & Singh, J. (2016). Pediatric antipsychotic use and outcomes monitoring. Journal of Child Adolescent Psychopharmacology.

Santosh, P. J., Sattar, S., & Canagaratnam, M. (2011). Efficacy and tolerability of pharmacotherapies for attention-deficit hyperactivity disorder in adults. *CNS Drugs, 25*, 737–763.

Santosh, P. J., & Singh, J. (2016). Drug treatment of autism spectrum disorders and their comorbidities in children. *BJPsych Advances, 22*, 151–161.

Santosh, P. J., Taylor, E., Swanson, J., et al. (2005). Refining the diagnoses of inattention and over activity syndromes: A re-analysis of the multimodal treatment study of attention deficit hyperactivity disorder (ADHD) based on ICD10 criteria for hyperkinetic disorder. *Clinical Neuroscience Research, 5*, 307–314.

Scahill, L., McCracken, J. T., King, B. H., et al. (2015). Extended-release guanfacine for hyperactivity in children with autism spectrum disorder. *American Journal of Psychiatry, 172*, 1197–1206.

Schwantes, S., & O'Brien, H. W. (2014). Pediatric palliative care for children with complex chronic medical conditions. *Pediatric Clinics of North America, 61*, 797–821.

Sekar, A., Bialas, A. R., de Rivera, H., et al. (2016). Schizophrenia risk from complex variation of complement component 4. *Nature, 530*, 177–183.

Shaw, P., Eckstrand, K., Sharp, W., et al. (2007). Attention-deficit/hyperactivity disorder is characterized by a delay in cortical maturation. *Proceedings of the National Academy of Sciences of the United States of America, 104*, 19649–19654.

Shaw, P., Stringaris, A., Nigg, J., & Leibenluft, E. (2014). Emotion dysregulation in attention deficit hyperactivity disorder. *American Journal of Psychiatry, 171*, 276–293.

Shea, S., Turgay, A., Carroll, A., et al. (2004). Risperidone in the treatment of disruptive behavioral symptoms in children with autistic and other pervasive developmental disorders. *Pediatrics, 114*, e634–e641.

Simonoff, E., Pickles, A., Charman, T., et al. (2008). Psychiatric disorders in children with autism spectrum disorders: Prevalence, comorbidity, and associated factors in a population-derived sample. *Journal of the American Academy of Child and Adolescent Psychiatry, 47*, 921–929.

Singh, K., Connors, S. L., Macklin, E. A., et al. (2015). Sulforaphane treatment of autism spectrum disorder (ASD). *Proceedings of the National Academy of Sciences of the United States of America, 111*, 15550–15555.

Skene, P. J., Illingworth, R. S., Webb, S., et al. (2010). Neuronal MeCP2 is expressed at near histone-octamer levels and globally alters the chromatin state. *Molecular Cell, 37*, 457–468.

Deepmala, Slattery, J., Kumar, N., et al. (2015). Clinical trials of *N*-acetylcysteine in psychiatry and neurology: A systematic review. *Neuroscience and Biobehavioral Reviews, 55*: 294–321.

Smeets, E., Julu, P., van Waardenburg, D., et al. (2006). Management of a severe forceful breather with Rett syndrome using carbogen. *Brain Development, 28*, 625–632.

Smoller, J. W., Ripke, S., Lee, P. H., et al. (2013). Identification of risk loci with shared effects on five major psychiatric disorders: A genome-wide analysis. Cross-disorder group of the psychiatric genomics consortium. *Lancet, 381*, 1371–1379.

Staley, D., Wand, R., & Shady, G. (1997). Tourette disorder: A cross-cultural review. *Comprehensive Psychiatry, 38*, 6–16.

Stefanelli, G., Gandaglia, A., Costa, M., et al. (2016). Brain phosphorylation of MeCP2 at serine 164 is developmentally regulated and globally alters its chromatin association. *Scientific Reports, 6*, 28295.

Storebø, O. J., Ramstad, E., Krogh, H. B., et al. (2015). Methylphenidate for children and adolescents with attention deficit hyperactivity disorder (ADHD). *Cochrane Database of Systematic Reviews, 11*, CD009885.

Stuhec, M., Munda, B., Svab, V., & Locatelli, I. (2015). Comparative efficacy and acceptability of atomoxetine, lisdexamfetamine, bupropion and methylphenidate in treatment of attention deficit hyperactivity disorder in children and adolescents: A meta-analysis with focus on bupropion. *Journal of Affective Disorders, 178*, 149–159.

Sukhodolsky, D. G., Bloch, M. H., Panza, K. E., et al. (2013). Cognitive-behavioural therapy for anxiety in children with high-functioning autism: A meta-analysis. *Pediatrics, 132*, e1341–e1350.

Swanson, J. M., Kraemer, H. C., Hinshaw, S. P., et al. (2001). Clinical relevance of the primary findings of the MTA: Success rates based on severity of ADHD and ODD symptoms at the end of treatment. *Journal of the American Academy of Child and Adolescent Psychiatry, 40*, 168–179.

Sztainberg, Y., Chen, H. M., Swann, J. W., et al. (2015). Reversal of phenotypes in MECP2 duplication mice using genetic rescue or antisense oligonucleotides. *Nature, 528*, 123–126.

Tai, D. J., Liu, Y. C., Hsu, W. L., et al. (2016). MeCP2 SUMOylation rescues Mecp2-mutant-induced behavioural deficits in a mouse model of Rett syndrome. *Nature Communications, 7*, 10552.

Tarvainen, M. P., Niskanen, J. P., Lipponen, J. A., et al. (2014). Kubios HRV–heart rate variability analysis software. *Computer Methods and Programs in Biomedicine, 113*, 210–220.

Taylor, E., Schachar, R., Thorley, G., et al. (1987). Which boys respond to stimulant medication? A controlled trial of methylphenidate in boys with disruptive behaviour. *Psychological Medicine, 17*, 121–143.

Turner, T. N., Sharma, K., Oh, E. C., et al. (2015). Loss of δ-catenin function in severe autism. *Nature, 520*, 51–56.

Urbano, M., Okwara, L., Manser, P., et al. (2014). A trial of D-cycloserine to treat stereotypies in older adolescents and young adults with autism spectrum disorder. *Clinical Neuropharmacology, 37*, 69–72.

Urbano, M., Okwara, L., Manser, P., et al. (2015). A trial of d-cycloserine to treat the social deficit in older adolescents and young adults with autism spectrum disorders. *Journal of Neuropsychiatry and Clinical Neurosciences, 27*, 133–138.

Ure, K., Lu, H., Wang, W., et al. (2016). Restoration of Mecp2 expression in GABAergic neurons is sufficient to rescue multiple disease features in a mouse model of Rett Syndrome. *Elife, 5*, pii: e14198.

Venkata, J. A., & Panicker, A. S. (2013). Prevalence of attention deficit hyperactivity disorder in primary school children. *Indian Journal of Psychiatry, 55*, 338–342.

Verdellen, C., van de Griendt, J., Hartmann, A., et al. (2011). European clinical guidelines for Tourette syndrome and other tic disorders. Part III: Behavioural and psychosocial interventions. *European Child and Adolescent Psychiatry, 20*, 197–207.

Volkow, N. D., & Swanson, J. M. (2013). Clinical practice: Adult attention deficit-hyperactivity disorder. *New England Journal of Medicine, 369*, 1935–1944.

Walkup, J. T., Albano, A. M., Piacentini, J., et al. (2008). Cognitive behavioral therapy, sertraline, or a combination in childhood anxiety. *New England Journal of Medicine, 359*, 2753–2766.

Wells, M. F., Wimmer, R. D., Schmitt, L. I., et al. (2016). Thalamic reticular impairment underlies attention deficit in Ptchd1(Y/-) mice. *Nature, 532*, 58–63.

Whitford, K. L., Marillat, V., Stein, E., et al. (2002). Regulation of cortical dendrite development by Slit-Robo interactions. *Neuron, 33*, 47–61.

Whittington, C., Pennant, M., Kendall, T., et al. (2016). Practitioner review: Treatments for Tourette syndrome in children and young people—a systematic review. Journal of Child Psychology and Psychiatry.

WHO. (1992). *International statistical classification of diseases and related health problems, 10th revision*. Geneva: World Health Organization.

Willsey, A. J., Sanders, S. J., Li, M., et al. (2013). Coexpression networks implicate human midfetal deep cortical projection neurons in the pathogenesis of autism. *Cell, 155*, 997–1007.

Wingate, M., Kirby, R. S., Pettygrove, S., et al. (2014). Prevalence of autism spectrum disorder among children aged 8 years—autism and developmental disabilities monitoring network, 11 sites, United States, 2010. Developmental disabilities monitoring network surveillance year 2010 principal investigators; Centers for disease control and prevention (CDC). *MMWR. Surveillance Summary, 63*, 1–21.

Wink, L. K., Adams, R., Wang, Z., et al. (2016). A randomized placebo-controlled pilot study of *N*-acetylcysteine in youth with autism spectrum disorder. *Molecular Autism, 7*, 26.

Witteveen, J. S., Willemsen, M. H., Dombroski, T. C., et al. (2016). Haploinsufficiency of MeCP2-interacting transcriptional co-repressor SIN3A causes mild intellectual disability by affecting the development of cortical integrity. *Nature Genetics*, 1–11.

Wood, J. J., Ehrenreich-May, J., Alessandri, M., et al. (2015). Cognitive behavioral therapy for early adolescents with autism spectrum disorders and clinical anxiety: A randomized, controlled trial. *Behavior Therapy, 46*, 7–19.

Yahata, N., Morimoto, J., Hashimoto, R., et al. (2016). A small number of abnormal brain connections predicts adult autism spectrum disorder. *Nature Communications, 14*(7), 11254.

Yatawara, C. J., Einfeld, S. L., Hickie, I. B., et al. (2015). The effect of oxytocin nasal spray on social interaction deficits observed in young children with autism: A randomized clinical crossover trial. *Molecular Psychiatry*, 1–7.

Chapter 19
Electro Convulsive Therapy in the Treatment of Severe Psychiatric Disorders in Children and Adolescents

Yuval Bloch and Neera Ghaziuddin

Abstract Severe mental disorders endanger the lives and development of children and adolescents. For many of these patients' other forms of therapy including psychotherapy and pharmacotherapy are not efficient, due to a significant time lag before these interventions may be effective. In many cases, the patient may have already failed several pharmacological trials and psychotherapeutic interventions. This chapter will discuss electroconvulsive therapy (ECT) in the treatment of severe psychiatric disorders in children and adolescents, in particular treatment resistant mood disorders, catatonia, psychotic spectrum disorders, and self-injurious behaviors. A course of ECT includes a few brief well-monitored electrically-induced brain convulsive activity of the anesthetized patient, often followed by a rapid at times lifesaving response. Stigma and ignorance about the use of ECT especially in treating children and adolescents is a widely prevalent problem; thus depriving many sufferers from the probable benefits of this therapeutic modality. The use of ECT is complex and demands taking into account ethical questions, patients' rights, and following legal regulations that vary between different places in the world. ECT requires a well-coordinated professional team with expertise in the field. It demands updated equipment, prudent patient selection, a comprehensive treatment plan, and psychiatric, cognitive, and physical monitoring during and after the treatment course. This chapter presents current evidence about the use of ECT, underscoring clinical knowledge and guidelines in the field.

Y. Bloch (✉) · N. Ghaziuddin
University of Michigan, Ann Arbor, USA
e-mail: yuvalbloch10@gmail.com

N. Ghaziuddin
e-mail: neerag@umich.edu

Y. Bloch · N. Ghaziuddin
"Shalvata" Mental Health Center, Hod Hashron, Israel

Y. Bloch · N. Ghaziuddin
Sacker School of Medicine, Tel Aviv University, Tel Aviv, Israel

S. Malhotra and P. Santosh (eds.), *Child and Adolescent Psychiatry*,
DOI 10.1007/978-81-322-3619-1_19

Keywords ECT · Children and adolescents · Severe mental disorder · Treatment · Electro convulsive therapy

Abbreviations

ECT	Electro convulsive therapy
BL	Bilateral electrode placement while performing ECT
UL	Unilateral electrode placement (usually right) while performing ECT

19.1 Introduction

Severe psychiatric disorders such as treatment resistant mood disorders, catatonia, psychotic spectrum disorders, and self-injurious behaviors are major risk factors for the well being and future development of children and adolescents (Fergusson and Woodward 2002; Jonsson et al. 2011; Weissman et al. 1999). Suicide is a major risk associated with many severe psychiatric disorders, which in addition to accidents and other causes of violent death, constitutes the most common cause of mortality among the adolescent age group (Mortality and Causes of Death 2015). These severe forms of psychiatric disorders cause significant suffering to minors and their families with grave immediate and longer term consequences such as substance abuse, school failure, family conflict, and behavioral problems (Fergusson and Woodward 2002). There is substantial evidence that childhood onset of several psychiatric disorders is a marker of severity (Birmaher et al. 2014; Jaaskelainen et al. 2015). To counteract these adverse outcomes, it is imperative to identify and treat to achieve remission (defined as minimal or absent symptoms) so that the young person is able to return to his/her baseline function (Birmaher et al. 2014; Dunn and Goodyer 2006). However, many adolescents with severe mood and other disorders do not have a robust response (defined as a 50 % improvement) or stable remission, following combined treatment with psychotherapy and pharmacotherapy (Birmaher et al. 2014; Brent and Birmaher 2002; Fava 2003). Considering that suicide is the most severe and a tragic complication of these severe disorders, there is scarce evidence that modern psychiatry has any pharmacological or psychotherapeutic interventions which can result in robust response (2012).

The interest in electro modulation therapies, specifically electroconvulsive therapy (ECT) as putative of biological therapies was likely the result of limited success with conventional treatments in this subgroup (D'Agati et al. 2010; Donaldson et al. 2014; Ghaziuddin et al. 2004; Lima et al. 2013).

Electroconvulsive therapy (ECT) is currently considered a well-accepted, effective, and safe procedure in adult psychiatric patients (Group 2003; Tharyan and Adams 2005) and is considered a first-line treatment option in adult patients with a depressive or a bipolar (depressed and manic) disorder who are at imminent risk due to inadequate food or fluid intake, are catatonic, and/or acutely suicidal. In these severely ill groups, ECT has been found to exert significant benefit beyond specific diagnosis (Fink 2001). Therefore, ECT is now considered a standard therapeutic procedure for the treatment psychotic depression, depressive disorder refractory to adequate antidepressant drug treatment, and in patients with acute mania with severe psychomotor agitation who may be unresponsive to standard treatments. Adverse effects of ECT are notably minimal, especially if adequate precautions necessary for effective ECT are used (appropriate total amount of electricity, pulse width and duration of the electrical current, adequate oxygenation during treatment, avoiding or minimizing pharmacotherapy during ECT) (American Psychiatric Association. Task Force on Electroconvulsive 1990; Fink 2000, 2001, 2014; Song et al. 2015). There are no absolute contraindications to the use of ECT in adult patients, although relative risks may include an elevated intra-cranial pressure, active pulmonary infection, or a recent myocardial infarction (Ghaziuddin et al. 2004). ECT-related anterograde amnesia is a transient deficit probably as a result of a reversible but short-lived inhibition of protein synthesis in the hippocampal and the medial temporal lobes. This appears to be the underlying mechanism of a transitory deficit in the consolidation and retention of new memory (McClintock et al. 2014). Retrograde memory loss, although potentially problematic, is usually patchy and in most cases also time limited (Sackeim et al. 2008). Well-designed neuropsychological studies have consistently shown that several months after completion of ECT, the ability to learn new information and to remember returns to baseline functioning (Bodnar et al. 2015). Advances in clinical research, largely limited to adults, involving ECT has focused on methods to achieve optimal efficacy, maintain improvement after the completion of a course of ECT to prevent relapse, and minimize overall side effects with special emphasis on cognitive side effects.

Based on these impressive outcomes in relation to response to treatment and benign side effects of ECT in adults, child and adolescent psychiatrists are faced with the question whether this knowledge and data may be applied to children and adolescents with severe psychiatric disorders. Indeed, our current knowledge does support the use of ECT in this age group, although there are no double blind controlled trials.

Due to the evidence of chronicity of psychiatric disorders, risk of completed suicide and other serious psychosocial impairment in children and adolescents, it is important that patients in this age group are not denied a lifesaving treatment modality. In fact, some experts may consider that it would be unethical to deny access across the age span to this highly effective treatment (Taylor 1983). Continuity of psychiatric illness, from adolescence to adulthood, is supported by persistence of illness into adult hood. For instance, in a prospective follow-up 40–70 % of depressed adolescents suffered from a depressive episode as adults (Weissman et al. 1999). Similarly, the diagnosis of schizophrenia is stable over the course of development (Bromet et al. 2011), while patients with catatonia are at risk for developing chronic physical and psychiatric morbidity and are at an increased risk of dying from suicide (Sienaert et al. 2014).

While recognizing the similarity between severe psychiatric disorders in youth (children adolescents) and adults, it is also important to recognize that "children are not small adults." There are notable adult/youth differences which include that although tricyclic antidepressants are highly effective for the treatment of adult depression, no valid therapeutic effect has been found in children and adolescents (Hazell et al. 2000). Along the same lines, adults unlike adolescents and even young adults below 24 years, do not exhibit an increase in suicidal ideation in response to treatment with SSRIs (Miller et al. 2014).

In summary, although level 1 evidence (at least one controlled trial) for the use of ECT in adolescents is currently lacking, abundant evidence, based on descriptive studies, case reports, expert committees and adult data support that ECT is an effective treatment for a subgroup of severly ill children and adolescents.

19.2 ECT in Children and Adolescents—A Controversial Issue

It is difficult to fully comprehend the controversy that surrounds the use of ECT in youth. Robertson et al., in book "Use of ECT in Children and Adolescents" describe with quotations, terms which have been used to describe the use of ECT in youth. Highly emotive and misinformed description have included "depravity of the psychiatrist who use or promote the use of ECT in children" (Frank 2007), and "I am shocked and dismayed…." (Hale 2009), and "To impede this medical steamroller called shock treatment will require public outrage, organized resistance from survivor groups and psychiatric reformers, lawsuits, and state legislation" (Breggin 2007). These exaggerated statements about possible harm sharply contrast with any evidence that might support that the porcedure is harmful to children or adolescents.

Based on currently available knowledge and data, the indications for the use ECT in adolescents do not differ from those in adults (Ghaziuddin et al. 2004). However, what is remarkable about the use of ECT in adolescents, let alone in pre pubertal children, are inconsistent practices, negative attitudes, and marked controversy even within the field of child psychiatry which suggest that most child and adolescent psychiatrist are not familiar with the use of modern ECT (Ghaziuddin et al. 2004; Lima et al. 2013; Rabheru 2001; Walter and Rey 2003).

The study and the effective use of ECT is limited by a vicious circle; the stigma and fear restrain research and restrict its use thereby maintaining the paucity of data that could calm fears and contribute to the proper use of ECT. Since its appearance in the late 1930s, the initial resistance to ECT was fear related to its putative deleterious effects of what was perceived as an inadequately understood procedure on the human brain. Reports of misuse, inaccurate media portrayal, and active propaganda of policymakers (McDonald and Walter 2001) have undoubtedly contributed to the public concern. Not surprisingly, these criticisms become louder and more extreme when it comes to the treatment of children and adolescents (Lima et al. 2013). Therefore, any attempt to restrict this treatment must examine the ethics of depriving a lifesaving treatment for critically ill children and adolescents and question the risk versus benefits of treatment for a severe psychiatric illness.

19.3 Rate of ECT Use in Children and Adolescents

ECT is rarely used in children and adolescents. Its use is extremely rare in prepubertal children and only a few cases have been reported, while it is relatively more frequently used in adolescents. There are no recent adolescent data, however, based on the numbers reported for United States in 1980, approximately 500 (1.5 %) of 33,384 patients who received ECT were in the age range of 11–20 years (Thompson and Blaine 1987). A hospital chart survey in New South Wales, Australia, revealed that between 1990 and 1995, only 42 (0.93 %) patients treated with ECT were younger than age 18 (Walter and Rey 1997). In a survey of all members of the royal College of Psychiatrists in UK, only 12 patients younger than 18 were identified as having received ECT during 1996 (Duffett et al. 1999). At the Hospital de la Salpetriere in Paris, seven adolescents aged 15–18 years had received ECT during 1986–1988 (Paillere-Martinot et al. 1990). In Israel 36 of all 600 adolescents (6 %) hospitalized in a psychiatric hospital between 1991 and 1997 were treated with ECT, in comparison to 570 adults (Stein et al. 2004). In northern India, a recent chart review found that 39 patients (5.9 %) among those who received ECT were under 18 years of age (Grover et al. 2013).

The exact frequency about the current use of ECT in minors could only be determined, if a nationwide mandatory reporting system would be established (Stein et al. 2006).

19.3.1 Studies of ECT in Children and Adolescents

There are no randomized or controlled trials of ECT in children and adolescents. Our present knowledge is largely based on case reports, retrospective chart reviews, systematic epidemiologic reviews, a few studies which have used comparison groups, and some prospective albeit open labeled recently completed prospective studies. Despite the limitations of the available literature, findings suggest robust positive outcomes including a marked reduction in suicidal thoughts and behaviors. Therefore, the field of ECT research in minors is well positioned to conduct controlled study of ECT, although comparison with sham treatment would not be ethically permissible because of the robust data to support its efficacy. The following is a summary of our current knowledge based on meticulous review of currently available literature.

The most widely used practice parameters about the use of ECT in children and adolescents were published by the American Academy of Child and Adolescent Psychiatry (AACAP) which guide modern practice of ECT in children and adolescents (Ghaziuddin et al. 2004). According to these guidelines ECT is indicated in adolescent patients who meet the following three criteria: (1) Diagnosis: Severe, persistent major depression or mania with or without psychotic features; schizoaffective disorder; or, less often, schizophrenia. ECT may also be used to treat catatonia or neuroleptic malignant syndrome. (2) Severity of Symptoms: Symptoms must be severe, persistent, and significantly disabling. They may include life-threatening symptoms such as refusal to eat or drink, severe suicidality, uncontrollable mania, or florid psychosis. (3) Lack of Treatment Response: Failure to respond to at least two adequate trials of appropriate psychopharmacological agents accompanied by other appropriate treatment modalities. Both duration and dosage determine the adequacy of medication trials. It is important to note that whenever there is imminent danger of acute (at times life-threatening) deterioration, ECT should be recommended without endangering the patient by waiting for an adequate and/or additional medication trials.

19.3.2 Short-Term Efficacy

Bertagnoli and Borchardt (1990) summarized all published reports between 1947 and 1990. However, most studies were noted to have methodological problems, including a lack of diagnostic clarity and heterogeneous diagnoses among patients who had received ECT. Other disadvantages of these earlier publications are retrospective study design, small sample size, and the lack of objective outcome criteria. While acknowledging these shortcomings, it is noteworthy that with the exception of a single report of lack of efficacy by Guttmacher and Cretella (1988), ECT was found to be effective in all published reports, no serious side effects were reported, nor is there any report of fatality associated with ECT.

In another review, Rey and Walter (1997) systematically searched medical and psychological databases until 1996 (including publications in English and in other languages) which yielded 60 reports describing 396 patients. Only five were younger than 12 years. Each author evaluated the quality of the reports independently, and the independent ratings were then compared. When there was disagreement, reports were jointly reexamined and consensus was reached. They concluded that the overall quality of the studies was poor. Almost one-half provided no diagnosis, or there was insufficient information about the symptoms to make a definite diagnosis. Response to treatment was almost invariably described in an impressionistic and not in quantitative terms. Short-term outcome (outcome immediately after the last treatment to 6 months posttreatment) was poorly described in 35 %, while information on longer term outcome (6 or more months after ECT) was provided only in around 40 %. Despite these limitations, the analysis of the short-term efficacy of ECT yielded surprisingly optimistic results; improvement rates following ECT ranged from 80 to 100 % for mania, 60–80 % for bipolar and unipolar depression and 75 % for patients with catatonic conditions, irrespective of the underlying psychiatric morbidity. Additionally, overall improvement following ECT was shown in approximately 90 % of adolescents with depression resistant to pharmacotherapy (Rey and Walter 1997).

In another epidemiological survey of a 5 years' experience in an area with approximately 6 million inhabitants, Walter and Rey (1997) found significant response in one-half of 42 adolescents who had received 47 ECT courses, although ECT was administered as a treatment of "last resort" after failure of pharmacotherapy (Walter and Rey 1997).

Another four studies were identified by Ghazuiddin et al. (2004) when they conducted a Medline search using key words ECT children, and adolescents. These publications included two retrospective studies (Cohen et al. 1997; Walter and Rey 1997), and one prospective open design study (Strober et al. 1998) with 72 combined number of adolescents in the reports. Another case report was identified involving two adolescents with mania who had received ECT (Hill et al 1997). Based on these publications, the overall efficacy of ECT was 60–100 % in depression and 75–100 % in mania.

A review by Stein et al. (2006) added four retrospective open studies (Bloch et al. 2001; Duffett et al. 1999; Stein et al. 2004; Walter and Rey 2003) and two case reports (Cohen et al. 2000; Russell et al. 2002), which all together included 132 adolescents and 2 pre pubertal children. The improvement rates were between 60 and 80 % for major depression, and around 60 % for bipolar disorder. The report by Russell et al. (2002) described a prepubertal child diagnosed with severe depression with catatonic features, where a protracted course of ECT was found to save the life of the child. Another report described the efficacy of ECT efficacy in a neurologically compromised adolescent with bipolar disorder following craniotomy for an intracranial neoplasm (Ghaziuddin et al. 1999), suggesting that ECT may be safely administered in selected adolescents with some types of neurological complications.

Some studies have utilized a comparison group, which provides a qualitative reference about the efficacy of ECT in this age group (Bloch et al. 2001, 2008). Kutcher and Robertson (1995), for instance, compared treatment outcome in a group of hospitalized adolescents ($n = 22$) who were diagnosed with BP disorder (acute mania or depression) and were either treated with ECT ($n = 16$) or received standard care ($n = 6$). All 22 adolescents were initially referred for ECT, however, 6 had declined and thus received pharmacotherapy while remaining hospitalized (26). Cases that were treated with ECT had a positive response and their length of hospitalization was one-half that of the group that had received standard care (73.8 vs. 176 days). The shorter hospital stay could be translated to a considerable cost saving expressed in Canadian dollars which amounted to $58,608 spent for the ECT group, compared with $143,264.00 spent on group that had received standard care. The authors concluded that ECT was both effective and a less expensive treatment option.

Bloch et al. (2001) compared records of 24 consecutively treated adolescents hospitalized between 1991 and 1995, with a group of 33 adults who had started ECT on the same day (Bloch et al. 2001). Findings included that the technique used in adolescents was essentially the same as in adults and that ECT was equally effective in both age groups. However, in terms of the primary diagnosis adolescents were more likely to belong to the "psychotic spectrum," while adults were more commonly on the "affective spectrum."

Stein et al. (2004) compared retrospective data for two groups which included adolescents and randomly selected adults (adolescents = 36; adults = 57) who were all treated with ECT at the same center (Stein et al. 2004). They found that while the majority of adolescents were treated for affective disorder, including life-threatening symptoms such as catatonia or suicidality, adults on the other hand, were more likely to be treated for schizophrenic disorders. The authors also noted that 61 % of adolescents had improved in response to ECT, and 58 % did not need hospitalization during the following year, whereas rates for adults were 83 and 49 %, respectively; and, adolescents were more likely to be hospitalized for a longer period prior to being treated with ECT and were less likely than adults to complete treatment (80 % adults vs. 60 % adolescents had completed treatment). Overall findings of this study indicated that in addition to other mentioned differences, clinicians are more cautious about using ECT in adolescents (based on longer hospitalization prior to ECT).

Recent publications are a considerable improvement and some have utilized prospective methodology and more detailed evaluations including structured assessments. For instance, Baeza et al. in 2010 presented retrospective data involving 13 adolescents diagnosed with schizophrenia spectrum disorder (Baeza et al. 2010). The majority of the patients (53.8 %) achieved response which was defined as a 20 % reduction in positive symptoms measured on the Positive and Negative Symptom Scale (PANSS) scale (Kay et al. 1987), but not on the negative subscale. Ghaziuddin et al. (2011) described retrospective data involving 33 adolescents who were all treated under standardized conditions at the same institution between 1989 and 2008, were diagnosed with MDD and achieved a 60 % remission rate. Zhang et al. (2012) have published to date the largest study of ECT in adolescents and young adults (Zhang et al. 2012). This study involved 112 adolescents and young adults ranging in age from 13 to 20 years who were hospitalized due to an acute psychotic episode and had been ill for less than a year. They were matched on age and sex and randomized on a ratio of 2:1 to receive either an antipsychotics and ECT ($n = 78$) or an antipsychotic alone ($n = 34$). The ECT treated group had a significantly shorter hospital stay, a lower PANSS score and improved quality of sleep. However, there was no improvement in negative symptoms. This study by Zang and colleagues is unusual in using ECT as an add-on for augmenting treatment during the early and acute phase of a psychotic disorder and may guide new directions in using ECT and other forms of brain stimulation in this subgroup.

It is important to stress that the literature relating to ECT in pre adolescents is extremely sparse and is based on even fewer case reports, which mainly involve life-threatening clinical scenarios related to catatonia or deliberate self-harm.

In conclusion, while acknowledging the retrospective and open-labeled data, multiple publications from a number of authors worldwide support that ECT has a significant short-term benefit in at least 60 % adolescents who were treated for affective or psychotic disorders. In addition, there is evidence of similar benefit from more recent publications, which have employed standardized assessments such as the Clinical Global Inventory (CGI) (Green et al. 1994), Children's Depression Rating Scale (CDRS; Poznanski et al. 1984) and PANSS (Kay 1990). Finally, the efficacy of ECT is also supported by studies that have used comparison adolescent groups who were treated with standard treatment. Along the same lines, studies that have compared the efficacy of ECT in adolescents to adults indicate that the treatment is generally equally effective in both age groups and more robust response reported for adults in some studies is probably related to diagnostic differences and possibly referral patterns (adolescents appear to be more sick and possibly more chronically ill). In respect to referral reasons, adolescents in contrast to adults are more likely to be referred for ECT for acute life-threatening conditions, whereas adults are referred due to treatment resistance (Rey and Walter 1997; Bloch et al. 2008).

19.3.3 Short-Term Side Effect

ECT is considered a safe procedure and the majority of side effects observed appears to be minor in nature. Common minor side effect which appears immediately following ECT session are headache (5.9–65 %), confusion (18 %), subjective memory loss (5 %), nausea or vomiting (2–14 %), muscle aches (12 %) agitation (0.5–9 %). These complaints are invariably mild and transitory and do not require premature discontinuation of treatment (Rey and Walter 1997; Stein et al. 2006; Walter and Rey 1997).

As far as for major concerns surrounding ECT, there has never been a reported death in a child or an adolescent directly related to ECT. The overall risk is considered low to the procedure, however, there is a small potential risk related to anesthesia in ECT, which based on experience with adults is estimated at 2 deaths/100,000 treatments. Other significant side effects related to the anesthesia and the convulsion include prolonged apnea, cardiac arrhythmia, and damage to teeth (extremely rare with modern ECT). A prolonged seizure induced during ECT is a known complication, with an approximate 0.4–10 % prevalence in adolescents and is defined as a seizure that lasts longer than 120 s. A prolonged seizure can be rapidly terminated with an intravenous benzodiazepine and may be prevented during subsequent treatment by adequate oxygenation and hydration, treating electrolyte imbalance if any, using a lower amount of electrical current and terminating the seizure with a benzodiazepine at one-minute seizure duration. Delayed or tardive seizures have also been reported, which are known to appear hours or days after an ECT treatment. These are rare and appear to resolve without any adverse outcome during follow-up, although there is a reported case of administering an anticonvulsant agent for several months after the event (de la Serna et al. 2011). Treatment-induced mania, hypomania, or subclinical hypomania (increased irritability, erratic behaviors that are inconsistent with past behavior) have been reported. Most experts agree that ECT should be continued and emergence of such episodes should not be considered an indication to stop ECT.

Confusional states are frequent during the first few hours following an ECT session. This is an immediate effect of ECT treatment and is correlated with the number of ECT sessions received (Shapira et al. 1991), the amount of the current in relation to the seizure threshold (Calev et al. 1991; Shapira et al. 1991), and the nature of the current used (may last a few minutes with use of brief pulse current, or several hours with sinusoidal current which is almost never used in modern ECT) (Weiner et al. 1986). Transient, mostly mild, subjective memory disturbances may occur following ECT in adolescents (Ghaziuddin et al. 2000; Rey and Walter 1997; Stein et al. 2006), but these subside shortly after completion of the treatment. Subjective memory complaints reported just after ECT were found by Kutcher and Robertson (1995) to be less than 5 % (75), 22 % by Walter and Rey (Rey and Walter 1997), and approximately 50 % by Cohen et al. (2000).

Some general observations in regards to the frequency of side effects depend on: (1) The ECT technique such as the wave form (greater with sine wave compared with brief pulse), electrode placement (greater with bilateral frontotemporal ECT) and the amount of electrical current (higher dosage is associated with more side effects (see later under memory disturbance). (2) It has also been noted that any systematic examination, versus a global impression, is more likely to yield a higher number of side effects (Bloch et al. 2001; Ghaziuddin et al. 2000; Stein et al. 2004).

19.3.4 Long-Term Clinical Outcome

Majority of studies have identified positive outcome in multiple areas of functioning following ECT. For instance, improved functioning at 6 months or more following ECT was noted in 72–80 % of the patients who initially responded favorably to ECT, regardless of the psychiatric diagnosis. More recently, Cohen et al. (2000) noted that 9 of 10 adolescents treated with ECT for mood disorders were fully remitted when evaluated after 3.5 ± 1.7 years with exception of one patient who suffered from mild hypomanic symptoms. Stein et al. (2004) assessed the effect of ECT in 36 adolescent inpatients. Remission in the short term was a predictor for better outcome. Twenty-two cases, who had improved with ECT, all of them were discharged to their home by the end of the treatment, 15 remitters (68 %) were not rehospitalized in the subsequent year, while in the group of the ECT nonremitters only 4 among 14 were not rehospitalized at the end of the year.

Taieb et al. (2002) compared 11 adolescents treated with BL ECT (depression = 6, mania = 5) with 34 matched psychiatric controls (matched on age, gender, educational level, and diagnosis), following both groups for a mean duration 5.2 years. Findings included: (1) All adolescents at follow-up, with exception of 2 in the control group, had developed BP disorder; (2) 15/22 had experienced an additional episode of mood disorder; (3) the impact on school functioning was related to the severity of mood disorder rather than to treatment with ECT. In addition to demonstrating the deleterious effect of the severity of the mood disorder on functioning, the study findings also underscored the high rates of switch from unipolar to BP mood disorder in this age group.

19.3.4.1 Cognitive Side Effects

Memory deficits following ECT and fear of this side effect have played a major role in the practice of ECT. Although there are no large-scale studies in children and adolescent, at least three studies have reported the absence of residual memory impairment when testing was completed a few months after the last session of ECT (Cohen et al. 2000; de la Serna et al. 2011; Ghaziuddin et al. 2000, 2011). Ghaziuddin et al. (2011) compared pre- and post-ECT cognitive functions in a small group of adolescents ($n = 6$) 4–81 weeks after the initiation of ECT; participants had been treated with an index course of ECT, followed by a continuation course (6 months after the end of the index course) and/or maintenance ECT (additional treatment that extended beyond 6 months after the end of the index course). Paired comparison (within subject, pre and post-testing results) found a significant gain in delayed memory, whereas other functions (intellectual function, verbal fluency, and motor speed) were not significantly affected. In another study, Ghaziuddin et al. retrospectively assessed cognitive functions in 16 adolescents prior to ECT, approximately one week after and 8 months after ECT. Some dysfunction, including attention and concentration deficits and long-term memory impairment was reported one week after the ECT course; however, there was no evidence of cognitive dysfunction in these domains when testing was completed several months after the procedure (Ghaziuddin et al. 2011).

Another study did not find any differences in anterograde long-term memory when cognitive functions of 10 adolescents treated with BL ECT 5.2 years following ECT were compared with matched psychiatric controls (matched on age, gender, diagnosis, educational level, place of hospitalization). Mean age of the group was 17.6 years and two participants had received more than one course of ECT. The indication for ECT was severe mood disorders with psychotic features (major depressive disorder with melancholic characteristics = 5, manic episode = 3, mixed episode = 2). Cognitive functions were assessed using the California Verbal Learning Test, Squire's Subjective Memory Questionnaire, and the attention-concentration index from the Weschler Scale. Although 6 of 10 patients had reported memory impairment just after ECT, only one reported subjective memory impairment at the time of the assessment. All subjects (the patients receiving ECT and the control group) were assessed for diagnosis, symptoms, social adaptation, and educational attainment. No significant difference was found on these variables, except for educational attainment (Taieb et al. 2002). Similarly, another study involving adolescents did not find any cognitive deficits between controls and adolescents with schizophrenia, when tested two years after completion of ECT (de la Serna et al. 2011).

In one study, among eight adolescents interviewed by telephone after the last ECT session, none reported subjective memory impairment at 8 months to 3 years after the final ECT session (Moise and Petrides 1996). In another study by Cohen et al., one patient continued to complain of subjective memory impairment two years after ECT (Cohen et al. 2000). More recently, nine adolescents diagnosed with a psychosis spectrum disorder were assessed just before ECT and at 2-year follow-up; there was no significant difference in cognitive variables between adolescents who had received ECT and controls at the 2-year follow-up (de la Serna et al. 2011).

To summarize there is strong preliminary evidence that the cognitive deficits and recovery of these deficits in adolescents treated with ECT are similar to that of psychiatric controls and that the cognitive functioning is likely to return to its baseline level within several months after ECT. It is also pertinent to be cognizant of the difficulty in ascertaining the effect of disease on cognition, versus the effect of ECT. Clearly, large-scale, systematic, and prospective studies are necessary before drawing definite conclusions.

19.4 ECT Procedure

19.4.1 Indications and Contraindications

ECT is indicated for children or adolescents who meet the diagnostic criteria for severe Axis I psychiatric disorders (e.g., mood disorders, psychosis, catatonia, neuroleptic malignant syndrome, or severe self-injurious behaviors) and/or have failed to respond adequately to conventional treatments. Although both illness-severity and the failure to respond are important patient-selection criteria, the severity of illness-criteria may take precedence in cases when waiting for treatment response may jeopardize safety and/or cause additional decline. The classical diagnostic indications include severe mood disorders and catatonia. However, there is emerging experience in successfully treating patients with schizophrenia spectrum disorders (SSD) and deliberate self-harm (especially those with an associated autistic spectrum disorders). A dimensional conceptualizing of symptoms, versus a categorical approach when specific symptoms are associated with certain diagnoses, is useful in these conditions. For instance, in cases of severe self-injurious behaviors, it is often unclear whether the symptoms are related to an affective, catatonic or to a psychotic process. However, there is emerging data that this symptom, irrespective of comorbid psychiatric diagnosis is known to have a favorable response to ECT (Wachtel et al. 2013). ECT also has a place in the treatment of SSD when there is lack of response to antipsychotics, unable to tolerate antipsychotics or there are other symptoms (affective, suicidal thoughts and behaviors), which are known to response to ECT. ECT is the treatment of choice in catatonia when there is inadequate response to benzodiazepines. Irrespective of the diagnoses, it would be reasonable to proceed quickly to ECT whenever there is imminent danger to life either due to severe suicidal behavior, refusal to eat or drink or any other life-threatening or life-impairing psychiatric symptom.

19.4.1.1 Contraindications

Although there are insufficient data specific to adolescents, currently available data involving adults suggest that there are no absolute contraindications to the use of ECT. However, there are a few relative contraindications which apply to all age groups. These include tumors of the central nervous system associated with elevated cerebrospinal fluid levels, active chest infection, and a recent myocardial infarction. A seizure disorder is not a contraindication for ECT and, in fact, ECT may be equally effective with a comorbid seizure disorder, when indicated for a psychiatric illness. Pregnancy is also not a contraindication for ECT. Finally, no comorbid Axis I or an Axis II psychiatric disorder should be considered as a reason to deny this treatment, when the patient is additionally diagnosed with a condition known to respond to ECT

19.4.1.2 Assessment

Psychiatric Assessment

A detailed and a comprehensive psychiatric evaluation, reviewing both current and lifetime psychiatric diagnoses and treatment is an essential first step. It is advised (and in many countries it is obligatory) that the assessment will be performed by more than one psychiatrist. In addition to reaching the diagnoses, the assessment must include previous treatment failures and current assessment of danger, target symptoms, premorbid cognitive function and the patient's overall level of functioning. These evaluations should attempt to delineate a comprehensive treatment plan including pharmacotherapy and psychotherapy, family intervention, and managing the educational expectation during and after ECT. In general, it is prudent to discontinue all previous psychotropic medications during an ECT course. This may be explained by the lack of improvement noted in response to current medications and concern for exacerbated side effects when certain medications are combined with ECT. Antipsychotics and antidepressants may lower the convulsive threshold and my affect cardiac conduction while anticonvulsant agents may prevent the induction of an effective seizure. In contrast, benzodiazepines can be safely administered because the anticonvulsive effect of this group of medications can be easily reversed with flumazenil administered just prior to ECT. Lithium was suspected to be associated with greater postictal delirium and delayed seizures, however, it is currently administered concurrently with ECT by postponing the dose prior to a treatment and, thereby, lowering the blood levels at the time of the procedure. Therefore, each concurrently prescribed medication should be carefully evaluated to decide whether to discontinue or to continue the agent and the risks and benefits associated with either decision.

It is highly recommended that the psychiatrist should select a standardized rating scale/scales to monitor response to treatment. The clinical global impression scale (CGI) (Poznanski et al. 1984) is a simple clinician-rated instrument to evaluate the general functioning of the patient. In addition, more symptom-specific standardized rating scales may be used such the Children's Depression Rating Scale-Revised

(CDRS-R; Green et al. 1994), the Hamilton Rating Scale (HRSD; Robbins et al. 1985) for measuring depressive symptoms; the Brief Psychiatric Rating Scale-Child (BPRS-C; Overall and Pfefferbaum 1982) to measure behavior and psychotic symptoms; and the Bush Francis Catatonia Rating Scale (BFCRS; Wong et al. 2007) to measure signs and symptoms of catatonia. These measures should be repeated at regular intervals, possibly every one to two weeks over the treatment course.

Cognitive assessment

The two main goals of cognitive testing are: (1) Measure the base line cognitive functioning of the patient. (2) Monitor the cognitive side effects following treatment. Standard clinical practice includes the examination of baseline cognitive functions followed by reexamination approximately 3–6 months post-ECT. This practice allows the identification of strengths and deficits and educational curriculum of the adolescent may be adjutsted, if necessary, until there is full recovery. The baseline assessment is complicated by the severity of symptoms of patients who are referred for ECT. In many cases, the patient may have difficulty completing the tests and the interpretation of these tests is also problematic due to the impact of disturbed motivation and attention among other illness-related cognitive functions.

Based on the adult literature, cognitive domains that are generally tested at baseline and at post-ECT time points include attention, processing speed, working memory, short-term and long-term memory. A notable observation is a large gap frequently identified between the subjective loss of memory reported by patients and findings from objective evaluations. The assessment of autobiographical memory (AM)-tests which assess personal memories of events that occurred prior to ECT has been found to be useful in some adult studies but remains under debate. In addition to neuropsychological test batteries, commonly employed tools used in clinical and research practice, to measure change over time, include the Mini Mental Status Examination (MMSE), MacQueen et al. (2007), and the Montreal Cognitive Assessment (MoCA) (Russell et al. 2003).

Medical Assessment

Every patient considered for ECT must receive a comprehensive general medical evaluation. This is intended to assess for any medical conditions that may coexist, and also determine the risk of anesthesia during ECT. Beyond a careful medical history and physical and neurological examinations, an assessment by an anesthesiologist is essential. Appropriate laboratory investigation must be completed and may include a complete blood cell count, differential white blood cell count, thyroid function tests, liver function tests, urinalysis and toxicology screen, and an electrocardiogram. The use of electro encephalogram, and computed tomography or magnetic resonance imaging of the brain should be considered if necessary. All female patients must have a serum or a urine pregnancy test, which is usually repeated at regular interval through the treatment course.

Informed Consent

Every attempt must be made to educate the adolescent and parents regarding the ECT procedure and its risks and benefits. Written informed consent for ECT must be obtained from a parent or another legal guardian. In addition, the consent or assent of the adolescent should be obtained, although, some children and adolescents may be too ill to fully understand the procedure, therefore unable to participate in meaningful consent. In rare instances involving adolescents, legal advice may be sought if the parents are agreeable but the patient refuses treatment. Parents and adolescents should be informed that they may withdraw consent for ECT at any time. Most states in the United States and institutions require consensus between 2 to 3 psychiatrists before proceeding with the treatment. ECT is probably the only medical treatment in the entire field of medical practice which is regulated by these criteria.

19.4.1.3 ECT Procedure

Anesthesia

Anesthesia should be administered by qualified personnel experienced in treating adolescents. The medications administered during anesthesia include methohexital to achieve sedation, succinylcholine is used for muscle relaxation and intravenous atropine or glycopyrrolate may be administered immediately before ECT to protect from vagally induced bradycardia and arrhythmias. However, at the present time, there is a lack of consensus as to whether atropine or glycopyrrolate should be administered routinely. Patients are ventilated with 100 % oxygen before administration of the electrical stimulation.

Administering ECT

Standard procedures for administering ECT to children and adolescents include hospitalization for initiating the index treatment course, an overnight fast, a specially designated unit where staff are trained in ECT, administration of anesthesia including care of an unconscious patient to assist with recovery. Treatment is usually initiated at two or three times per week, but the schedule may be adjusted based on illness-severity and degree of confusion.

Psychiatrists vary in their preference for bilateral (BL) versus unilateral (UL) electrode placement (applied to the non-dominant parietal area). Some due to its faster and more predictable onset of action may prefer BL, while UL may be the preferred method because it is associated with less memory impairment in the immediate posttreatment period. In a critically ill patient (refusal to eat or drink, severe suicidality, florid psychosis, catatonia), it is preferable that treatment commences with BL electrode placement. There is also evidence to suggest that bilateral ECT may be more effective for manic patients (Mohan et al. 2009). Additionally, changing from unilateral to bilateral treatment may be indicated if there is inadequate response (D'Cunha et al. 2015; Krystal et al. 2000).

The total number of ECT's administered during a treatment course should be determined by clinical response, although a usual course may consist between 10 and 18 treatments. Preliminary response to treatment is usually measured after the first five or six treatments, however, ongoing assessment is essential. Use of brief pulse and an adequate dose of electricity is recommended. An adequate convulsive dose should be used to induce an EEG seizure lasting 30–90 s. It is advisable to select a lower electrical charge for the initial treatment, which also permits identifying the seizure threshold by using a gradually increasing current dosage. Seizure duration is monitored with simultaneous EEG recording and/or observing the motor activity of a seizure using the cuff method.

Patient Management After ECT

ECT is an effective treatment of an acute episode of a mood disorder. However, there is no evidence that effective treatment of an episode would prevent future relapse. Therefore, ECT should be regarded as an intervention to be used during the acute phase of the illness and additional interventions, such as pharmacotherapy and psychotherapy, are usually necessary to maintain a positive outcome. Psychotherapy may be added after the recovery of the cognition and the type of therapy should be determined based on residual symptoms. While acknowledging the paucity of data specific to adolescents treated with maintenance ECTM-ECT), M-ECT appears to be a useful strategy to prevent relapse and maintain remission (Ghaziuddin et al. 2011).

19.5 Take Home Message

Properly administered ECT is an important part of the "tool box" of current child and adolescent psychiatry. Applying ECT to minors demands expertize, following updated guidelines and team work. The main indications are similar to those applied in adults: Severe treatment resistant or life-threatening mood disorders, catatonia or severe deliberate self-harm. Ethical issues include proper explanation to the adolescent and his/her family, informed consent and assent when possible and consultation with independent child psychiatrists are important components of the procedure. Modern technique minimizes the risk of side effects including cognitive side effects. The process should be monitored medically and psychiatrically at each stage of the treatment.

References

A report of the U.S. surgeon general and of the national action alliance for suicide prevention: national strategy for suicide prevention: goals and objectives for action, 2012, Washington (DC).

American Psychiatric Association. Task Force on Electroconvulsive, T. (1990). The practice of ECT: Recommendations for treatment, training and privileging. Convulsive Therapy, 6(2), 85–120. Retrieved from http://www.ncbi.nlm.nih.gov/pubmed/11659302

Baeza, I., Flamarique, I., Garrido, J. M., Horga, G., Pons, A., Bernardo, M., et al. (2010). Clinical experience using electroconvulsive therapy in adolescents with schizophrenia spectrum disorders. *Journal of Child and Adolescent Psychopharmacology, 20*(3), 205–209. doi:10.1089/cap.2009.0066.

Bertagnoli, M. W., & Borchardt, C. M. (1990). A review of ECT for children and adolescents. *Journal of the American Academy of Child and Adolescent Psychiatry, 29*(2), 302–307. doi:10.1097/00004583-199003000-00022.

Birmaher, B., Gill, M. K., Axelson, D. A., Goldstein, B. I., Goldstein, T. R., Yu, H., et al. (2014). Longitudinal trajectories and associated baseline predictors in youths with bipolar spectrum disorders. *American Journal of Psychiatry, 171*(9), 990–999. doi:10.1176/appi.ajp.2014.13121577.

Bloch, Y., Levcovitch, Y., Bloch, A. M., Mendlovic, S., & Ratzoni, G. (2001). Electroconvulsive therapy in adolescents: similarities to and differences from adults. *Journal of the American Academy of Child and Adolescent Psychiatry, 40*(11), 1332–1336. doi:10.1097/00004583-200111000-00014.

Bloch, Y., Sobol, D., Levkovitz, Y., Kron, S., & Ratzoni, G. (2008). Reasons for referral for electroconvulsive therapy: A comparison between adolescents and adults. *Australas Psychiatry, 16*(3), 191–194. doi:10.1080/10398560801886039.

Bodnar, A., Krzywotulski, M., Lewandowska, A., Chlopocka-Wozniak, M., Bartkowska-Sniatkowska, A. et al. (2015). Electroconvulsive therapy and cognitive functions in treatment-resistant depression. *The World Journal of Biological Psychiatry*, 1–6. doi:10.3109/15622975.2015.1091501

Breggin, P. (2007). ECT damages the brain: Disturbing news for patients and shock doctors alike. *Ethical Human Psychology and Psychiatry: An International Journal of Critical Inquiry, 9*, 83–86.

Brent, D. A., & Birmaher, B. (2002). Clinical practice. Adolescent depression. *The New England Journal of Medicine, 347*(9), 667–671. doi:10.1056/NEJMcp012249.

Bromet, E. J., Kotov, R., Fochtmann, L. J., Carlson, G. A., Tanenberg-Karant, M., Ruggero, C., et al. (2011). Diagnostic shifts during the decade following first admission for psychosis. *American Journal of Psychiatry, 168*(11), 1186–1194. doi:10.1176/appi.ajp.2011.11010048.

Calev, A., Cohen, R., Tubi, N., Nigal, D., Shapira, B., Kugelmass, S. et al. (1991). Disorientation and bilateral moderately suprathreshold titrated ECT. *Convulsive Therapy, 7*(2), 99–110. Retrieved from http://www.ncbi.nlm.nih.gov/pubmed/11941109

Cohen, D., Flament, M., Taieb, O., Thompson, C., & Basquin, M. (2000). Electroconvulsive therapy in adolescents. *European Child & Adolescent Psychiatry, 9*(1), 1–6. Retrieved from http://www.ncbi.nlm.nih.gov/pubmed/10795849

Cohen, D., Paillere-Martinot, M. L., & Basquin, M. (1997). Use of electroconvulsive therapy in adolescents. *Convulsive Therapy, 13*(1), 25–31. Retrieved from http://www.ncbi.nlm.nih.gov/pubmed/9152585

Cohen, D., Taieb, O., Flament, M., Benoit, N., Chevret, S., Corcos, M., et al. (2000b). Absence of cognitive impairment at long-term follow-up in adolescents treated with ECT for severe mood disorder. *American Journal of Psychiatry, 157*(3), 460–462. doi:10.1176/appi.ajp.157.3.460.

D'Agati, D., Bloch, Y., Levkovitz, Y., & Reti, I. (2010). rTMS for adolescents: Safety and efficacy considerations. *Psychiatry Research, 177*(3), 280–285. doi:10.1016/j.psychres.2010.03.004.

D'Cunha, C., Plakiotis, C., Macfarlane, S., Moss, F., Reddy, M., Singh, D., et al. (2015). The clinical and service outcomes of unilateral and bilateral ECT electrode placements in Australian aged psychiatry services. *The Journal of ECT,*. doi:10.1097/YCT.0000000000000268.

de la Serna, E., Flamarique, I., Castro-Fornieles, J., Pons, A., Puig, O., Andres-Perpina, S., et al. (2011). Two-year follow-up of cognitive functions in schizophrenia spectrum disorders of adolescent patients treated with electroconvulsive therapy. *Journal of Child and Adolescent Psychopharmacology, 21*(6), 611–619. doi:10.1089/cap.2011.0012.

Donaldson, A. E., Gordon, M. S., Melvin, G. A., Barton, D. A., & Fitzgerald, P. B. (2014). Addressing the needs of adolescents with treatment resistant depressive disorders: A systematic review of rTMS. *Brain Stimulation, 7*(1), 7–12. Retrieved from http://www.ncbi.nlm.nih.gov/pubmed/24527502

Duffett, R., Hill, P., & Lelliott, P. (1999). Use of electroconvulsive therapy in young people. *The British Journal of Psychiatry, 175*, 228–230. Retrieved from http://www.ncbi.nlm.nih.gov/pubmed/10645323

Dunn, V., & Goodyer, I. M. (2006). Longitudinal investigation into childhood- and adolescence-onset depression: Psychiatric outcome in early adulthood. *British Journal of Psychiatry, 188*, 216–222. doi:10.1192/bjp.188.3.216.

Fava, M. (2003). Diagnosis and definition of treatment-resistant depression. *Biological psychiatry, 53*(8), 649–659. Retrieved from http://www.ncbi.nlm.nih.gov/pubmed/12706951

Fergusson, D. M., & Woodward, L. J. (2002). Mental health, educational, and social role outcomes of adolescents with depression. *Archives of General Psychiatry, 59*(3), 225–231. Retrieved from http://www.ncbi.nlm.nih.gov/pubmed/11879160

Fink, M. (2000). ECT has proved effective in treating depression. *Nature, 403*(6772), 826. doi:10.1038/35002776.

Fink, M. (2001). ECT has much to offer our patients: It should not be ignored. *The World Journal of Biological Psychiatry, 2*(1), 1–8. Retrieved from http://www.ncbi.nlm.nih.gov/pubmed/12587179

Fink, M. (2014). What was learned: Studies by the consortium for research in ECT (CORE) 1997-2011. *Acta Psychiatrica Scandinavica, 129*(6), 417–426. doi:10.1111/acps.12251.

Frank, L. (2007). Electroshocking children. http://psychiatrybuster.blogspot.com/2007/06/electroshocking-children-by-leonard-roy.html

Ghaziuddin, N., DeQuardo, J. R., Ghaziuddin, M., & King, C. A. (1999). Electroconvulsive treatment of a bipolar adolescent postcraniotomy for brain stem astrocytoma. *Journal of Child and Adolescent Psychopharmacology, 9*(1), 63–69. Retrieved from http://www.ncbi.nlm.nih.gov/pubmed/10357519

Ghaziuddin, N., Dumas, S., & Hodges, E. (2011). Use of continuation or maintenance electroconvulsive therapy in adolescents with severe treatment-resistant depression. *The Journal of ECT, 27*(2), 168–174. doi:10.1097/YCT.0b013e3181f665e4.

Ghaziuddin, N., Kutcher, S. P., Knapp, P., Bernet, W., Arnold, V., Beitchman, J., … AACAP. (2004). Practice parameter for use of electroconvulsive therapy with adolescents. *Journal of the American Academy of Child & Adolescent Psychiatry, 43*(12), 1521–1539. Retrieved from http://www.ncbi.nlm.nih.gov/pubmed/15564821

Ghaziuddin, N., Laughrin, D., & Giordani, B. (2000). Cognitive side effects of electroconvulsive therapy in adolescents. *Journal of Child and Adolescent Psychopharmacology, 10*(4), 269–276. Retrieved from http://www.ncbi.nlm.nih.gov/pubmed/11191687

Green, B., Shirk, S., Hanze, D., & Wanstrath, J. (1994). The Children's Global Assessment Scale in clinical practice: an empirical evaluation. *Journal of the American Academy of Child and Adolescent Psychiatry, 33*(8), 1158–1164. doi:10.1097/00004583-199410000-00011.

Group, U. E. R. (2003). Efficacy and safety of electroconvulsive therapy in depressive disorders: A systematic review and meta-analysis. *Lancet, 361*(9360), 799–808. doi:10.1016/S0140-6736(03)12705-5.

Grover, S., Malhotra, S., Varma, S., Chakrabarti, S., Avasthi, A., & Mattoo, S. K. (2013). Electroconvulsive therapy in adolescents: A retrospective study from north India. *The Journal of ECT, 29*(2), 122–126. doi:10.1097/YCT.0b013e31827e0d22.

Guttmacher, L. B., & Cretella, H. (1988). Electroconvulsive therapy in one child and three adolescents. *The Journal of Clinical Psychiatry, 49*(1), 20–23. Retrieved from http://www.ncbi.nlm.nih.gov/pubmed/3422073

Hale, E. (2009). Child shock therapy. *Sunday Herald Sun* January 25.

Hazell, P., O'Connell, D., Heathcote, D., & Henry, D. (2000). Tricyclic drugs for depression in children and adolescents. The *Cochrane Database* of Systematic Reviews (3), CD002317. doi:10.1002/14651858.CD002317

Hill, M. A., Courvoisie, H., Dawkins, K., Nofal, P., & Thomas, B. (1997). ECT for the treatment of intractable mania in two prepubertal male children. *Convulsive Therapy, 13*(2), 74–82. Retrieved from http://www.ncbi.nlm.nih.gov/pubmed/9253527

Jaaskelainen, E., Haapea, M., Rautio, N., Juola, P., Penttila, M., Nordstrom, T., et al. (2015). Twenty years of schizophrenia research in the Northern Finland birth cohort 1966: A systematic review. *Schizophrenia Research and Treatment, 2015*, 524875. doi:10.1155/2015/524875.

Jonsson, U., Bohman, H., von Knorring, L., Olsson, G., Paaren, A., & von Knorring, A. L. (2011). Mental health outcome of long-term and episodic adolescent depression: 15-year follow-up of a community sample. *Journal of Affective Disorders, 130*(3), 395–404. doi:10.1016/j.jad.2010.10.046.

Kay, S. R. (1990). Positive-negative symptom assessment in schizophrenia: Psychometric issues and scale comparison. *Psychiatric Quarterly, 61*(3), 163–178. Retrieved from http://www.ncbi.nlm.nih.gov/pubmed/2075220

Kay, S. R., Fiszbein, A., & Opler, L. A. (1987). The positive and negative syndrome scale (PANSS) for schizophrenia. *Schizophrenia Bulletin , 13*(2), 261–276. Retrieved from http://www.ncbi.nlm.nih.gov/pubmed/3616518

Krystal, A. D., Holsinger, T., Weiner, R. D., & Coffey, C. E. (2000). Prediction of the utility of a switch from unilateral to bilateral ECT in the elderly using treatment 2 ictal EEG indices. *The Journal of ECT, 16*(4), 327–337. Retrieved from http://www.ncbi.nlm.nih.gov/pubmed/11314870

Kutcher, S., & Robertson, H. A. (1995). Electroconvulsive therapy in treatment resistant bipolar youth. *Journal of Child and Adolescent Psychopharmacology, 5*, 167–175.

Lima, N. N., Nascimento, V. B., Peixoto, J. A., Moreira, M. M., Neto, M. L., Almeida, J. C., et al. (2013). Electroconvulsive therapy use in adolescents: A systematic review. *Annals of General Psychiatry, 12*(1), 17. doi:10.1186/1744-859X-12-17.

MacQueen, G., Parkin, C., Marriott, M., Begin, H., & Hasey, G. (2007). The long-term impact of treatment with electroconvulsive therapy on discrete memory systems in patients with bipolar disorder. *Journal of Psychiatry & Neuroscience: JPN, 32*(4), 241–249. Retrieved from http://www.ncbi.nlm.nih.gov/pubmed/17653292

McClintock, S. M., Choi, J., Deng, Z. D., Appelbaum, L. G., Krystal, A. D., & Lisanby, S. H. (2014). Multifactorial determinants of the neurocognitive effects of electroconvulsive therapy. *The Journal of ECT, 30*(2), 165–176. doi:10.1097/YCT.0000000000000137.

McDonald, A., & Walter, G. (2001). The portrayal of ECT in American movies. *The Journal of ECT, 17*(4), 264–274. Retrieved from http://www.ncbi.nlm.nih.gov/pubmed/11731728

Miller, M., Pate, V., Swanson, S. A., Azrael, D., White, A., & Sturmer, T. (2014). Antidepressant class, age, and the risk of deliberate self-harm: A propensity score matched cohort study of SSRI and SNRI users in the USA. *CNS Drugs, 28*(1), 79–88. doi:10.1007/s40263-013-0120-8.

Mohan, T. S., Tharyan, P., Alexander, J., & Raveendran, N. S. (2009). Effects of stimulus intensity on the efficacy and safety of twice-weekly, bilateral electroconvulsive therapy (ECT) combined with antipsychotics in acute mania: A randomised controlled trial. *Bipolar Disorders, 11*(2), 126–134. doi:10.1111/j.1399-5618.2009.00668.x.

Moise, F. N., & Petrides, G. (1996). Case study: Electroconvulsive therapy in adolescents. *Journal of the American Academy of Child and Adolescent Psychiatry, 35*(3), 312–318. doi:10.1097/00004583-199603000-00012.

Mortality, G. B. D., & Causes of Death, C. (2015). Global, regional, and national age-sex specific all-cause and cause-specific mortality for 240 causes of death, 1990–2013: A systematic analysis for the Global Burden of Disease Study 2013. *Lancet, 385*(9963), 117-–171. doi:10.1016/S0140-6736(14)61682-2

Overall, J. E., & Pfefferbaum, B. (1982). The brief psychiatric rating scale for children. *Psychopharmacology Bulletin, 18*(2), 10–16. Retrieved from http://www.ncbi.nlm.nih.gov/pubmed/7111598

Paillere-Martinot, M. L., Zivi, A., & Basquin, M. (1990). Use of electroconvulsive therapy in adolescence. *Encephale, 16*(5), 399–404. Retrieved from http://www.ncbi.nlm.nih.gov/pubmed/1979944

Poznanski, E. O., Grossman, J. A., Buchsbaum, Y., Banegas, M., Freeman, L., & Gibbons, R. (1984). Preliminary studies of the reliability and validity of the children's depression rating scale. *Journal of the American Academy of Child Psychiatry, 23*(2), 191–197. Retrieved from http://www.ncbi.nlm.nih.gov/pubmed/6715741

Rabheru, K. (2001). The use of electroconvulsive therapy in special patient populations. *The Canadian Journal of Psychiatry, 46*(8), 710–719. Retrieved from http://www.ncbi.nlm.nih.gov/pubmed/11692973

Rey, J. M., & Walter, G. (1997). Half a century of ECT use in young people. *American Journal of Psychiatry, 154*(5), 595–602. doi:10.1176/ajp.154.5.595.

Robbins, D. R., Alessi, N. E., Colfer, M. V., & Yanchyshyn, G. W. (1985). Use of the Hamilton rating scale for depression and the Carroll self-rating scale in adolescents. *Psychiatry Research, 14*(2), 123–129. Retrieved from http://www.ncbi.nlm.nih.gov/pubmed/3857652

Russell, J. C., Rasmussen, K. G., O'Connor, M. K., Copeman, C. A., Ryan, D. A., & Rummans, T. A. (2003). Long-term maintenance ECT: A retrospective review of efficacy and cognitive outcome. *The Journal of ECT, 19*(1), 4–9. Retrieved from http://www.ncbi.nlm.nih.gov/pubmed/12621270

Russell, P. S., Tharyan, P., Arun Kumar, K., & Cherian, A. (2002). Electro convulsive therapy in a pre-pubertal child with severe depression. *Journal of Postgraduate Medicine, 48*(4), 290–291. Retrieved from http://www.ncbi.nlm.nih.gov/pubmed/12571387

Sackeim, H. A., Prudic, J., Nobler, M. S., Fitzsimons, L., Lisanby, S. H., Payne, N., et al. (2008). Effects of pulse width and electrode placement on the efficacy and cognitive effects of electroconvulsive therapy. *Brain Stimulation, 1*(2), 71–83. doi:10.1016/j.brs.2008.03.001.

Shapira, B., Calev, A., & Lerer, B. (1991). Optimal use of electroconvulsive therapy: Choosing a treatment schedule. *Psychiatric Clinics of North America, 14*(4), 935–946. Retrieved from http://www.ncbi.nlm.nih.gov/pubmed/1771155

Sienaert, P., Dhossche, D. M., Vancampfort, D., De Hert, M., & Gazdag, G. (2014). A clinical review of the treatment of catatonia. *Front Psychiatry, 5*, 181. doi:10.3389/fpsyt.2014.00181.

Song, G. M., Tian, X., Shuai, T., Yi, L. J., Zeng, Z., Liu, S., et al. (2015). Treatment of adults with treatment-resistant depression: Electroconvulsive therapy plus antidepressant or electroconvulsive therapy alone? Evidence from an indirect comparison meta-analysis. *Medicine (Baltimore), 94*(26), e1052. doi:10.1097/MD.0000000000001052.

Stein, D., Kurtsman, L., Stier, S., Remnik, Y., Meged, S., & Weizman, A. (2004). Electroconvulsive therapy in adolescent and adult psychiatric inpatients—A retrospective chart design. *Journal of Affective Disorders, 82*(3), 335–342. doi:10.1016/j.jad.2004.01.009.

Stein, D., Weizman, A., & Bloch, Y. (2006). Electroconvulsive therapy and transcranial magnetic stimulation: Can they be considered valid modalities in the treatment of pediatric mood disorders? *Child and Adolescent Psychiatric Clinics of North America, 15*(4), 1035–1056, xi. doi:10.1016/j.chc.2006.05.012

Strober, M., Rao, U., DeAntonio, M., Liston, E., State, M., Amaya-Jackson, L. et al. (1998). Effects of electroconvulsive therapy in adolescents with severe endogenous depression resistant to pharmacotherapy. *Biological Psychiatry, 43*(5), 335–338. Retrieved from http://www.ncbi.nlm.nih.gov/pubmed/9513748

Taieb, O., Flament, M. F., Chevret, S., Jeammet, P., Allilaire, J. F., Mazet, P. et al. (2002). Clinical relevance of electroconvulsive therapy (ECT) in adolescents with severe mood disorder: Evidence from a follow-up study. *European Psychiatry, 17*(4), 206–212. Retrieved from http://www.ncbi.nlm.nih.gov/pubmed/12231266

Taylor, P. J. (1983). Consent, competency and ECT: A psychiatrist's view. *Journal of Medical Ethics, 9*(3), 146–151. Retrieved from http://www.ncbi.nlm.nih.gov/pubmed/6620319

Tharyan, P., & Adams, C. E. (2005). Electroconvulsive therapy for schizophrenia. The *Cochrane Database of Systematic Reviews* (2), CD000076. doi:10.1002/14651858.CD000076.pub2

Thompson, J. W., & Blaine, J. D. (1987). Use of ECT in the United States in 1975 and 1980 *American Journal of Psychiatry, 144*(5), 557–562. doi:10.1176/ajp.144.5.557.

Wachtel, L. E., Schuldt, S., Ghaziuddin, N., & Shorter, E. (2013). The potential role of electroconvulsive therapy in the 'Iron Triangle' of pediatric catatonia, autism, and psychosis. *Acta Psychiatrica Scandinavica, 128*(5), 408–409. doi:10.1111/acps.12158.

Walter, G., & Rey, J. M. (1997). An epidemiological study of the use of ECT in adolescents. *Journal of the American Academy of Child and Adolescent Psychiatry, 36*(6), 809–815. doi:10.1097/00004583-199706000-00018.

Walter, G., & Rey, J. M. (2003). Has the practice and outcome of ECT in adolescents changed? Findings from a whole-population study. *The Journal of ECT, 19*(2), 84–87. Retrieved from http://www.ncbi.nlm.nih.gov/pubmed/12792456

Weiner, R. D., Rogers, H. J., Davidson, J. R., & Squire, L. R. (1986). Effects of stimulus parameters on cognitive side effects. *Annals of the New York Academy of Sciences, 462*, 315–325. Retrieved from http://www.ncbi.nlm.nih.gov/pubmed/3458412

Weissman, M. M., Wolk, S., Goldstein, R. B., Moreau, D., Adams, P., Greenwald, S., … Wickramaratne, P. (1999). Depressed adolescents grown up. *JAMA, 281*(18), 1707–1713. Retrieved from http://www.ncbi.nlm.nih.gov/pubmed/10328070

Wong, E., Ungvari, G. S., Leung, S. K., & Tang, W. K. (2007). Rating catatonia in patients with chronic schizophrenia: Rasch analysis of the Bush-Francis Catatonia Rating Scale. *International Journal of Methods in Psychiatric Research, 16*(3), 161–170. doi:10.1002/mpr.224.

Zhang, Z. J., Chen, Y. C., Wang, H. N., Wang, H. H., Xue, Y. Y., Feng, S. F., et al. (2012). Electroconvulsive therapy improves antipsychotic and somnographic responses in adolescents with first-episode psychosis—A case—Control study. *Schizophrenia Research, 137*(1–3), 97–103. doi:10.1016/j.schres.2012.01.037.

Part VI
Non-Pharmacological Treatments

Chapter 20
Play as a Medium for Assessment and Therapy in Child and Adolescent Mental Health Practice

Rachel Z. Ritvo

Abstract Play reflects the child's internal world and facilitates trial action, problem solving and practice. Observing the process of play as closely as the content of play facilitates assessment of developmental status and mental status. Axline's eight basic principles for open-ended play interviews facilitate the child's playing freely. "Working in displacement" and "turning-passive-to-active" facilitate communication within the play metaphor. Games with rules can enhance self-reflection, problem solving, relationship building and the ability to sustain attention. Developmentally normative cognitive and language limitations of children between four and eleven years make play a preferred path to therapeutic change.

Keywords Play therapy · Psychodynamic therapy · Child mental status exam · Games

20.1 Introduction

Child mental health care is a multidisciplinary field benefiting from the expertise of child and adolescent psychiatrists and all the allied professionals. The use of play is one of the features of our work that unites us across disciplines and distinguishes us from adult mental health practitioners. The ability to engage the child patient in play is an essential skill of child mental health professionals.

What makes play so important? Play is a natural form of expression in children. Developmentally, well into adolescence, children lag behind adults in their capacity to use language to fully communicate their experiences, their thoughts and their feelings. Because play comes naturally to children, it puts the child at ease with the psychiatrist and facilitates forming a therapeutic relationship.

R.Z. Ritvo (✉)
Department of Psychiatry and Behavioral Sciences, School of Medicine and Health Sciences, George Washington University, Washington, D.C., USA
e-mail: rzritvomd@gmail.com

S. Malhotra and P. Santosh (eds.), *Child and Adolescent Psychiatry*,
DOI 10.1007/978-81-322-3619-1_20

Consistent with the psychological principle of over-determination, play provides a modality of communication that carries large quantities of information condensed into each action. Play emerges from the child's internal world and reflects the child's psyche. I use "psyche" very broadly here. Play will reflect a child's cognitive capacities just as it will reflect the child's emotional regulation, anxieties or core conflicts. This reflection of the child's mind, the child's psyche, makes play a most useful vehicle for child psychiatric assessment. By training oneself to observe the child's play within the relatively standardized environment of your office, you, the clinician, can get important information about the child's developmental status, relational capacities, language capacity, fund of knowledge, frustration tolerance and more. Just as the child's face is unique to that child, each child's play will be uniquely their own. My late father, a psychoanalyst and child psychiatry professor, called the individual patterns of a child's play the child's "play signature" (Ritvo 1993).

Play is pretend. "The opposite of play is not work. It is reality" (Yanof 2013). It's "as if" quality makes play an excellent modality for therapeutic work. The child and therapist can explore, communicate and act together without irreversibly changing the world outside. Play is safe and safety is a fundamental building block of effective therapy. Play allows for problem solving, trial actions and practice, leading to growth and change in the mind's capacity to cope with experiences in life outside the therapy room.

20.1.1 Play Assessment

I have two purposes in drawing attention to play as an assessment tool. Firstly, if we do not at least do some portion of our assessment of the child patient in a mode of communication that is natural and puts the child in a position of ease and competence, we will not get a full understanding of this child, of what it is like to be this child or of this child's particular strengths and cognitive style. Secondly, focusing on play as an assessment tool allows us to concentrate on developing our observational skills without worrying about mastering the techniques of play therapy interventions.

Despite the long, nearly 100 year, history of using play in child psychiatric practice, there is relatively little published on standardizing the process of play observation. The late Paulina Kernberg and her colleague Saralea Chazan at the State University of New York, Downstate did a very respectable job of developing the Children's Play Therapy Instrument (CPTI) for analyzing play-interviews (Kernberg et al. 1998). They developed their instrument for a research study of the play of traumatized children in ongoing therapy. Although I do not use the entire instrument, I find their approach to "observing play activity" to be useful in practice and teaching (Chazan 2002).

The Children's Play Therapy Instrument is divided into three sections: Descriptive Analysis; Structural Analysis and; Functional Analysis. In my work teaching child psychiatry trainees, it is the Descriptive Analysis that I emphasize to sharpen the clinician's observational skills. Any video of a child at play can be used to teach the observational approach. In our training program at Children's National Medical Center in Washington, D.C. we invite a child from our inpatient ward to play with me while the interview is observed through a one-way mirror and recorded. Immediately after the interview, the observing trainees and I review what we have seen. The following week we can review it again from the recording and look at the process moment to moment in the manner described by Kernberg and Chazan.

Descriptive Analysis begins with *segmentation*. Whether looking at a video or reviewing an encounter in one's head while writing process notes or charting, parsing the session into segments is the first step. Segmentation provides an overview of the progression and flow of the child's activity within the session. The segments may be:

(a) *play*: recognized for absorption or focus, expression of engagement, there may be an invitation to play, and the directing of action.
(b) *pre-play*: "setting-up" which precedes play or can occur as a pause in the middle of a play. Some children may spend the whole session "setting-up" so that the sorting, aligning and designing have become the play.
(c) *non-play*: the realm of daily actions such as reading, conversing with the therapist, or eating.
(d) *interruptions/disruptions*: behaviors that reflect mounting tension within the session that cannot be tolerated by the child so that he/she seeks relief by leaving the room, or abruptly stopping the play.

Once the session has been segmented, the observer can choose segments for a complete descriptive analysis, which considers: the type of play activity entered into; who initiates the play; how it progresses or fails to progress; how it ends; and, the sphere in which it takes place.

The CPTI identifies thirteen *categories of play activity* (sensory, gross motor, exploratory, manipulative, sorting-aligning, cause-effect, problem-solving, construction, literal imitation, traumatic, fantasy, game play, art). Some occur infrequently but are quite striking when you see them so that it is reassuring to know that they are seen in other children as well. For instance, *sorting-aligning* is an activity in which toy objects are sorted or lined-up with no further elaboration or symbolic meaning. I have seen this from time to time and, as you might expect, it shows up in children with obsessional tendencies.

Children tend to play from their strengths and talents. Those who choose gross motor activities are likely either to be athletic or hyperactive. The choice of fantasy play may signal creativity and emotional strength or, if it becomes loose and disjointed, it may signal difficulties in organizing experience and affect regulation. As you consider a segment of a play session, think about the choice of play activity the child makes, presuming you have made the room suitable for a range of choices covering all or most of the thirteen categories of play. Think about how the child's choice fits into the assessment puzzle this particular child presents for you.

Once the category of play has been identified, the next step is *script description*. The observer notes the *initiation* of the play. Is the child eager, hesitant, collaborative, or self-absorbed? After taking note of how the play is initiated, the observer proceeds to consider the play *facilitation*. Is the activity maintained by the child or by the therapist? Does *inhibition* occur during the segment? Does the inhibition come from the child of the therapist? Script description concludes with observing the "ending" of the segment. Was there play *satiation*? Did the play end because the child felt it was complete? Or did the child simply lose interest, or become frustrated or interrupt the play abruptly?

Satiation is an idea associated with Erik Erikson. For many children it represents resolution of the problem they are struggling to master. Traumatized children typically cannot resolve the trauma and keep up a frantic repetitive play. Chazan (2002) also adopted from Erikson the concept of "Spheres of Play Activity." Erikson (1972) described three spheres of play. In the *autosphere* the child uses his or her own body for entertainment such as the way infants and toddlers play with and suck on their toes. The *microsphere* refers to play with toy objects such as a doll-sized tea set or action figures. Play in the *macrosphere* refers to the use of full sized objects and the exploration of objects in the environment. The child who plays with the stapler to staple papers or to take it apart and reassemble is playing in the macrosphere. This nomenclature is not used frequently in the current literature but I find it useful to note and I encourage my students to pay attention to the child's choice of sphere and shifts between spheres.

Structural Analysis of the play session pulls out the information needed for the mental status exam and developmental assessment. You may wish to organize it differently from Chazan to suit your own needs. They group their structural observations in four categories: *affective; cognitive; narrative and; developmental.* Affective assessment looks at overall hedonic tone, spectrum of affects, regulation and moderation of affect, transitions between affective states, appropriateness of affect to content, child's affect toward the therapist, and the therapist's affective tone toward the child.

Chazan looks at cognitive functioning through an object relations theory lens. I think this is an area where this instrument could be revised to track more closely a cognitive neuroscience view of cognitive development. The cognitive categories in the CPTI are: the complexity of the role representations; the stability of the representations; the use of play objects; and, the style of representation ranging from reality based to bizarre.

I think of narrative ability as a subset of cognitive functioning. Is this child strong or weak in language abilities? With older children I consider whether they do or do not have age appropriate narrative abilities and also evaluate their expository abilities, poetic talent and their skills for categorizing and list making. Chazan looks at play segments as narratives and analyzes them for topic of play, theme, level of relationship (self-centered, dyadic, triadic, complex), quality of relationships portrayed and overall use of language.

Like the cognitive assessment, the developmental assessment can be tailored to the clinician's theoretical perspective. I was trained in the psychoanalytic school of psychology, as were Kernberg and Chazan. The categories they recommend begin with a consideration of the age appropriateness of the child's play. Is it immature, age appropriate or advanced? What is the social/interactive level of the play? Is it isolated and unaware of the therapist, parallel, reciprocal or cooperative? Themes of the play help the observer to determine the psychosexual level of the child: oral; anal; phallic; Oedipal or; latency. The play can also be examined for evidence of the child's progress on separation—individuation and gendered expression.

Just as the Structural Analysis helps us organize our understanding of the structure of the child's psyche, the Functional Analysis requires the clinician to reflect on the coping strategies or defenses deployed through the course of the play. How does the child function psychologically, as internal and external events unfold? A behaviorist might make a different sort of functional analysis. Here again theory affects what you are looking for and the meaning you place on what you see in the play.

20.1.2 Play Therapy

Up to this point we have been exploring the use of play as a tool for exposing the child's concerns and capacities to the clinician and organizing what we see to allow us to make a thorough assessment of the child's mental state and developmental capacities. I would now like to turn our attention to play as an experience that leads to change, to healing, to growth. I want to take a look at generic features of play therapy that can apply no matter what therapeutic school of therapy you are undertaking.

Framing is a term used to refer to the context constructed for a psychotherapy session. What is the set-up for using play in the clinical encounter? By creating a physical and social frame the therapist constructs for the child a context for the play that defines it both as play and as therapy. Having a separate playroom for work with children is a luxury few of us have. It does allow a freedom that is very beneficial for non-directive therapies but it is not necessary to using play for assessment or treatment. If you look at the list of play activities Chazan gave us, you can get a feel for the sort of play equipment that you would like to have to allow the child to choose the activity that suits that child: paper and pencil; scissors; tape; a ball; blocks; figures either human or animal that could represent a family; an aggressive figure such as a lion or shark; a deck of cards and, perhaps, also a doctor's kit and some toy plates and food.

More challenging for many starting clinicians is creating the relational frame of the play session. Because we are more accustomed as adults and as health care professionals to taking a directive stance toward children, (e.g., the routine pediatric visit in which the child is a passive respondent), I work with my students to teach them the non-directive stance. Once the non-directive stance is mastered they can then work on developing the clinical judgment to decide where along the continuum from non-directive to directive they want to be for a particular child, at a particular moment, with a particular clinical task.

I have found that the most succinct and vivid description of non-directive principles is Virginia Axline's guide to client centered play therapy (Axline 1947). First published in 1947, this book is still in print and is now available as an e-book. Axline presents eight basic principles that guide the therapist in all non-directive therapeutic encounters.

Establishing Rapport is the first principle. The therapist builds a warm, friendly relationship with the child. *Accepting the Child Completely,* requires the therapist to be patient and avoid criticism or reproof. The third principle requires the therapist to *Establish a Feeling of Permisiveness.* This is at the core of non-directive approaches. The child is made to feel free to express him/herself freely in words or actions. Axline's fourth principle, *Recognition and Reflection of Feelings,* recommends that the therapist note the feelings the child is expressing and find a manner of reflecting the feelings back to the child in a way that does not tell the child what to feel but rather promotes insight. *Maintaining Respect for the Child* does not just mean being polite or kind but rather refers to respecting the child's agency. Axline means for the therapist to have a conviction that the child has the ability to solve his/her own problems if given an opportunity. She says, "The responsibility to make choices and to institute change is the child's." Consistent with this respect for the child's agency is the non-directive tenet *The Child Leads the Way.* The therapist does not attempt to direct the child's actions or conversation but rather follows the child's lead. Consistent with giving the child agency is the precept that *Therapy Cannot Be Hurried;* when the child is ready to express his/her feelings in the presence of the therapist, he/she will do so.

The eighth principle, the *Value of Limits,* focuses on an approach to limit setting that is consistent with the social framing of the therapy. Limit setting is an issue at every point along the non-directive to directive spectrum of play with child patients. Rather than giving the child a list of limits at the outset, it is best to address the limits as situations arise. Time constraint is experienced as a limitation in all therapies that have a start time and a stop time. The child might wish to stay longer but the therapist must work to keep to the schedule.

The therapy, the space, time and the therapist, are framed as a safe place and relationship in which free expression of thought and emotion is possible. In psychodynamic therapies, limits protect the "as if" nature of play and delineate the boundary between pretend and reality. When the child leaves at the end of the session, the room is restored to its pre-session, tidy state. Therefor the therapist does stop the child from actions that would actually do damage to the office, the patient or the therapist. To maintain respect for the child, the therapist avoids precipitating a power struggle or becoming physically coercive. It takes training to become expert in containing the child without coercing or bribing. The therapist works to reflect the child's feelings and shore up failing defenses that impel the child past the limit (Bellinson 2009).

The child leaving the therapy room is a common situation. Many times it is a disruption that can be accommodated. For example, the child might need to use the lavatory or wants to check on the parent in the waiting room. At other times it may be dangerous or bothersome to others in the clinic and needs to be contained.

One of the most dramatic "near" departures I have experienced allows me to demonstrate reflecting on what might impel the child and my temperate use of a physical constraint. I title this vignette "Headlines Read, 'Boy Lost in Psychiatrist's Ceiling!'

> Always a climber, Jody, a 9-year-old later diagnosed as Bipolar II, had stacked a small, sturdy play room chair, on top of a larger, sturdy playroom chair, on top of a sturdy playroom table. Then, while I was still wondering what he had in mind, Jody, with what seemed like lightening speed, clambered up this tower and began removing the ceiling tile where it met the room-partitioning wall. He was pulling himself up on that wall as I restrained him by wrapping myself around his feet. As I wondered aloud "Am I the policeman? Where is your own policeman? Where is your red light, Jody?" he was announcing with relish "Headlines read, 'Boy lost in psychiatrist's ceiling.

My goal was to use the minimum physical restraint necessary to keep him from going further while wondering aloud why he could not stop himself.

Having set the frame for the therapy, we can now turn our attention to the *play process* that unfolds within this frame. What do the child and therapist do and say? There are three features of the play process that are particularly useful for the therapist to understand and to become skilled at using: *Working in the Displacement; Turning Passive to Active and; The Running Commentary.*

Displacement has historically been studied as a defense mechanism. In a defensive displacement there is a transfer of emotions, ideas, or wishes from the original object or target to a more acceptable substitute object or target. For children, much of their learning and problem solving occurs in displacements. If we observe a young child playing at diapering a baby doll that play is a displacement from the child's own experience of being changed and diapered. Whereas when a toddler sits in the highchair and tries to feed herself, that is not a displacement. Displacement is most obvious in fantasy play in which the child creates stories that are metaphors for the child's own feelings, worries and experiences.

Displacement modulates the emotional intensity of the topic the child is struggling to master. As the emotional intensity is modulated, dampening mid-brain and limbic system activity, cortical function can increase and the child can "figure things out." Displacement allows the child to gain a more objective perspective on what is otherwise an intensely subjective experience. This turning of subjective into objective experience facilitates cognitive functioning.

In the displacement, the child often develops a metaphor and even an extended metaphor for the issue the child is tackling. Like metaphor, displacement allows a person to take what is known in one context and apply it in a similar but different context. Linguists propose that metaphor uses what is known concretely to understand what cannot easily be known concretely. For example, the idea of family has many different features. In the metaphors "family is a rock to stand on" or "family is a safety net" we bring out the meaning of support that is part of the idea of family.

Judith Yanof, in her 2013 article "Play Techniques in Psychodynamic Psychotherapy", gives an excellent guide to the technique of working in the play displacement (Yanof 2013). I have adapted one of her examples:

> Ryan, a 5-year old with frequent episodes of significant emotional dysregulation, played with a family of clay figures. They were sitting peacefully in their living room when a knock came on the door. It was a creature from "another planet" who was "weird" with two heads and a tail. Ryan explained that the creature was a baby orphan and wanted the family to care for him. Dr. Y was directed to play the family and to help the creature and give him food. But the creature ate up ALL the food and took the family's car and drove it until it crashed. He ignored all the rules. He spoke a different language and could not understand the family's rules. Losing control of himself the creature destroyed the house. He tried to fly and fell into a pit. At this moment Ryan started to tear the creature into pieces, a pile of body parts, which he tossed about.

Here Ryan has given us a great deal of information about how he "goes to pieces," which was his presenting complaint, dysregulation. As a 5 year old, Ryan could not possibly have the conceptual language to communicate so much in words alone. In the metaphor of the creature, he was "alien" and an orphan, small and helpless as a baby, hungry and devouring and vulnerable to falling apart.

In clinical practice we put play episodes such as this into the context of the history, the current life experiences and the developmental and psychological formulation of the case. Is Ryan presenting an experience from his past or from his current life or both? Are the relationships from the past or are they, perhaps, a reference to the current transference relationship with the therapist? He is showing us his fears, his conflicts and his lack of solutions.

How does a therapist work with Ryan in the displacement of the space-creature to assist him in mastering his feelings and holding onto his coherent self? The therapist could comment about the play from outside, as an observer, still using the patient's play metaphor. *"The family doesn't seem to have enough food to keep this creature from feeling hungry. What should they do?"* Or, the therapist can comment from inside the play as one of the characters in the patient's story. *In the father's voice Dr. Y might say "It looks like he hasn't had food for days. The poor creature is starving!"* A third technique is to comment by creating a new character or by telling a related story. *Just as Ryan is pulling the creature apart the father calls a doctor who speaks "creature language" and says kindly but firmly "Pull yourself together son. I have just the skills to help you."*

Most importantly, the therapist avoids prematurely puncturing the displacement and insisting the action is about the child. The therapist would not say: *"Ryan, I think you feel so angry you feel like breaking your house apart."* A direct interpretation like this can be felt as accusatory if it is given before the child is ready to let go of the defensive function of the displacement. The therapeutic effect does not require this final step of self-acknowledgement. It is possible to do the entire work of the therapy inside the displacement.

Mastery of self, of skills and of the environment both social and physical is the major task of childhood. Play, as a form of trial action, frequently is used by the child to turn from the role of being the passive partner in an experience to being the active partner to facilitate mastery and to maintain self-esteem. As children grow and develop within the family and their culture, they actively pursue mastering the activities they see others execute. Children play at activities they may never actually do themselves for a very long time. For example, a 16 month old plays at diapering a baby doll. The drive to relive and rework an experience by shifting from the passive role (the baby being diapered) to the active role (diapering the doll-baby) is a normal, healthy path to learning. Children naturally bring this passive to active play into the therapy setting.

The typical passive to active game in therapy draws on Yanof's second approach to working in displacement; the therapist takes on a role as a character in the patient's pretend play. A common example is the "Teacher Game". Here I borrow from a clinical vignette published by a Louisiana State University professor, Drell (1992).

> Laura, age 7, was brought for therapy because she and her mother were locked in an interminable civil war. They argued over everything and vied for father's attention. Laura introduced a game in which she was a mean teacher and Dr. D was the "ever-trying-to-please student." As they went over play math assignments some unknown, undetectable error would cause the teacher to berate the student. As soon as he protested she sent him to the principal's office in the corner with the threat that parents would be called.

Failing to observe Dr. Yanof's rule of not puncturing the displacement, Dr. Drell tried to link the play to similar situations with her mother since there were no problems at school. Laura told him to "*quit the "psychiatry stuff*""!

> Dr. D then kept his comments in character balking at going to the office and muttering under his breath. Suddenly, several sessions later, the principal (played by Laura) switched to taking the student's side and fired the teacher. And a new teacher with lesson plans and a calmer manner was played. But even the new teacher fell into harsh criticism. And Dr. D continued to comment in character. Laura went through several cycles of teachers each getting nicer. Eventually there was a teacher who was firm and orderly but now Dr. D complained she was boring. Laura, as teacher, added art so he would have some fun. The last teacher made Dr. D her pet and they collaborated on the projects she assigned. At this point the parents found Laura much improved in her behavior at home and the therapy concluded.

Playing the active role of the unreasonable teacher, Laura could safely and unabashedly express her own bossy, controlling feelings and gradually learn to contain them. Playing the passive role, the therapist performs an act of empathy and facilitates clarification of feelings and articulation of conflicts. Dr. Drell was expressing the helplessness and unfairness Laura felt with her mother but also that the mother felt with Laura. In the voice of the student he could describe inner conflict, "I want to be good but this teacher is making me angry. She is so unfair."

We know from developmental studies that the ability to put feelings and psychic realities into words is learned by children when an adult labels and identifies their feelings accurately. Playing the passive role for the child, the therapist has many opportunities to connect feeling and words. The child absorbs this like a sponge.

There is a great deal more to say about the use of play in clinical work with children and with adolescents. However, we do not have space to discuss the ins and outs of the therapeutic use of games with rules or construction projects or spontaneous games of catch. But there is a technique for addressing these activities when they occur in the therapy room. Your goal is to show non-judgmental attentive interest and to draw the patient's awareness to observing their own subjective experience. The running commentary creates a second layer to the play experience. The child and the therapist are involved in both an action layer and in a conversational, reflective layer.

Jill Bellinson, a psychologist and psychoanalyst at the William Alanson White Institute in New York, has written several beautiful articles on using board games in psychodynamic play therapies. In her recent article in the Child and Adolescent Psychiatric Clinics of North America (Bellinson 2013), she gives some very nice examples of how to comment on a child's actions from an interested but non-judgmental position. The therapist models putting into language observable connections between feelings and actions. Putting the experience into words promotes growth of self-awareness and self-understanding. Of course, the child may correct or refine the observation.

Bellinson distinguishes four kinds of therapist comments on the child's behavior in the play. She describes playing with a child who is making up rules or reacting to playing a board game, but these responses are easily generalized to other situations.

1. Interpretations of awareness:
   "It took a lot of throws to get the number you wanted"
   "You landed on the Extra-turn square when I thought your number came out on the one before."
   "You have drawn that very carefully to keep all the blue marker inside the black line."
2. Interpretations of feelings:
   "It hurts you so much when you have to go backward."
   "You hate it when I have a lucky turn."
3. Interpretations of circumstances:
   "You missed it three times and now your going to make sure you get it by searching the deck."
   "One "lose a turn card" was ok for you but two is too many."
   "You really like to spin in that chair and you don't get dizzy!"
4. Interpretations of outcome:
   "You just couldn't feel ok about how you drew the nose and you tore up the whole picture."
   "You built the tallest tower, using all the blocks and now you want to show Mommy."

This kind of non-judgmental interested commentary can be practiced easily with any children that you meet in your day to day life outside the office. If you hit the right note or tone, the child will respond with engagement and pleasure in your company. If you get it wrong, they will let you know.

Play is a natural form of expression in children. Play provides for communication that carries large quantities of information condensed into each action. Careful descriptive analysis of play helps the clinician recognize and organize this information. From this information the clinician can complete a mental status examination, a developmental assessment and make a psychological formulation.

Play therapy is performed along a continuum of non-directive to directive frames. Psychodynamic play therapy utilizes the child's tendency toward displacement, the transfer of emotions, ideas, or wishes from the original object or target to a more acceptable substitute object. Or to put it in plain English, working through analogies and metaphors because when one is not directly referring to oneself it is easier to try out feelings and to problem solve. Children also benefit from reversing their passive experiences into one's in which the child plays out the role of the active initiator. Even board games can be worked with in a non-judgemental, self-exploratory manner that allows the child to grow. The ability to engage the child patient in play is an essential skill of child mental health professionals.

References

Axline, V. M. (1947). *Play therapy*. New York: Ballantine.

Bellinson, J. (2009). You can't do that—Or can you? Historical and clinical perspectives on limit setting in child psychotherapy. *Journal of Infant, Child and Adolescent Psychotherapy, 8*(2), 87–95.

Bellinson, J. (2013). Games children play: Board games in psychodynamic psychotherapy. *Child and Adolescent Psychiatric Clinics of North America, 22*(2), 283–293.

Chazan, S. E. (2002). *Profiles of play: Assessing and observing structure and process in play therapy*. Philadelphia: Jessica Kingsley Publishers.

Drell, M. (1992). Clinical vignettes: The teacher game. *AACAP News, 23*, 17.

Erikson, E. (1972). Play and actuality. In M. Piers (Ed.), *Play and development*. New York, : W.W. Norton.

Kernberg, P. F., Chazan, S. E., & Normandin, L. (1998). The children's play therapy instrument: Description, development, and reliability studies. *Journal of Psychotherapy Practice and Research., 7*(3), 196–207.

Ritvo, S. (1993). Play and illusion. In A. J. Solnit, D. J. Cohen, & P. Neubauer (Eds.), *The many meanings of play: A psychoanalytic perspective* (pp. 234–251). New Haven: Yale University Press.

Yanof, J. A. (2013). Play technique in psychodynamic psychotherapy. *Child and Adolescent Psychiatric Clinics of North America, 22*(2), 261–282.

Chapter 21
Poor Scholastic Performance: Psychosocial Perspectives in Assessment and Management

Rakesh Kumar Chadda and Bichitra Nanda Patra

Abstract Poor scholastic performance has immediate as well as lifelong adverse effects on a child and adolescent's self-esteem and future growth. Psychosocial factors are one of the important causative factors for poor scholastic performance in the under privileged societies, and often remain unidentified. Poor scholastic performance is associated with poor concentration in studies and high dropout rate from schools, and thus has high social costs. A comprehensive assessment covering psychosocial and biological factors is needed to identify the exact cause and plan effective management at the earliest so as to avoid long-term complications. This chapter mainly focusses on psychosocial issues in assessment and management of poor scholastic performance.

Keywords Academic performance · Specific learning disability · Schooling · Developmental · School dropout

Key Points

- Children and adolescents with poor scholastic performance need a detailed evaluation.
- Poor scholastic performance can be due to variety of causes varying from developmental problems to undiagnosed physical illnesses and psychosocial factors.
- Cause needs to be identified at the earliest and corrected, since otherwise the problem can have long-term adverse consequences.

R.K. Chadda (✉) · B.N. Patra
Department of Psychiatry, All India Institute of Medical Sciences, New Delhi 110029, India
e-mail: drrakeshchadda@gmail.com

B.N. Patra
e-mail: patrab.aiims@gmail.com

S. Malhotra and P. Santosh (eds.), *Child and Adolescent Psychiatry*,
DOI 10.1007/978-81-322-3619-1_21

21.1 Introduction

Education is crucial for multifaceted development. Every child should be getting an opportunity to use one's potentials to the best. Poor scholastic performance has adverse effects on the self-esteem and future growth of the children and adolescents. Prevalence of poor scholastic performance is quite high, to the extent of about 20 % (Thacker 2007). It is very important to identify the children with poor scholastic performance at the earliest, and also those, who are at risk, so that early interventions may be instituted.

Starting of schooling involves the process of separation from parents and adjustment to new environment, and adaptation to new social contacts. The child has to deal with the issues of competition, assertion, and intimacy. A mastery of all these characteristics is important for an optimal performance at school. A child's physical, cognitive, and emotional adjustment is important for success and acceptance at school, and a disturbance in adjustment at any of these areas may affect scholastic performance of the child.

India has made extraordinary progress over the past decade in increasing access to elementary education. Over 98 % of children in India are estimated to have access to primary schooling within 1 km of their residence, and almost 92 % to an upper primary school within 3 km of their residence (http://ssa.nic.in/quality-docs/RTE%20SSA%20Final%20Report.pdf). In India, out of 20.41 crores of children aged 6–13 years, 60.41 lakhs (2.97 %) are out of school. However, there has been a progressive decrease in this group of children from 6.94 % in 2006 to 4.28 % in 2009 to 2.97 % in 2014. But unfortunately, the rate of school dropout in India is very high. The number of children with special needs who are out of school is much higher at 28.07 % (http://ssa.nic.in/pabminutes-documents/NS.pdf).

Poor scholastic performance is one of the important reasons for school dropout, and may be the real unidentified culprit, while the dropout is attributed to the other more socially acceptable factors like lack of facilities or resources or the teachers' attitude.

21.2 Causes of Poor Scholastic Performance

Poor scholastic performance may occur due to a variety of causes including pregnancy and birth complications, developmental disturbances, sensory impairments, nutritional deficiencies, physical illnesses, and psychosocial and environmental factors and specific psychiatric illnesses. Details are discussed as below.

Pregnancy and birth complications: Pregnancy and birth related complications and low birthweight leading to developmental delays are one of the important causes of scholastic backwardness (Karande et al. 2007).

Developmental disorders: Developmental disorders especially subnormal intelligence and specific learning disabilities are important causes of scholastic backwardness. Undiagnosed intellectual disability and borderline or low average intelligence can also adversely affect the scholastic functioning. Specific developmental disorders of reading, writing or speech can affect studies and learning and thus have a potential to lead to scholastic backwardness (Karande et al. 2007; Haneesh et al. 2013).

Sensory impairments: Sensory impairments especially undiagnosed visual and hearing impairments can affect learning, leading to scholastic backwardness (Haneesh et al. 2013; Shashidhar et al. 2009).

Nutritional deficiencies: Similarly nutritional deficiencies including malnutrition, anaemia, and deficiencies of vitamins A, B_1, B_2, B_6, D_3 and niacinamide can also contribute by affecting the physical health and growth, and further affecting the scholastic performance (Haneesh et al. 2013; Rashmi et al. 2015; Nair et al. 2003).

Physical illnesses: Both common as well as chronic physical illnesses, if not properly managed, increase the risk for scholastic backwardness. Physical illnesses like bronchial asthma, allergic rhinitis, and worm infestation are quite common in children, and if untreated, may affect scholastic performance. Children suffering from chronic medical illnesses like epilepsy, diabetes, hematological disorders, leukemia, and congenital hypothyroidism need regular long-term treatment, affecting their functioning at school. Some children may suffer from idiopathic short stature and growth hormone deficiency, which can also lead to scholastic backwardness. HIV infection is another emerging problem with a potential to affect scholastic skills (Haneesh et al. 2013; Florence et al. 2008).

Psychosocial and environmental factors: Psychosocial stressors in the family like disturbed relations with parents, family conflict, broken homes and parental neglect may all affect the child's school performance. Adequate supervision by the parents is often required for optimal academic performance, which if lacking, can affect it adversely, leading to scholastic backwardness. Physical or sexual abuse also worsens the scholastic performance (Nair et al. 2003; Shenoy and Kapur 1996; Mogasale et al. 2012; Khurana 1980).

Sociocultural and environmental factors like low priority being given to education in the family, education level of parents, lack of basic facilities and overcrowding at home, absence of space for studying at home, and alcohol and drug abuse in the family may be in the background of scholastic backwardness. Many times, the child is burdened with the domestic work and does not get adequate time for studies.

Environmental factors, peer group, change of school, and language issues can also adversely affect scholastic performance. Sometimes a child is put in a high profile school which may not be keeping in with the general sociocultural background of the child, and adds to the child's burden. This is likely to affect the child's scholastic performance. Similarly overuse of computers, mobile phones and internet, and excessive watching of television may also adversely affect the child's school performance (Nair et al. 2003; Shenoy and Kapur 1996).

Psychiatric illnesses: Any psychiatric illness like anxiety disorders, childhood depression, conduct disorders, attention deficit hyperactivity disorder (ADHD), Tourette disorder, or autism spectrum disorders occurring in childhood, can lead to scholastic backwardness.

Anxiety may prevent the child to respond to the questions asked by the teacher or prevent the child to ask questions to clarify his or her problems in the class. The affected child may also have constant concerns about the way others view him/her, and affect peer relations at school. All these can adversely affect child's academic performance at school.

A child suffering from depression may feel low and start losing interest and motivation in studies. Both anxiety and depression can also affect concentration in the studies.

Children affected by ADHD and conduct disorders also suffer scholastic backwardness, because of the innate nature of these illnesses. Some children may have conflictual feelings about success and may fear the success, and its consequences. Tourette disorder may lead to reduced socialisation, and can be incapacitating. Autism spectrum disorders can cause scholastic backwardness by affecting communication (Haneesh et al. 2013; Karande and Kulkarni 2005).

21.3 Psychosocial Factors Important for Academic Functioning

Certain psychosocial factors are essential for optimal scholastic functioning. Some of these have been referred to in the previous section. Psychosocial factors may be grouped into child and parent related factors, and are discussed as below.

21.3.1 Child Related Factors

- Motivation for studies. An optimal level of motivation is essential for satisfactory scholastic performance. If it is lacking, it is likely to cause scholastic backwardness.
- Ability to apply oneself to studies at school and complete school's assignments.
- Regular attendance at school.
- Average intelligence. An average IQ is required for an optimal performance, and above average intelligence is required for academic excellence.
- Absence of any sensory deficits.
- Absence of any chronic physical illnesses.
- Ability to cope with stressful life events.
- Perception of support from parents, teachers, and peers (Rashmi et al. 2015; Shenoy and Kapur 1996; Karande et al. 2013).

21.3.2 Parent-Related Factors

- Parental encouragement and supervision
- A stable marital relationship in the parents

- Positive attitude for education
- Provision of healthy environment and space to the child
- Child not to be over burdened with the domestic responsibilities (Haneesh et al. 2013; Rashmi et al. 2015; Nair et al. 2003; Shenoy and Kapur 1996)

Refractory errors, not having help for study at home, not doing home work regularly, not solving question bank papers, and studying only before the examinations have been identified to be associated with poor scholastic performance in adolescents (Florence et al. 2008). Psychological disturbances, families lacking basic amenities, alcohol dependence in father, inconsistent disciplining and poor parental interaction, frequent school changes, and fewer hobbies have been reported to contribute to the poor scholastic performance in 5–8 year old children (Shenoy and Kapur 1996). Vision impairment, hearing impairment, physical disability, subnormal IQ and specific learning disabilities have been identified as common causes of scholastic backwardness in primary school children in Karnataka (Mogasale et al. 2012) (Table 21.1).

Similar findings have also been reported from other Asian countries. In a study from Malaysia conducted on 1470 children, poor academic achievement was identified in 14 % of the children (Ong et al. 2010). Cognitive ability, male gender, prematurity and lower socioeconomic status were associated with poor academic achievement. Children's nutritional status, household socioeconomic background, and parental child feeding beliefs and practices have also been found to affect the children's academic achievement (Lee et al. 2014; Mohd Nasir 2012). Living with one parent, parental divorce, and parents showing no interest in their child's education and school system, low income, and smoking have also been identified as important contributors to poor scholastic performance in a study from the Middle East (Kamal and Bener 2009). The study also reported that frequent absence from school, incomplete homework, and hyperactivity, inattentiveness and disruptiveness in classroom were associated with poor scholastic performance. Most frequent psychological disorders contributing to school failure were examination phobia, anxiety, anger, fear and learning disability. The most prevalent health disorders included visual disturbances, asthma, anemia and hearing deficiency (Kamal and Bener 2009).

21.4 Epidemiology

Poor scholastic performance may be a manifestation of another underlying problem. The specific developmental disorders of scholastic skill (SDDSS), also known as specific learning disability (SLD) or disorder affect up to 10 % of the school children in the US (Altarac and Saroha 2007). Another study from the UK found specific arithmetic, arithmetic and reading, and specific reading difficulties in 1.3, 2.3, and 3.9 % of the children studied (Lewis et al. 1994). Reading disabilities have been reported more frequently in boys than in girls across various epidemiological studies (Rutter et al. 2004).

Table 21.1 Common causes of poor scholastic performance in India

Authors	Setting	Disorder studied	Methodology	Causes/factors associated with poor scholastic performance (in %)
Khurana (1980)	Psychiatric outpatient ($N = 100$)	Learning disabilities	Clinical evaluation, Kamat's test of intelligence and Bhatia's battery of performance tests of intelligence	Impaired relationship with parents-81 Impaired relationship in school-57 Battering-51
Shenoy and Kapur (1996)	School setting($N = 1535$)	Scholastic backwardness	Application of child behavior questionnaire, overall performance	Regular drinking in father-42 Inconsistent disciplining-55 Poor interaction in family-16 Frequent school changes-84
Nair et al. (2003)	School setting($N = 1892$)	Poor scholastic performance	Questionnaire survey method under supervision of pediatrician and psychologist	Not studying daily lessons: 51.8–82 Poor concentration in class: 35–61.7 Problems in the family: 5–20.3
Karande and Kulkarni (2005)	–	Poor scholastic performance	Review	Medical causes, below average intelligence, specific learning disability, ADHD, autism, Tourette syndrome, emotional problems, poor sociocultural home environment, conduct disorders, oppositional defiant disorders, early signs of emerging depression or psychosis and environmental causes

(continued)

Table 21.1 (continued)

Authors	Setting	Disorder studied	Methodology	Causes/factors associated with poor scholastic performance (in %)
Karande et al. (2007)	Consecutive clinic sample ($N = 50$)	Specific learning disorders and ADHD	Assessment by pediatrician, psychiatrist and psychologist	Significant perinatal history-30 Refractive errors-34 Hearing loss-16 Microcephaly-10 Soft neurological signs-54
Shashidhar et al. (2009)	School setting ($N = 1230$)	Poor scholastic performance	Questionnaire and marks of last annual exam	Refractory error-4.219[a] No help at home-3.623[a] Not doing homework regularly-5.235[a] Not solving question bank papers-3.39[a] Studying only before exam-3.8[a]
Mogasale et al. (2012)	Primary school children ($N = 1101$)	Scholastic backwardness	Multi-staged stratified randomized cluster sampling	Vision impairment-1.8 Hearing impairment-0.5 Physical disability-1 Subnormal IQ-2 Specific learning disability: 15.17

(continued)

Table 21.1 (continued)

Authors	Setting	Disorder studied	Methodology	Causes/factors associated with poor scholastic performance (in %)
Haneesh et al. (2013)	Clinic sample ($N = 110$)	Scholastic backwardness	Clinical assessment aided with parents' and teaches' information Binet Kamat test for IQ	Mental retardation-27 Borderline intelligence-36 Microcephaly-11 Under nutrition-33 Stunted growth-28 Chronic medical problems-26 Visual defect 6 Hearing 5 Speech defects 11
Karande et al. (2013)	Clinic based study ($N = 246$)	Poor school performance	Clinical and psychoeducational assessments (retrospective)	Specific learning disabilities-73 Borderline intellectual functioning-8.94 Language barrier-8.54 Mental retardation-4.88 ADHD-40.6 Chronic medical condition-13.25
Rashmi et al. (2015)	Rural school ($N = 582$)	Scholastic performance	Test scores of the previous two classes	Malnutrition

[a]Odds ratio

There have been a number of studies from India on the magnitude of poor scholastic performance and learning disorders. One of the earliest studies conducted in 1980s reported prevalence of learning disability as 20.61 % among school children studying in fourth and fifth standard (Venugopal and Raju 1988). In another study on primary school children from a rural area, 12.97 % of the children with IQ of 90 or more were found to have poor achievement in arithmetic and on teacher's assessment. Children identified to have poor achievement had impaired perceptual maturity and conceptual grasp, and deficits in information processing (Agarwal et al. 1991). A large study from Bangalore on school children in the age group of 5–8 years reported prevalence of learning problems as 17.1 % and of scholastic backwardness as 10.23 %. Prevalence of the both was marginally higher in boys as compared to the girls. Rates of specific difficulties such as reading, writing, and arithmetic were 4.69, 5.15, and 15.96 %, respectively (Shenoy and Kapur 1996; Shenoy et al. 1998). A review of Indian studies conducted over two decades on prevalence of learning disability has reported a prevalence of 3–10 % of various specific learning disabilities (including scholastic abilities) among student population in the states of Karnataka, Kerala, and Tamil Nadu (Ramaa 2000).

A recent study conducted on scholastic backwardness on 1101 children found a prevalence of 24 % (Mogasale et al. 2012). The prevalence of specific learning disabilities was 15.17 %. Dysgraphia, dyslexia, and dyscalculia were specifically observed in 12.5, 11.2, and 10.5 % of the children, respectively. The study had used a six-level screening approach to identify scholastic backwardness. A stepwise exclusion of the subjects was done by excluding the common causes of scholastic backwardness like impaired vision and hearing, chronic medical conditions and subnormal intelligence among these children, and the remaining children were subjected to specific tests for reading, comprehension, writing, and mathematical calculation.

The results have however been highly variable, depending on the place of the study and the methodology used. A recent study from the city of Chandigarh in North India has reported a very low (1.58 %) prevalence of specific developmental disorder of scholastic skills in students of classes VII to XII. The study included a screening by teachers followed by detailed evaluation of the positives by NIMHANS Index for specific learning disability (Arun et al. 2013). A low prevalence of 0.5 % has also been reported in another study (Bansal and Berman 2011). One incidence study from India has reported incidence of specific developmental disorder of scholastic skills among school children at 1.8/1000/year (Malhotra et al. 2009).

The wide variations in the prevalence rates could be due to differences in the demographic profile of the general population, general standards of the school, population studied and methodology.

Table 21.2 summarizes some of the studies on prevalence of poor scholastic performance and learning problems.

Table 21.2 Epidemiology of poor scholastic performance

Authors	Setting	Disorder studied	Methodology	Prevalence (in %)
Venugopal and Raju (1988)	School children ($N = 137$)	Learning disability	Application of screening questionnaire	20.61
Agarwal et al. (1991)	Rural primary school children ($N = 1336$)	Learning disability	Teacher's assessment and arithmetic test	12.97
Shenoy and Kapur (1996)	School children ($N = 1535$)	Scholastic backwardness	Teacher and parent rating checklist	10.23 (10.99 in boys and 9.38 in girls 9.38)
Shenoy et al. (1998)	School children ($N = 1535$)	Learning problem	Teacher and parent rating checklist	17.1 (17.9 in boys and 16.3 in girls)
Ramaa (2000)	Student population in the States of Karnataka, Kerala and Tamil Nadu	Specific learning disabilities (including scholastic abilities)	Review	3–10
Bansal and Berman (2011)	School children ($N = 982$)	Learning disorder	Applied childhood psychopathology measurement schedule cross sectionally	0.5
Mogasale et al. (2012)	Urban primary school children ($N = 1101$)	Scholastic backwardness	Six level screening approach followed by specific tests for reading, comprehension, writing and mathematical calculation	24
Arun et al. (2013)	Urban school children ($N = 2402$)	Specific developmental disorder of scholastic skills	Teacher's screening instrument followed by detailed evaluation by NIMHANS Index	1.58
Malhotra et al. (2009)	School children ($N = 963$)	Specific developmental disorder of scholastic skills	Screening by teachers and parents followed by recontacted after 6 years	1.8/1000/year[a]

[a]Incidence

21.5 Psychological Comorbidities

In the current examination conscious age, children are often categorized on the basis of their academic performance. Failure in examinations is viewed as a catastrophe. This results in stress and psychiatric problems in the child. At times, due to difficulty in coping with the examination stress and poor academic performance, many children develop psychological problems. Around one fourth of the children with scholastic backwardness have been reported to have psychological disturbances (Shenoy and Kapur 1996). About 20 % of adolescents with learning disabilities recollect being teased by classmates about their disability and being insulted by the teachers (Karande et al. 2009). A positive correlation between psychological disturbance and poor school achievement has also been reported from a Chinese study (Ekblad 1990).

Children with dyslexia are exposed to a higher risk of anxiodepressive and behavioural disorders. The affected children experience three times more behavioural disorders, and one-third of children with behavioural problems turn out to be affected by dyslexia. Though the literature reveals inconsistent findings about depression among children with dyslexia, evidence of a persistent increase in the rate of anxiety disorders has been observed. The environmental factors have an impact in precipitating these psychiatric comorbidities (Huc-Chabrolle et al. 2010). Youth with learning disabilities (LD) have been suggested to be at an increased risk for suicidal behavior (Bender et al. 1999). Students with LD express more loneliness, more victimization, and less social satisfaction (i.e., school integration) than their non-LD matched peers (Martínez and Semrud-Clikeman 2004).

Data from the National Longitudinal Study of Adolescent Health, which has followed up a nationally representative sample of adolescents in grades 7–12 in US, has found diminished scholastic achievement to be associated with attention problems, delinquency, and substance use, but not with depression (McLeod et al. 2012). Another study on the subject found neuropsychiatric comorbidity in 62.2 % of the children with learning disorders (Margari et al. 2013). The comorbid disorders in specific learning disorders subgroup included ADHD (33 %), anxiety disorders (28.8 %), developmental coordination disorder (17.8 %), language disorder (11 %) and mood disorders (9.4 %) (Margari et al. 2013).

Delayed school progression is associated with general mental health problems in adolescence, though this relationship is confounded by other factors (Tempelaar et al. 2014). Poor school performance has also been reported to be associated with increased rates of schizophrenia, schizoaffective disorder and other psychoses (MacCabe et al. 2008), though it may be difficult to differentiate the poor scholastic performance from the prodromal phase.

21.6 Assessment

Poor scholastic performance may be due to varied causes of medical and psychological nature. A detailed medical and developmental history should be taken and thorough physical and neurological examination should be conducted to identify the medical causes, if any, for the poor school performance. The possibility of having a chronic physical or psychiatric illness which might lead to prolonged school absenteeism and subsequent scholastic backwardness should be considered. Information should be obtained from multiple sources like the parents, class teacher, and school counselor to substantiate the diagnosis. Detailed information about psychosocial and environmental stressors should be taken. These may include alcohol use in parents, relationship with parents, marital disharmony in parents, adverse comparison with siblings, fear of teacher and examination, and battering by parents and teacher (Haneesh et al. 2013; Khurana 1980). For this the child should be interviewed in a nonjudgmental manner.

The inability to read and comprehend is a major obstacle to learning that may have long-term educational, social, and economic implications. Teaching children with reading difficulties is a big challenge for the teachers as well as the parents. It is also a great source of stress for the affected child. Because dyslexia can be both familial and heritable, the affected younger siblings can be identified earlier. A child should be observed for early indications of dyslexia if he or she has a family history of learning disabilities. An early history of language difficulties such as delay or difficulty in developing speech and language, learning rhymes, or recognizing letters and sound/symbol connections, may be an early indication of dyslexia (Handler et al. 2011).

If a child has any of the risk factors as discussed in the earlier sections, the child should be monitored for the learning difficulties. Identification at the initial stage can help in instituting early intervention and can so improve the prognosis.

To rule out medical causes of poor scholastic performance, hearing and visual acuity should also be tested, and must be attended to, if any problem was identified. As intellectual disability is a well-known cause of poor scholastic performances, IQ assessment by a clinical psychologist should also be done. A detailed psychiatric assessment should be done to screen for any psychiatric disorder.

In India, school teachers have a limited awareness and knowledge about LD (Kamala and Ramganesh 2013). It is recommended that all school teachers should be sensitized to suspect, and trained to screen for LD, when the child is in primary school. School managements should become proactive to setup resource rooms and employ special educators to ensure that these children receive regular and affordable remedial education. Teachers, parents, and the school management need to ensure that these children get the mandatory provisions both during school and board examinations (Karande et al. 2011).

21.7 Management

21.7.1 Management of the Identified Medical or Psychiatric Comorbidity, if Any

Treatment should be started as soon as the problem is identified. If any medical problem is identified, it should be treated promptly. If any visual or hearing impairment is detected, it should be corrected. Psychiatric comorbities, if diagnosed, should be managed using the standard psychotherapeutic or pharmacological approaches. Any sociocultural, familial, or environmental factors interfering with the scholastic performance identified during the assessment should be addressed. If need be, the class teacher of the student may also be contacted.

If a specific learning disorder is identified, remedial education is indicated (Coste-Zeitoun et al. 2005). One should not wait for implementing remedial measures, until the children are formally diagnosed with dyslexia or experience repeated failures (Vaughn et al. 2010). The treatment is tailored to the individual child's cognitive function profile and severity of manifestations (Louis and Emerson 2014). Using specific teaching strategies and materials, the special educator formulates an individualized education program to reduce or modify the child's deficiencies in specific learning areas such as reading, writing, and mathematics, as identified during the child's educational assessment. During the remedial education sessions, the child undergoes systematic and highly structured training exercises to learn that words can be segmented into smaller units of sound (phoneme awareness), and that these sounds are linked with specific letters and letter patterns (phonics). The child also requires practice in reading stories, both to apply newly acquired decoding skills to reading words in context and to experience reading for meaning. The management of specific learning disorders is the more time demanding setting of secondary school is based more on providing provisions rather than remediation. The provisions include exemption from spelling mistakes, availing extra time for written tests, dropping a second language and substituting it with work experience, dropping algebra and geometry and substituting them with lower grade of mathematics and work experience; and are meant to help the child cope up in a regular mainstream school. With appropriate remedial education and provisions, most children can be expected to achieve academic competence (Karande and Kulkarni 2005).

21.7.2 Special Education

If the child is having intellectual disability or severe form of neurobehavioral deficits, he/she may need an open school or a special school. Recently, the Government of India has come out with the concept of 'inclusive education', in which such children (especially the less severe cases) can be educated in a regular mainstream school (Karande and Kulkarni 2005). Parents of children with "language barrier" should be advised to educate their children in their own language medium schools or to attend a facility for language stimulation (Silverstein et al. 2002).

Individualized education programme (IEP) has been shown to be effective for slow learners in school. The programme can be imparted on a daily basis or twice in week for 2–4 months. The training programme has been found to improve academic functioning as per the final test results and the parents' reporting. It also improves the self-esteem of the children which is the first step towards successful remedial education. IEP can be integrated with the normal school curriculum (Krishnakumar et al. 2006, 2011).

Response to intervention (RTI) approach is another management method for LD. It includes eight central features and six common attributes. The central features include high-quality classroom instruction, research-based instruction, classroom performance measures, universal screening, continuous progress monitoring, research-based intervention, progress monitoring during intervention, and fidelity measures. The common attributes include use of concepts of multiple tiers, transition from instruction for all to increasingly intense interventions, implementation of differentiated curricula, instruction delivered by staff other than the classroom teacher, varied duration, time, and frequency of intervention, and categorical or non-categorical placement decisions (Grigorenko 2007).

Children at risk for reading difficulties can be identified in kindergarten (five years of age), and intervention programs started as a part of preventive measures. Classroom-based intervention programs that emphasize phonological awareness, vocabulary and reading strategies, if introduced early, have been found to benefit such children (Lesaux and Siegel 2003).

Schools also need to implement systemic models of prevention including primary, secondary, and tertiary prevention. Primary prevention would include provision of high-quality education for all children. Secondary prevention includes targeted, scientifically-based interventions for children who are not responding to primary prevention. As part of the tertiary prevention, provision of intensive individualized services needs to be created and interventions introduced for those children who do not respond to high-quality instruction or subsequent intervention efforts (Grigorenko 2007).

Parent involvement and advocacy, with assistance from pediatricians and knowledgeable school personnel, is necessary to ensure that appropriate resources available from various sectors are well coordinated and provided for children with learning disorder to improve their school performance and ongoing educational experience (Lambros and Leslie 2005).

21.8 Initiatives at the State Level

Long back, the Government of India had also constituted a committee under a famous educationist, Professor Yash Pal. The committee in its report "learning without burden" (1993) strongly raised the issue of noncomprehension in the class room. A significant fraction of children who drop out may be those who refuse to compromise with noncomprehension. These children may be potentially superior to those who just memorise and do well in examination, without comprehending very much. The National Curriculum Framework-2005 has pointed out "A majority of children have a sense of fear and failure in mathematics. Hence, they give up early on, and drop out of serious mathematical learning". Keeping in view of these problems, a nationwide subprogram to the Sarva Shiksha Abhiyan (SSA), '*Padhe Bharat, Badhe Bharat*' is planned to improve language development by creating an enduring interest in reading and writing with comprehension, and to create a natural and positive interest in mathematics related to the physical and social world (http://ssa.nic.in/pabminutes-documents/Padhe%20Bharat%20Badhe%20Bharat.pdf).

In the recent past, the Government of India has introduced some special provisions in examination system for children with LD. Such provisions have been shown to improve the academic performance at the board examinations (Kulkarni et al. 2006). Since 1999, the National Educational Boards, which conduct the Indian Certificate of Secondary Education (ICSE) and the Central Board of Secondary Education (CBSE) examinations, have also formally granted children with LD the benefit of availing the necessary provisions. Since 2010, the Government of India has also implemented the Right of Children to Free and Compulsory Education 2009 (RTE Act) which makes education free and compulsory to all children, including those with disabilities (Karande et al. 2011).

Sarva Shiksha Abhiyan (SSA) of the Government of India provides for a grant up to Rs. 1200/- per child per year for inclusion of disabled children. The interventions under SSA for inclusive education are identification, functional, and formal assessment, appropriate educational placement, preparation of individualized educational plan, provision of aids and appliances, teacher training, resource support, removal of architectural barriers, research, monitoring and evaluation, and a special focus on girls with special needs. SSA ensures that every child with special needs, irrespective of the kind, category, and degree of disability, is provided meaningful and quality education (http://ssa.nic.in/inclusive-education/overview-on-inclusiveeducation/Overview%20synopsis.pdf/view). As a part of the inclusive education, training modules have been developed for resource teachers for disabled children. With the help of training modules, teachers are sensitized to identify and pick up the children with early signs or symptoms of disability causing poor scholastic performance (http://ssa.nic.in/inclusive-education/training-module-for-resource-teachers-for-disable-children).

21.9 Conclusion

Poor scholastic performance in children and adolescents can be due to a number of causes including psychosocial, developmental and physical abnormalities. The children need to be assessed in details to find out the exact cause. Some of the causes like refractory errors or nutritional deficiencies can be easily corrected.

There is a need to sensitise the teachers to identify the common causes in the children with poor scholastic performance. The State needs to take adequate steps to introduce counselling facilities in all the schools so that the child can be offered psychosocial help in the school itself. Parents should be informed by the school at the earliest if the child is not performing satisfactorily, and advised to take remedial measures. A multilevel approach at the level of schools, counsellors, pediatricians, mental health professionals, parents, and the State is required.

References

Agarwal, K. N., Agarwal, D. K., Upadhyay, S. K., & Singh, M. (1991). Learning disability in rural primary school children. *Indian Journal of Medical Research, 94*, 89–95.

Altarac, M., & Saroha, E. (2007). Lifetime prevalence of learning disability among US children. *Pediatrics, 119*(Suppl 1), S77–S83.

Arun, P., Chavan, B. S., Bhargava, R., Sharma, A., & Kaur, J. (2013). Prevalence of specific developmental disorder of scholastic skill in school students in Chandigarh,India. *The Indian Journal of Medical Research, 138*, 89–98.

Bansal, P. D., & Berman, R. (2011). Psychopathology of school going children in the age group of 10–15 years. *International Journal of Applied and Basic Medical Research, 1*, 43–47.

Bender, W. N., Rosenkrans, C. B., & Crane, M. (1999). Stress, depression, and suicide among students with learning disabilities: Assessing the risk. *Learning Disability Quarterly Journal, 22*, 143–156.

Coste-Zeitoun, D., Pinton, F., Barondiot, C., Ducot, B., Warszawski, J., & Billard, C. (2005). Specific remedial therapy in a specialist unit: Evaluation of 31 children with severe, specific language or reading disorders over one academic year. *Revue Neurologique, 161*, 299–310.

Ekblad, S. (1990). The children's behavior questionnaire for completion by parents and teachers in a Chinese sample. *Journal of Child Psychology and Psychiatry, 31*, 775–791.

Florence, M. D., Asbridge, M., & Veugelers, P. J. (2008). Diet quality and academic performance. *Journal of School Health, 78*, 209–215.

Grigorenko, E. L. (2007). Learning disabilities. In A. Martin & F. R. Volkmar (Eds.), Lewis's Child and Adolescent Psychiatry: A Comprehensive Textbook (4th ed., pp. 410–148). Lippincott Williams & Wilkins.

http://ssa.nic.in/pabminutes-documents/Padhe%20Bharat%20Badhe%20Bharat.pdf. Accessed July 08, 2015

http://ssa.nic.in/quality-docs/RTE%20SSA%20Final%20Report.pdf. Accessed July 10, 2015.

http://ssa.nic.in/pabminutes-documents/NS.pdf. Accessed July 10, 2015

http://ssa.nic.in/inclusive-education/training-module-for-resource-teachers-for-disable-children. Accessed July 10, 2015

http://ssa.nic.in/inclusive-education/overview-on-inclusiveeducation/Overview%20synopsis.pdf/view. Accessed July 12, 2015

Handler, S. M., Fierson, W. M., et al. (2011). Learning disabilities, dyslexia, and vision. *Pediatrics, 127*, e818–e856.

Haneesh, K., Krishnakumar, P., Sukumaran, S. K., & Riyaz, A. (2013). Risk factors for scholastic backwardness in children. *Indian Pediatrics, 50*, 655–658.

Huc-Chabrolle, M., Barthez, M. A., Tripi, G., Barthélémy, C., & Bonnet-Brilhault, F. (2010). Psychocognitive and psychiatric disorders associated with developmental dyslexia. *L'Encéphale, 36*, 172–179.

Kamal, M., & Bener, A. (2009). Factors contributing to school failure among school children in very fast developing Arabian Society. *Oman Medical Journal, 24*, 212–217.

Kamala, R., & Ramganesh, E. (2013). Knowledge of specific learning disabilities among teacher educators in Puducherry, Union Territory in India. *International Journal of Humanities and Social Science, 6*, 168–175.

Karande, S., Doshi, B., Thadhani, A., & Sholapurwala, R. (2013). Profile of children with poor school performance in Mumbai. *Indian Pediatrics, 50*, 427.

Karande, S., & Kulkarni, M. (2005). Poor school performance. *Indian Journal of Pediatrics, 72*, 961–967.

Karande, S., Mahajan, V., & Kulkarni, M. (2009). Recollections of learning-disabled adolescents of their schooling experiences: A qualitative study. *Indian Journal of Medical Sciences, 63*, 382–391.

Karande, S., Satam, N., Kulkarni, M., Sholapurwala, R., Chitre, A., & Shah, N. (2007). Clinical and psychoeducational profile of children with specific learning disability and co-occurring attention-deficit hyperactivity disorder. *Indian Journal of Medical Sciences, 61*, 639–647.

Karande, S., Sholapurwala, R., & Kulkarni, M. (2011). Managing specific learning disability in schools in India. *Indian Pediatrics, 48*, 515–520.

Khurana, S. (1980). Non intellectual factors in learning disability. *Indian Journal of Psychiatry, 22*, 256–260.

Krishnakumar, P., Geeta, M. G., & Palat, R. (2006). Effectiveness of individualized education program for slow learners. *Indian Journal of Pediatrics, 73*, 135–137.

Krishnakumar, P., Jisha, A. M., Sukumaran, S. K., & Nair, M. K. (2011). Developing a model for resource room training for slow learners in normal schools. *Indian Journal of Psychiatry, 53*, 336–339.

Kulkarni, M., Karande, S., Thadhani, A., Maru, H., & Sholapurwala, R. (2006). Educational provisions and learning disability. *Indian Journal of Pediatrics, 73*, 789–793.

Lambros, K. M., & Leslie, L. K. (2005). Management of the child with a learning disorder. *Pediatric Annals, 34*, 275–287.

Lee, Y. Y., & Wan Abdul Manan, W. M. (2014). Nutritional status, academic performance and parental feeding practices of primary school children in a rural district in Kelantan, Malaysia. Progress in Health Science, *4*, 144–152.

Lesaux, N. K., & Siegel, L. S. (2003). The development of reading in children who speak English as a second language. *Developmental Psychology, 39*, 1005–1019.

Lewis, C., Hitch, G. J., & Walker, P. (1994). The prevalence of specific arithmetic difficulties and specific reading difficulties in 9- to 10-year-old boys and girls. *Journal of Child Psychology and Psychiatry, 35*, 283–292.

Louis, P. T., & Emerson, I. A. (2014). Evaluating the cognition, behavior, and social profile of an adolescent with learning disabilities and assessing the effectiveness of an individualized educational program. *Iranian Journal of Psychiatry and Behavioral Sciences, 8*, 22–37.

MacCabe, J. H., Lambe, M. P., Cnattingius, S., Torrång, A., Björk, C., Sham, P. C., et al. (2008). Scholastic achievement at age 16 and risk of schizophrenia and other psychoses: a national cohort study. *Psychological Medicine, 38*, 1133–1140.

Malhotra, S., Kohli, A., Kapoor, M., & Pradhan, B. (2009). Incidence of childhood psychiatric disorders in India. *Indian Journal of Psychiatry, 51*, 101–107.

Margari, L., Buttiglione, M., Craig, F., Cristella, A., de Giambattista, C., Matera, E., et al. (2013). Neuropsychopathological comorbidities in learning disorders. *BMC Neurology, 13*, 198.

Martínez, R. S., & Semrud-Clikeman, M. (2004). Emotional adjustment and school functioning of young adolescents with multiple versus single learning disabilities. *Journal of Learning Disabilities, 37*, 411–420.

McLeod, J. D., Uemura, R., & Rohrman, S. (2012). Adolescent mental health, behavior problems, and academic achievement. *Journal of Health and Social Behavior, 53*, 482–497.

Mogasale, V. V., Patil, V. D., Patil, N. M., & Mogasale, V. (2012). Prevalence of specific learning disabilities among primary school children in a South Indian city. *Indian Journal of Pediatrics, 7*, 342–347.

Mohd Nasir, M. T., Norimah, A. K., Hazizi, A. S., Nurliyana, A. R., Loh, S. H., & Suraya, I. (2012). Child feeding practices, food habits, anthropometric indicators and cognitive performance among preschoolers in Peninsular Malaysia. Appetite, *58*, 525–530.

Nair, M. K. C., Paul, M. K., & Padmamohan, J. (2003). Scholastic performance of adolescents. *Indian Journal of Pediatrics, 70*, 629–631.

Ong, L. C., Chandran, V., Lim, Y. Y., Chen, A. H., & Poh, B. K. (2010). Factors associated with poor academic achievement among urban primary school children in Malaysia. *Singapore Medical Journal, 51*, 247–252.

Ramaa, S. (2000). Two decades of research on learning disabilities in India. *Dyslexia, 6*, 268–283.

Rashmi, M. R., Shweta, B. M., Fathima, F. N., Agrawal, T., Shah, M., & Sequeira, R. (2015). Prevalence of malnutrition and relationship with scholastic performance among primary and secondary school children in two select private schools in Bangalore rural district (India). *Indian Journal of Community Medicine, 40*, 97–102.

Rutter, M., Caspi, A., Fergusson, D., Horwood, L. J., Goodman, R., Maughan, B., et al. (2004). Sex differences in developmental reading disability: new findings from 4 epidemiological studies. *The Journal of the American Medical Association, 291*, 2007–2012.

Shashidhar, S., Rao, C., & Hegde, R. (2009). Factors affecting scholastic performances of adolescents. *Indian Journal of Pediatrics, 76*, 495–499.

Shenoy, J., & Kapur, M. (1996). Prevalence of scholastic backwardness among five to eight year old children. *Indian Journal of Psychiatry, 38*, 201–207.

Shenoy, J., Kapur, M., & Kaliaperumal, V. G. (1998). Psychological disturbance among 5- to 8-year-old school children: a study from India. *Social Psychiatry and Psychiatric Epidemiology, 33*, 66–73.

Silverstein, M., Iverson, L., & Lozano, P. (2002). An English-language clinic-based literacy program is effective for a multilingual population. *Pediatrics, 109*, E76.

Tempelaar, W. M., Otjes, C. P., Bun, C. J., Plevier, C. M., van Gastel, W. A., MacCabe, J. H., et al. (2014). Delayed school progression and mental health problems in adolescence: a population-based study in 10,803 adolescents. *BMC Psychiatry, 14*, 244.

Thacker, N. (2007). Poor scholastic performance in children and adolescents. *Indian Pediatrics, 44*, 411–412.

Vaughn, S., Cirino, P. T., Wanzek, J., Wexler, J., Fletcher, J. M., Denton, C. A., et al. (2010). Response to intervention for middle school students with reading difficulties: effects of a primary and secondary intervention. *School Psychology Review, 39*, 3–21.

Venugopal, M., & Raju, P. (1988). A study on the learning disabilities among IV and V standard students. *The Indian Journal of Psychological Medicine, 11*, 119–123.

Chapter 22
Low Cost Solutions for Learning Disabilities

Malavika Kapur

Abstract Learning difficulties are encountered in the school settings across the globe. Economic recession in the Western world and absence of quality education for the majority of children in the developing world forces us to re-examine our educational practices across cultures. Yet the nature of these problems, their causes and ways to intervene are entirely different in the developed and the developing nations. Much of the literature on the management of learning difficulties is anchored to western research. These are mostly inapplicable in the Asian/African context. Since the 1980s the author and her team in Bangalore have developed tools of assessment and strategies of intervention packages for specific learning disabilities based on western as well as indigenous strategies that are modified to suit the Indian context in terms of language, schooling and culture. But these are meant for children from schools with adequate infrastructure. The Asian reality at the grass roots level reveals that the majority of the schools suffer from paucity of teachers and infrastructure. Most intervention strategies developed in the West target specific deficits with specific intervention strategies based on certain theoretical constructs. The author examines some of the intervention strategies developed in India and highlights the results. The author also proposes to demonstrate effective models of empowering children to learn through play and providing effective low cost intervention for learning difficulties caused by poor school practices. These models are based on holistic and eclectic approaches with outcome evaluation of the intervention with a pre- and post-design. This is especially a model that can be replicated across the world especially in the developing counties and in countries hit by recession in the recent times.

M. Kapur (✉)
National Institute of Advanced Studies, Indian Institute of Science Campus,
Bengaluru 560012, India
e-mail: malavikakapu@yahoo.co.in

S. Malhotra and P. Santosh (eds.), *Child and Adolescent Psychiatry*,
DOI 10.1007/978-81-322-3619-1_22

Keywords Learning disability (LD) · LD in school population · Specific learning disability (SLD) · Context of adequate schooling · Context of school system failure · Efficacy of play way methods

Abbreviations

LD	Learning disability
SLD	Specific learning disability
MBD	Minimal brain dysfunction
NIMHANS SLD BATTERY	NIMHANS index learning disability
NIMHANS	National Institute of Mental Health and Neuro Sciences
CPM	Coloured progressive matrices test
SFB	Seguin form board
PASS	Planning, attention, arousal, simultaneous and successive
COGENT	Cognitive enhancement training
Malin's WISC	Wechsler's intelligence scale for children

22.1 Definitions

The term Learning Disabilities emerged from a need to identify and serve students who continually fail in school yet are not intellectually disabled. The concept of learning disabilities has undergone distinct phases of development in its history. The study of learning disabilities began in the early 1940s. The term they used for these children was "brain-injured" children. They established several criteria to classify these children. They were: perceptual disorders, perseveration, conceptual or thinking disorders, behavioural disorders, soft neurological signs, a history of neurological impairment with no history of mental retardation.

In 1960s a shift in terminology occurred with the introduction of the term "Minimal Brain Dysfunction (MBD)". The term brought in the concept of minor brain injury and linked to with learning problems. The National Advisory Committee on handicapped children USA in 1968 submitted the first definition. Since then a number of definitions have been proposed but none of them are totally acceptable. The latest definition proposed by DSM 5 (2013) is as follows: Specific learning disorders are diagnosed when the individual's achievement on individually administered, standardized tests in reading, mathematics or written expression is substantially below that expected for age, schooling and level of intelligence. The learning problems significantly interfere with academic achievement or activities of daily living.

Torgensen (1991) opined that the standard definition of LD has four major problems.

i. The definitions do not indicate that LDs are a heterogeneous group.
ii. The definition fails to recognize that the condition persists into adulthood.
iii. It does not specify that there is inherent problem in the way information is processed regardless of the cause.
iv. The definition does not recognize that individuals with other disabilities or environmental limitations may concurrently have learning disability.

22.2 Characteristics of Learning Disabilities

1. Discrepancy factor—A discrepancy exists between a child's ability and academic performance across one or all skill areas.
2. Academic learning difficulty—Academic problems exist in the area of reading, writing, spelling and mathematics.
3. Perceptual disorder—Perceptual problems include inability to recognize, discriminate and interpret sensation. It can be in the area of auditory channel or/ and visual channel.
4. Metacognitive deficits—Metacognitive abilities involve the ability to use self-regulatory mechanisms such as planning moves, evaluating effectiveness of ongoing activities, checking the outcome and remediation of the errors.
5. Memory problems—Most students complain of poor memory. Students with learning disabilities fail to use strategies that nondisabled students readily use.
6. Phonological deficits—students with reading, spelling difficulties often have poor phonological skills.
7. Motor disorders—Children with this problem are clumsy, unable to skip or hop. Some exhibit fine motor difficulties such as in cutting with scissors.
8. Attention problems and hyperactivity—Many researchers have documented that many learning-disabled children have short attention span, distractibility and impulsivity. Some are restless and hyperactive.
9. Social emotional problems—The prevalence rate of psychological disturbance is high among learning-disabled children compared to the normal population. Continuous failures in academics results in poor self-concept and self-esteem.
   This section reveals that the features are varied in nature. Obviously there would be multiple causes leading to the varied symptoms of SLD.

22.3 Attributed Causes of Learning Disabilities

There is no single cause to explain the origin of learning disabilities. Nor are any of them proven empirically. A variety of factors have been linked with its occurrence. However. coexistence does not mean it is the cause

1. Genetic—It is found that learning disabilities run in families.
2. Language—Poor phonological processing is seen in children with reading and spelling disabilities.
3. Biochemical—Possible chemical imbalance that lead to inefficient or faulty brain functioning.
4. Biological—Head trauma that causes brain Injuries, foetal distress during birth and so on.
5. Unfavourable uterine environment—Drugs, smoking, alcohol that adversely affect development of the foetal brain in the uterus.
6. Environmental deprivation—A lack of stimulation at critical times of development that prevents optimal brain function.

These are some of the common correlates. There are also other factors, such as the problem of laterality, size of the left hemisphere and the size of the neurons in the left hemisphere.

22.4 Biological Approaches to Learning Disabilities

1. The inferred pathologies in the following systems (Hallahan et al. 1985) are described. These are: Perceptual Systems, perceptual motor functioning, neurological Organization and oculo motor functioning.

Causes are attributed to: genetic, head injury, chemical deficits, allergens and toxic substances.

Yet there is no firm evidence for any of these are really the causes and are merely speculations and applicable only in small number of cases.

2. **Neuropsychological Approaches**

   Initially began with the speculation of brain damaged, when not found, led to use of another term, 'minimal brain damage'. When there was no evidence of brain damage, minimal brain dysfunction was hypothesized. These are of two types: acquired and developmental.

Taylor (1988) described the processes as: somato sensory/motor skills, language and auditory processing, visuo-spatial/constructional skills, memory and learning skills, attention and psychomotor efficiency and abstract reasoning and problem-solving skills.

3. **Psycholinguistic Approaches**

   Mann and Liberman (1984) proposed LD as deficiency in a variety of language functions namely, in reading, writing and spelling.
4. **Psycho-Educational Approaches** (Kaufmann 1985) consist of: Insensitivity to student as an individual, too high or too low expectations, uncertain classroom

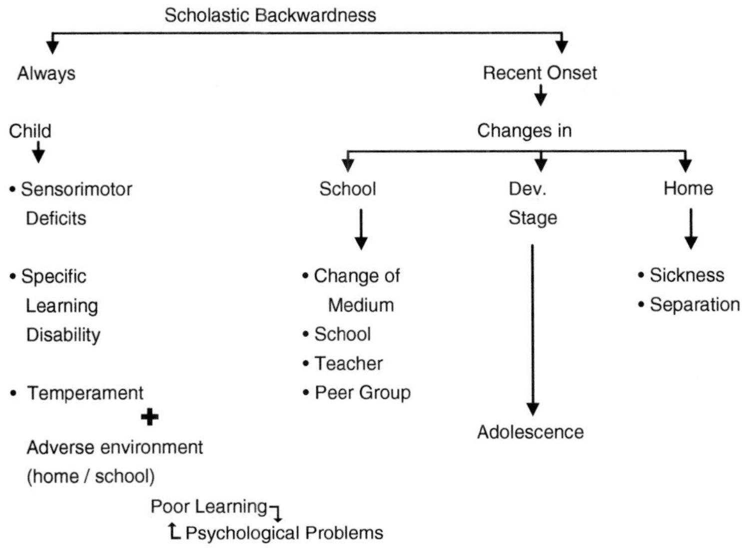

Fig. 22.1 Scholastic backwardness

situation, uninteresting instructional tasks, reinforcement of undesirable behaviour, undesirable models and teacher centred rather than child-centred methods.

It may be seen from the above that the causes of SLD are multifactorial, while the theories focus on specific areas or systems. These are like the proverbial blunders of the story of the blind men and the elephant.

Nature of SLD

The children with learning difficulties present with scholastic backwardness. These children need to be examined as given below, relying on the history of the disorder, the nature of onset and detailed assessment of the child, the family and the school (Figs. 22.1 and 22.2).

The above flow chart highlights that a detailed psychological assessment is essential in case of learning difficulties. These include;

i. The psychosocial contexts in which the problems occur such as poor home environment or ineffectual school system.
ii. The assessment of individual profile of assets and liabilities in learning in the child as this forms the basis on which the remedial work is initiated.
iii. Most of the remedial measures overlook the above two factors as the theoretical anchors of the practitioner does not permit recognition to the multifactorial nature of the problem and the heterogeneity of the group of the learning disabled.

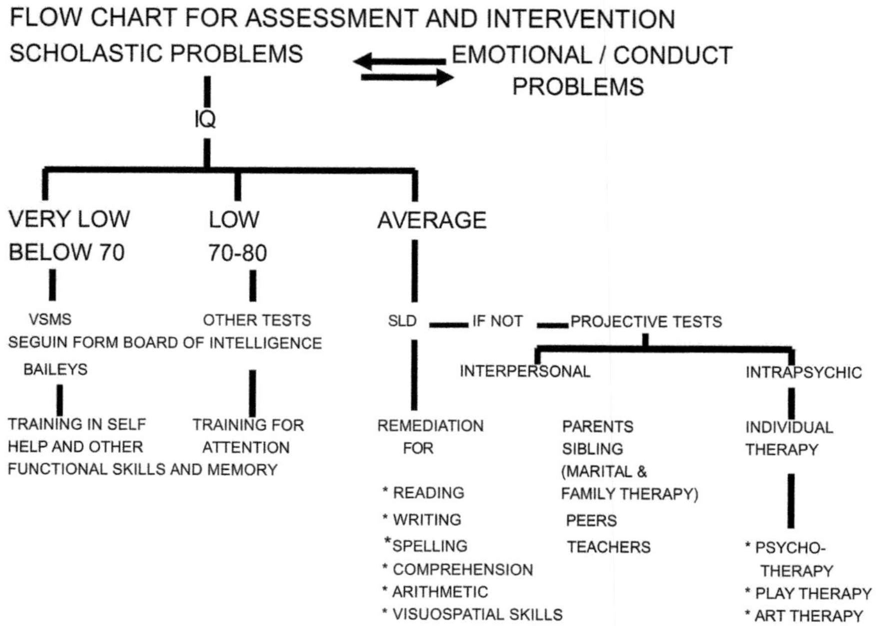

Fig. 22.2 Flow chart for assessment and intervention

22.5 Interventions for Learning Disabilities

1. **Interventions or Remediation for SLD in the West**

The initial training methods focused on multi-sensory stimulation, and subsequently, training focused on phonological awareness as some argue that phonological awareness is the core deficit seen in reading disorders. Some other researchers argue there are deficits in receiving and perceiving auditory inputs. Working memory and semantic memory deficits were implicated in math disorders.

Initial training methods focused on multi-sensory stimulation (Lindamomd-Bell method; Orton—Gillingham method). Subsequent training focused on phonological awareness. Researchers argue that phonological awareness is the core deficit seen in reading disorder (Shaywitz and Shaywitz 2005). Other researchers argue there are deficits in receiving and perceiving auditory input is impaired (Tallal 1998). Working memory and semantic memory deficits noted in math disorders (Greary 2000). Several studies have claimed functional changes within the network supporting phonological processing after training (Shaywitz and Shaywitz 2005). Training in processing and sequencing rapid auditory inputs associated with improved reading (Tallal 1998; Troier and Whitney 2003). And was found to improve cognitive functions across several age groups. Findings indicate improved cognitive functions in addition to improved reading and spelling (Das et al. 2006; Hayward et al. 2007).

2. **Studies of SLD in the Indian Context**

Prevalence, nature and assessment
While western studies report a prevalence of 10 %, prevalence in India is reported to be 5–12 % of school population with the prevalence being higher in rural areas (Srinath et al. 2005). Prevalence in India—being 5–12 % of school-going population is reported by others too (Thapa 2008; Bhola and Kapur 2000). Prevalence is higher in rural areas (Yadav and Agrawal 2008). Increased prevalence of reading disorder in classes 2–5, greater incidence of writing disorder in classes 6 and above has been reported (Tripathi and Kar 2008). Phonological awareness is neither evident nor crucial for development of reading skills in Indian languages (Prakash and Rekha 1992; Prakash et al. 1993; Prema and Karanth 2003). Language deficits appear to be higher than phonological awareness deficits in both younger (Sharma 2000) and older children (Shankaranarayana 2003).

While most workers in India in the area prefer to work with the western models, there has been reasonable amount of research based on Indian work on assessment and remediation. The NIMHANS Index Learning Disability is a battery of tests evolved out of empirical data (Uma et al. 2011). The NIMHANS battery consists of: Attention test (Single and double colour and number cancellation), Language tests (Reading, writing, spelling and comprehension), Arithmetic tests (Addition, subtraction, multiplication, division) (single and double digits and fractions), Visuo-motor skills (Bender Gestalt Test BGT) and Developmental Test of Visuo Motor Integration and Memory tests (Auditory and Visual).

In addition there is a pre-academic skill assessment section in level—I while level—II consists of the above tests. The validity of the NIMHANS index was examined and found to be adequate (Uma et al. 2011).

Neuropsychological Profile of Learning Disability in the Indian Population-Preliminary Results studied by Krishna et al. (2007) in a sample of 60 children in classes 3–7 from English medium schools—who presented with learning difficulties in Child and Adolescent Mental Health Unit at NIMHANS, Bangalore. They were assessed on NIMHANS SLD battery, Malin's WISC and NIMHANS Neuropsychological battery.

The four patterns of deficits found were: Reading, Spelling, Writing and Arithmetic, with subgroups with any of the two, three or four deficits. The neuropsychological deficits were of two types suggestive of diffuse cortical or fronto-temporal dysfunction. The results showed that the age and the kind of neuropsychological deficits influenced the type of disability. Age and the nature of neuropsychological aspects, suggests some biological underpinnings of learning disability.

3. **Remedial Measures in India**

While several studies have used remedial packages developed in the west and these are theoretically driven (Das 1999).

Training on sight words, phonics and language skills was associated with better reading (Rozario 2003). Training auditory visual channel, spelling rules, comprehension skills, oral expression and visuo-motor perceptual aspects improved language based SLD (Srikanth and Karanth 2003). Remedial measures for 7–11-year olds was better than remedial training as usual for word attach and word identification skills (Padegar and Saranath 2008).

Neuropsychological Remediation for Children with Specific Learning Disorder for Arithmetic

Sukumaran (2003) in his doctoral thesis focused on specific disorder of arithmetic. The study consisted of two phases. In phase I norms were developed for a test of arithmetic ability that was based on a neuropsychological model. The test was administered on a sample of 284 children studying in III to VI. Standard wise cut off scores were obtained to identify Specific Learning Disorder for Arithmetic. In the second phase a remedial program for the Specific Learning Disorder for Arithmetic was developed. The remedial program consisted of two components, i.e. neuropsychological remediation and content-based arithmetic skills training given sequentially. The sample consisted of 17 children studying in standards III to VI with a diagnosis of Specific Learning Disorder for Arithmetic as identified by the NIMHANS Index for SLD. There were 10 children in the treatment group and 7 children in the control group. The children in the treatment and control groups were comparable in severity of arithmetic disorder at the pre-remediation assessment. The treatment group received neuropsychological remediation while the control group received remedial sessions for improvement of handwriting skills. These were daily individual sessions, which ranged from 15 to 20 min. Arithmetic remediation was given in small groups of 2–3 children. Children from the treatment and control groups were regrouped based on the nature of arithmetic deficit as seen on the Test of Arithmetic Ability.

The post remediation assessment showed significant improvement in arithmetic skills in the treatment group but not in the control group. This indicates that a combination of neuropsychological remediation together with content-based arithmetic skills training is efficacious. The neuropsychological tasks of attention, verbal and visual memory could have contributed to the improvement of arithmetic skills in the treatment group. Improvement of attention may have led to an overall improvement of attention to details and relevant information needed for successful problem solving. Improvement of visual memory could have led to a decrease of visuo-spatial difficulties experienced by the children.

Improvement of verbal memory could have improved encoding and rehearsal of verbal information. Thus improvement of neuropsychological components appears to contribute positively to improvement in arithmetic skills in children with Specific Learning Disorder for Arithmetic.

Comparing two Intervention Programmes for Reading Disorder (Sadasivan et al. 2009a, b). The sample consisted of two groups of 10 children with reading disorder in age range of 10–13 years. Group 1 received 20 sessions of phonological awareness intervention while group 2 received 20 sessions of neuropsychological intervention. Both groups were assessed before, immediately after and 3 months after intervention, were comparable in the outcomes. Both groups assessed on reading subtest, phonological awareness measures and neuropsychological measures.

Much of the phonological work is only for children studying in English medium schools. This may not be applicable for phonetic languages as the Indian languages. In the Indian studies, apart from a few that merely replicate Western remediation strategies, the others are innovative and appropriate to the Indian school context.

Good practice guidelines for India have been brought out by John et al. (2013). These are characterized by the following features.

a. The assessments take into account of heterogeneity in the SLD population.
b. The remediation measures of SLD are more comprehensive and consequently more effective.
c. There is willingness to accommodate multiple theories while handling individual cases.
d. The relation of SLD to the inherent linguistic structures of the Indian languages have been explored.

To summarize, several Indian studies have replicated theoretically driven western tools and found them useful, but these are not understood very well by children whose medium of instruction is not English and inadequate school system.

22.6 Approaches to Learning Difficulties—Asian Reality and Challenges

Learning difficulties could be a function of developmental problems which would lend itself to the western methodologies. Or could be due to poor school systems that are rampant in many of the developing countries. The corollaries are as follows:

Specific Learning Disabilities in the individual child due to developmental problems despite average intelligence, normal schooling and absence of sensory motor deficits require **individual intervention**.

Learning difficulties due to deficient school system in most of the children requiring **universal intervention with child-centred play way method**.

With the former group the focus is on assessment and intervention package that is applicable for children with 'genuine' SLD, despite good educational support, there are large sections of those who come from socio-economically and educationally backward backgrounds who may appear to have skill deficits, similar to SLD. While the children with SLD require **individualized** intervention to target specific skill deficits the latter group needs **'universal'** intervention. The following report shows an experiential work with 2000 children in rural and tribal regions in Karnataka in one district (Kapur 2007) of a model of universal intervention.

1. **Interventions may be of two kinds: Specific and Universal**

In the specific interventions individually tailored programmes to remedy the skill deficit profile of the child with special focus on phonetic languages.

In the universal intervention, the aim is to modify the school system adopting child-centred Universal Intervention through PLAY WAY methods.

An example of Universal intervention

A study by Kapur (2007) was carried out in H.D. Kote in Karnataka in one of the 19 clusters of schools. This programme on integrated approach consisted of training of 21 Primary Health Care doctors, 65 Health workers and 96 Anganwadi workers on mental health and child development. One cluster of school of the 19 clusters was taken for the intervention study. This cluster had 15 rural schools with 1200 children from class 1–9, with 41 teachers. In addition 9 Ashram schools for 800 tribal and scheduled caste primary school children were also taken.

The programme aimed at promotion of Psychosocial Development. It was characterized by directly working with children, one hour a day over 24 sessions and the activities consisted of free art, craft, music, dance, drama and play. Evaluation was carried out before and after the intervention on tests of attention, intelligence, creativity, language, number skills and memory.

Results in the rural schools (N:1200)

Revealed that Performance there was significant improvement with reduced time on Seguin Form Board (SFB) test and significant improvement on simple attention and complex attention in colour cancellation tests in Children in Class 1 and 2.

There was improvement in performance of Children in Class 3–7, on simple and complex attention on number cancellation tests. Significant improvement was seen on intellectual function on Coloured Progressive Matrices Test (CPM) (Raven 1965) There was improved performance on Creativity test (Mehdi 1985), Vocabulary test (NIMHANS SLD Battery 2002) and Arithmetic test (NIMHANS SLD Battery 2002).

Results in the tribal schools (N:800)

Significant Improvement of Tribal Children in Class 1 and 2 on Intelligence measured on Seguin Form Board (SFB), simple and complex attention on colour cancellation test (NIMHANS SLD Battery) along with Vocabulary, Creativity (Mehdi 1985), Number skills and Memory (Barnabas et al. 2011).

Significant Improvement occurred in Children in Class 3–7 on simple and complex attention on number cancellation tests, on Coloured Progressive Matrices test, Creativity test (Mehdi), Vocabulary test (NIMHANS SLD Battery), Arithmetic test (NIMHANS SLD Battery) and Memory test (Barnabas et al. 2011).

Improvement in Performance of Rural and Tribal Children using Play Way, child-centred methods an hour a day over 15–20 sessions in the regular class room setting, statistically significant improvement on quantitative assessment on psychological test on attention, intelligence, creativity, vocabulary arithmetic and memory. Additional improvement observed qualitatively on school performance, extracurricular activities, class room participation and enhanced interest in learning. This study is an unparalleled demonstration effectiveness of child-centred play in promotion of psychosocial development as especially suited to developing nations that is universally applicable.

2. **Low Cost Universal Solutions for Asian Countries**

The assessment tools are not available in the developing nations, especially in the regional languages and English as taught in the local context. The following strategies can be employed to develop the material locally.

a. Assessment of language and Arithmetic skill deficit profiles using standard text books in the Asian languages from class 1–7
b. Performance gap of 2 years/2 grades and above indicates LD
c. Nature of language, arithmetic and visuo-spatial skill deficit profile is to be obtained

Remediation of Language may be carried out in the following steps:

First: Read an entire illustrated simple story aloud, showing the text and running a finger below the words and sentences
Second: Ask questions to check the comprehension at the end
Third: Ask them to enact the story
Fourth: Read again till they repeat by heart
Continue till they CAN READ independently

Remediation of Arithmetic
Chinese Abacus (from internet) and games that use numbers, ludo, snakes and ladders, chess, etc. Concrete objects such as sticks or beads can be used for basic counting starting from where the child understands the basic concepts—simple addition, subtraction, multiplication and division and then build on it.

22.7 Synopsis

Learning difficulties are frequently encountered in the school setting across the globe. It is essential to distinguish two kinds of learning difficulties.

First is those difficulties arising out of inadequate school systems resulting in learning problems in all the children and the second is those arising out of inherent specific learning difficulties of individual children where there has been adequate school inputs.

Consequently the remedial work needs to be carried out for all the children in the inadequate school system. In contrast, individual remediation is required for those who have individual profiles of specific deficits. Common strategies can be adopted for the children who are in the poor school system. But children with idiosyncratic deficit profiles in reading, writing and mathematics individually or in combination, require individually tailored remediation strategies. In addition, they may have difficult temperament, may in addition have psychological problems such as hyperactivity attention deficit disorder, conduct and emotion disorders.

In addition to remediation, supportive measures and counseling the child and the family and sometimes of even the concerned teacher may be needed. The specific learning disabled group is a very heterogeneous group requiring multiple strategies to solve the problem.

22.8 Conclusions

Specific packages based on specific theories may be of limited use to the child with SLD because of the overlapping deficits.

A holistic and eclectic packages based on individual child's skill deficits profiles are essential for good outcome.

Scholastic problems have multiple causes and hence simplistic solutions do not work. Multiple approaches tailored to each child's deficit profile needs to be adopted in a holistic manner. However, if there are failed school systems, the method of dealing with them need to be an universal intervention through child-centred play.

22.9 Implications

In the developing countries, the assessment and diagnosis of specific learning disability needs to be made on the background of similar profile being a function of poor schooling as well.

Assessments need to take into account of the cultural context in which the problem arises. The tools assessments are not culture free. Even Progressive Matrices in not culture free in rural India.

Specific learning disability is one group of multiple learning disorders that cannot be accommodated within a single theoretical frame work. The closest one can hypothesize is that it is a developmental disorder causing multiple deficits. However, the absence of a theory is no barrier for effective assessment and remediation.

References

Barnabas, I., Subba, K., Kapur, M., Uma, H., & U.K. Sinha. (2011). Tests of memory for children. In H. Uma, A. Oomen, & M. Kapur (Eds.), *Psychological assessment of children in the clinical setting* (3rd edn., p. 48). Bangalore Publication, NIMHANS.

Bhola, P., & Kapur, M. (2000). Prevalence of emotional disturbance in indian adolescent girls. *Indian Journal of Clinical Psychology, 27*, 217–222.

Das, J. P. (1999). *PASS reading enhancement programme*. Edmonton Canada: Developmental Disabilities, University of Alberta.

Das, J. P., Hayward, H. C., Samantaray, S., & Panda, J. J. (2006). Cognitive enhancement training (COGENT): What is it? How does it work with a group of disadvantaged children. *Journal of Cognitive Education and Psychology, 5*, 328–335.

Diagnostic and Statistical Manual of Mental Disorders, DSM-5. (2013). American Psychiatric Association, USA.

Geary, D. C., Hamson, C. O., & Hoard, M. K. (2000). Numerical and arithmetical cognition: A longitudinal study of process and concept deficits in children with learning disability. *Journal of Experimental Child Psychology, 77*, 236–263.

Hallahan, D. P., Kauffmann, J. M., & Lloyd, J. W. (1985). *Introduction to learning disabilities*. Englewood Cliffs, NJ, USA: Prentice Hall.

Hayward, H. C., Das, J. P., & Janzen, T. (2007). Innovative programme for improvement in reading through cognitive enhancement. *Journal of Learning Disabilities, 40*, 443–457.

John, A., Sadasivan, A., Sukumaran, B., Bhola, P., David, N. J., & Manickam, L. S. S. (2013). Practice guidelines: Learning disability. *Indian Journal of Clinical Psychology., 40*(1), 65–68.

Kapur, M. (2007). Learning from Children What to Teach Them. New Delhi Sage Publications Private Limited.

Kauffmann, J. M. (1985). *Characteristics of children's behaviour disorders* (3rd ed.). Columbus, Charles E. Merril.

Krishna, R., Oommen, A. & Rao, S. L. (2007). Neuropsychological profile of learning disability in the indian population-preliminary results. Indian Journal of Clinical Psychology, *34*, 69–75.

Mann, A. V., & Liberman, I. Y. (1984). Phonological awareness and verbal short-term memory. *Journal of Learning Disabilities, 17*, 592–599.

Mehdi, B. (1985). *Non verbal test of creative thinking* (2nd ed.). Agra: Psychological Corporation.

National Advisory Committee on Handicapped Children. (1968). First Annual Report of the US Office of Education, Washington D.C.; US, Department of Health, Education and Welfare.

Padegar, S., & Sarnath, J. (2008). A theory-driven approach to the diagnosis and remediation of learning problems in children. In G. A. K. Thapa, M. Van Der, & J. Pandey (Eds.), *Perspectives on learning disabilities in india: current practices and prospects* (pp. 238–254). New Delhi: Sage Publications Private Limited.

Prakash, P., & Rekha, B. (1992). Phonological awareness and reading acquisition in Kannada. In A. K. Srivastava (Ed.), *Researches in child and adolescent psychology* (pp. 47–52). New Delhi: NCERT.

Prakash, P., Rekha, R., Nigam, R., Karanth, P. (1993). Phonological awareness, orthography and literacy. In R. Scholes (Ed.), *Literacy and language* (pp. 138 149). Mahwah, NJ: Lawerence Erlbaum Associates.

Prema, K. S., & Karanth, P. (2003). Assessment of learning disability: Language based tests. In P. K. J. Rozario (Ed.), *Learning disabilities in India: Willing the mind to learn* (pp. 138–149). New Delhi: Sage Publications Private Limited.

Raven, J. C. (1965). *The coloured progressive matrices*. London: H. K. Lewis and Company Limited.

Rozario, J. (2003). Assessment of learning disabilities. In P. Karanth & J. Rozario (Eds.), *Learning disabilities in India: Willing the mind to learn*. New Delhi: Sage Publications Private Limited.

Sadasivan, A., Gillon, G., & Rucklidge, J. (2009a). The effects of phonological awareness intervention on neuropsychological functioning in children with reading disabilities. *New Zealand Speech and Language Therapy Journal, 64*, 12–25.

Sadasivan, A., Gillon, G., Rucklidge, J., & Kapur, M. (2009b). Neuropsychological intervention for specific learning disorder—An innovative approach. *Malaysian Journal of Special Education, 2011*.

Shankaranarayana, A. (2003). Cognitive profiles of children learning to read English as a second language. In P. Karanth & J. Rozario (Eds.), *Learning disabilities in India: Willing the mind to learn* (pp. 77–90). New Delhi: Sage Publications Private Limited.

Sharma, A. (2000). *Language skills in children with learning disability.* Unpublished Dissertation, Mangalore University, Mangalore.

Shaywitz, S. E., & Shaywitz, B. A. (2005). Dyslexia (Specific reading disability). *Biological Psychiatry, 57*, 1301–1309.

Srikanth, N., & Karanth, P. (2003). Speech language pathologists and the remediation of reading disabilities. In P. Karanth & J. Rozario (Eds.), *Learning disabilities in India: Willing the mind to learn.* New Delhi: Sage Publications Private Limited.

Srinath, S., Girimaji, S. G., Gururaj, P., Sheshadri, S., Subbakrishna, D. K., Bhola, P., et al. (2005). Epidemiological study of child and adolescent psychiatric disorders in urban and rural areas of Bangalore. *Indian Journal of Medical research, 122*, 67–79.

Sukumaran, B. (2003). *Neuropsychological remediation for children with specific learning disorder for arithmetic.* Unpublished Doctoral Thesis. NIMHANS, Bangalore.

Tallal, P. (1998). Children with language impairment can be accurately identified using temporal processing measures: A response to Zhang and Tomblin. *Brain and Language, 65*, 395–403.

Taylor, G. H. (1988). Psychological testing; relevance for assessing children's learning disabilities. *Journal of Consulting and Clinical Psychology, 56*(6), 795–800.

Thapa, K. (2008). Learning disabilities: Issues and concerns. In K. Thapa, G. Aalsvoort, M. Van Der, & J. Pandey (Eds.), *Perspectives on learning disabilities in india: Current practices and prospects* (pp. 23–47). New Delhi: Sage Publications Private Limited.

Torgenson, J. K. (1991). Learning disabilities: Historical and conceptual issues. In B. Y. L. Wong (Ed.), *Learning about learning disabilitie.* (pp 3–31). San Diego, CA: Academic Press.

Tripathi, N., & Kar, B. R. (2008). Teachers' perception of learning-related problems in school-going children. In K. Thapa, G. Aalsvoort, M. Van Der, & J. Pandey (Eds.), *Perspectives on learning disabilities in india: current practices and prospects* (pp. 200–220). New Delhi: Sage Publications Private Limited.

Troier, G. A., & Whitney, S. D. (2003). A close look at the efficacy of fast forward language for children with academic weaknesses. *Contemporary Educational Psychology, 3*(4), 465–495.

Uma, H., Oomen, A., & Kapur, M. (2011). *Psychological assessment of children in the clinical setting* (3rd edn.). Bangalore Publication, 48, NIMHANS.

Yadav, D., & Agarwal, V. (2008). A base-line study of learning disabilities: Its prevalence, teacher awareness and classroom practices. In K. Thapa, G. Aalsvoort, M. Van Der, & J. Pandey (Eds.), *Perspectives on learning disabilities in India: Current practices and prospects* (pp. 221–238). New Delhi: Sage Publications Private Limited.

Part VII
Service, Training and Policy

Chapter 23
Child Mental Health Policy: The Time Is Now

Myron L. Belfer

Abstract Policy is essential for the rational and sustained development of child mental health services. Unfortunately, only approximately 7 % of all countries have an identifiable child mental health policy. The World Health Organization has developed a series of comprehensive policy guidelines including one for child and adolescent mental health. Policy has often developed as an outcome of the need to respond to crises impacting a country. The economic evidence is available to reinforce an argument for implementing child mental health policies globally. Rich and poor countries show a discrepancy between access to services in rural versus urban and wealthy versus poor populations. There are now several model policies often embracing a rights-based or inclusion approach. Asia has participated in the movement for the development of policy to support child mental health services particularly in schools. For policy to develop there is the need for "political will" which can be fostered through broad-based advocacy and the ability to make the economic and social arguments to demonstrate the importance of child mental health policy.

Keywords Policy · World Health Organization · Child mental health services · Political will · Economic argument for services · Mental health in schools

M.L. Belfer (✉)
Department of Psychiatry, Boston Children's Hospital, 300 Longwood Avenue, Boston, MA 02115, USA
e-mail: Myron_Belfer@hms.harvard.edu

M.L. Belfer
Harvard Medical School, Boston, MA 02115, USA

S. Malhotra and P. Santosh (eds.), *Child and Adolescent Psychiatry*,
DOI 10.1007/978-81-322-3619-1_23

23.1 Introduction

For more than 70 years there have been those arguing for more attention to the mental health of children across the globe. The rhetoric at first focused on the plight of children after the great wars of the twentieth century and as a result of the industrial revolution. In each subsequent era there has been a call for attention to the mental health of children. Most recently, with the emphasis on education, ADHD captures worldwide attention, autism is falsely seen as an epidemic and psychopharmacology as a panacea. There is without a doubt a need to address the mental health needs of children but a rational framework for understanding those needs, fitting the interventions to the diverse global cultures and ensuring sustainability of programs remains a challenge as great now or perhaps greater than at the outset of the concern with child mental health in the modern era (Kieling et al. 2011; World Health Organization 2003). The cruelest irony is that countries and regions with the largest child and adolescent populations lag significantly in the development of child and adolescent mental health policy (Belfer and Saxena 2006; Belfer 2007). Policy should not be seen to be dependent on the economic status of a country but rather on the consciousness to provide for some of its most vulnerable citizens.

There are many factors that have stymied the development of child mental health services including lack of resources both financial and professional, difficulty with access, stigma, unfounded myths about etiology, and a host of other factors (Kieling et al. 2011). Perhaps most critical has been the absence of child mental health policy (Belfer and Saxena 2006). The promulgation of policy serves to engage stakeholders, ensure accountability, garner financial resources and offers a roadmap for development. The World Health Organization in 2005 (World Health Organization 2005) and others subsequently have documented the absence of child mental health policy worldwide (Shatkin and Belfer 2004). In addition, to the lack of overall policy there has been a failure to address what should be the core values incorporated in policy (Belfer and Saxena 2006). This gap exists despite a significant contribution from the World Health Organization in the form of guidelines for policy development that not only outlined key elements of policy but discussed financing and other key aspects that would be difficult to confront in resource poor settings (World Health Organization 2005).

23.2 Impediments to Policy Development

Child mental health services are of necessity inter-sectorial (Harper and Cetin 2008). It is the very nature of the different sectors impacted by child mental disorders and poor child mental health that has impeded progress in policy development. Worldwide there has been competition for resources between the many sectors: adult mental health services versus child mental health services; educational services versus mental health services; disability-related services versus those focused on mental disorders. In addition, service development has often been impeded by a perceived either/or focus on prevention or services. This is clearly a false and unnecessary dichotomy.

Governments see the development of child mental health policy as opening the way to increased health expenditures and often assume that the evidence for interventions are insufficient to warrant the investment. This now runs counter to the increased evidence that effective interventions are available and that the treatment of disorders leads to less unemployment, youth suicide, and delinquent behavior (Kieling et al. 2011; Conti and Heckmann 2010; Scott et al. 2001). Non-governmental organization (NGOs), often unwittingly, let governments "off the hook" when they provide services in countries where the government fails to provide support for mental health (Belfer and Saxena 2006). The NGO services are rarely sustainable and thus when the NGO departs the populations are left unserved. Furthermore, NGOs too often operate outside the governance structures of government thus escaping regulation. When confronted with the absence of mental health policy many governments point to their ratification of the UN Convention on the Rights of the Child (Carlson 2001). While this is a significant accomplishment for many societies, the Convention is rarely fully operationalized and those provisions that would support the development of child mental health related services and interventions are neglected.

Child mental health-related policies are often found in policies associated with various segments of government serving children. For instance, policies on children who are abused and neglected are found in policies promulgated for social service agencies, policies for delinquent children are found in criminal justice policies, and a large number of child mental health related policies are found in educational policy (Krug et al. 2002; Burns et al. 1995). This fragmentation leads to an inability to focus attention on the whole child and too often is reflected in fragmented and competitive services.

It is often argued that child mental health policy cannot be developed because there is a lack of appropriate epidemiological data. However, this argument now needs to be put aside as it has been shown repeatedly that in country after country there are no epidemiological surprises when comparable, well-established methodologies are utilized (Verhulst 2004). Furthermore, solid epidemiological data has shown that over 50 % of adult mental disorders begin before the age of 14 (Kessler et al. 2010).

The World Health Organization developed a series of mental health policy and service guidelines including one for child and adolescent mental health (World Health Organization 2005). These policy and service guidelines provide virtually all the information necessary to develop mental health policy including crucial data on financing and governance.

23.3 Policy Behind the Curve

Too much emphasis on policy development has been on more traditional child mental health service needs. In many countries it is the desire of vested interests to see policy support through regulation, financial incentive or training increasing numbers of highly trained specialists. The emergence of "big pharma" and other interests with financial incentives have too often distorted child mental health policy (Eisenberg and Belfer 2009; Turner et al. 2008). This emphasis fails to recognize the imperative to develop more public health approaches to mental health supported by strong public policy. In populous countries, particularly low- and middle-income countries there will never be enough highly trained professionals to meet the mental health needs of the youth population. Thus, there is a need to find ways to incorporate child mental health in public health initiatives.

It is remarkable that when it has been shown that consumer advocacy can be so effective in establishing policy or highlighting a particular mental health need such as services for autistic children consumer input into policy and support for consumer involvement in policy lags in almost all countries (Bennetts et al. 2011; Funk et al. 2006).

It has been known for decades that early intervention to support children and to intervene in observable mental disorders is cost-effective. Yet, this economic data fails to be recognized. Heckman (2008) and Doyle (Doyle et al. 2009) have provided compelling financial arguments for investing in a public health approach beginning at a very early age.

23.4 Progress in Policy Development

Critical moments and decisions in a country's history have sometimes led to dramatic changes in mental health policy including that related to children. The increased attention given to the plight of children after natural disasters spurs governments to create programs and policies to provide care, protection and healing (Munir et al. 2004). In China the "One Child Policy" and a concern for "left behind children" has led to an examination of existing child mental health policies (Zheng and Zheng 2015; Cheng and Sun 2015). However, it would be a mistake to consider this a problem isolated to China (Tomsa and Jenaro 2015). In almost every low income country literally many thousands of people leave behind their children to go to work in other countries and see their children infrequently (Mazzucato et al. 2015). In high-income countries and in many societies in the process of evolution the choice is to have only one or no children thus leading to the same potential consequences being addressed in China.

Turkey as a result of two devastating earthquakes and the advocacy of professional societies was able to establish a mental health law (Doyle et al. 2009). This was a significant achievement, but its implementation in regards to child mental health lags. In China, through NGO support the "iDream" program has been implemented in Chengdu to give children and adolescents a sense of "hope" for the future through facilitating access to individuals who have achieved success after adversity.[1] In Alexandria, Egypt there is a unique program of linkage that requires real estate developers to either take on the support of a public education facility or build such a facility.[2] This has resulted in the development of a model facility to serve developmentally disabled youth including the latest in diagnostic resources and helped to support a school mental health consultation program.

Brazil's implementation of Guardianship Councils has given a voice to parents/caregivers seeking to obtain services for their children (Duarte et al. 2007). The Councils are available for all children under the age of 21 and does not emphasize an "at risk" group. These quasi-judicial bodies can resolve access to service issues. The role of the Councils is to make referrals and guarantee the delivery of service.

Chile in its efforts to improve the health and wellbeing of children has demonstrated through Chile Crece Contigo (CCC) a model for providing services to young children.[3] This is a model crosscutting initiative involving the Ministry of Social Development, Ministry of Health and Ministry of Education. While not focused on mental health its aim is to promote equal development opportunities for children ages 0–4 and prevent diseases through accessible preschool education programs, preventive health checks, parental leave and increased child support. The program now covers approximately 80 % of the 0–4 population.

China has approved a sweeping and inclusive mental health policy but it has not specific provisions for child mental health (Xiang et al. 2012a, b). As much as there is the need for independent child mental health policy undoubtedly addressing adult mental health needs child mental health will be improved to some extent. This should be recognized as well in other societies. Importantly, in China, like many other countries with a long-term planning process, the current health-related strategic plan calls for a major investment in child mental health services even in the absence of policy. China also highlights a very common global problem that is the discrepancy between access to services in rural versus urban populations (Muennig 2014). This is a phenomenon in rich and poor, well-resourced and sparsely resourced countries. How China addresses the problem may serve as a model for other countries.

The World Health Organization, through its Mental Health Gap Action Programme (mhGAP) initiative is providing models of care that can be scaled up by countries (The Lancet 2010). With evidence of the feasibility of these programs and their associated training components governments will have the evidence to promote policy development in the area of child mental health.

---

[1]Personal communication, Malcolm Au, Shanghai, China

[2]Personal communication, Amira Seif Eldin, MD, Alexandria, Egypt

[3]www.crececontigo.gob.cl.

23.5 Asia: Unique Challenges and Opportunities

Asia is a diverse region but shares certain common characteristics. Professionals tend to be highly trained and very conversant with the latest findings in the scientific literature. Clinicians who work in the public sector are faced with seeing large numbers of patients thus limiting their ability to provide more psychosocial interventions. The development of allied professions has lagged with certain notable exceptions. Thus, for instance, there is the challenge to train more social workers. Focusing on policy, there is no shortage of very well-trained professionals capable of developing policy in health, mental health and other areas. In fact, some limited policies not focused on mental health have incorporated innovative, sustainable funding models. What appears to be missing is the "political will" to do more to develop child mental health policy (Richmond and Kotelchuck 1983). There are many possible reasons for this lack of "political will." There are other pressing social problems demanding attention, a lack of understanding of how child mental health problems can be addressed, a failure to understand how addressing child mental health problems may have a positive impact on social stability, and economic achievement.

China, India, Singapore, Indonesia, Korea and other countries show evidence of active concern with child mental health and have moved to implement training and service programs that in several cases incorporate innovative ideas. South Korea pioneered an innovative form of taxation to support child mental health (World Health Organization 2003). Singapore has developed the REACH (Response, Early Assessment and intervention in Community mental Health) program, a model school consultation program, on a national level.[4]

Of course the challenge is to be able to meet the needs of countries with hundreds of millions, even billions of citizens. In these instances across Asia it is evident that increased public health focused approaches will be needed along with a significant increase in the training of those in nonmedical disciplines who can work in the community in rural, underserved areas.

23.6 Conclusion

Developing child mental health policy should be on the public agenda in every country. All of the evidence necessary to make the argument for "stand-alone" child mental health policy has been developed. Advocacy at the highest levels of government, and the engagement with consumers to bolster advocacy and increasing awareness of child mental health needs as a part of advocacy can advance the cause of developing child mental health policy and fostering "political will" to do so (Richmond and Kotelchuck 1983).

---

[4]www.reachforstudents.com.

References

Atlas: Child and adolescent mental health resources, global concerns: Implications for the future. World Health Organization (2005).

Belfer, M. L. (2007). Critical review of world policies for mental healthcare for children and adolescents. *Current Opinion in Psychiatry, 20*, 349–352.

Belfer, M. L., & Saxena, S. (2006). WHO child atlas project. *The Lancet, 367*, 551–552.

Bennetts, W., Cross, W., & Bloomer, M. (2011). Understanding consumer participation in mental health: Issues of power and change. *International Journal of Mental Health Nursing, 20*(3), 155–164.

Burns, B. J., Costello, E. J., Angold, A., et al. (1995). Children's mental health services use across services sectors. *Health Affairs, 14*, 147–159.

Caring for children and adolescents with mental disorders: setting WHO directions. Geneva: World Health Organization (2003).

Carlson, M. (2001). Child rights and mental health. *Child and Adolescent Psychiatric Clinics of North America, 10*, 825–839.

Cheng, J., & Sun, Y. H. (2015). Depression and anxiety among left-behind children in China: A systematic review. *Child Care Health Development, 41*(4), 515–523.

Conti, G., & Heckmann, J. J. (2010). The educational-health gradient. *American Economic Review, 100*, 234–238.

Doyle, O., Harmon, C. P., Heckman, J. J., & Tremblay, R. E. (2009). Investing in early human development: Timing and economic efficiency. *Economics and Human Biology, 7*, 1–6.

Duarte, C. S., Rizzini, I., Hoven, C. W., Carlson, M., & Earls, F. (2007). The evolution of child rights councils in Brazil. *International Journal of Child Rights, 15*, 269–282.

Eisenberg, L., & Belfer, M. (2009). Prerequisites for global child and adolescent mental health. *Journal of Child Psychology and Psychiatry, 50*(1–2), 26–35.

Funk, M., Minoletti, A., Drew, N., Taylor, J., & Saraceno, B. (2006). Advocacy for mental health: Roles for consumer and family organizations and governments. *Health Promotion International, 21*(1), 70–75.

Harper, C., & Cetin, F. C. (2008). Child and adolescent mental health policy: Promise to provision. *International Review of Psychiatry, 20*, 217–224.

Heckman, J. J. (2008). The case for investing in disadvantaged young children. In *Big ideas for children: Investing in our nation's future,* Washington, DC, First Vision.

Kessler, R. C., McLaughlin, K. A., Green, J. G., et al. (2010). Childhood adversities and adult psychopathology in the WHO World Mental Health Surveys. *British Journal of Psychiatry, 197*, 378–385.

Kieling, C., Baker-Henningham, H., Belfer, M., Conti, G., Ertem, I., Omigbodun, O., et al. (2011). Child and adolescent mental health worldwide: Evidence for action. *The Lancet, 378*, 1515–1525.

Krug, E. G., Dahlberg, L. L., Mercy, J. A., Swi, A., & Lozano, R. (2002). *World report on violence and health*. Geneva: World Health Organization.

Mazzucato, V., Cebotari, V., Veale, A., White, A., Grassi, M., & Vivet, J. (2015). International parental migration and the psychological well-being of children in Ghana, Nigeria, and Angola. *Social Science Medicine, 132*, 215–222.

Muennig, P. (2014). What China's experiment in community building can tell us about tackling health disparities: Community building and mental health in mid-life and older life: Evidence from China. *Social Science Medicine, 107*, 217–220.

Munir, K., Ergene, T., Tunaligil, V., & Erol, N. (2004). A window of opportunity for the transformation of national mental health policy in Turkey following two major earthquakes. *Harvard Review of Psychiatry, 12*, 238–251.

Richmond, J. B., & Kotelchuck, M. (1983). Political influences: Rethinking national health policy. In C. H. McGuire, R. P. Foley, A. Gorr, & R. W. Richards (Eds.), *The handbook of health professions education*. San Francisco: Jossey-Bass.

Scott, S., Knapp, M., Henderson, J., et al. (2001). Financial cost of social exclusion: Follow-up study of anti-social children into adulthood. *British Medical Journal, 322*, 191–195.

Shatkin, J. P., & Belfer, M. L. (2004). The global absence of child and adolescent mental health policy. *Child and Adolescent Mental Health, 9*, 104–108.

The Lancet. (2010). Mental Health: WHO minds the GAP. *Lancet, 376*, 1274.

Tomsa, R., & Jenaro, C. (2015). Children left behind in Romania: anxiety and predictor variables. *Psychol ogical Reports, 116*(2), 485–512.

Turner, E. H., Matthews, A. M., Linardatos, E., Tell, R. A., & Rosenthal, R. (2008). Selective publication of antidepressant trials and its influence on apparent efficacy. *NEJM, 358*, 252–260.

Verhulst, F. C. (2004). Epidemiology as a basis for the conception and planning of services. In H. Remschmidt, M. L. Belfer, & I. Goodyer (Eds.), *Facilitating pathways: Care, treatment, and prevention in child and adolescent mental health* (pp. 3–15). Berlin: Springer.

World Health Organization. (2005). *Mental health policy and service guidance package: Child and adolescent mental health policies and plans*. Geneva: World Health Organization.

Xiang, Y.-T., Sartorius, N., Ungvari, G. S., & Chiu, H. F. K. (2012a). Mental health in China: Challenges and progress. *The Lancet, 380*, 1715–1716.

Xiang, Y.-T., Yu, X., Ungvari, G. S., Lee, E. H. M., & Chiu, H. F. K. (2012b). China's National Mental Health Law: A 26-year work in progress. *The Lancet, 379*, 780–781.

Zheng, Y., & Zheng, X. (2015). Current state and recent developments in child psychiatry in China. *Child and Adolescent Mental Health, 9*, 10.

Chapter 24
Telepsychiatry in Child and Adolescent Mental Healthcare

Savita Malhotra, Subho Chakrabarti and Ruchita Shah

Abstract Telepsychiatry, also termed as telemental health or e-mental health is defined as the use of information and communication technology (ICT) to provide or support psychiatric services across distances. Telepsychiatric services using different technology media, such as videoconferencing, internet, and telephone improve the accessibility of treatment, may reduce its cost, and are found to be useful and satisfying for diagnosis or treatment of specific disorders in children. There is need to carry out methodologically sound high-quality research before telepsychiatry becomes viable as an adjunct to the traditional methods of healthcare delivery. Traditional models of telepsychiatry programmes, such as direct patient management, consultation models, or collaborative care models would be impractical in developing countries like India, as they rely on availability of specialists at one end, and qualified psychiatrists are either unavailable or already over burdened. The authors present an innovative two-pronged '*tele-enabling*' approach has been designed and developed at Postgraduate Institute of Medical Education and Research (PGIMER), Chandigarh, India to overcome this difficulty. The tele-enabling model involves (a) use of a newly developed online, logical diagnostic, and management decision support system by a team of non-specialists, i.e. general physicians and para-professionals; and (b) training, supervision, and monitoring of these non-specialists by the psychiatrists at the hub via videoconferencing and additional use of telephone and email. In this chapter, literature related to telepsychiatry for children and adolescents is reviewed and the working of the tele-enabling model is discussed.

S. Malhotra (✉) · S. Chakrabarti · R. Shah
Department of Psychiatry, Post Graduate Institute of Medical Education and Research, Chandigarh 160012, India
e-mail: savita.pgi@gmail.com

S. Chakrabarti
e-mail: subhochd@yahoo.com

R. Shah
e-mail: drruchitashah@gmail.com

S. Malhotra and P. Santosh (eds.), *Child and Adolescent Psychiatry*,
DOI 10.1007/978-81-322-3619-1_24

Keywords Telepsychiatry · E-mental health · Digital health · Low resource countries · Service delivery · Remote areas

List of Abbreviations

ADHD	Attention deficit hyperactivity disorder
CBT	Cognitive behaviour therapy
FTF	Face-to-face
ICT	Information and Communication Technology
IT	Information Technology
LAMI	Low and middle income
PCP	Primary care physicians
SAARC	South Asian Association for Regional Cooperation
SMS	Short messaging system
VC	Videoconferencing

24.1 Need for Child and Adolescent Telepsychiatry

Child and adolescent mental health problems have high prevalence and cause significant functioning impairment and disability in emotional, social, interpersonal, and academic domains of a child's life. A review of epidemiological studies worldwide revealed that approximately one-fourth of youth experience a mental disorder during the past year, and about one-third across their lifetimes (Merikangas et al. 2009). The prevalence of child and adolescent mental disorders is more serious in low and middle income (LAMI) countries, merely due to the large numbers of children and adolescents who constitute nearly 35–50 % of the population (Patel et al. 2008). A recent systematic review and meta-analysis from India (Malhotra and Patra 2014) found the prevalence rate of these disorders in the community to be at 6.46 %, i.e. about 29 million children and adolescents suffer from psychological problems that need treatment. Further, children and adolescents' mental illnesses differ in terms of symptom presentations, comorbidities, assessment procedures, treatment strategies and response to treatment from those of adults. Therefore, a substantial number of specifically trained professionals from various disciplines (e.g., psychiatrists, psychologists, educationists) are required to cater to the mental healthcare needs of this population. However, the WHO Atlas on Child and Adolescent Mental Health Resources has revealed an almost total failure of countries, especially LAMI nations, in developing adequate policy, training, and services for child and adolescent mental health (Belfer and Saxena 2006). Sharan and Malhotra (2007) observed that there are only 100–125 psychiatrists in India who specifically cater to this population, i.e. approximately 1 child psychiatrist for 290,000 children and adolescents needing treatment. Most of these professionals are settled in urban areas, working in universities or in the private sector. This situation further limits the access to the already meagre services both geographically and economically to a very small section of children and their families. On the other hand, the primary care physicians (PCP) at the grass root level either have very limited or no requisite knowledge, skills and expertise to deal with these problems. The situation is no different in other LAMI nations. Such a mental health gap between demand and services though narrower, also exists in the predominantly rural and geographically inaccessible states of developed nations (e.g., Starling et al. 2003; Hilty et al. 2006a, b; Myers et al. 2006; Starling and Foley 2006). Integration of mental healthcare into primary care services and school-based services, and education and training of the PCPs, teachers and other workers has been considered crucial towards narrowing this gap. The conventional means and efforts for achieving the same though laudable are fraught with several logistic difficulties especially in the developing nations where less than 2 % of the health budget is dedicated to mental healthcare (Sinha and Kaur 2011). Further, these programmes fail to provide with the requisite dedicated and continued support from mental health professionals beyond initial training simply because of their scarcity, care is restricted only to severe mental health problems; neglecting important areas, such as common childhood disorders, adolescent counselling and stress management. Therefore, a need to develop alternative means to deliver comprehensive, good quality and sustained mental health services to children and adolescents, especially for those residing in rural and geographically isolated regions has been a pressing issue worldwide, more so in the developing countries. On the other hand, the information and communication technology (ICT) sector has been growing rapidly and has today, percolated into all the spheres of our lives, supporting our social needs to banking and business needs. The large-scale reach of these technologies (such as internet and satellite services), its exponentially increasing acceptability and appeal amongst both general public and professionals, ever-increasing familiarity with technology-based applications and its percolation in day-to-day life all make optimum and innovative use of ICT for healthcare delivery possible and promising (Malhotra et al. 2013a). It would only be appropriate that these technological advancements are utilised towards fulfilling the healthcare needs of the large underserved population.

24.2 History of Child and Adolescent Telepsychiatry

The history of telepsychiatry with child and adolescent telemental health dates back to late 50s and early-60s with use of telephones and televisions for two way communication for educational and clinical purposes. In fact, telemedicine, broadly defined as the use of telecommunications technologies for medical diagnosis, patient care, research and education via any form of electronic communication, first originated through its telepsychiatry application (Hyler and Gangure 2002). In 1959, the first telepsychiatry/telemedicine unit established in Nebraska Psychiatric Institute in Omaha used 2-way, closed-circuit microwave television to transmit demonstrations with neurologic patients as part of the education of medical students at the state mental hospital 112 miles away (Liebson 1997). Within a decade of its first telepsychiatric application, in 1968, two different groups of workers in the U.S. used 2-way interactive television for evaluation of both adults and children, and for consultation to the referring physician to provide patient care collaboratively (Liebson 1997). Over the next two to three decades, telepsychiatry programmes were described from various developed nations besides the U.S., viz, Canada, Australia and some European nations (Fahey et al. 2003; Starling et al. 2003; Hilty et al. 2004, 2006a, b; Myers et al. 2006; Starling and Foley 2006). Most of these programmes initially used some form of two way live or real-time audio-video interaction (Hilty et al. 2004, 2006a, b; Myers et al. 2006;). Over the last about 20 years there has been a definite growth in telepsychiatry. Besides programmes in the US, Australia and other developed nations, there have been recent sporadic efforts from developing nations, including those from Asia (Thara et al. 2008; Malhotra et al. 2013a; Rahman 2006; Wynchank and Fortuin 2010; Qadir 2014). Most of these latter programmes are part of broader telemedicine systems, and are restricted to email consultations and real-time or video-recorded educational programmes, though a handful have been set up as sole telepsychiatry units using innovative methods (Thara et al. 2008; Malhotra et al. 2013a, b; Malhotra and Chakrabarti 2013). Besides the establishment of telepsychiatry programmesprogrammes in LAMI nations, there have been developments in the field in at least four major ways. First, there has been a rapid expansion in the modalities of information and communication technologies used, including email, short messaging system (SMS), online chat rooms and interactive online programmes. The second area has been expansion in the scope of telepsychiatric services beyond mere real-time face-to-face consultation and includes individual therapy, group therapy, consultation to the primary care physicians (PCP), education and training. Third, programmes targeting special populations such as children and adolescents in remote areas, children in day care centres, school-based programmes, juvenile homes and detention centres have been established. Fourth, many of the programmes explored and used newer models for providing care through telepsychiatry (discussed in later sections) (Hilty et al. 2006a, b).

Despite all these recent developments, historically, telepsychiatry has met with major obstacles including cost and physicians' resistance to the use of a technology they consider unproven (Liebson 1997) and were uncomfortable with. Most of the earlier programmes did not survive beyond the pilot phase (Perednia and Allen 1995). Most importantly, though telepsychiatry is more than half a century old, studies evaluating these programmes (including those specifically for children and adolescents) are mainly restricted to their acceptability and feasibility. Extremely few studies assess effectiveness, outcomes and cost-efficiency of these programmes. Overall, methodologically sound and rigorous research is almost non-existent in the field of child and adolescent telepsychiatry (reviewed in later sections).

24.3 Definitions

Telepsychiatry or telemental health or e-mental health is defined as the use of information and communication technology (ICT) to provide or support psychiatric services across distances. There are two major modes of communication using ICT, synchronous or live and asynchronous or store-forward. Synchronous services provide live, two-way interactive transmission between patient and provider at distant locations. The interactive forms of communication include telephone, online communication (e.g., chat forums), and video-conferencing, and these have the advantages of real-time interaction whereby response is immediate. However, reference to synchronous technology usually means use of videoconferencing. Store-and-forward mode of communication involves acquiring medical data and then transmitting this clinical information via email or Web applications for later review by a specialist. As against synchronous forms of communication, asynchronous communication involves non-real time or 'store-and-forward' interaction and does not require the presence of both parties at the same time. The information can be transferred in the form of data, audio, video clips, or recordings. Email is the most commonly used form of asynchronous communication in telemedicine services and has the advantages of being relatively inexpensive and does not need any extra hardware support.

24.4 Models of Telepsychiatry Care for Children and Adolescents

Several models of telepsychiatry care have been described in the literature (Hilty et al. 2006a; Szeftel et al. 2011). There are three major models, namely, (a) direct care, (b) consultation care and (c) collaborative care.

24.4.1 Direct Care

The direct care model also known as the traditional referral, or replacement model, uses the psychiatrist at the nodal centre as the principal provider of mental health services to the patients at remote sites. In this model, the child psychiatrist carries out the initial assessment as well as provides treatment directly to the patient. Also, he continues to follow up the patient as in regular practice, albeit from a distance usually via videoconferencing. The clinic staff at the remote end facilitates the process of consultation with the telepsychiatrist. Also, the child psychiatrist may have meetings with the staff. It has been suggested that this model may work well for children with more limited impairments, where a coordinated team of professionals is not required. This model of care is more resource intensive as the telepsychiatrist provides with all the care. Hence, direct care model would not be ideal in most situations where there is already a dearth of child psychiatrists (Sharan and Malhotra 2007). In addition, the tele-consultant may be from a different culture and may not be familiar with several important aspects of the child's culture such as, childrearing practices, norms of child behaviour, and views of illness causation (Savin et al. 2011). These factors are extremely important in determining the diagnostic possibilities, understanding symptom genesis and perpetuation, and also in treatment. This problem has often been highlighted in Western studies involving ethnic minorities, such as Hispanics and Indian--Americans (Savin et al. 2011). In addition, since the telepsychiatrist belongs to an urban locale, he might not be cognizant of rural realities. Also, clients and their families might perceive the barriers of culture and language with the specialist located in a university. Also, as the duty of care lies with the telepsychiatrist alone, there may be difficulty in extending care during times of emergency (Malhotra et al. 2013a). Direct care has also been used by private practice telepsychiatrists based in large cities who are paid by the hour as compared to state or university funded programmes which follow the other models (Glueck 2011). Some psychiatrists also provide first consultation in the clinic followed by direct care over videoconferencing.

24.4.2 Consultation Care Model

The consultation care model includes the primary care physician (PCP) as the principal provider of mental health services, after the initial psychiatric consultation. In this model, the tele-psychiatrist plays a circumscribed role of assessing, diagnosing and making treatment recommendations without providing ongoing follow up care. The implementation of recommendations and follow up is the responsibility of the PCP and his team at the remote site. The model can function in two broad ways—patient-centred and consultee-centred (PCP centred). In the former, the focus is on the patients and families, while in the latter, the focus is on the local providers who will continue with the delivery of care. In a variation of the consultee-centred model, the psychiatrist may provide consultation to the PCP based on clinical report without seeing patients, i.e. doctor–doctor consultation. This is followed as the only strategy in telepsychiatry programmes which are part of larger telemedicine programmes, especially in developing countries as store-forward technology (use of email) can be applied without any additional costs. In the consultation care model, the initial consultation may be followed by telephonic or email communication between the psychiatrist and the local provider

(Hilty et al. 2006a; Szeftel et al. 2011). This model has the advantage of providing local care through PCPs with whom the treatment-seeking families would be more comfortable. Also, it saves an enormous amount of time of the child psychiatrists. However, the major disadvantages are that there is heavy reliance on the PCPs psychological orientation and knowledge, motivation and confidence, as well as his relation with the consultant telepsychiatrist. Treatment recommendations may or may not be implemented effectively depending on these factors. Also, PCPs have expressed that the content of patient as well as consultee-centred consultation, such as explanation regarding diagnosis and medications given by the telepsychiatrist determines whether recommendations are followed or not (Boydell et al. 2007). In addition, it has been suggested that this model of care may lead to frustration and lowered job satisfaction in the tele-consultant as he is not involved in further care of the patient.

24.4.3 Collaborative Care Model

The collaborative-care model involves mental health services jointly provided by the PCP and the psychiatrist, using frequent communication between providers (Hilty et al. 2006a). In this model, after the initial consultation, the psychiatrist follows patients in conjunction with the PCP. It also involves collaboration with a local treatment team that may include case managers, social workers, counsellors and even teachers. The role of the psychiatrist goes beyond that of providing diagnosis and treatment recommendations. He should also play an administrative role. With the aid of a clinic facilitator located remotely, the telepsychiatrist builds a comprehensive team for each child. Also, he provides the other team members with necessary knowledge and guidance on case to case basis. This model is ideal especially for children and adolescents, as most childhood disorders, such as developmental disabilities require a multi-disciplinary approach (Szeftel et al. 2011). The psychiatrist, along with his team at the remote site can provide comprehensive services to children and their families. Also, the PCP is responsible for the follow up care, which the telepsychiatrist seeing patients less often than in direct care. Communication via telephone and email between PCP or other providers and the telepsychiatrist is usual, and it assists the treatment. Continued support of the psychiatrist can instil confidence in the local provider as well as patient/his parents. This model has been considered by far, the most ideal as it provides specialist care through utilisation of local resources, as well as trains the PCPs in child mental healthcare.

Many of the telepsychiatry programmes have integrated basic care principles from more than one model (for, e.g. Hilt et al. 2015). For example, to serve children and their families in the rural state of Wyoming in the United States, an academic centre coordinated a consult system of (1) televideo consults for high-needs children, (2) remote medication reviews for beyond-guidelines prescribing, and (3) elective community provider telephone-based consults (Hilt et al. 2015). There has been no direct comparison of these models in terms of treatment outcomes or cost effectiveness. However, in an on-going consultation-based telepsychiatry programme combined with specific educational interventions, appears to facilitate the enhancement of skills and knowledge of PCPs, it was found that over time, PCPs significantly improved medication dosing and referred patients more for treatment planning rather than diagnostic difficulties, and their satisfaction also improved over time (Hilty et al. 2006a).

24.5 Research in Child and Adolescent Telepsychiatry

Telepsychiatry research across various populations (i.e. children, adults and elderly) and various settings has been reviewed extensively (for recent reviews, see Hilty et al. 2013; Chipps et al. 2012; Malhotra et al. 2013a). Overall, telepsychiatry literature pertains to reliability of psychiatric and neuropsychological assessments, satisfaction with and acceptability of telepsychiatry, and outcome studies focusing on clinical outcome (i.e. improvement in symptoms and functioning), quality of life and treatment adherence. However, research specifically addressing child and adolescent telemental health is extremely meagre, with most publications being programme descriptions or feasibility studies. Only two randomised clinical trials have been conducted in this field (Elford et al. 2000; Nelson et al. 2003) and there are a few outcome studies with a pre-post intervention design. Recently, Malhotra et al. (2013b, c, 2014b, 2015a, b, c, in press) have reported validation of a newly developed clinical decision support system used through telepsychiatry for psychiatric disorders seen in children and adolescents. Child and adolescent telepsychiatry research pertaining specifically to videoconferencing has been well reviewed by Pesamaa et al. (2004), Diamond and Bloch (2010), Myers et al. (2011), and all the three reviews reflect similar observations regarding paucity of research. Also, overall child and adolescent (and, also in general) telepsychiatry literature is mainly restricted to videoconferencing with few reports on use of asynchronous telepsychiatry for clinical, training and educational purposes.

24.5.1 Feasibility, Acceptability and Satisfaction

A number of studies have reported on patient and caregiver satisfaction, as well as provider satisfaction with the overall positive conclusion that there is high satisfaction and acceptability with VC (Elford et al. 2001; Kopel et al. 2001; Hilty et al. 2006a, b; Myers et al. 2006, 2007). Myers et al. (2008) have also reported high utilisation rates for telepsychiatry services. Other descriptive studies have suggested feasibility and acceptability of telepsychiatry for providing child and adolescent mental healthcare (Cloutier et al. 2008; Myers et al. 2010). A case series has also suggested that a sub-set of children and adolescents preferred use of VC over FTF because of the novelty of the consultation and the extra distance involved (both psychological and physical) made it easier for adolescents to talk regarding their drug problems (Pakyurek et al. 2010). However, problems with audio-visual quality with lack of technical support have been perceived as major hurdles to satisfaction. Also, few studies reported that parents would have preferred to see the psychiatrist in person. Although this has been attributed to parents discomfort with or feeling intimidated by the technology, preference for in-person consultation with the doctor for personal satisfaction cannot be ruled out (Savin et al. 2011). Only one study (Wagnild et al. 2006) reported a low rate (26 %) of satisfaction with VC among psychiatrists. Rather, there is the possibility of publication bias for positive reports of satisfaction with VC. This has been pointed out previously by Pesamaa et al. (2004).

24.5.2 Reliability of Assessment

Only one study has directly compared VC to FTF assessments in children. Elford et al. (2000) assessed reliability of psychiatric assessments through videoconferencing (VC) in 23 patients aged 4–16 years by conducting a randomised controlled trial. The patients accompanied by their parents completed two psychiatric assessments, one via videoconferencing and other, face-to-face (FTF) in a randomised order. In 96 % of cases the diagnosis and treatment recommendations made by VC were same as in FTF. The authors also reported that there was no difference in patient and parent satisfaction between the two modalities. Keilman (2005) compared the quality and acceptability of telemedicine consultations to face-to-face interactions in children with history of abuse, referred by a state child welfare agency. However, these comparisons were based on subjective assessments. Myers et al. (2004) compared diagnosis, demographics and costs for 159 youths seen in telepsychiatry clinic to 210 seen in routine outpatient clinics and found that these groups were comparable on the study variables. This study did not assess reliability of telepsychiatric evaluations, and can be construed as a feasibility study.

24.5.3 Treatment Outcome

Nelson et al. (2003) evaluated a 8 week cognitive behaviour therapy (CBT) intervention for childhood depression in 28 youths who received the intervention either FTF or via VC. The participants were evaluated on depression inventories pre-and post-treatment. CBT treatment was effective and comparable across the two conditions. This study also successfully demonstrated the feasibility of conducting a randomised controlled trial in child telepsychiatry. Stoep and Myers (2013) reported on the methodology for conducting a randomised controlled trial evaluating the effectiveness of telepsychiatry in improving outcomes of children with Attention deficit and hyperactivity disorder (ADHD) living in underserved communities. Recently, Myers et al. (2015) have reported on this randomised controlled trial conducted over 223 children referred by 88 primary care providers (PCPs) in 7 communities. Children randomised to the experimental telehealth service model received 6 sessions over 22 weeks of combined pharmacotherapy, delivered by child psychiatrists through videoconferencing, and caregiver behaviour training, provided in person by community therapists who were supervised remotely. Children randomised to the control service delivery model received treatment with their PCPs augmented with a telepsychiatry consultation. Children in both service models improved with children assigned to the telehealth service model showing significantly more improvement on several measures. A retrospective analysis for a follow up period of 3 months was conducted by Yellowlees et al. (2008) on the diagnostic and clinical outcomes for 139 children who were evaluated via videoconferencing. Authors found that ADHD and mood disorders were the most common diagnostic categories and that there was a significant symptom improvement over the follow up period. Individual case reports have described delivery of telepsychiatric care (VC) for children with anorexia nervosa (Goldfield and Boachie 2003), depression (Alessi 2002), post-traumatic stress disorders (Alessi 2003) and ADHD (Hilty et al. 2000). Hilt et al. (2015) reported on a state-wide child telepsychiatry consult system which included televideo consults, medication reviews and provider-telephone consults. They found that there was a significant decrease in the number of children aged less than five using psychotropic medications, children using psychotropic doses >150 % of the maximum approved and children slated by caseworkers for a psychiatric residential treatment facility admission.

24.5.4 Follow up of Recommendations

Follow up of treatment recommendations made during 100 randomly selected telepsychiatry consultations was carried out to evaluate the implementation of recommendations by interviewing the case managers (Boydell et al. 2007). Results indicated that cooperation of both child and parent, clear communication of recommendations, involvement of school and local health providers, stability of agencies, and availability of services were the main factors instrumental in successful implementation of recommendations.

24.5.5 Change in Clinicians Knowledge and Skills

Some studies have reported on tele-education initiatives for training of clinicians in rural areas in child psychiatry. These studies have reported improvement of knowledge and skills of PCP and decreased professional isolation (Fahey et al. 2003).

24.5.6 Cost Effectiveness

Hilt et al. (2015) calculated a positive financial return on investment for combined consultation services in Wymoing as state expenditures on psychotropics for youth decreased during this time frame by approximately $209,500, much greater than the $29,375 cost of performing mandatory medication reviews through telepsychiatry. Using standard cost-accounting procedures for 132 patients who received 257 telepsychiatric consultations a 6 month period, Spaulding et al. (2010) found that an average cost of a telepsychiatry consult in was only $30.99 compared to $168.61 for an in-person consultation. In a small study by Elford et al. (2001), the cost of telepsychiatric consultation was comparable to cost of travelling for the 30 patients.

24.5.7 Telepsychiatry in Special Populations—Intellectual Disability, Juvenile Justice System, School Mental Health

Use of telemental health and its feasibility and acceptability has been described in special populations, such as children in juvenile detention centres (as reviewed in Kaliebe et al. 2011). Patient, provider and facility related advantages have been highlighted. However, a Myers et al. (2006) has highlighted that though the youth are satisfied with the consultations, they are concerned about breach of confidentiality. It has been suggested that telepsychiatry is well suited for children with developmental disabilities, as travelling to a tertiary centre may be difficult, the stress from travel may complicate a child's presentation during clinical evaluation, critical community providers can be involved in the process and child may be more comfortable in familiar surroundings like his school (as reviewed by Szeftel et al. 2011). School telemental health services in form of clinical care to a child in the school, education and training of teachers have been described in literature (reviewed by Grady et al. 2011). Use of telepsychiatry has also been described for children who were victims of abuse (Keilman 2005).

24.6 Child and Adolescent Telepsychiatry: Asian Scenario

Telepsychiatry services in Asia have mainly been part of established telemedicine programmes. Use of store-forward technology has been the most common, where a referring physician sends an email with a brief report on patient's history and seeks advice on further evaluation, diagnosis and management from a teaching hospital-based psychiatrist. The psychiatrist devotes requisite time to reply to the queries, but is usually not a full-time telepsychiatrist. Occasionally, real-time patient consultation may be conducted at a scheduled time. The telemedicine infrastructure is utilised for education and training of students in other South Asian Association for Regional Cooperation (SAARC) nations, by relaying pre-recorded lectures from experts at hub site. In India, besides these initiatives, a telepsychiatry project from Chennai, India (Thara et al. 2008) offers service to 156 villages by means of a bus that has been custom-built to contain a consultation room and a pharmacy. After a teleconsultation, a prescription is advised by the psychiatrist located at the nodal centre to the telepsychiatry clinic facilitator in the bus and dispensed by the on-board pharmacy. However, this requires a dedicated psychiatrist to provide consultation and a customised vehicle to provide out-reach services. Majumdar (2007) reported on telepsychiatry services to tsunami affected persons in Nagapattinam district in the state of Tamil Nadu, India. A study form Rawalpindi, Pakistan demonstrated the feasibility of using 'store and forward', through use of internet and a dedicated email address to train and supervise staff in the diagnosis and management of children and adolescents aged 16 years or less at no extra cost (Rahman 2006). Real-time videoconferencing for psychiatric care and capacity building in remote areas has also been attempted in Pakistan (Aga Khan Development Network eHealth Resource Centre 2015). Another report from Pakistan (Qadir 2014) describes use of telepsychiatry for assessment and rehabilitation of 615 psychiatric patients from a remote district where no psychiatrist was available, although it is not clear if it catered to children and adolescents also. The services were part of a telemedicine programme; though no other details were mentioned. Besides India and Pakistan, telepsychiatry programmes have been conceived as part of telemedicine in Nepal (No author 1998) and Bangladesh (Nessa et al. 2010), though further developments have not been reported in the literature. There has been no dedicated telepsychiatry programme or initiative except the one reported by Rahman (2006). All the programmes report on the feasibility of telepsychiatry (including child and adolescent telepsychiatry). Effectiveness, outcomes and cost-benefits have not been studied.

Overall, in Asia most of the existing programmes are part of wider telemedicine networks and use provider-centred consultation care model or training and education through asynchronous technology (mainly using email) that needs no extra revenue. Though these programmes target the providers, their success largely depends on the PCP's motivation and pro-activeness. Also, the major disadvantage is that the PCPs are not exposed to assessment and interviewing skills displayed by the psychiatrist in a patient-centred consultation model. Hence, after seeking consultation, they may not feel confident to carry out the assessment or treatment just on the basis of prescription. This approach should therefore, be combined with sensitization of PCP, their continued medical education and a mechanism for mental health screening and referral (Hilty et al. 2006). A handful of programmes from Asia have reported dedicated telepsychiatry programmes using live videoconferencing for all consultations and follow up, i.e. providing direct care. However, the major concern with such an approach has been that it simply redistributes and burdens the existing resources rather than creating additional capacity. Also, there are concerns regarding satisfaction of patients and their caregivers, satisfaction of the providers, and quality of audio-visual communication affecting various aspects of the telepsychiatric consultation. Further, it has been suggested that videoconferencing might preclude certain opportunities for observation, e.g. an adolescent boy holding his mother's hand under the table, out of the sight of the telepsychiatrist or the activities of a toddler who refuses to sit in front of the camera (Szeftel et al. 2011). Moreover, though videoconferencing is considered as the best modality, use of live technologies is capital intensive. On the other hand, the collaborative care model where the PCP takes the responsibility of patient care and the psychiatrist makes recommendations, but is not directly responsible for care, have the advantages of utilising the existing resources at primary level, providing education, training and guidance to the PCPs and other staff members, and improving the overall quality of services besides improving accessibility. In the West, where consultation and collaborative models have been implemented in a systematic manner, these have been found to improve the PCP's confidence and skills in managing the patients (Hilty et al. 2006), and showed a gradual transition from requesting assistance in diagnostic process to increased requests for assistance with developing or modifying management plans. Thus, such a strategy has the potential to create and strengthen resources at local level, and this is expected to be beneficial and cost-effective in the long run. Moreover, it resolves the important issue of duty of care, where the psychiatrist is not available and able to assume responsibility (as in an emergency situation) (Sharan and Malhotra 2007).

The author (SM) envisaged that software packages with codified medical knowledge, i.e. clinical decision support systems as an aid to assessment, diagnosis, and management should be designed that would train, aid and enable PCPs to provide services. Clinical decision support systems for diagnosis and management have been shown to improve practitioner performance and adherence to clinical practice guidelines. However, such a CDSS for child and adolescent psychiatric disorders should be comprehensive with adequate coverage of common childhood disorders, culturally sensitive, based on evidence and guidelines, and be user-friendly. Therefore, a model that involves the use of a diagnostic and management application by PCPs and other non-psychiatrists, such as pediatricians locally, combined with minimal supervision and support from psychiatrists located at the hub, via synchronous and asynchronous modes, seems to be ideal. Such a model based on the principles of collaborative care model of telepsychiatric care and decision informatics or "E Psychiatrist" has been designed and developed at Postgraduate Institute of Medical Education and Research, Chandigarh, India with funding support from Department of Science and Technology, Govt. of India (Malhotra et al. 2013a; Malhotra and Chakrabarti 2013).

24.6.1 "E Psychiatrist": A Tele-enabling Model of Telepsychiatric Care

The model of psychiatric care for the underserved in remote and geographically isolated regions has been termed as the "E Psychiatrist"; a '*tele-enabling*' model

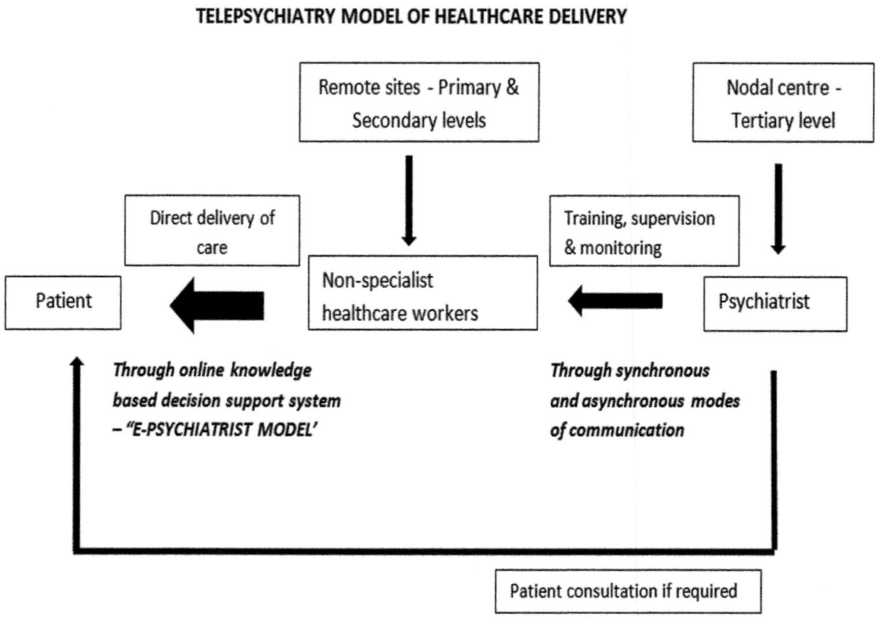

Fig. 24.1 Tele-enabling model of healthcare delivery using telepsychiatry

by the developers. The department at PGIMER is the nodal centre, with three peripheral sites located in neighbouring sub himalayan hill states in northern India, namely Bilaspur in Himachal Pradesh, Srinagar in Uttarakhand and Srinagar in Jammu and Kashmir. At each remote site, a telepsychiatry centre was established in district level hospital which was supervised by the medical officer at the remote site and the psychiatrists at the nodal centre. The staff recruited included a general physician or a psychiatrist if available, psychologists or social worker and computer operators at these sites. The service delivery model applies a logical decision support system (for diagnosis and management) with facilities for real-time as well as store-forward (web-based) video recording, teleconferencing, and creation of electronic medical records (see Fig. 24.1).

A novel, web-based application covering 19 childhood and adolescent psychiatric disorders with diagnostic sub-system linked logically to management sub-system has been developed. The diagnostic system consists of a 'core' diagnostic tool based on the standardised classificatory systems with criteria-based approach, has a screening module for all disorders for a comprehensive assessment, followed by detailed questioning for specific disorders as indicated by responses to screening. The system guides the interviewer in rating responses. Based on in-built thresholds and hierarchies, it auto-generates a multi-axial diagnosis. The diagnostic system is linked to the management decision support system through psychiatric diagnosis, severity, medical disorders (if present) and age and gender specifics. The latter system includes pharmacological and psychological management for all the disorders, besides modules for investigations and referrals. All the modules except pharmacological intervention have been developed bilingually (Hindi and English), and have been kept simple, brief, and practical. The application includes a system for longitudinal follow up in continuation with previous visits and generates a temporally linked electronic medical record for each patient. The different components of the CDSS, including those for children and adolescents and adults have been tested separately and it has been found to have acceptable level of diagnostic accuracy, sensitivity and specificity, inter-rater reliability and feasible to use even when used by non-specialists (Malhotra et al. 2013b, c, 2014, 2015a, b, c, in press). The application can be accessed online, is password protected and is hosted on developer-owned servers. The non-psychiatrists at remote sites, i.e. a physician and psychologists or social workers need to be trained in using the application. The training was carried out using real—time videoconferencing over two weeks without need for trainees to be present physically at the hub site (Malhotra et al. 2012). Following training, the non-psychiatrists at remote sites have used the Application for over 1000 patients, with good inter-rater reliability tested for a sub-sample (unpublished). The application is expected to act as a self-educating tool, improving the skills and confidence of the non-psychiatrists with repeated use. The feedback from the staff at all the centres validated this expectation. Further, videoconferencing with supplementary use of internet and telephone has been applied to conduct booster training sessions, provide support, supervision and monitoring to the staff placed remotely. Also, the application has provision to be updated and revised by the experts at the nodal site and stores a huge database.

24.7 Ethical and Legal Issues

There are several ethical and legal challenges in practice of telepsychiatry, which raise legitimate concerns regarding its use by clinicians (Kramer and Luxton 2016). These issues relate to not only VC, but to also other forms of communication. The most important of these are issues related to privacy and confidentiality, and issues of responsibility and liability especially during emergency situations. Electronic transmission of patient data has raised concerns regarding loss of confidentiality. However, new methods, such as data encryption, authentication procedures, authorization procedures, auditing and tracking programmes, and firewalls have increased data security. In addition to data security, VC poses a unique challenge. The presence of non-clinical technicians, camera operators and schedulers has the potential to create privacy related issues. These individuals may be located at either the hub centre or at the site of a service provider physically or through technology. Moreover, if their presence is through technology and not physically, they may not be visible to the child or adolescent client.

It is always a good practice to let the patient know about any such individual present and take his informed consent for the telepsychiatric consultation, to avoid breach of trust and confidentiality. Rather, informed consent is one of the most important risk management strategies in telepsychiatric care (Kramer and Luxton 2016). Specific legal requirements regarding valid informed consent varies from state to state. Hence, the telepsychiatrist must apprise himself of the same and abide by these requirements. However, in the absence of specific law or regulation, as in developing countries, the clinicians practicing telepsychiatry, must include elements of confidentiality and limits to confidentiality when using electronic communications, emergency plan, process for documentation and storage of information, potential for technical failure and procedures for coordination of care with other professionals, protocol for contact between sessions, and conditions under which telemental health services are terminated and a referral for face-to-face care made (Turvey et al. 2013). An additional issue in case of children is that of age of consent, and legal provisions of a given state must be followed.

Hyler and Gangure (2004) have highlighted difficulties faced by the telepsychiatrist in an emergency situation, e.g. a suicidal patient tries to cut her wrist during the telepsychiatric consultation and she is alone in the room due to privacy issues. It has been strongly advised that there must be some system in place so that the telepsychiatrist can contact the staff at the remote site. Also, it is recommended that the primary care providers be present with the patient for at least part of the session. The telepsychiatrist should introduce himself to the local provider and the patient, explain his expertise, and outline the process and limits of service. Also, he must clarify that he is not assuming any shared responsibility or duty of care once the consultation is over. Also, it is equally important to consider and establish a plan for addressing technical, medical, and clinical emergencies (Kramer and Luxton 2016). This should include knowledge of local requirements and plan regarding duty to warn/protect and mandatory reporting, specific emergency procedures (if they exist) for any site and transportation issues. The model of care as outlined in the section on tele-enabling model (Sect. 24.6.1) would resolve the issue of duty of care as the local providers would assume the responsibility. Different states have different licensing procedures and regulatory bodies. These procedures specific to the local (satellite) site should be followed.

Overall, the use of telepsychiatry can be an appropriate adjunct or an alternative to deliver mental health services if its application is compliant with policies on medical ethics and confidentiality. In developing countries, use of telepsychiatry is rapidly growing in both government and private sectors. Therefore, there is a definite need for policies and guidelines to protect the interests of both the patients and telepsychiatrists. For the time being, clinicians practicing telepsychiatry in developing nations where specific laws or policies do not exist, should take into consideration and follow local laws pertaining to ICT and cybercrime, and medical negligence as well as internationally prescribed guidelines.

24.8 Conclusions and Future Directions

To summarise,

- Child and adolescent telepsychiatry has been shown to be feasible, acceptable and effective to a large extent. Evidence regarding cost-effectiveness is limited.
- Overall, the evidence is from its use across various settings in the developed nations.
- Direct care model, consultative and collaborative models of telepsychiatric care are applied singly or in combination.
- In LAMI nations, telepsychiatry is gaining foothold and holds huge promise
- The newly developed tele-enabling model that empowers non-psychiatrists in treating psychiatric disorders in children and adolescents seems to be suitable for resource-strained developing nations
- Ethical and legal issues relate to confidentiality, duty of care, emergency situations, and licensing and regulatory procedures and mandates. Clinicians wanting to practise telepsychiatry must follow the local (satellite) laws and regulations. In absence of clear rules, laws pertaining to ICT and cybercrime, and medical negligence as well as internationally prescribed guidelines should be considered while practising telepsychiatry.

Overall, telepsychiatry in child and mental health care is gradually finding its place in the Asian continent through its various applications. In the current scenario of enormous shortage of manpower and huge urban--rural discrepancies in availability of these resources on one hand, and rapidly growing Information Technology (IT) sector on the other, telepsychiatry has a huge potential to take quality mental health services to the doorsteps of the people. Also, with the exponential rise in the use of internet and internet-based applications by lay people, there is a greater likelihood of increasing acceptability of telepsychiatry and hence, increasing use. The need of the hour, therefore, is to locally develop and test implementable models of telepsychiatric care for children and adolescents that take into consideration the ground realities and resources of a given nation or state. As the field is expected to grow rapidly, it also becomes absolutely essential that laws, and regulatory policies and procedures are evolved and implemented in the Asian countries.

References

Aga Khan Development Network eHealth Resource Centre. (2015). *eHealth programme expands: telepsychiatry services for Northern Pakistan*. Available at: http://www.aku.edu/aboutaku/news/Pages/ehealth-programme.aspx. Last accessed on December 19, 2015.

Alessi, N. E. (2002). Telepsychiatric care for a depressed adolescent. *Journal of the American Academy of Child and Adolescent Psychiatry, 41*(8), 894–895.

Alessi, N. E. (2003). Quantitative documentation of the therapeutic efficacy of adolescent telepsychiatry. *Telemedicine Journal and e-health, 9*(3), 283–289.

Belfer, M. L., & Saxena, S. (2006). WHO child atlas project. *Lancet, 367*, 551–552.

Boydell, K. M., Volpe, T., Kertes, A., & Greenberg, N. (2007). A review of the outcomes of the recommendations made during paediatric telepsychiatry consultations. *Journal of Telemedicine and Telecare, 13*, 277–281.

Chipps, J., Brysiewicz, P., & Mars, M. (2012). Effectiveness and feasibility of telepsychiatry in resource constrained environments? A systematic review of the evidence. *African Journal of Psychiatry, 15*, 235–243.

Cloutier, P., Cappelli, M., Glennie, J. E., & Keresztes, C. (2008). Mental health services for children and youth: A survey of physicians' knowledge, attitudes and use of telehealth services. *Journal of Telemedicine and Telecare, 14*(2), 98–101.

Diamond, J. M., & Bloch, R. M. (2010). Telepsychiatry assessments of child or adolescent behavior disorders: A review of evidence and issues. *Telemedicine Journal and e-health, 16*(6), 712–716.

Elford, R., White, H., Bowering, R., Ghandi, A., Maddiggan, B., St, John K., et al. (2000). A randomized, controlled trial of child psychiatric assessments conducted using videoteleconferencing. *Journal of Telemedicine and Telecare, 6*(2), 73–82.

Elford, R., White, H., St, John K., Maddigan, B., Ghandi, M., & Bowering, R. (2001). A prospective satisfaction study and cost analysis of a pilot child telepsychiatry service in Newfoundland. *Journal of Telemedicine and Telecare, 7*(2), 73–81.

Fahey, A., Day, N. A., & Gelber, H. (2003). Tele-education in child mental health for rural allied health workers. *Journal of Telemedicine and Telecare, 9*(2), 84–88.

Glueck, D. A. (2011). Telepsychiatry in private practice. *Child and Adolescent Psychiatric Clinics of North America, 20*(1), 1–11.

Goldfield, G. S., & Boachie, A. (2003). Delivery of family therapy in the treatment of anorexia nervosa using telehealth. *Telemedicine Journal and e-health, 9*, 111–114.

Grady, B. J., Lever, N., Cunningham, D., & Stephan, S. (2011). Telepsychiatry and school mental health. *Child and Adolescent Psychiatric Clinics of North America, 20*(1), 81–94.

Hilt, R. J., Barclay, R. P., Bush, J., Stout, B., Anderson, N., & Wignall, J. R. (2015). A statewide child telepsychiatry consult system yields desired health system changes and savings. *Telemedicine Journal and e-health, 21*(7), 533–537.

Hilty, D. M., Ferrer, D. C., Parish, M. B., Johnston, B., Callahan, E. J., & Yellowlees, P. M. (2013). The effectiveness of telemental health: A 2013 review. *Telemedicine Journal and e-health, 19*(6), 444–454. doi:10.1089/tmj.2013.0075.

Hilty, D. M., Marks, S. L., Urness, D., Yellowlees, P. M., & Nesbitt, T. S. (2004). Clinical and educational telepsychiatry applications: A review. *Canadian Journal of Psychiatry, 49*(1), 12–23.

Hilty, D., Sison, J., Nesbitt, T., & Hales, R. (2000). Telepsychiatric consultation for ADHD in the primary care setting. *Journal of the American Academy of Child and Adolescent Psychiatry, 39*, 15–16.

Hilty, D. M., Yellowlees, P. M., Cobb, H. C., Bourgeois, J. A., Neufeld, J. D., & Nesbitt, T. S. (2006a). Models of telepsychiatric consultation—Liaison service to rural primary care. *Psychosomatics, 47*(2), 152–157.

Hilty, D. M., Yellowlees, P. M., & Nesbitt, T. S. (2006b). Evolution of telepsychiatry to rural sites: changes over time in types of referral and in primary care providers' knowledge, skills and satisfaction. *General Hospital Psychiatry, 28*, 367–373.

Hyler, S. E., & Gangure, D. P. (2002). Technological advances in telepsychiatry. *Primary Psychiatry, 9*(9), 24–28.

Hyler, S. E., & Gangure, D. P. (2004). Legal and ethical challenges in telepsychiatry. *Journal of Psychiatric Practice, 10*(4), 272–276.

Kaliebe, K. E., Heneghan, J., & Kim, T. J. (2011). Telepsychiatry in juvenile justice settings. *Child and Adolescent Psychiatric Clinics of North America, 20*(1), 113–123. doi:10.1016/j.chc.2010.09.001.

Keilman, P. (2005). Telepsychiatry with child welfare families referred to a family service agency. *Telemedicine Journal and e-health, 11*(1), 98–101.
Kopel, H., Nunn, K., & Dossetor, D. (2001). Evaluating satisfaction with a child and adolescent psychological telemedicine outreach service. *Journal of Telemedicine and Telecare, 7*(2), 35–40.
Kramer, G. M., & Luxton, D. D. (2016). Telemental health for children and adolescents: An overview of legal, regulatory, and risk management issues. *Journal of Child and Adolescent Psychopharmacology, 26*(3), 198–203.
Liebson, E. (1997). Telepsychiatry: thirty-five years' experience. *Medscape Psychiatry & Mental Health eJournal*, *2*(4). Available at: http://www.medscape.com/viewarticle/431064
Majumdar, A. K. (2007). Advances in telemedicine and its usage in India. In *15th International Conference on Advanced Computing and Communications*, IEEE.
Malhotra, S., & Chakrabarti, S. (2013d). Telepsychiatry: A new paradigm for mental healthcare. *Journal of Postgraduate Medicine and Research.* Available at: http://www.jaypeejournals.com/eJournals/ShowText.aspx?ID=2844&Type=FREE&TYP=TOP&IN=_eJournals/images/JPLOGO.gif&IID=222&isPDF=YES. Last accessed December 15, 2015.
Malhotra, S., Chakrabarti, S., Gupta, A., Mehta, A., Shah, R., Kumar, V., et al. (2013a). A self-guided relaxation module for telepsychiatric services: Development, usefulness, and feasibility. *International Journal of Psychiatry in Medicine, 46*(4), 325–337.
Malhotra, S., Chakrabarti, S., Gupta, A., Mehta, A., Sharma, M., Kumar, V., et al. (2012). Training non-specialists in clinical evaluation using video conferencing: feasibility and effectiveness. In *Proceedings of 8th International Telemedicine Conference*, India (pp. 66–67).
Malhotra, S., Chakrabarti, S., & Shah, R. (2013b). Telepsychiatry: Promise, potential, and challenges. *Indian Journal of Psychiatry, 55*(1), 3–11.
Malhotra, S., Chakrabarti, S., Shah, R., Gupta, A., Jassal, G. D., Upadhyaya, S. K., et al. (2013c). Computerised system of diagnosis and treatment in telepsychiatry: Experience and feasibility study of diagnostic module. *Indian Journal of Psychiatry, 55*, S47.
Malhotra, S., Chakrabarti, S., Shah, R., Gupta, A., Mehta, A., Nithya, B., Kumar, V. (2014b). Development of a novel diagnostic system for a telepsychiatric application: A pilot validation study. *BMC Research Notes,* 7, 508. Available from http://www.biomedcentral.com/1756-0500/7/508. doi:10.1186/1756-0500-7-508
Malhotra, S., Chakrabarti, S., Shah, R., Mehta, A., Gupta, A., & Sharma, M. (2015a). A novel screening and diagnostic tool for child and adolescent psychiatric disorders for telepsychiatry. *Indian Journal of Psychological Medicine, 37*(3), 288–298.
Malhotra, S., Chakrabarti, S., Shah, R., Sharma, M., Sharma, K. (2015c). An online clinical decision support system for child and adolescent psychiatric disorders: Validity, reliability, and feasibility of the diagnostic sub-system. In: *Proceedings of AACAP's 62nd Annual Meeting.* Available at: https://aacap.confex.com/aacap/2015/webprogram/Paper24524.html
Malhotra, S., Chakrabarti, S., Shah, R., Sharma, M., Sharma, K. P., Malhotra, A., Upadhyaya, S. K., Margoob, M. A., Dar, M., Jassal, G. D. (in press). Telepsychiatry clinical decision support system used by non-psychiatrists in remote areas: Validity and reliability of Diagnostic module. *Indian Journal of Medical Research.*
Malhotra, S., Chakrabarti, S., Shah, R., Sharma, M., Sharma, K., & Singh, H. (2015b). Diagnostic accuracy and feasibility of a net-based application for diagnosing common psychiatric disorders. *Psychiatry Research, 230*(2), 369–376.
Malhotra, S., & Patra, B. (2014). Prevalence of child and adolescent psychiatric disorders in India: a systematic review and meta-analysis. *Child and Adolescent Psychiatry and Mental Health, 8*, 22. doi:10.1186/1753-2000-8-22.
Merikangas, K. R., Nakamura, E. F., & Kessler, R. C. (2009). Epidemiology of mental disorders in children and adolescents. *Dialogues in Clinical Neuroscience, 11*(1), 7–20.
Myers, K. M., Palmer, N. B., & Geyer, J. R. (2011). Research in child and adolescent telemental health. *Child and Adolescent Psychiatric Clinics of North America, 20*(1), 155–171. doi:10.1016/j.chc.2010.08.007.

Myers, K. M., Sulzbacher, S., & Melzer, S. M. (2004). Telepsychiatry with children and adolescents: Are patients comparable to those evaluated in usual outpatient care? *Telemedicine Journal and e-health, 10*(3), 278–285.

Myers, K. M., Valentine, J. M., & Melzer, S. M. (2007). Feasibility, acceptability, and sustainability of telepsychiatry with children and adolescents. *Psychiatric Services*, 58, 1493–1496.

Myers, K. M., Valentine, J. M., & Melzer, S. M. (2008). Child and adolescent telepsychiatry: Utilization and satisfaction. *Telemedicine Journal and e-health, 14*, 131–137.

Myers, K., Valentine, J., Morganthaler, R., & Melzer, S. M. (2006). Telepsychiatry with incarcerated youth. *The Journal of Adolescent Health, 38*, 643–648.

Myers, K. M., Vander Stoep, A., McCarty, C. A., Klein, J. B., Palmer, N. B., Geyer, J. R., et al. (2010). Child and adolescent telepsychiatry: variations in utilization, referral patterns and practice trends. *Journal of Telemedicine and Telecare, 16*(3), 128–133.

Myers, K., Vander Stoep, A., Zhou, C., McCarty, C. A., & Katon, W. (2015). Effectiveness of a Telehealth Service Delivery Model for Treating Attention-Deficit/Hyperactivity Disorder: A community-based randomized controlled trial. *Journal of the American Academy of Child and Adolescent Psychiatry, 54*(4), 263–274. doi:10.1016/j.jaac.2015.01.009. Epub 2015 Jan 29.

Nelson, E. L., Barnard, M., & Cain, S. (2003). Treating childhood depression over videoteleconferencing. *Telemedicine Journal and e-health, 9*, 49–55.

Nessa, A., Al Ameen, M., Ullah, S., & Kwak, K. (2010). Applicability of Telemedicine in Bangladesh: Current Status and Future Prospects. *The International Arab Journal of Information Technology, 7*, 138–146.

No author. (1998). Nepal sets up telepsychiatry program. *Telemedicine and virtual reality, 3*(4), 46.

Pakyurek, M., Yellowlees, P., Hilty, D. (2010). The child and adolescent telepsychiatry consultation: can it be a more effective clinical process for certain patients than conventional practice? *Telemedicine journal and e-health, 16*, 289–292.

Patel, V., Flisher, A. J., Nikapota, A., & Malhotra, S. (2008). Promoting child and adolescent mental health in low and middle income countries. *Journal of Child Psychology and Psychiatry, 49*, 313–334. doi:10.1111/j.1469-7610.2007.01824.x.

Perednia, D. A., & Allen, A. (1995). Telemedicine technology and clinical applications. *JAMA, 273*, 483–488.

Pesamaa, L., Ebeling, H., Kuusimaki, M. L., Winblad, I., Isohanni, M., & Moilanen, I. (2004). Videoconferencing in child and adolescent telepsychiatry: A systematic review of the literature. *Journal of Telemedicine and Telecare, 10*(4), 187–192.

Qadir, M. A. (2014). *Telemedicine: A success story of assessment and rehabilitation of psychiatric patients in Rajanpur District of Southern Punjab, Pakistan*. Available at: http://www.medetel.eu/download/2014/parallel_sessions/presentation/day3/Telemedicine_A_Success_Story.pdf

Rahman, A. (2006). E-mental health in Pakistan: A pilot study of training and supervision in child psychiatry using the internet. *Psychiatric Bulletin, 30*, 149–152.

Savin, D., Glueck, D. A., Chardavoyne, J., Yager, J., & Novins, D. K. (2011). Bridging cultures: Child psychiatry via videoconferencing. *Child and Adolescent Psychiatric Clinics of North America, 20*(1), 125–134.

Sharan, P., & Malhotra, S. (2007). Telepsychiatry: The bridge across the access gap in child and adolescent mental health. *Journal of Indian Association for Child and Adolescent Mental Health, 3*, 18–20.

Sinha, S. K., & Kaur, J. (2011). National mental health programme: Manpower development scheme of eleventh five-year plan. *Indian Journal of Psychiatry, 53*(3), 261–265.

Spaulding, R., Belz, N., DeLurgio, S., & Williams, A. R. (2010). Cost savings of telemedicine utilization for child psychiatry in a rural Kansas community. *Telemedicine Journal and e-health, 16*(8), 867–871.

Starling, J., & Foley, S. (2006). From pilot to permanent service: Ten years of paediatric telepsychiatry. *Journal of Telemedicine and Telecare, 12*(3), 80–82(3).

Starling, J., Rosina, R., Nunn, K., & Dossetor, D. (2003). Child and adolescent telepsychiatry in New South Wales: Moving beyond clinical consultation. *Australasian Psychiatry*, 11, S117–S121.

Stoep, A. V., & Myers, K. (2013). Methodology for conducting the children's attention-deficit hyperactivity disorder telemental health treatment study in multiple underserved communities. *Clinical Trials, 0*, 1–10.

Szeftel, R., Mandelbaum, S., Sulman-Smith, H., Naqvi, S., Lawrence, L., Szeftel, Z., et al. (2011). Telepsychiatry for children with developmental disabilities: Applications for patient care and medical education. *Child and Adolescent Psychiatric Clinics of North America, 20*(1), 95–111.

Thara, R., John, S., & Rao, K. (2008). Telepsychiatry in Chennai, India: The SCARF experience. *Behavioral Sciences & the Law, 26*, 315–322. doi:10.1002/bsl.816.

Turvey, C., Coleman, M., Dennison, O., Drude, K., Goldenson, M., Hirsch, P., et al. (2013). ATA practice guidelines for video-based online mental health services. *Telemedicine Journal and e-health, 19*, 722–730.

Wagnild, G., Leenknecht, C., & Zauher, J. (2006). Psychiatrists' satisfaction with telepsychiatry. *Telemedicine Journal and e-health, 12*(5), 546–551.

Wynchank, S., & Fortuin, J. (2010). Telepsychiatry in South Africa—Present and future. *South African Journal of Psychiaatry, 16*(1).

Yellowlees, P. M., Hilty, D. M., Marks, S. L., Neufeld, J., & Bourgeois, J. A. (2008). A retrospective analysis of a child and adolescent e-mental health program. *Journal of American Academy of Child and Adolescent Psychiatry, 47*, 103–107.

Chapter 25
Bridging the Mental Health Gap in India: Issues and Perspectives

Pratap Sharan and Saurabh Kumar

Abstract Almost 20 % of children and adolescents suffer from some form of mental illness, but a very small proportion of them are able to access mental health services that results in a huge treatment gap. The situation is particularly grim in India where almost 30 % of population of the country consists of children in the age group between 0 and 14 years. There could be several possible reasons for this gap ranging from stigma associated with mental illnesses, lack of resources for mental health and apathy on part of policy makers to counter this problem. Although several steps have been taken like formulation of national mental health policy and programme(s) to increase coverage for mental health in India, a lot remains to be done. In the chapter, we emphasize that access to mental health care is a human right and describe the current mental health resource situation for children and adolescents in India, and highlight certain alternate modes of service delivery like school mental health services, provision of services at primary care and use of technology to reach remote areas. We also emphasizes the need for multidisciplinary training of child and adolescent mental health professionals, introduction of topics related to child and adolescent mental health in psychiatry, pediatrics and undergraduate curriculum as well as task sharing/task shifting approaches.

Keywords Child · Adolescent · Treatment gap · Mental health policy · Primary health care · School mental health

P. Sharan (✉) · S. Kumar
Department of Psychiatry, All India Institute of Medical Sciences,
New Delhi 110029, India
e-mail: pratapsharan@gmail.com

S. Kumar
e-mail: saurabhksingh.singh@gmail.com

S. Malhotra and P. Santosh (eds.), *Child and Adolescent Psychiatry*,
DOI 10.1007/978-81-322-3619-1_25

Abbreviations

ADHD	Attention deficit hyperactivity disorder
CAP	Child and adolescent psychiatry
DALY	Disability adjusted life year
INTERCAMHS	International Alliance for Child and Adolescent Mental Health and Schools
LMIC	Low- and middle-income countries
NOS	Not otherwise specified
NIMHANS	National Institute of Mental Health and Neurosciences
NGO	Non-government organization
NMHP	National Mental Health Program
OPD	Out Patient Department
PGIMER	Postgraduate Institute of Medical Education and Research

25.1 Introduction

India is home to a huge population of children and adolescents, with age group between 0 and 14 years forming approximately 30 % of the entire population of the country (Office of Registrar General & Census Commissioner India 2011). The number of adolescents estimated to be in India is approximately 243 million, which is almost one quarter of the country's population (Unicef India 2011). It is of utmost importance that health need of this population is met to ensure that they get the opportunities to fulfill their potential. World Health Organization (WHO) puts mental health at par with physical health for any individual's overall well-being. Mental illnesses can cause significant morbidity and mortality and put an enormous burden on countries financial resources. It is pertinent in this regard that almost 50 % of mental disorder start during childhood and adolescence and persist into adulthood (Kessler et al. 2007). Occurrence of mental disorders at an early age prevents the child from achieving a sense of identity and self worth, forge meaningful relationships and achieve a productive life.

The data collected by WHO for the 'Atlas'on the global child and adolescent mental health service reflects a huge deficit of resources particularly in low- and middle-income countries (LMIC) (World Psychiatric Association, International Association for Child, Adolescent Psychiatry and Allied Professions and World Health Organization 2005). Only a small proportion of child and adolescent population in LMIC access any type of mental health services—children and adolescents form only 12 % of the patient population in mental health outpatient facilities and less than 6 % in all other types of mental health facilities (World Psychiatric Association, International Association for Child, Adolescent Psychiatry and Allied Professions and World Health Organization 2005). The situation is alarming if we consider the fact that approximately 88 % of the worlds adolescent population live in LMIC (Unicef India 2011). The situation, if anything is worse in India, with estimates suggests that almost 29 million children and adolescents suffer from mental disorders, while only 1 receive any form of care (Malhotra and Patra 2014; Shastri 2008). It is stated that lack of resources, failure to recognize those in need and lack of evidence base to guide treatment could be some of the reasons for the gross deficiencies in the services (Belfer 2007).

This chapter talks about the need for robust epidemiological studies to determine the prevalence of mental illnesses in this population as well as identify various risk factors and protective factors, which can help in planning proper services to address the health care requirements of children and adolescents. We will also emphasize that access to care is a human right issue, and that a policy framework is needed for planning a robust health service delivery system. This chapter highlights the relative paucity of mental resources for children and adolescents and possible ways like school health services or using technology to develop alternative modalities to deliver needed services.

25.2 Extent of Mental Health Problems

Current data suggest that mental health disorders account for 7.4 % of all disability adjusted life years (DALY) worlwide (Whiteford et al. 2013). The data on DALYs specifically due to child and mental health disorders are not available. Several authors have pointed out the limitations of DALYs, while measuring disease burden especially in children as DALYS are age biased with greatest weight being given to individuals who are 25 years of age or above as they are believed to be more important in fulfilling the societal role (e.g. 1 year at age 2, has only 20 % of weight at age 25) (Anand and Hanson 1997). Further, DALY's have not been computed for many disorders that are common during childhood and adolescence.

Epidemiological studies conducted in developed countries suggest that approximately one in every five child suffers from mental illnesses (Unicef India 2011). Indian studies have reported wide variations in prevalence of mental disorders in children and adolescents, ranging from 0.5 (Nandi 2000) to 29.4 % (Singh et al. 1983). In a recent meta-analysis, the prevalence was reported as 6.5 % in community samples and 23.3 % in the school-going population (Malhotra and Patra 2014). The differences in the rates can be attributed to methodological differences, e.g. diagnostic criteria, instruments and informants or sampling methods (Merikangas et al. 2009). General population studies conducted in India show markedly lower rates of depression, substance use disorders and disruptive behaviour disorders and a greater rate of sub-syndromal (e.g. behaviour disorder NOS) and mono-symptomatic conditions (e.g. enuresis and stuttering) compared to Western studies (Belfer 2008).

The exact aetiology of mental disorders might still be elusive but several potential risk factors have been identified during childhood, which results in higher occurrence of mental disorders. Some of the more common risk factors are child abuse (both physical and sexual), loss of parents (due to death or separation), adverse familial environment and substance abuse (Fergusson and Horwood 2001). A cross-sectional study conducted in India identified living in urban areas compared to rural areas, and physical and sexual abuse were significantly correlated with common mental disorders in youth, whereas being able to talk about the problems was identified as a protective factor (Fernandes et al. 2013). A longitudinal UK-based study found that emotional disorders were specifically related to physical illness, change in number of parents, number of children staying together and poor mental health of the mother. Similarly, conduct disorder was seen more commonly in children from low socioeconomic strata and if they were living in a rented accommodation or in reconstituted family. Mothers' low level of education and changes in her mental health over time were also significant risk factors (McGinnity et al. 2005). There is dearth of such longitudinal studies in India.

There is an urgent need to carry out more methodologically sound community-based epidemiological studies to address the lack of national statistics on mental health in children. Ideally, these studies should be prospective in nature to map out the natural course of disorders and lifetime co-morbidity. Prospective studies would also help in establishing the role of multiple risk factors and their interaction over time producing multiple outcomes. There would be many challenges in conducting research on epidemiology on children and adolescents in India such as age group ascertainment, selection of instruments, standardization and validation of instruments, translation of instruments, research design (single stage or multiple stages), research methodology (sampling methods, etc.), types of disorders to be included, setting (school or household), number of informants (parents, teachers), validation, etc (Sharan and Sagar 2008). These challenges need to be taken up and studies have to be carried out in a nationally representative sample of children and adolescents, as lack of data on various facets of mental illnesses like its prevalence, course, etiological factors and degree of health services utilization has impeded efforts in establishing mental health policy for this population.

Development of a legal and policy framework may provide the needed impetus for addressing existent service gaps. The next two sections discuss various laws, which deal with children and adolescents and the need for separate mental health policy for children.

25.3 Mental Health Services as Human Rights Issue

Human rights refer to the freedom and entitlements concerned with the protection of the inherent dignity and equality of every human being and are not just moral entitlements but are guaranteed by law (UN Office of the High Commissioner for Human Rights 2000). The United Nation convention on rights of children to which India is a signatory clearly enunciates the various duties of the state in ensuring the protection of human rights of all children. It also lays special emphasis on the rights of vulnerable population. Children suffering from mental illnesses are prone to abuses, violence and to gross neglect. Mental health legislations are important for ensuring that rights of mentally ill persons.

The Mental Health Care Bill, 2013 has several specific provisions for children and adolescents (Ministry of Health and Family Welfare 2013). The admission of minors under the age of 18 years requires evaluation by two independent professionals (one psychiatrist and one psychiatrist/mental health professional/medical practitioner) to ascertain that the admission is in the best interests of the minor (from the perspective of health, well-being or safety). Minors should be kept separately from the adults in an environment suitable to their developmental needs and the admission should be notified to the concerned board within 72 h. If the minor has to be kept admitted beyond 30 days, permission has to be taken from mental health review commission. The bill prohibits electro-conclusive therapy to minors though several authors have contended that this treatment modality may be useful in certain cases. The bill has generated a debate, but it correctly emphasizes the human rights perspective. Similarly, the Disability Amendment Act, 2012 has widened the scope of affirmative action by including new disorders like specific learning disability in its ambit (Ministry of Social Justice & Empowerment 2012).

The Juvenile Justice (Care and Protection of Children) Act, 2000 (amended in 2011) caters to juveniles in conflict with law and to children in need of care and protection (Ministry of Women and Child Development 2014). The basic spirit of juvenile justice system is that this population cannot be treated at par with adults committing crime as their immaturity prevents them from understanding the consequences of their deed and every corrective step should be taken so that they can be rehabilitated in the community to which they belong. The act ensures that juveniles are not sent to prison but to correctional facilities. The offence committed by a juvenile should be tried in juvenile courts and the Act has provisions for the establishment of juvenile welfare boards in all districts. The law requires that the principal magistrate of Juvenile justice board has special knowledge or training in child psychology, which reflects the intention of the government that such children are seen as having mental health issues requiring specialized care. Though systemic data on mental health issues in children in conflict with law in India is lacking, there are several international studies that points towards higher incidence of internalizing (i.e. depression and anxiety) and externalizing disorders (i.e. conduct disorder, oppositional defiant disorder, ADHD), psychosis-related symptoms as well as substance abuse and dependence in juvenile delinquent populations (Colins et al. 2009).

The quality of correctional facilities in the country, however, is an area of continuing concern. Most of them are closed institutions that deprive the children and adolescents of their liberty and expose them to norms of inmate subcultures for long periods. Inmates are at higher risk of developing psychological problems (Gupta 2011). Studies show that at least two-thirds of males and three-fourths of females in juvenile homes meet the criteria for one or more psychiatric disorders and about 20 % of them have serious mental illness (Teplin et al. 2002). It is difficult to ascertain whether these disorders were consequence of detention or led to the detention. Either ways, the moot point is that these children have special mental health needs and they should be diverted from criminal justice system by developing robust in-home and community-based services to prevent serious crises. Different services like crisis stabilization, family support, respite and in-home psychiatric care should be provided. With effective and evidence-based treatment and supports, these children and youth can experience success in the home, school and community (Skowyra and Cocozza 2007). Child and adolescent mental health specialists thus have an important role in advising the legal authorities regarding the need for continued support for such children in correctional homes.

Child abuse (both physical and sexual) has been shown to be an important determinant of mental illness. The Government of India has recently passed the Protection of Children from Sexual Offenses Act 2012, which defines various punishments to be given in case of such offenses. There are several other legislations like The Child Labour (Prohibition and Regulation) Act, 1986 and Right to Education Act 2009, which have mental health implications. We can see that India has many legislations for protecting the rights of children but faulty or partial implementation limit the purpose for which they were formulated.

25.4 Developing a Comprehensive Mental Health Policy

The National Policy for Children 1974 was the first policy document concerning the needs and rights of children that recognized them as an important asset to the nation. It emphasized that children should figure prominently in any efforts being made towards developing human resources and national programmes should be developed to help them grow in all domains so that children become assets in nation building. The government adopted a resolution on the National Policy for Children in 2013. It aims to address mental, emotional, cognitive, social and cultural development of the child in totality (Ministry of Women and Child Development 2013); however, it fails to specify how mental health issues of children and adolescents will be addressed.

An effective mental health policy is central to any country's effort towards providing mental health services to its population. The data from Child Mental Health Atlas shows that most LMIC lack separate mental health policy for children. Among the 66 reporting countries, only 6.3 % of African as against 66.7 % of European countries reported the presence of a child and adolescent mental health programme; and 0 % of low-income and 78 % of high-income countries reported having a document related to policy on child and adolescent mental health (World Psychiatric Association, International Association for Child, Adolescent Psychiatry and Allied Professions and World Health Organization 2005).

India formulated a national mental health policy in 2014, which recognizes children as vulnerable population requiring special care but it does not address their needs specifically. Hence, it would be desirable to have a specific mental health policy for children to address their development-related issues, because developmental stages determine the vulnerability to develop disorders, affect the manner in which disorders manifest and determine how best treatment should be approached. Most childhood and adolescent mental disorders persist into adulthood, so development of early and specific interventions can reduce the possibility of long-term impairment and the financial burden associated with them. It will not be an overstatement to suggest that failure to develop such a policy is an important reason for the enormous unmet need of children and adolescent with mental health issues and persistence of barriers to their care (WHO 2005).

Guidance on how to develop a child and adolescent mental health policy in LMIC is available as a part of the WHO's Mental Health Policy and Service Guidance Package (WHO 2005). Policies must explicitly focus on providing high-quality care in settings where children are most comfortable like family settings and educational settings. The services in primary health care also need to be upgraded as they are often the first contact point of the children in need of intervention. Services at specialist mental health care should be able to take comprehensive care of more seriously ill children and should be equipped with all type of services required to help and guide these children. It should be mentioned that young people are often dependent on others to advocate on their behalf. It is the duty of mental health professionals along with people in other spheres like in legal and media fields to pitch for the formulation and implementation of mental health policy for children and adolescents. Through joint efforts, only a political will and sustainable financing can be ensured for such policy (Belfer 2007).

Legal and policy frameworks have to be implemented—and this calls for resources (financial, manpower, institutional) that is lacking in LMIC countries. The next section will focus on resources and possible evidence-based alternatives that can be adopted to reduce treatment gap at the population level.

25.5 Resources

25.5.1 Financial

The national mental health policy adopted in 2014 by India emphasizes the need to increase allocation of funds for mental health services. It states that "spending on health by the government is not expenditure but a social investment and a social right"; (Ministry of Health and Family Welfare 2014) but the fact remains that India spends only 0.06 % of its total health budget on mental health (WHO 2011). There could be several reasons for this dismal allocation: low priority of mental health needs, absence of need based policy assessment, non-recognition of mental illnesses, low resources and failure to optimize available resources (McDaid et al. 2008).

Due to limited government spending on mental health care in LMIC, the patient or the family has to bear most of the economic burden. Compared to developed countries where funds for mental health services are provided through combination of taxation, social health insurance and private insurance, many LMIC like India are dependent on out-of-the-pocket payments (Saxena et al. 2003). Evidences suggest that out-of-pocket payment may not be an ideal mode of funding as it can deter patients from service utilization and can lead to inequitable distribution of services in favour of people who can afford it leading to marginalization of poor patients (Saxena et al. 2003). A careful balance should be struck between different methods of financing and wherever possible government should try to ensure mandatory universal access to mental health services either through tax-based system or social insurance cover. In cases of countries where government cannot bear out the cost single handedly it should try to establish an effective public private partnership by involving private insurance companies.

25.5.2 Human Resources

Any health care system cannot achieve its objective without trained and adequate human resource as they are at the heart of delivering the services. The overwhelming shortage of adequate manpower in the field of mental health services is well known. In India the number of psychiatrist, psychologist, nurses and social workers per 100,000 people are 0.31, 0.04, 0.16 and 0.03, respectively (WHO 2011). The current training infrastructure produces about 320 psychiatrists, 50 clinical psychologists, 25 psychiatric social workers and 185 psychiatric nurses annually—which are too few to fill the deficit (Sinha and Kaur 2011). The other facet of the problem is that even the available resources are distributed in skewed fashion with about nine states accounting for more than one-third of the population having more than 90 % deficit (Thirunavukarasu and Thirunavukarasu 2010). Under the 11th 5-year plan, the Government of India has increased financial support for developing qualified mental health professionals. The scheme will establish 11 centres of excellence and support various government colleges and state run mental hospitals in starting or increasing the uptake of postgraduate students. The scheme is expected to yield 104 psychiatrists, 416 clinical psychologists, 416 psychiatric social workers and 820 psychiatric nurses annually in addition to current trainee turnover (Sinha and Kaur 2011). However, there is no provision for increasing manpower that would address the mental health needs of children and adolescents.

Few organized facilities for psychiatric care of children and adolescents are there in India. If we assume that 1 facility is required per 100,000 children, it is estimated that India needs at least 10,500 facilities for children and adolescents (Shastri 2009). Compared to this requirement, we have only 164 child guidance clinics, suggesting that mental health needs of large population of children are unmet (Shastri 2009). There are very few centres in government sector with exclusive inpatient treatment and dedicated faculty to provide child and adolescent mental health services. The child guidance clinics in most hospitals are once a week affair, where services are provided either by general adult psychiatrists or a visiting mental health professional (psychiatrist/psychologist) in Pediatrics OPD (Beaglehole et al. 2008).

There is a lack of uniformity in training in child and adolescent psychiatry across the postgraduate training facilities in India ranging from no training in most places to 3 or 4 month training in certain centres. Although the need for super specialization courses in Child and Adolescent Psychiatry (CAP) was identified as early as in 1979, in a workshop on postgraduate training of psychiatrists held at NIMHANS, only two institutions in the country are offering super-specialty training. Super specialists in the field may play many key roles such as, ensuring advanced evidence-based standards of care, refining the research agenda and creating educational models for further training in the specialty.

Task shifting, i.e. developing a new cadre of mental health professionals with either less training or narrowly tailored training can be another strategy for overcoming manpower shortage (Government of India 2014). One example is training medical officers to develop expertise in diagnosing mild non-complicated cases so that specialist could focus on more complex cases. National Institute of Mental Health and Neurosciences (NIMHANS) has been providing training in child and adolescent psychiatry (CAP) for a period of 3 months to qualified psychiatrists, clinical psychologists, psychiatric social workers and pediatricians from several parts of the country (Beaglehole et al. 2008).

Including child and adolescent psychiatry training in undergraduate medical education is also important. Currently, the undergraduates are provided separate training in pediatrics in their final year of teaching. It would be advisable to design curricula for integrating the training in child and adolescent psychiatry along with pediatrics and would require collaborations between these departments.

25.5.3 Developing Alternate Modalities for Service Delivery

There is a huge shortage of specialized mental health facilities in general and child and adolescent facilities in particular and it would take enormous time and resources to fill the gap. To circumvent this problem we need to develop other mechanisms through which mental health services could be provided.

25.5.4 Integration of Child and Adolescent Mental Health Services with Primary Health Care

It has been advocated for long that mental health services should be integrated into primary health care system and indeed this is one of the objectives of the National Mental Health Program. Currently, there are about 24,500 primary health care centres in India (Giel et al. 1982) with a large reach in rural populations of the country. There is a high prevalence of mental disorders amongst children and adolescents attending primary health care services. In a study carried out at four different countries including India, the frequency of mental disorders was found to be between 12 and 29 % amongst children attending primary health care (Kelleher et al. 2006). Despite this high prevalence, the primary health workers were able to recognize only between 10 and 22 % of the cases. This reflects that there is inadequate skill amongst these providers to fully address the social and emotional needs of children. Another facet of the problem is that even if primary health workers recognize mental health problems and refer clients to mental health systems, less than half of the families' follow through on the referrals (World Health Organization, World Organization of National Colleges, Academies and Academic Associations of General Practitioners/Family Physicians 2008). At least partly the lack of follow through could be due to the shortage of mental health services, the distance between primary and specialist care facilities and lack of communication between the two types of facilities. This problem can be tackled by collaborative or shared care model in which joint consultations and interventions are held between primary care workers and mental health specialists or by providing adequate training to primary care workers with secondary components like systems for referrals in complicated cases. The WHO states that integrated care would enhance access to services and decrease violation of human rights of patients suffering from mental illness. The services would be more cost-effective and would generate better health outcome (Ministry of Health and Family Welfare 2011). In 2014, the Government of Karnataka launched a programme with the name 'Manochaitanya' with an aim of integrating mental health care in all public health care institutions including primary health centres of the state. Hopefully, this programme would incorporate elements for monitoring and evaluation and provide a model for other states.

A lot of groundwork including an extensive policy and relevant legislation would be needed to ensure successful integration. Despite good intentions, only 127 districts out of 626 districts in India have implemented the District Mental Health program and even in these districts a large number of primary health care doctors have not been trained (Jacobs et al. 2012). The reasons for shortfalls in this process include poor infrastructure, overburdened primary health systems, inappropriate training, inadequate financing, professional apathy and lack of human resources (Venkatesh et al. 2015). These shortcomings need be addressed to meet the huge treatment gap in mental health services.

One of the biggest barriers in accessing mental health facilities by families is social stigma. They find it extremely difficult to accept that their child has a mental health problem. The situation is further worsened by fear of using psychotropic medications on their children. Several studies have shown that stigma towards people with mental illness is very high. In one of the community-based studies done in southern part of India, it was found that the prevalence of stigma towards mentally ill people was present in almost 75 % of people (Thara and Srinivasan 2000). There could be several reasons for this stigma like lack of marriage proposals especially for women, fear of rejection by society or the need to hide the fact from others (Thornicroft et al. 2010). Although stigma associated with mental illnesses occurs all over the world, several studies have pointed out that it to be commoner in low resource countries and in vulnerable populations like poor people, women and ethnic minorities (Thornicroft et al. 2016). Studies have also shown that there is paucity of literature from LMIC groups about effective interventions to reduce stigma. Authors have also cautioned that the strategies that have been shown to be beneficial in developed nations should not be overgeneralized and specific cultural considerations should be kept in mind while devising any strategy (Mascayano et al. 2015). For example, in Indian context it has been suggested that public stigma could be reduced best if it is promoted that people with severe mental illness like schizophrenia can achieve a level where they can perform the roles expected from them socially or by traditions of Dharma rather than by promoting generic stereotyped messages like 'people with mental illnesses are not dangerous' (Weare 2004).

25.5.5 School Mental Health Services

Schools are spaces of learning for children and adolescents and are the place where they spend much of their waking time. Schools can be ideal places for early detection and intervention for mental health issues in a child as such issues reflects in their performance. Historically, professional consultations occur in school only when a child has been diagnosed with a disorder. Ideally, the integration should happen at all levels from universal promotion and prevention of mental well-being to tertiary intervention, which will result in optimization of the learning environment.

The International Alliance for Child and Adolescent Mental Health and Schools (INTERCAMHS) provides the following broad approach to school mental health services (Bharat et al. 2008):

(a) Universal initiatives: This will reach all the students and would mainly be involved in identifying and addressing the risk factors for developing mental illness and promotion of mental well-being. This could also be utilized to identify children with more in-depth needs.
(b) Selective interventions: Around 10–15 % of children who are at greater risk for developing mental illness due to identified risk factors can be benefited by it. The mental health professional can guide the school for the interventions required.
(c) Indicated intervention: It would typically reach about 10–15 % of the student body providing intensive services to youths exhibiting emotional and behavioural problems, but who do not meet diagnostic criteria.
(d) Treatment for 3–12 % of children who might have diagnosable mental illness.

NIMHANS has been at forefront in India in providing school health services. The child psychiatry unit of NIMHANS started the teachers' orientation programme in 1976 and over the years several such programmes have been carried out both in the city of Bangalore and the surrounding rural areas including institutions for special children (e.g. hearing impaired and orthopedically challenged). Through these programmes, teachers were trained in basic mental health issues and problems of children and adolescents and with skills to identify these problems. These programmes were complemented by 1 year skill training in counselling skills for interested teachers (Thara and Patel 2010).

NIMHANS also developed student enrichment programmes for rural adolescents in which guidance was provided to students in various skills like effective study methods, principles of mental health, understanding self and others, interpersonal relations and planning for the future. Based on the concept of 10 generic life skills introduced by WHO, NIMHANS developed a Cascade Model of Life Skills Education and trained people over 5 days to become master trainers in life skills, who would further train other teachers. The programme is run in 265 government secondary schools of four districts of Karnataka. Navodaya Schools (Southern Region) have also initiated the LSE in their schools (Thara and Patel 2010).

There is a draft guideline for school mental health programme in India (Thara and Patel 2010); However, its successful implementation would require that

- It is made an inherent part of the National Mental Health Program
- It is integrated with ongoing programmes of the Departments of Education and Health
- It encourages active involvement of multiple stakeholders—teachers, families and community leaders
- It has a large preventive component that includes training for school staff in recognizing stresses that may lead to mental health problems as well as early signs of emotional problems
- It is supported by presence of good referral system for children with diagnosed mental disorders which is coordinated by written protocols, monitored for adherence and evaluated for effectiveness
- It is supported with provision of private, confidential and comfortable physical space at the school site for mental health services
- It is supported by a health professional team (or roles) consisting of a pediatrician, school counsellor, special educator and a mental health professional

As the next step, elements of the School Mental Health Program should be extended to include children and adolescents who are not attending schools for various reasons.

25.5.6 Collaboration with Non-Government Organizations (NGO)

The government and public enterprises have a primary role in provision of mental health services, but as it is clear that there is huge scarcity of such services—this gap can be partly bridged by NGOs. The NGOs can help in ensuring implementation of NMHP in their respective areas, either by providing services themselves by adopting PHCs in areas where government services are lacking; or can serve as training centres for mental health professionals in the community (Malhotra et al. 2013). There are a few documented examples of NGOs that work specifically in child and adolescent mental health in India. Some like Sangath, based in Goa, focus on child development and adolescent and youth health. Sangath provided Goa with its first multidisciplinary child development clinic.

25.5.7 *Use of Technology*

A key part of mental health care reform could be using technology to circumvent the human resource gap especially in remote and geographically isolated areas. One of the advancement in this field has been growth of telepsychiatry. It is defined as the use of information and communication technology to provide mental health services across distances (Department of Science and Technology, no date). Several studies have shown its viability in improving access to mental health services and also as an educational tool to enhance the skills of non-specialist in managing mental illnesses (Department of Science and Technology, no date).

Postgraduate Institute of Medical Education and Research (PGIMER), Chandigarh have recently completed a 4-year project (August 2010–September 2014) entitled "development and implementation of a model telepsychiatry application for delivering mental health care in remote areas (using a medical knowledge-based decision support system)". The PGIMER acted as a nodal centre for three peripheral centres at Srinagar, J&K, Srinagar, Uttrakhand and Bilaspur in Himachal Pradesh. It developed net-based computerized application for diagnosis and treatment of common psychiatric disorders and had separate version for adults and children [52]. The project has shown that services can be provides in far flung areas very effectively through technology. The field of telepsychiatry is very promising; however, some issues of legal and ethical nature like privacy, confidentiality, security of electronic data, duty of care and role in emergency situation, need to be addressed in greater detail (Department of Science and Technology, no date).

25.6 Conclusions

Considering the fact that a large proportion of Indian population consists of children and adolescents and a significant number of them have serious mental health issues, it is of extreme importance that we scale up our mental health services to meet the needs of the population. Addressing mental health needs of these children is important for their overall growth and failure to do so is depriving them of their basic human rights. Pressure groups needs to be created to advocate for the rights of these children and reinforce the commitment of governments, international organizations and other stakeholders to increase the allocation of financial and human resources for care of child and adolescent mental health issues. We need to develop alternate models of providing the services like integrating child mental health services with primary health care services to widen our reach. Organizations like NIMHANS have taken the initiative by showing how effectively these services can be provided in school settings and similarly PGIMER has shown how to use technology to reach far flung areas. Awareness created through the partnerships can lead to reduced stigma and discrimination faced by children and adolescents with mental health and behavioural issues. Finally, there is a need for a specific policy for children and adolescent mental health and relevant legislation to help bring mental health at par with physical health in India.

Key Points

- Approximately one in every five child suffers from mental illnesses.
- There is a huge service gap vis-à-vis the mental health needs of this population, which could be due to lack of resources (human and financial), lack of political will or due to stigma associated with mental illness.
- There should be robust legal and policy framework to guide services to those in need.
- Government should try to ensure mandatory universal access to mental health services either through tax-based system or social insurance cover.
- Integrating mental health services to primary health care, school mental health programmes, collaboration with NGO's and use of technology can help in reducing this gap.

References

Anand, S., & Hanson, K. (1997). Disability-adjusted life years: A critical review. *Journal of Health Economics, 16*(6), 685–702.

Beaglehole, R., Epping-Jordan, J., Patel, V., Chopra, M., Ebrahim, S., Kidd, M., et al. (2008). Improving the prevention and management of chronic disease in low-income and middle-income countries: a priority for primary health care. *The Lancet, 372*(9642), 940–949.

Belfer, M. L. (2007). Critical review of world policies for mental healthcare for children and adolescents. *Current Opinion in Psychiatry, 20*(4), 349–352.

Belfer, M. L. (2008). Child and adolescent mental disorders: The magnitude of the problem across the globe. *Journal of Child Psychology and Psychiatry, 49*(3), 226–236.

Bharat, S., Kumar, K. V., & Mukesh, Y. P. (2008). Clinical practice guidelines for school mental health program. *Indian Journal of Psychiatry, CPG*, 307–321. http://www.indianjpsychiatry.org/cpg2008.asp. Accessed May 16, 2016.

Colins, O., Vermeiren, R., Schuyten, G., & Broekaert, E. (2009). Psychiatric disorders in property, violent, and versatile offending detained male adolescents. *American Journal of Orthopsychiatry, 79*(1), 31–38.

Department of Science and Technology. (no date). *Development and implementation of a model telepsychiatry*. Available at: www.dst.gov.in/. Accessed May 16, 2016.

Fergusson, D. M., & Horwood, J. L. (2001). The christchurch health and development study: Review of findings on child and adolescent mental health. *Australian and New Zealand Journal of Psychiatry, 35*(3), 287–296.

Fernandes, A. C., Hayes, R. D., & Patel, V. (2013). Abuse and other correlates of common mental disorders in youth: A cross-sectional study in Goa, India. *Social Psychiatry and Psychiatric Epidemiology, 48*(4), 515–523.

Giel, R., de Arango, M. V., Climent, C. E., Harding, T. W., Ibrahim, H. H. A., Ladrido-Ignacio, L., et al. (1982). Childhood mental disorders in primary health care: Result of observations in four developing countries. *Journal of the American Academy of Child Psychiatry, 21*(2), 215.

Government of India. (2014). Primary Health Centre. Open Government Data (OGD) Platform India. Available at: https://data.gov.in/keywords/primary-health-centres. Accessed May 16, 2016.

Gupta, A. (2011). The juvenile justice (care and protection) act, 2000—A critique. *SSRN Electronic Journal* 07/2011. doi:10.2139/ssrn.1884927

Jacobs, B., Ir, P., Bigdeli, M., Annear, P. L., & Van Damme, W. (2012). Addressing access barriers to health services: An analytical framework for selecting appropriate interventions in low-income Asian countries. *Health Policy and Planning, 27*(4), 288–300.

Kelleher, K. J., Campo, J. V., & Gardner, W. P. (2006). Management of pediatric mental disorders in primary care: Where are we now and where are we going? *Current Opinion in Pediatrics, 18*(6), 649–653.

Kessler, R. C., Amminger, G. P., Aguilar-Gaxiola, S., Alonso, J., Lee, S., & Ustun, T. B. (2007). Age of onset of mental disorders: A review of recent literature. *Current Opinion in Psychiatry, 20*(4), 359–364.

Malhotra, S., Chakrabarti, S., & Shah, R. (2013). Telepsychiatry: Promise, potential, and challenges. *Indian Journal of Psychiatry, 55*(1), 3–11.

Malhotra, S., & Patra, B. (2014). Prevalence of child and adolescent psychiatric disorders in India: A systematic review and meta-analysis. *Child and Adolescent Psychiatry and Mental Health, 8*(1), 22.

Mascayano, F., Armijo, J. E., & Yang, L. H. (2015). Addressing stigma relating to mental illness in low-and middle-income countries. *Frontiers in Psychiatry, 6*. doi:10.3389/fpsyt.2015.00038

McDaid, D., Knapp, M., & Raja, S. (2008). Barriers in the mind: Promoting an economic case for mental health in low-and middle-income countries. *World Psychiatry, 7*(2), 79–86.

McGinnity, Á., Meltzer, H., Ford, T., & Goodman, R. (2005). *Mental health of children and young people in Great Britain, 2004*. Basingstoke: Palgrave Macmillan.

Merikangas, K. R., Nakamura, E. F., & Kessler, R. C. (2009). Epidemiology of mental disorders in children and adolescents. *Dialogues in Clinical Neuroscience, 11*(1), 7–20.

Ministry of Health and Family Welfare. (2011). *Government of India. Regional Workshops on National Mental Health Programme—A report*. Available at: http://mohfw.nic.in/…/ComprehensiveReport%20Part%201-78786581.pdf/. Accessed May 16, 2016.

Ministry of Health and Family Welfare. (2013). *The mental health care bill, 2013—PRS*. Available at: www.prsindia.org/. Accessed May 16 2016.

Ministry of Health and Family Welfare. (2014). *National mental health policy*. Available at: www.mohfw.nic.in/index1. Accessed May 16, 2016.

Ministry of Social Justice & Empowerment. (2012). *Draft rights of persons with disabilities bill 2012*. Available at http://socialjustice.nic.in/. Accessed May 16 2016.

Ministry of Women and Child Development. (2013). *The National Policy for Children, 2013—CHILDLINE India Foundation*. Available at: www.childlineindia.org.in/. Accessed May 16 2016.

Ministry of Women and Child Development. (2014). *The juvenile justice (care and protection of children) bill, 2014—PRS*. Available at: www.prsindia.org/. Accessed May 16, 2016.

Nandi, D. N. (2000). Psychiatric morbidity of a rural Indian community: Changes over a 20-year interval. *The British Journal of Psychiatry, 176*(4), 351–356.

Office of Registrar General & Census Commissioner India. (2011). *Census of India Website*. Available at: http://censusindia.gov.in/. Accessed May 16, 2016.

Saxena, S., Sharan, P., & Saraceno, B. (2003). Budget and financing of mental health services: Baseline information on 89 countries from WHO's project atlas. *Journal of Mental Health Policy and Economics, 6*(3), 135–143.

Sharan, P., & Sagar, R. (2008). Editorial: The need for national data on epidemiology of child and adolescent mental disorders. *Journal of Indian Association of Child and Adolescent Mental Health 4*(2), 22–27.

Shastri, P. (2008). Future perspective of planning child guidance services in India. *Indian Journal of Psychiatry, 50*(4), 241–243.

Shastri, P. C. (2009). Promotion and prevention in child mental health. *Indian Journal of Psychiatry, 51*(2), 88.

Singh, A. J., Shukla, J. D., Verma, B. I., Kumar, A., & Srivastava, R. N. (1983). An epidemiological study in childhood psychiatric disorders. *Indian Paediatrics, 20*, 167–172.

Sinha, S. K., & Kaur, J. (2011). National mental health programme: Manpower development scheme of eleventh five-year plan. *Indian Journal of Psychiatry, 53*(3), 261–265.

Skowyra, K. R., & Cocozza, J. J. (2007). Blueprint for change: A comprehensive model for the identification and treatment of youth with mental health needs in contact with the juvenile justice system. Available at: www.modelsforchange.net/…/Blueprint_for_Change_. Accessed May 16, 2016.

Teplin, L. A., Abram, K. M., McClelland, G. M., Dulcan, M. K., & Mericle, A. A. (2002). Psychiatric disorders in youth in juvenile detention. *Archives of General Psychiatry, 59*(12), 1133–1143.

Thara, R., & Patel, V. (2010). Role of non-governmental organizations in mental health in India. *Indian Journal of Psychiatry, 52*(7), 389–395.

Thara, R., & Srinivasan, T. N. (2000). How stigmatising is schizophrenia in India? *International Journal of Social Psychiatry, 46*(2), 135–141.

Thirunavukarasu, M., & Thirunavukarasu, P. (2010). Training and National deficit of psychiatrists in India—A critical analysis. *Indian Journal of Psychiatry, 52*(7), 83–88.

Thornicroft, G., Alem, A., Santos, R. A., Barley, E., Drake, R. E., Gregorio, G., et al. (2010). WPA guidance on steps, obstacles and mistakes to avoid in the implementation of community mental health care. *World Psychiatry, 9*(2), 67–77.

Thornicroft, G., Mehta, N., Clement, S., Evans-Lacko, S., Doherty, M., Rose, D., et al. (2016). Evidence for effective interventions to reduce mental-health-related stigma and discrimination. *The Lancet, 387*(10023), 1123–1132.

UN Office of the High Commissioner for Human Rights. (2000). Human rights: A basic handbook for UN staff. Available at: http://www.refworld.org/docid/483eac7b2.html. Accessed May 16, 2016.

Unicef India. (2011). Adolescence—An age of opportunity. UNICEF. Available at: http://unicef.in/PressReleases/87/. Accessed May 16, 2016.

Venkatesh, B. T., Andrews, T., Mayya, S. S., Singh, M. M., & Parsekar, S. S. (2015). Perception of stigma toward mental illness in South India. *Journal of Family Medicine and Primary Care, 4*(3), 449–453.

Weare, K. (2004). The international alliance for child and adolescent mental health and schools (INTERCAMHS). *Health Education, 104*(2), 65–67.

Whiteford, H. A., Degenhardt, L., Rehm, J., Baxter, A. J., Ferrari, A. J., Erskine, H. E., et al. (2013). Global burden of disease attributable to mental and substance use disorders: Findings from the Global Burden of Disease Study 2010. *The Lancet, 382*(9904), 1575–1586.

WHO. (2005). *Mental health policy, plans and programmes*. World Health Organization. Available at: http://www.who.int/mental_health/policy/services/. Accessed May 16, 2016.

WHO. (2011). *Mental health atlas*. Available at: www.who.int/mental_health/publications/mental_health_atlas_2011/en. Accessed May 16, 2016.

World Health Organization, World Organization of National Colleges, Academies and Academic Associations of General Practitioners/Family Physicians. (2008). *Integrating mental health into primary care: A global perspective*. World Health Organization. Available at: www.who.int/mental_health/resources/mentalhealth_PHC_2008.pdf. Accessed May 16, 2016.

World Psychiatric Association, International Association for Child, Adolescent Psychiatry and Allied Professions and World Health Organization. (2005). *Atlas: Child and adolescent mental health resources: Global concerns: implications for the future*. Geneva: World Health Organization.

Chapter 26
Teaching in Child Psychiatry: A Transcultural Perspective

Anula Nikapota

Abstract This chapter focuses on training needs in a transcultural context. Hence, a curriculum that could meet needs for global child mental health is presented with the rationale for the proposal. This includes a discussion on cultural differences and different service contexts. The purpose is to train clinicians who can meet need and are also empowered to contribute to service development and research.

Keywords Training · Culture · Global needs · Service systems

26.1 Introduction

This chapter will highlight significant issues relating to transcultural training and teaching in child psychiatry. The term transcultural training is used here to describe training that is relevant across the globe and hence across many different country situations.

Let us set the context. Children and adolescents under the age of 17 years form a significant part of a countries population varying from 25 to 35 % or more increasing to 50 % under 15 years in some countries. 90 % of the world's 2.2 billion children live in LAMIC country situations with very diverse cultural settings, and limited service provisions if at all for child mental health. Of this proportion, a significant number will live in the Asian continent. It is acknowledged that child psychiatric morbidity worldwide is about 20 % with variations in rate and morbidity. Recognition of child mental health as an integral part of child health, and of the needs of children with disorders has increased steadily over the last 35 years leading to the increased child development and child psychiatric

A. Nikapota (✉)
Emeritus Consultant Child and Adolescent Psychiatry, South London and Maudsley NHS Trust, Institute of Psychiatry Kings College London, South London, UK
e-mail: anula.nikapota@kcl.ac.uk

S. Malhotra and P. Santosh (eds.), *Child and Adolescent Psychiatry*,
DOI 10.1007/978-81-322-3619-1_26

services in many countries (WHO 2005), and training in child psychiatry in a variety of settings in countries with established and extensive child psychiatric services such as UK, USA, Canada, Australia, Singapore and other settings where child psychiatric services have developed but where the need far outweighs resource such as in Nigeria and India. It is hence appropriate to consider issues relating to a training curriculum to meet global need.

Such a training curriculum is designed for higher specialist training. It will also facilitate various changes and exchanges that are occurring all over the world. For example, training needs lead to a sharing of expertise from one country and cultural context to another. Trainers from one culture must relate to trainees and service systems in another culture. Centres of excellence will have transcultural groups of students whose training needs must be met. The global movement of clinicians has resulted in clinicians working in one context who may have grown up in another, and hence require cultural adaptation to work successfully. In fact, all clinicians will meet culturally diverse groups in their practice. Cultural diversity has increased as a result of people movement from one country to another for a variety of reasons resulting in multicultural populations. One must not forget that cultural diversity also exists within national boundaries with communities who share different beliefs and value systems as in India for example. The need for thinking about culture and training in culture and diversity has been accepted by many training schemes medical and non-medical particularly in the West. Curriculum content for training in cultural competence has been outlined by the American Academy of Child and Adolescent Psychiatry (Mian et al. 2010). Content includes the definition of the concept of cultural competence, the need to understand cultural identity and related differences in normal development and pathology and the skills and competence for working in a culture appropriate manner within systems of health care. A culture sensitivity process model used for medical education in the UK is presented as most appropriate for child psychiatry (Karnik and Dogra 2010). Kirmayer et al. (2008) discusses the success and experience of teaching cultural psychiatry to trainees in Canada. In an article that discusses the conceptual basis of cross-cultural medical education Betancourt (2003) argues the appropriateness of skills-based teaching rather than a categorical approach to ethnicity and culture when teaching medical graduates and also looks at how best to evaluate such training. These are all very appropriate developments but are insufficient for the purpose of multicultural training for global need, which has to go beyond a training in cultural competence, or cross-cultural psychiatry.

26.2 Training of Clinical Specialists for Global Child Mental Health

The training of clinical specialists to work in a transcultural context has to prepare trainees for a multifaceted role, which include advocacy for policy and service development, involvement in service planning, take an advisory role re-child protection and risk situations, undertake teaching, training and clinical supervision, as well as direct clinical work and developing liaison with other disciplines especially pediatrics and community medicine. Research activity is also part of the role. The challenge for such a training curriculum is that it should have relevant content for trainees whether in HIC or LAMIC, where there will be varying levels of resource as well as vulnerabilities and risk. The end goal of the training must be that it will empower specialist trainees cope with diverse service contexts in different countries and cultures. Empowering trainees means the curriculum has to be built round the role of a clinical specialist as defined above. The issues that face child psychiatry development in high need situations has been well described with reference to India, and the role for child psychiatrists described resonates closely with this definition (Malhotra 2003).

The essential components of the curriculum is first a transcultural/multiculturally relevant knowledge base in child mental health, which includes content on child development and child mental health problems. Conceptual understanding of what constitutes a child mental health problem may vary leading, where CAMH services exist to approaches for help for children with a variety of organic or neuropsychiatric conditions with associated behaviour difficulties. Hence, the content on child mental health problems needs to include content on epilepsy, learning disability and other neuropsychiatric conditions.

This knowledge base must include teaching on appropriate assessments, effective and feasible interventions, issues relating to consent and confidentiality, child protection, legal frameworks for children. A very important component will relate to service planning including inputs for promotion and prevention.

Some teaching on research methodology and research ethics is also essential. The bulk of research on child development, child psychiatric disorders and interventions are carried out in HIC in the West. There are an increasing number of research projects initiated and carried out by clinicians in different parts of the world. However these are often published in journals that are not indexed. There is a discrepancy in the number of journals indexed from different parts of the world (Mari et al. 2010). Currently only about 10 % of publications in indexed journals originate from LAMIC countries.

The teaching on child development and child psychiatric disorders will include discussion of the role of culture contributing to different value systems in child care, culture related differences in perception and recognition of behaviour problems and disorders. Although there is still insufficient cross-cultural research, there is sufficient to emphasis the fact that culture is an integral part of the mediating influences on parenting, child care and child development. Hence, cultural aspects should be an integral part of teaching in all curricula. Discussion must also identify gaps in current knowledge that may relate to a particular culture. Factoring in discussion time into teaching schedules is important and has good results (Nikapota 2008). Trainees need to be aware of early important research relating to culture and child development. In her work on Samoan adolescents, Margaret Mead highlighted the fact that difference is not a deficit (Mead 1928). This view is as important now as it was then as there is still a tendency for replication of findings across countries rather than exploration to ensure what is not only similar but also may be different. The alternate developmental trajectories arising from value systems based on independence as opposed to interdependence, value systems that reflect differences between Western and traditional Asian thinking, are well described by Greenfield et al. (2003). The socioecological theory of development (Bronfronbrenner and Morris 2006) illustrates the interaction at micro, meso and macro levels between the developing child and psychosocial environment. This well illustrates the influence of the cultures of family, school and neighbourhood, wider society on the growing child. Attachment is accepted as a developmental process that occurs universally, but there may be qualitative differences in this process if there are multiple caretakers as in extended family systems as compared to one primary caregiver. Attachment styles have been noted as varying within and between cultures (Van Ijzendoorn and Kroonenberg 1988). Pumariega and Joshi (2010) review knowledge in this area with a view to illustrating the need for a fresh look at established assumptions with regard to developmental trajectories, in response to the increasing ethnic diversity in the USA.

26.3 Epidemiology: Available Evidence of Global Need

Trainees should be aware of the continuing debate re: the extent to which psychiatric diagnoses are valid across cultures. This is equally an issue for child psychiatry. Current epidemiological data demonstrates that there is considerable similarity in patterns of behaviour across cultures although there are differences in rates by age and gender (Crijnen et al. 1997; Rescorla et al. 2007). The evidence from epidemiological studies is that most common disorders occur across the globe. The cross-cultural research and in country epidemiological studies contributing to this data use almost invariably screening and diagnostic instruments developed in a Western context validated for use elsewhere. Nevertheless, there is now sufficient data across the globe for trainees to appreciate the significance of epidemiological evidence and the methodological issues relating to research in different cultural contexts (Bird 1996). A recent review by Srinath et al. (2010) documents studies in Asia with comments on the different methodological approaches used. Polanczyk et al. (2015) have presented a meta-analysis of studies resulting in world wide prevalence estimates for disorders in children and adolescents again highlighting the methodological differences that exist but also pointing to methodologies that are now available for epidemiological study in different cultures. Rutter scales (Rutter et al. 1970) the SDQ and DAWBA (Goodman et al. 2000a, b) and the Achenbach ASEBA scales (Achenbach and Rescoria 2001). Despite the many similarities, there are differences in prevalence related to culture as, for example, conversion disorder that may be very rarely seen in the West but is relatively common in LAMIC contexts (Pehlimanturk Berna and Utul Fatih 2008; Srinath et al. 1993). Sociocultural values and attitudes and cultural norms relating to socially acceptable behaviour influence expressions of distress, anger. Cultural attitudes will also influence the recognition of disorders such as attention deficit or conduct disorder. Conditions such as oppositional and conduct disorder, the diagnosis of which is influenced by cultural norms must be viewed from a cultural context (Nikapota and Rutter 2008). Canino and Algeria (2008) discuss the evidence in relation to a universalist or relativistic view of child psychiatric diagnoses. They conclude that thus far, the evidence favours an approach that combines universalist and relativistic views though further research on gene environment correlates may alter this view.

Research has also pointed to similarities in risk and vulnerability factors but there are added risks depending on context and altered baselines of vulnerability. Divorce is a risk factor in all contexts but the sociocultural implications and impact of divorce in different cultures such as among Asian families whether living in their home context or as migrant communities have still not been explored. Physical punishment is a risk factor but again there are differences relating to culture. Abusive situations are identifiable across the globe but trainees will need to be aware of the need to negotiate where societal values and attitudes may run counter to internationally recognised definitions of abuse. Genital mutilation in the practice of female circumcision is one such example. Context dependant risk includes civil conflict, war, disaster; HIV orphans; high levels of poverty, severe malnutrition, physical health morbidity and mortality. Resilience is a universal factor, which can be explained using a socioecological model. The different social factors that contribute to resilience in adversity are highlighted from available evidence in a comprehensive review by Ungar et al. (2013) illustrates ways of looking at situations designated risks such as child labour. This does not mean that child labour is desirable, but this type of discussion is invaluable for trainees to develop their own ideas in this regard and how they would inform policy. Kieling et al. (2011) review epidemiological research from a global perspective and conclude with recommendations for further research to strengthen the evidence base on the epidemiology of disorders, risk and resilience. Critical discussion on the main classification systems DSM V and ICD 10 has to be a part of teaching on epidemiology and diagnoses in relation to transcultural work.

Research skills. Teaching on research methodology could be basic but sufficient to allow participation in research, the development of simple hypotheses and ability to meet some of the research agenda for epidemiological data as mentioned above. Advancing research must encourage trainees to consider research following not only an etic perspective but be aware of emic concepts as well. Weisner (1996) points out that research training should include qualitative approaches not only quantitative as a means of increasing culturally relevant knowledge.

Therapeutic modalities taught should be learnt sufficiently well to be practised with confidence by trainees and include those that may be used in resource scarce settings. Psychoeducation is a key aspect and trainees should acquire skill in doing this for children and adults. Experiential role play is an excellent way of acquiring these skills. Simple methods such as the therapeutic value of helping children express emotion through play or artwork should be included along with teaching on behavioural techniques, cognitive behaviour therapy, basics of family therapy and interpersonal therapies. Increasing access for children and young people with anxiety and depression to talking therapies is a model of care suitable for use in many contexts (Bala and Maguire 2011). Psychopharmacology is an essential component, with teaching related also to availability of specific products in a particular context. It is useful to present the decision making that should accompany the decision to use physical treatments to facilitate effective use (Kutcher and Chehil 2008). Analytic child psychotherapy is not an option in most contexts and not in resource scare situations. However, using these skills to teach communication with children is valuable. Culture specific activities that are useful therapeutic adjuncts should be identified and included in teaching content.

Forensic and legal aspects re-child mental health. This topic includes child protection. Child protection: legal aspects and clinical services are still in a rudimentary stage in many countries. There can also be a reluctance to admit the existence of child abuse. The author recalls presenting cases of physical abuse to child domestic servants in Sri Lanka at a Pediatric conference and being asked by a senior pediatrician whether it was true that these children were seen in the country. It is useful for this topic to include input on developments in different countries, so trainees may appreciate where their own context stands in relation to child protection legal frameworks and services, and also how best to deal with situations where alternative child care is required within their own cultural context. The issue of dealing with abusive practices, which occur as part of established practice/rituals, has already been mentioned earlier.

Service Planning. Teaching on service planning with discussion about context specific issues of resource availability and need is essential. Service inputs may be promotive focusing on positive mental health where they may be universal or targeted in relation to a high need or vulnerable group. Prevention relates to morbidity. Preventive inputs may focus on vulnerability and risk to prevent disorders or on early identification and treatment for already existing problems. Both aspects can contribute to millennium goals such as extending education to all children by better identification of children with learning disabilities and improvement of maternal mental health (Patel et al. 2008).

The methodologies to monitor and evaluate service inputs needs to be a part of this teaching (Wolpert 2008). Tasks and systems related to service planning will be presented. These include advocacy with policy makers, planners (including politicians!) and colleagues from related disciplines such as pediatrics and psychiatry. Advocacy is an aspect of specialist activity, the need for which exists everywhere. The ability to structure service-related tasks within existing resources and structures should be a part of training activity. Discussion time is required during teaching to help clinicians explore how they could develop services and meet perceived and actual need in their own service contexts. Trainees not only require practice on service planning but also on teaching and training especially structuring task oriented training for teaching in primary care. Development of capacity through a cascading process and task shifting into primary care is required to increase access to services.

26.4 Teaching and Learning

Clinical skills. The adequate development of clinical skills for engagement with families, carrying out appropriate assessments and planning a therapeutic intervention has to be the part of the curriculum. One problem in resource scarce situations will be provision of adequate supervision time from a senior clinician or mentor. Clinical training must emphasise the need for a comprehensive and sensitive clinical history gathering and assessment. Child psychiatric assessment allows for cultural exploration. Trainees need to remind that cultural variation is important for clinical understanding and encouraged to view this variable in a positive sense. Families are usually the best informants when approached in a sensitive manner. The child psychiatric assessment and formulation is in fact well structured for exploration of a family's views, attitudes and practices (Nikapota 2009). Such exploration could be viewed very appropriately as an ethnographic exercise (Pumariega and Joshi 2010). Trainees should be made aware of the variation in family systems and childcare patterns across communities and cultures. Families may be nuclear, extended, or reconstituted. Head of family may be a family elder, father, or mother. The mother-headed family is common as a result of divorce, separation, or in groups where single parenthood may be the norm and in other contexts as a result of widowhood due to war. There may be significant variations in family size depending on family values and expectations. The author found when training international students in the UK, that it was necessary to illustrate for them the different family types they will meet. Many did not appreciate that a couple arriving at the clinic may not be married and the male partner may not be the father of the child. Differences in family structures and values is equally a need requiring appropriate training for international medical graduates doing child psychiatry in the US (Rao et al. 2010). Appreciation of different explanatory models of behaviour 'ours' and 'theirs' is also required for effective work.

Using available technology. The widespread use of the internet can be utilised to facilitate learning by access to internet-based materials, programmed teaching sessions, clinical supervision and participation in virtual discussion groups.

Teaching for empowerment. The end goal of teaching is empowerment. Hence, it is useful to include examples of innovative approaches to increase access in resource scarce situations and examples of alternative models of care, use of task shifting, cascading of training in HIC and LAMIC contexts. In Chandigarh India, there is an innovative computer-based diagnostic process, which is piloted for use by medical officers in remote areas under online supervision from a tertiary centre (Malhotra 2013). In Nigeria, a child psychiatric service uses the RCQ to screen for child psychiatric referrals from community clinics, thereby ensuring appropriate use of scarce services (Omigbodun et al. 1996). The Central Child Mental resource in Cambodia has developed outreach to community areas, and has used teaching on problem solving and coping skills in a pilot programme to prevent suicide and promote mental health among adolescent school youths (Jegannathan et al. 2014). Parenting interventions increasingly used in HIC settings can be adapted for use in different settings (Baker-Henningham et al. 2012). School programmes can facilitate early detection of children with emotional problems or learning delays (Fazel et al. 2014).

26.5 Conclusion

It may seem that the curriculum proposed in this chapter is too broad, seeking to address too many issues. Child mental health and working for promotion and prevention is broad going far beyond the specific remit of clinical services. This is highlighted by Patel and Rahman in a recent commentary (Patel and Rahman 2015). It is essential that specialist clinicians are trained to meet the global need. Training child psychiatrists to take a lead in meeting the global challenge is now a priority.

Acknowledgments Prof. S. Malhotra and Dr. Ian Gordon Munt who joined me in presenting the Seminar Transcultural Teaching at the ASCAPAP meeting New Delhi September 2013.

References

Achenbach, T. M., & Rescoria, L. A. (2001). *Manual for the ASEBA school-age forms and profiles*. Burlington, VT: University of Vermont, Research Centre for Children, Youth, Families.

American Psychiatric Association. (2013). *Diagnostic and statistical manual*. Washington, DC: American Psychiatric Association.

Baker-Henningham, H., Scott, S., Jones, K., & Walker, S. (2012). Reducing child conduct problems and promoting social skills in a middle-income country: Cluster randomised controlled trial. *British Journal of Psychiatry, 201*(2), 101–108.

Bala, P., & Maguire, C. (2011). Improving access to psychological therapies for children and young people. In W. Yule & O. Udwin (Eds.), *Improving access to CAMHS* 35-44. Association of Child and Adolescent Mental Health.

Betancourt, J. R. (2003). Cross cultural medical education: Conceptual approaches and frameworks for evaluation. *Academic Medicine, 78*, 560–569.

Bird, H. (1996). Epidemiology of childhood disorders in cross-cultural context. *Journal of Child Psychology and Psychiatry, 37*, 35–49.

Bronfronbrenner, U., & Morris, P.A. (2006). Ecology of human development. In *Handbook of child psychology* (6th ed., pp. 793–820). New York: John Wiley.

Canino, G., & Algeria, M. (2008). Psychiatric diagnosis. Is it universal or relative to culture? *Journal of Child Psychology and Psychiatry 49*, 237–250.

Crijnen, A., Achenbach, T., & Velhulst, F. (1997). Comparisons of problems reported by parents of children in 12 cultures: Total problems, externalising and internalising. *Journal of the American Academy of Child and Adolescent Psychiatry, 36*, 1269–1277.

Fazel, M. P. V., Patel, V., & Tol, W. (2014). Mental health interventions in schools in low-income and middle-income countries. *Lancet Psychiatry, 1*, 388–398.

Gogineni, R., Fallon, A., & Rao, N. (2010). International medical graduates in child and adolescent psychiatry: Adaptation, training, and contributions. *Child and Adolescent Psychiatric Clinics of North America, 19*, 833–853.

Goodman, R., Ford, T., Richards, H., Gatwood, R., & Melzer, H. (2000a). The development and well-being assessment: Description and initial validation of an integrated assessment of child and adolescent psychopathology. *Journal of Child Psychology and Psychiatry, 41*, 645–655.

Goodman, R., Ford, T., Simmons, H., Gatwood, R., & Metzer, H. (2000b). Using the strengths and difficulties questionnaire (SDQ) to screen for child psychiatric disorders in a community sample. *British Journal of Psychiatry, 177*, 534–539.

Greenfield, P. M., Keller, H., Fuligmi, A., & Maynard, A. (2003). Cultural pathways through universal development. *Annual Review of Psychology, 54*, 461–490.

Jegannathan, B., Dahlblom, K., & Kullgren, G. (2014). Outcome of a school-based intervention to promote life-skills among young people in Cambodia. *Asian Journal of Psychiatry, 9*, 78–84.

Karnik, N. S., & Dogra, N. (2010). The cultural sensibility model: A process-oriented approach for children and adolescents. *Child and Adolescent Psychiatric Clinics of North America, 19*, 719–737.

Kieling, C., Baker-Henningham, H., Belfer, M., Conti, G., Ertem, I., Omigbodun, O., et al. (2011) Child and adolescent mental health worldwide: Evidence for action. *Lancet, 378*, 1515–1525.

Kirmayer, L., Rousseau, C., Guzder, J., et al. (2008). Training clinicians in cultural psychiatry: A Canadian perspective. *Academic Psychiatry, 32*, 313–319.

Kutcher, S., & Chehil, S. (2008). Physical treatments. In E. A. Taylor, M. Rutter, & D. Pine et al. (Eds.), *Rutter's textbook of child and adolescent psychiatry* (pp. 1092–1105).

Malhotra, S. (2003). Socio-cultural diversity and ethnocentrism in child mental health. In G. J. Young, P. Ferrari, S. Malhotra, S. Tyano, & E. Caffo (Eds.), *IACAPAP Book series. Brain, culture and development* (pp. 3–14). London: Macmillan India.

Malhotra, S. (2013). An innovative approach. Telepsychiatry in child psychiatry. Workshop presentation ASCAPAP 2013 New Delhi India.

Mari, J. J., Patel, V., Kieling, C., Razzouk, D., Tyrer, P., & Herrman, H. (2010). Gap in the indexation of psychiatric journals of low- and middle-income countries. *Acta Psychiatrica Scandinavica, 121*(2), 152.

Mead, M. (1928). *Coming of age in Samoa: A psychological study of primitive youth for Western civilization*. New York: William Morrow.

Mian, A. I., Al-Mateen, C. S., & Cerda, G. (2010). Training child and adolescent psychiatrists to be culturally competent. *Child and Adolescent Psychiatric Clinics of North America, 19*, 823–831.

Nikapota, A. D. (2008). Transcultural training in child and adolescent psychiatry. In E. Gerralda & J. P. Raynaud (Eds.), *Culture and conflict in child and adolescent mental health* (pp. 205–222). USA: IACAPAP Book series Pub Jason Aronson.

Nikapota, A. D. (2009). Cultural issues in child assessment. *Child and Adolescent Mental Health, 14*(4), 200–206.

Nikapota, A. D., & Rutter, M. (2008). Sociocultural/ethnic groups and psychopathology. In E. A. Taylor, M. Rutter, D. Pine, et al. (Eds.), *Rutter's textbook of child and adolescent psychiatry* (pp. 199–211). Oxford: Blackwell.

Omigbodun, O., Guruje, O., Gater, R., Ikuesan, B., & Adebayo, E. (1996). Psychiatric morbidity in a Nigerian paediatric primary care service: A comparison of two screening instruments. *Social Psychiatry and Psychiatric Epidemiology, 31*, 186–193.

Patel, V., Flisher, A. J., Nikapota, A. D., & Malhotra, S. (2008). Promoting child mental health in low and middle income countries. *Journal of Child and Adolescent Psychiatry 49*, 313–334.

Patel, V., & Rahman, A. (2015). Editorial commentary: An agenda for global child mental health. *Child and Adolescent Mental Health, 20*(1), 3–4.

Pehlimanturk, B., & Utul, F. (2008). Cultural and clinical aspects of conversion disorders with special reference to Turkish Children and adolescents. In E. Garralda & J. P. Raynaud (Eds.), *Culture and conflict in child and adolescent mental health* (pp. 133–156). USA: IACAPAP Book series Pub Jason Aronson.

Polanczyk, G. V., Salum, G. A., Sugaya, L. S., Caye, A., & Rohde, L. A. (2015). A meta-analysis of the worldwide prevalence of mental disorders in children and adolescents. *Journal of Child Psychology and Psychiatry, 56*(3), 345–365.

Pumariega, A. J., & Joshi, S. V. (2010). Culture and development in children and youth. *Child and Adolescent Psychiatric Clinics of North America, 19*, 661–680.

Rao Gogineni, R., Fallon, A. E., & Rao, N. R. (2010). International medical graduates in child and adolescent psychiatry: Adaptation, training and contributions. *In Child and Adolescent Psychiatric Clinics of North America 19*, 833–853.

Rescorla, L., Achenbach, T., Ivanova, M., Dumenci, L., Almqvist, F., Bilenberg, N., et al. (2007). Behavioural and emotional problems reported by parents of children ages 6 to 16 in 31 societies. *Journal of Emotional and Behavioural Disorders, 15*, 130–142.

Rutter, M., Tizard, J., & Whitmore, K. (1970). *Education, health and behaviour*. London: Longmans.

Srinath, S., Bharat, S., Girimaji, S., & Seshadri, S. (1993). Characteristics of a child inpatient population with hysteria in India. *Journal of the American Academy of Child and Adolescent Psychiatry, 32*, 822–825.

Srinath, S., Kandasamy, P., & Golhar, T. S. (2010). Epidemiology of child and adolescent mental health disorders in Asia. *Current Opinion in Psychiatry, 23*(4), 330–336.

Ungar, M., Ghazinour, M., & Richter, J. (2013). What is resilience within the social ecology of human development? *Journal of Child Psychology and Psychiatry, 54*(4), 348–366.

Van Ijzendoorn, M., & Kroonenberg, P. (1988). Cross-cultural patterns of attachment: A meta-analysis of the strange situation. *Child Development, 59*, 147–156.

Weisner, T. S. (1996). Why ethnography should be the most important method in the study of human development. In R. Jessor, A. Colby & R. Schweder(Eds.), *Ethnography and human development. Context and meaning in social inquiry*. Chicago: University of Chicago Press, pp. 305–324.

WHO. (1994). *International classification of disease* (10th ed.). Geneva: WHO.

WHO. (2005). *Atlas: Child and adolescent mental health resources*. Geneva: WHO.

Wolpert, M. (2008). Organisation of services for children and adolescents with mental health problems. In E. A. Taylor, M. Rutter, D. Pine, et al. (Eds.), *Rutter's textbook of child and adolescent psychiatry* (pp. 1156–1166). Oxford: Blackwell.

CPI Antony Rowe
Chippenham, UK
2017-07-28 11:56